NEUROCHEMISTRY

Edited by **Thomas Heinbockel**

Neurochemistry
http://dx.doi.org/10.5772/57074
Edited by Thomas Heinbockel

Contributors

Grant Hatch, Donald Miller, Michael Pogorzelec, Hieu Nguyen, Ngoc On, Siddhartha Dalvi, Victoria Campos-Peña, Marco Meraz-Ríos, Rocío Gómez, Victor Tsetlin, Igor Kasheverov, Carlos Gutierrez-Merino, Christian Harteneck, Kristina Leuner, Evgeniya Pushchina, Anatoly Varaksin, Dmitry Obukhov, Chloé Hegoburu, Luc Denoroy, Anne-Marie Mouly, Sandrine Parrot, Jose Luna-Muñoz, Alejandra Martinez-Maldonado, Miguel Angel Ontiveros-Torres, Isidre Ferrer, Benjamín Florán-Garduño, Maria del Carmen Cardenas-Aguayo, Raul Mena-López, Maria del Carmen Silva-Lucero, Maribel Cortes-Ortiz, Berenice Jimenez-Ramos, Laura Gomez-Virgilio, Gerardo Ramirez-Rodriguez, Eduardo Vera-Arroyo, Rosana Sofia Fiorentino-Perez, Ubaldo Garcia, Agnieszka Jankowska-Kulawy, Anna Ronowska, Andrzej Szutowicz, Elena Zakharova, Alexander Dudchenko, Thomas Heinbockel

Published by InTech

Janeza Trdine 9, 51000 Rijeka, Croatia

Publishing Process Manager Iva Lipovic

Technical Editor InTech DTP team

Cover InTech Design team

First published April, 2014

Printed in Croatia

Additional hard copies can be obtained from orders@intechopen.com

Neurochemistry, Edited by Thomas Heinbockel

p. cm.

ISBN 978-953-51-1237-2

For EU product safety concerns:
IN TECH d.o.o., Prolaz Marije Krucifikse Kozulić 3, 51000 Rijeka, Croatia,
info@intechopen.com or visit our website at intechopen.com.

Meet the editor

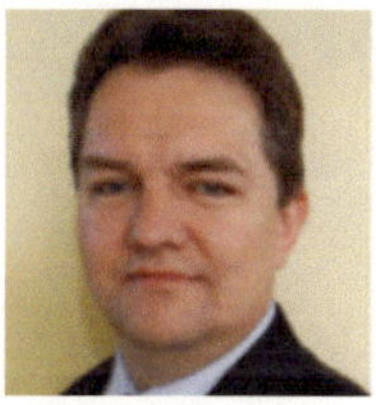

Thomas Heinbockel, Ph.D., is currently Associate Professor and Director of Graduate Studies in the Department of Anatomy, Howard University College of Medicine, Washington, DC, USA. His laboratory engages in multidisciplinary research to elucidate organizational principles of neural systems in the brain, specifically the limbic and olfactory system. His research has been directed at understanding brain mechanisms of information processing and their relation to neurological and neuropsychiatric disorders. Dr. Heinbockel studied biology at the Philipps-University, Marburg, Germany. His studies of the brain started during his M.S. thesis work at the Max-Planck-Institute for Behavioral Physiology, Starnberg/Seewiesen, Germany. Subsequently, he completed a Ph.D. in Neuroscience at the University of Arizona, Tucson, Arizona, USA. After graduating, he held a Research Associate position at the Institute of Physiology, Otto-von-Guericke-University School of Medicine, Magdeburg, Germany. Prior to his arrival at Howard University, Dr. Heinbockel held joint research faculty appointments in the Department of Anatomy and Neurobiology, and the Department of Physiology at the University of Maryland School of Medicine, Baltimore, Maryland, USA.

Contents

Preface

Neurochemistry is a flourishing academic field that contributes to our understanding of molecular, cellular and medical neurobiology. As a scientific discipline, neurochemistry studies the role of chemicals that build the nervous system, explores the function of neurons and glial cells in health and disease, discovers aspects of cell metabolism and neurotransmission, and reveals how degenerative processes are at work in the nervous system. Accordingly, this book contains chapters from a variety of topics that fall into the following broad sections: I. Neural Membranes and Intracellular Signaling, II. Neural Processing and Intercellular Signaling, III. Growth, Development and Differentiation, and IV. Neurodegenerative Diseases. The book presents comprehensive reviews in these different areas written by experts in their respective fields. Neurodegeneration and neuronal diseases are featured prominently and are a recurring theme throughout most chapters. This book will be a most valuable resource for neurochemists and other scientists alike. In addition, it will contribute to the training of current and future neurochemists and, hopefully, will lead us on the path to curing some of the biggest challenges in human health.

Section One of the book, I. Neural Membranes and Intracellular Signaling, starts with a discussion of the blood brain barrier by Dalvi et al. (chapter 1: 'The Blood Brain Barrier: Regulation of Fatty acid and Drug Transport') to introduce the reader to chemicals that enter the brain. The chapter has a strong focus on tight junctions. Dalvi et al. describe the various tight junction proteins and transport systems and provide a solid account of the role of fatty acids in blood brain barrier permeability.

In chapter 2 ('TRP Channels in Neuronal and Glial Signal Transduction'), Harteneck and Leuner provide a comprehensive review of transient receptor potential (TRP) channels and their relation to various neurological and psychiatric diseases. Many TRP channels are expressed in the brain and contribute to neuronal and glial functions. The authors offer detailed accounts of the many channel variants and their functional roles in CNS physiology.

In chapter 3 ('Cytosolic Calcium Homeostasis in Neurons: Control Systems, Modulation by Reactive Oxygen and Nitrogen Species, and Space and Time Fluctuations'), Gutierrez-Merino et al. review the critical role of calcium in neuronal activity and function of the nervous systems. The authors discuss cellular oxidative stress and metabolic deregulations in the process of neuronal death. Calcium transport systems control cytosolic calcium homeostasis within nanodomains of the neuronal plasma membrane associated with lipid rafts. The colocalization of ROS/RNS enzyme sources within nanodomains is of particular relevance for neurodegenerative insults and diseases.

In chapter 4, Section Two, II. Neural Processing and Intercellular Signaling, Tsetlin and Kasheverov ('Peptide and Protein Neurotoxin Toolbox in Research on Nicotinic Acetylcholine

Receptors') examine nicotinic acetylcholine receptors and the neurotoxins that helped researchers to identify their structure and function. The chapter takes the reader on a historical journey of the discovery of the receptor and its various peptide and protein neurotoxins.

In chapter 5 ('Synaptic Soluble and Membrane-Bound Choline Acetyltransferase as a Marker of Cholinergic Function in Vitro and in Vivo'), Zakharova and Dudchenko address the synapse as a unique, most dynamic and labile structure and discuss the use of synaptosomes to study neural transmission, specifically at cholinergic synapses. The authors explore the brain cholinergic system because of its role in cognitive, attention and motor functions as well as dysfunctions related to several neurological disorders.

Chapter 6 by Heinbockel ('Neurochemical Communication: The Case of Endocannabinoids') reviews the progress made in our understanding of a relatively novel neuronal signaling system, the endocannabinoid system which comprises endogenously produced cannabinoids and their specific receptors, cannabinoid receptors. This signaling system plays a critical role in neuronal communication in many brain areas and has been shown to crosstalk with other neurotransmitter system.

In chapter 7 ('High Temporal Resolution Brain Microdialysis as a Tool to Investigate the Dynamics of Interactions Between Olfactory Cortex and Amygdala in Odor Fear Conditioning'), Hegoboru et al. report how a specific experimental tool, in vivo microdialysis of major amino acid neurotransmitters, allows studying the interaction of two brain areas in a behavioral context.

Section Three, III. Growth, Development and Differentiation, houses two chapters. Chapter 8 by Pushchina et al. ('Participation of Neurochemical Signaling in Adult Neurogenesis and Differentiation') explores the organization and relationships of signal transduction systems that produce classic neurotransmitters or gaseous transmitters in the brain of fish and evaluates their participation in the processes of the postembryonic morphogenesis the CNS.

For quite some time, amyloid plaques in the body have been accepted as a cause of the neurodegeneration observed in Alzheimer's disease based on the hypothesis that the amyloid beta peptide is a toxic factor that impairs neuronal function and leads to cell death, see Section IV. In chapter 9 ('Physiological Role of Amyloid Beta in Neural Cells: The Cellular Trophic Activity'), Cárdenas-Aguayo et al. challenge this hypothesis by reviewing the physiological roles of amyloid beta and suggest that amyloid beta might even help to enhance synaptic plasticity and memory at appropriate concentration levels.

The last section, Section IV, is dedicated to Neurodegenerative Diseases. In chapter 10 ('Alzheimer Disease: the Role of Aβ in the Glutamatergic System'), Campos-Peña and Meraz-Ríos review the neurodegenerative process that occurs in Alzheimer's disease. The authors discuss the role of the glutamatergic system and the use of safe disease-modifying drugs in the treatment of Alzheimer's disease.

In chapter 11, the authors (Campos-Peña, Gómez, Meraz-Ríos) continue with a discussion of the 'Genetics of Alzheimer's Disease'. They review the evidence for a genetic basis of familial Alzheimer's disease, also known as early onset Alzheimer's disease which is associated with mutations in different genes. In contrast, sporadic Alzheimer's disease or late onset Alzheimer's disease is much more common and the cause for it might be a combination of lifestyle, environmental and some genetic factors which could favor the development of the disease.

In chapter 12 ('Accumulation of Abnormally Processed Tau Protein in Neuronal Cells as a Biomarker for Dementia'), Luna-Muñoz et al. inform the reader about the problem of early detection and better treatment of neurodegenerative disorders such as Alzheimer's and Parkinson's disease. They discuss the development of better therapeutic tools that are able to modify the disease progression based on reliable biomarkers to detect the disease at early stages to prevent the irreversible neuronal degeneration.

In the final chapter of the book (ch. 13, 'Energy–Dependent Mechanisms of Cholinergic Neurodegeneration'), Jankowska-Kulawy et al. point out that a characteristic feature of some neurodegenerative diseases is the preferential loss of cholinergic neurons which correlate with the degree of energy metabolism inhibition. Even though neurons constitute only 10% of all brain cells, they produce and consume about 80% of its energy. The authors raise the critical issue that effective functioning of neurons is dependent on the continuous supply of glucose and oxygen. The authors discuss energy homeostasis of the brain as a complex process because of the high sensitivity of neurons to metabolic stress, the isolation of the brain due to the existence of the blood brain barrier, the high energy requirements of the brain, and the existence of limited glycogen stores as a dynamic source of energy. Despite these constraints, dysfunction of mitochondria, the cellular source of energy, is the first step in neurodegeneration.

I am grateful to InTech – Open Access Publisher for initiating this book project and for asking me to serve as its editor. Many thanks go to Iva Lipović at InTech for guiding me through the publication process and for moving the book ahead in a timely fashion. Thanks are due to all contributors of this book for taking the time to first write a chapter proposal, compose their chapter and, lastly, make my requested revisions to it. Hopefully, all contributors will continue their neurochemistry research with many intellectual challenges and exciting new directions. I would like to thank my wife Dr. Vonnie D.C. Shields, Professor, Towson University, Towson, MD and our son Torben Heinbockel for allowing me to spend time on this book project during the past year. Finally, I am grateful to my parents Erich and Renate Heinbockel for their support over many years.

Thomas Heinbockel, Ph.D.
Associate Professor and Director of Graduate Studies
Department of Anatomy
Howard University College of Medicine
Washington, DC, USA

Section 1

Neural Membranes and Intracellular Signaling

Chapter 1

The Blood Brain Barrier — Regulation of Fatty Acid and Drug Transport

Siddhartha Dalvi, Ngoc On, Hieu Nguyen,
Michael Pogorzelec, Donald W. Miller and
Grant M. Hatch

Additional information is available at the end of the chapter

http://dx.doi.org/10.5772/57604

1. Introduction

1.1. The blood brain barrier

The blood brain barrier (BBB) is a selectively permeable cellular boundary between the brain and the peripheral circulation. The principal component of the BBB is the capillary or micro-vessel endothelial cell (Figure 1). The endothelial cells in the brain capillaries differ from those in the peripheral vasculature in several key features:

1. Presence of tight junctions (TJ) that limit the paracellular passage of macromolecules.
2. Restricted rate of fluid-phase endocytosis that limits the transcellular passage of macromolecules [1]
3. Presence of specific transporter and carrier molecules [2]
4. Lack of fenestrations [3]
5. Increased mitochondrial content [3]

Thus, the endothelial cells of the BBB are less "leaky" than those of the peripheral vessels. However, it has been shown that if the endothelial cells of the brain capillaries are removed from their natural environment and allowed to vascularize the peripheral tissue, they become more leaky [1]. In contrast, the endothelial cells from the periphery form tight junctions when allowed to vascularize the brain parenchyma. Morphologically, the tight junctions of the BBB

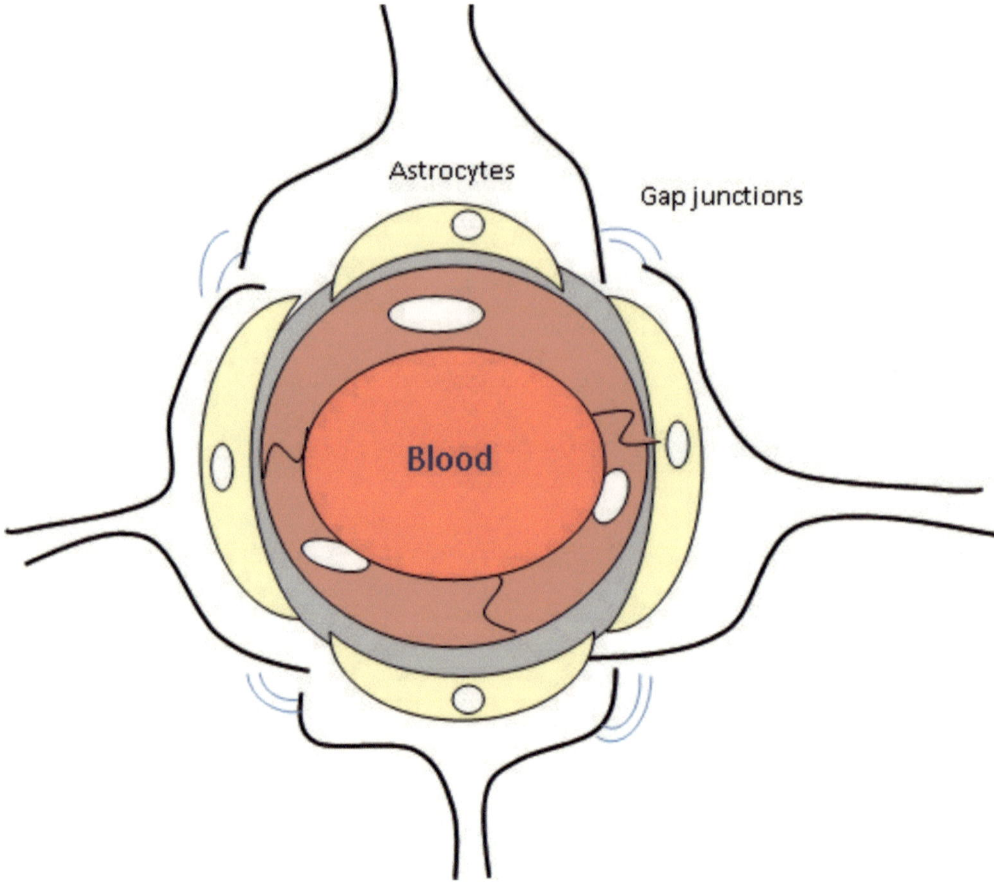

Figure 1. Neurovascular Unit of the blood brain barrier consists of the endothelial cells (pink) surrounded by basement membrane (gray), pericytes (yellow) and astrocyte foot processes. The tight junctions (black lines) formed between two endothelial cells restrict the paracellular diffusion of compounds.

resemble the tight junctions between epithelial cells rather than those between peripheral vascular endothelial cells [4].

The unique tight junctions of the BBB are responsible for producing very high transendothelial electrical resistance (TEER) of 1500 – 2000 Ωcm^2 [2,5,6]. Though the microvessel endothelial cells play a primary role in the formation of the BBB, several other cells are equally important in maintaining the integrity of the BBB. These cells, namely, the astrocytes, pericytes, neurons and other glial cells are said to form a "neurovascular unit" [7]. Integrity of the BBB is of utmost importance in maintaining the homeostasis of the brain microenvironment. Disruption of the BBB is seen in various states of inflammation (multiple sclerosis), neoplasia, infections (meningitis, encephalitis), trauma and Alzheimer disease [8,9]. It would be highly desirable to develop therapeutic strategies to reverse this disruption and tighten the BBB. At the same time, a transient opening of the BBB would be advantageous for delivery of drugs into the brain in conditions like epilepsy or Parkinson disease [2].

1.2. Functions of the BBB

The BBB is responsible for maintaining the appropriate ionic composition of the interstitial fluid of the brain that is required for optimum functioning of the neurons. To achieve this, the BBB functions as a *transport barrier* by facilitating the uptake of the required nutrients, while preventing the uptake of, or actively effluxing certain other molecules or toxic by-products of metabolism [10] The BBB also functions as a *metabolic barrier* by virtue of possessing intracellular and extracellular enzymes. For example, extracellular enzymes such as peptidases and nucleotidases break down peptides and ATP, respectively. Intracellular enzymes like cytochrome P450 (CYP450), primarily CYP1A and CYP2B degrade noxious substances and prevent their entry into the brain parenchyma [10].

1.3. Role of astrocytes in the BBB

It is now known that the astrocytes play a key role in the conditioning and development of the brain microvessel endothelial cells (BMEC). Astrocytes are one of the glial cells of the central nervous system (CNS) that play several important roles in the structure and function of the CNS. They are intimately associated with the BMEC such that their foot processes ensheath 99% of the external surface of the BMEC [11]. Astrocytes have been shown to alter the properties of cocultured brain endothelial cells in the following ways [11,12].

1. Increase in barrier-related marker enzyme activities, such as that of γ-glutamyl transpeptidase (GGT) and alkaline phosphatase.
2. Enhanced expression of a glucose transporter.
3. Elevation of trans-endothelial electrical resistance (TEER).
4. Tightening of the BBB as seen by decreased paracellular permeability of sucrose.
5. Increase in tight junction number, length and complexity.

It has also been shown that BMEC monolayers are less leaky if grown in the presence of astrocyte-conditioned medium (ACM) [1,11]. The precise molecular nature of the astrocyte-derived factors that is responsible for the tightness of the BBB have yet to be unequivocally elucidated. However, several factors have been postulated to play a role including glial cell-derived neurotrophic factor (GDNF), transforming growth factor-beta (TGF-β), and src-suppressed C-kinase substrate (SSeCKS) that leads to increased angiopoietin-1 secretion. The BMEC themselves are known to secrete factors that help in the maintenance of astrocyte health. One such putative factor is the leukemia-inhibitory factor (LIF), a cytokine known to be involved in astrocyte differentiation [11].

1.4. Role of pericytes in the BBB

The pericytes are specialized cells of mesenchymal lineage that have multiple organ-specific roles. For example, they are present in the kidney as mesangial cells, in the liver as perisinusoidal stellate cells and in the bone as osteoblasts [13,14]. The pericytes in the central nervous system are closely associated with the BMEC and play an important role in the maintenance of the BBB. Their functions include [14].

1. Cerebrovascular autoregulation and blood flow distribution
2. Differentiation of the BBB
3. Formation and maintenance of the tight junctions of the BBB.
4. Initiation of the extrinsic (tissue factor) pathway of blood coagulation following cerebrovascular injury
5. Brain angiogenesis via secretion of angiopoietin-1
6. Phagocytic and scavenging (macrophage-like) functions
7. Production of immunoregulatory cytokines like IL-1β, IL-6 and GM-CSF
8. Regulation of leukocyte transmigration, antigen presentation and T-cell activation.

2. Molecular components of the tight junctions

The tight junctions consist of both membrane proteins as well as cytoplasmic proteins [15] (Figure 2). The integral membrane proteins are Claudins, Occludin and Junctional adhesion molecules (JAM). There are also several cytoplasmic accessory proteins that form a plaque and function as adapter proteins to link the membrane proteins to the actin cytoskeleton of the cell [16,17]. These include Zonula occludens proteins (ZO-1, ZO-2, ZO-3), Cingulin, AF-6, 7H6 antigen and Symplekin. These tight junctional complexes are not static structures but rather very dynamic entities that can "bend without breaking", thereby maintaining structural integrity [8].

2.1. Claudins

The claudins are a large family of transmembrane phosphoproteins [15]. Twenty-four members have been characterized so far, claudins 1-24 [18,19]. Of these, claudins 1, 3, 5 and 12 have been shown to form the tight junctions of the BBB [9,17,20,21]. Claudin-5 appears to be specific to the tight junctions of the endothelial cells and is called the "endothelial claudin" [17]. Each claudin molecule has 4 transmembrane domains. The claudin on one cell binds homotypically to the claudin on the adjacent cell to form the seal of the tight junction. The claudins, along with occludin and the JAMs, form the tight Junctional strands that keep the cells together and prevent paracellular flux of macromolecules from the apical to the basolateral side of polarized cells like BMEC [18]. The cytoplasmic carboxy terminal of the claudins binds to the cytoplasmic ZO proteins [20]. Claudin-1 is an integral component of the tight junctions and its loss is associated with certain pathologic conditions like tumours, strokes and inflammatory diseases [21].

2.2. Occludin

Occludin is a 65-kDa transmembrane phosphoprotein and is distinct from the claudins. However, its subcellular localization parallels that of claudins and, like the claudins, it has

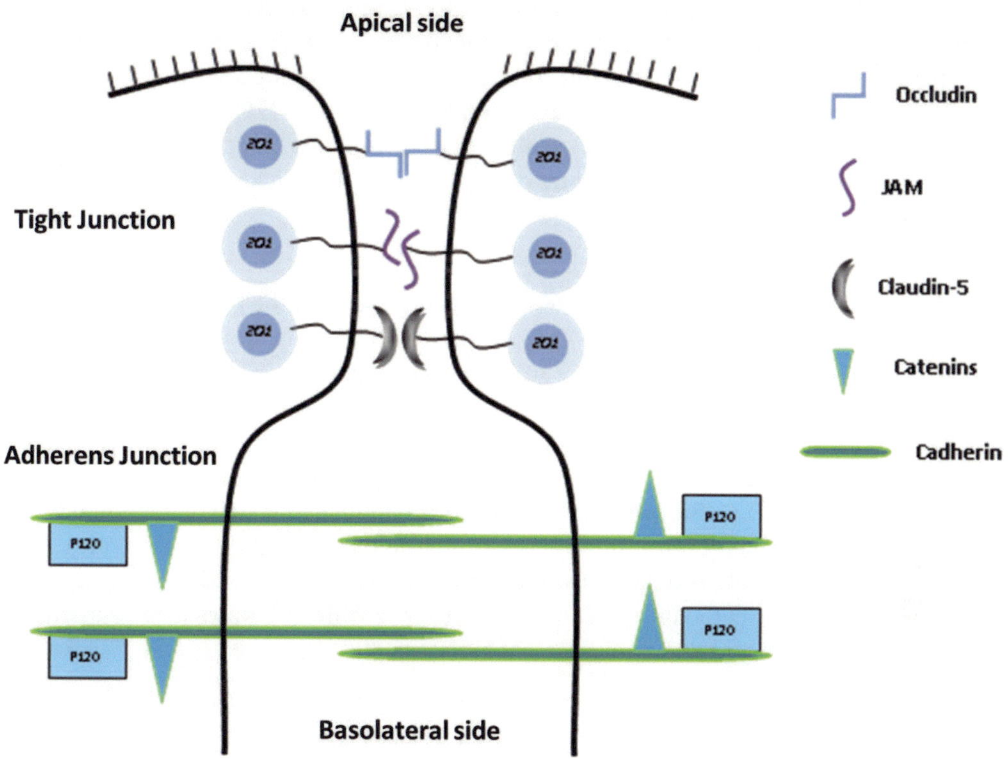

Figure 2. Schematic representation of proteins that are involved in the formation of the tight junction and adherens junctions in brain microvessel endothelial cells.

four transmembrane domains. The expression of occludin is higher in the adult BMEC compared to the peripheral endothelial cells. However, it is not expressed in the fetal or newborn human brain. Occludin plays an important structural, as well as a functional, role in the regulation of BBB permeability. As is the case with several other tight junction-associated proteins, phosphorylation or dephosphorylation of serine, threonine or tyrosine residues on the occludin molecule is crucial for its proper functioning [17,18,22,23]. For example, phosphorylation of occludin at serine and tyrosine residues correlates with tight junction assembly or tightening [8].

Occludin and the claudins interact intricately on the BMEC membrane. Together, they form channels that tightly regulate the paracellular flow of ions and other hydrophilic molecules. Thus, they are both essential in the formation, maintenance and regulation of the BBB [16,18].

2.3. Junctional Adhesion Molecules (JAM)

These molecules play an important role in the regulation of tight junction permeability in endothelial and epithelial cells [24]. These glycoproteins are members of the immunoglobulin superfamily of proteins. Three different JAMs have been characterized in humans, JAM-1,

JAM-2 and JAM-3, also referred to as JAM-A, JAM-B and JAM-C, respectively. Besides endothelial and epithelial cells, these molecules are also found on the surface of erythrocytes, leukocytes and platelets and are thought to contribute to various processes like leukocyte migration, platelet activation, angiogenesis and binding of reovirus [25]. The JAMs have short cytoplasmic tails that interact with cytoplasmic accessory proteins like ZO-1 and may require activation by phosphorylation, mediated by certain atypical protein kinases.

2.4. Cytoplasmic accessory proteins

Several cytoplasmic proteins appear to be essential components of the tight junctions. Among them, the zonula occludens proteins (ZO-1, ZO-2, ZO-3) play an important role. These 3 proteins have a molecular mass of 220, 160 and 130 kDa, respectively. They belong to a family of proteins called MAGUK (membrane-associated guanylate kinase-like protein) and form the submembranous plaque of the tight junction [2,15]. They are structurally complex proteins with several domains that make direct contact with claudins, occludin and JAM on one side and the actin cytoskeleton on the other [15]. Cingulin is a double-stranded myosin-like protein that serves as scaffolding and links the TJ accessory proteins with the cytoskeleton [8]. Actin, the cytoskeletal protein, plays a central role in the maintenance of the TJ. Actin-degrading macromolecules, such as cytochalasin-D, phalloidin and certain cytokines lead to disruption of the actin cytoskeleton and hence, of the tight junctions [8].

The tight junctional proteins can be modulated by several intracellular processes that involve calcium-signaling, phosphorylation, G-proteins, proteases and by TNF-α [4,8]. The tight junctional complexes also help localize the proteins and lipids of the apical and basolateral cell membranes in their respective compartments and prevent free mixing of these cell membrane macromolecules between the two domains. Thus, the BMEC owe much of their polarity to the TJ complexes [2,26].

3. Regulation of BBB permeability

Various factors play a role in regulating the permeability of the BBB as follows [2]:

1. Post-translational modifications of the TJ proteins. For example, phosphorylation and dephosphorylation mediated by protein kinases and phosphatases, respectively.
2. Alteration of the actin cytoskeleton.
3. Proteolytic degradation of certain TJ components like occludin, mediated by metalloproteinases.

4. *In vitro* models to study the BBB

In vitro models of the BBB have proven very effective to study the transport of endogenous macromolecules like fatty acids across the BMEC. They have also been used extensively in pharmaceutical research to study the passage of therapeutic molecules across the BMEC [5-7]. Several studies have shown that the BMEC lose many of their special properties when removed from their natural environment and show "dedifferentiation" behaviour. Thus, one potential limitation of in vitro BBB models is that the BMEC may not behave as site-specific specialized endothelial cells in vitro, but rather as common peripheral endothelial cells [7]. In spite of this shortcoming, several successful in vitro models of the BBB have been described [27]. Many of these have used human, bovine, and porcine or rat endothelial cells:

1. Alone [5,6,28-30], or

2. in combination with astrocyte conditioned medium supplemented with agents that elevate intracellular cAMP [1], or

3. Co-culture of endothelial cells on one side of a filter, with astrocytes on the other [31].

5. FA transport across the BBB and effects of FA on BBB permeability

Fatty acids (FA) are key components of membranes and exhibit many biological functions in a variety of tissues, including the key energy source for mitochondrial β-oxidation [32,33]. Cells acquire fatty acids through *de novo* synthesis, hydrolysis of triglycerides (TG) or uptake from exogenous sources [33]. Minimal amount of FA are derived from TG hydrolysis and most cells are dependent upon fatty acid uptake from the peripheral blood [32,34]. FA from the diet are absorbed by enterocytes in the small intestine and packaged into chylomicrons as TG. The liver also produces very low density lipoprotein (VLDL), a rich source of endogenously generated TG. Circulating chylomicrons and VLDL particles are hydrolyzed by lipoprotein lipase in the capillary lumen of tissues and the released FA from these lipoproteins may be taken up by tissues in the body [35]. FA that enter into cells are then esterified and stored as TG or transported to the mitochondria for β-oxidation. The importance of FA for the developing and adult brain has been recently reviewed [6]. FA transport from blood into parenchymal neurons is much more difficult than other cells since the tight junctions of the BBB severely restrict passage into the brain. FA must first move via transcellular transport across both the luminal (apical) and abluminal (basolateral) membranes of the endothelial cells and then across the plasma membrane of the neural cells [36-38].

The mechanism of FA transport into the brain remains controversial. Several studies support the notion that FA can move across membranes by diffusion [39,40]. Alternatively, others studies indicate that FA may enter into cells via specific protein-mediated transport [32,41,42]. In the diffusion model, once bound to the outer membrane leaflet, they quickly reach ionization equilibrium and the non-ionized form of fatty acids move across the membrane more rapidly than the ionized form [43]. The main problem with the FA diffusion model has always been whether diffusion is rapid enough to supply cells, which have a high long-chain FA metabolic requirement with sufficient amount of FA for β-oxidation [44]. In the protein-mediated transport model selective transport of FA occurs via specific protein transporters found on the cell membrane [33,41,45-47]. The mechanism of FA transport into the brain and the involvement of FA protein transporters has been reviewed [6]. We recently showed that the transport of various FA across confluent layers of HBMEC was, in part, mediated by fatty acid transport proteins (FATPs) [5,6]. Knock down of FATP-1 and CD36 resulted in reduced FA transport. In addition, transport appeared to be dependent upon fatty acyl chain length and degree of unsaturation.

The role of FA, such as arachidonic acid (AA), on BBB permeability is well documented and controversial. Studies have indicated that a rapid influx of AA into the brain occurs upon plasma infusion with AA [48,49]. In addition, a permeability-enhancing and neurotoxic effect of AA has been observed [50-52]. AA is a precursor for the formation of various bioactive molecules including prostaglandins, such as PGE_2, and leukotrienes. Several studies have indicated that the increase in BBB permeability is correlated with the formation of PGE_2 [29,30, 53-56]. The prostaglandin EP2 receptor was shown to be responsible for mediating the neuroinflammatory and neurodegenerative effects of PGE_2 in a mouse model of status epilepticus [57]. The permeability increase caused by AA in pial microvessels of rats was effectively blocked by a combination of indomethacin (COX inhibitor) and nordihyroguaria-retic acid (LOX inhibitor) but not singly by either agent [58]. In that same study, AA-mediated permeability increase was blocked by superoxide dismutase and catalase. These authors concluded that free radicals generated by either COX or LOX pathways were responsible for the permeability response to AA. In a mouse model of diabetic retinopathy 12-HETE and 15-HETE, products of the lipoxygenase pathway, were shown to be responsible for increasing the permeability of retinal endothelial cell barrier via an NADPH oxidase-dependent mechanism [59]. Interestingly, AA inhibited the cytokine-induced up-regulation of several genes involved in endothelial cell inflammation [60].

However, other studies have suggested that AA metabolites, such as PGE_2, have a protective role in the microvessels of the CNS and that PGE_2 prevents permeability increases. For example, the permeability increase caused by bradykinin was prevented or attenuated by exogenously added PGE_2 and iloprost, a prostacyclin analog [61]. In that study, COX-inhibitor drugs potentiated the permeability increases caused by bradykinin, thus suggesting an inhibitory role of PGE_2 in increasing endothelial cell permeability. In addition, PGE_2, acting via EP4 receptors, inhibited the increase in BBB permeability in a mouse model of experimental autoimmune encephalomyelitis [62]. Moreover, PGE_2, acting via EP2 receptors, has neuropro-tective properties and limits ischemic damage in mice stroke models [63]. It has been postulated in these studies [61,62] that engagement of EP2 and EP4 receptors by PGE_2 leads to an increase in cAMP levels. This cAMP accumulation has been shown to potentiate cadherin-mediated cell-cell contact and enhance endothelial barrier function. Thus, PGE_2 may promote BBB integrity via direct action on endothelial cells [62].

Several studies have demonstrated that microvessel endothelial cells from various organs have the capacity to produce a range of eicosanoids, notably, PGE_2, PGI_2 and $PGF_{2\alpha}$. In most of these studies the endothelial cells were stimulated with the calcium ionophore A23187 in addition to exogenously added AA [64-66]. However, in one study endothelial cells exposed to plasma from preeclamptic women showed increased production of prostaglandins [67]. In addition,

http://dx.doi.org/10.5772/57604

bovine brain microvessel endothelial cells (BBMEC) exposed to TNF-αreleased large amounts of PGE_2 over a 12-hour period [29].

Previous work has shown that docosahexanoic acid (DHA) is converted to its vasodilator metabolite, 17S-HDoHE in endothelial cells [68]. DHA is a precursor in the formation of several bioactive molecules in human blood cells and in glial cells [69]. However, in those experiments, the cells were exposed to stimulants like zymosan A or the calcium ionophore, A23187 to facilitate the release of DHA metabolites. These metabolites have been shown to have several biological effects like inhibition of inflammation and platelet aggregation, mediation of vasodilation, anti-arrhythmic effects and lowering of triglyceride levels [70].

6. Drug transport across the BBB

The tight junction complex that connects brain microvascular endothelial cells in the BBB as well as the epithelial cells of the choroid plexus that form the blood-cerebral spinal fluid barrier (BCSFB) serve as a physical barrier preventing the paracellular diffusion of endogenous and exogenous compounds. The presence of these tight junctions is essential for maintaining the proper environment required for neuronal transmission. However, paracellular diffusion of nutrients and metabolites between the blood and the extracellular compartment of the brain is also highly restricted. Consequently, the uptake of essential molecules, such as glucose and amino acids, to meet the metabolic requirements of the brain occurs through specific transporter proteins located on the plasma membrane of the endothelial cells. In addition to transporters that facilitate the entry of various solutes into the brain, the brain endothelial cells also express numerous efflux transporters [71]. These transporters are members of the ATP-binding cassette (ABC) protein family and utilize energy from adenosine triphosphate (ATP) hydrolysis to actively remove compounds from the cells against a concentration gradient.

From a drug transport perspective, there are several transporters that are critically involved in the movements of drugs across the BBB. These include organic anion-transporting polypeptide 1A2 (OATP1A2/SLO1A2), organic anion transporter 3 (OAT3/SLC22A8), monocarboxylate transporter 1 (MCT1/SLC16A1), from the solute transporter family, and P-glycoprotein (P-gp; MDR1/ABCB1), breast-cancer-resistance protein (BCRP/ABCG2) and multidrug-resistance-associated proteins 1-9(MRP1-9/ABCC1-9) from the ABC transporter family [72]. The localization of these transporters in both the BBB and BCSF barrier are shown in Figure 3 with each individual transporter is being discussed in greater detail below.

6.1. Organic Anion Transporting Polypeptide (OATP)

Organic anion transporting polypeptides (OATPs) are members of the solute carrier organic anion transporter family (SLCO) [73]. The OATPs accommodate the transport of a wide variety of amphipathic solutes, including bile salts, anionic peptides, steroid conjugates, thyroid hormones and an increasing number of pharmaceutical drugs and xenobiotics [74]. Members of the OATP family, of which there are currently 11 known to be expressed in humans

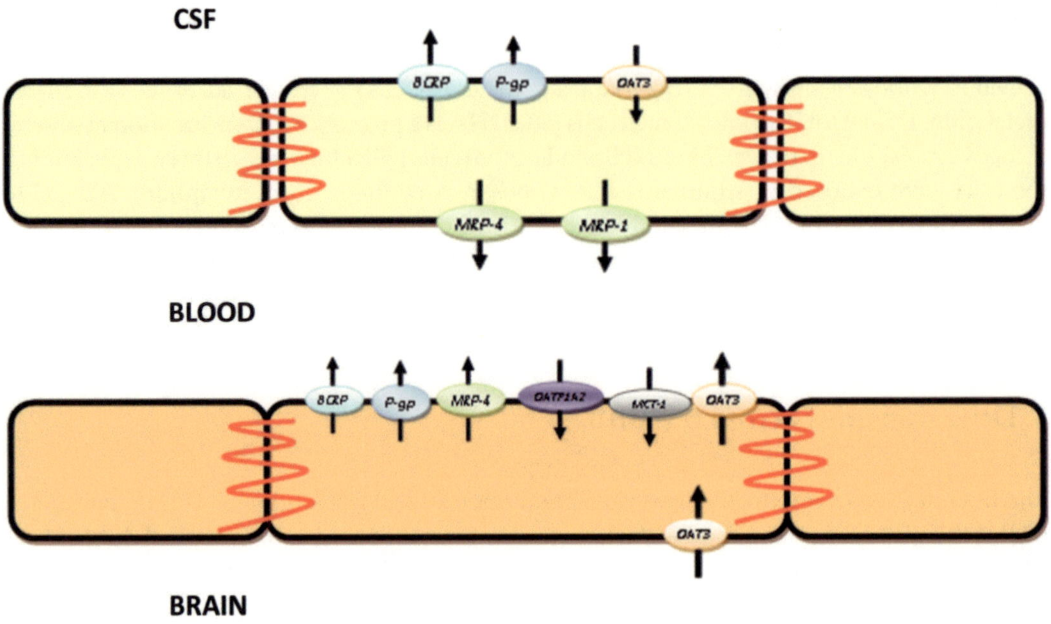

Figure 3. The localization of transporters in the blood brain barrier (BBB) and blood cerebral spinal fluid barrier (BCSFB) of CNS.

(OATP1A2, 1B1, 1B3, 1C1, 2A1, 2B1, 3A1, 4A1, 4C1, 5A1, and 6A1), share a great deal of amino acid sequence identity and transport solutes in a sodium independent manner [75].

Of the various OATPs, both OATP1A2 and OATP1A4 are expressed in the BBB. Organic anion transport protein 1A2 was the first member of the OATP family to be reported in humans, while OATP1A4 is a more recently discovered homolog of hepatic [76]. At the protein level, OATP1A2 (previously designated OATP-A) is expressed in many organs including the liver, intestine, kidney, lung, testes, and the brain. Within the brain, this transporter is localized in the frontal cortex and specifically confined to the endothelial cells of the BBB [74]. Its localization on the luminal side of brain microvessel endothelial cells suggests that OATP1A2 aids in the entry of various solutes and therapeutic agents into the brain [74]. While OATP1A4 is mainly concentrated in the liver, the transporter has also been detected within the brain microvessel endothelial cells [74]. In contrast to OATP1A2, immunohistochemical localization studies indicate that OATP1A4 is expressed on both the apical and basolateral side of the endothelial cells of the BBB and thus, mediates the uptake of compounds from both the brain and the blood compartments [77].

6.2. Organic Anion Transporter (OAT)

Organic anion transporters (OATs) belong to the SLC22A gene family. Similarly to OATPs, the OATs transport a broad range of chemically unrelated endogenous and exogenous compounds. There are at least 10 families of OATs designated by Arabic numbers (eg. OAT1).

OAT1 is predominantly expressed in the kidney although a very small amount is also found in the brain particularly concentrated in regions such as cortex, hypothalamus, hippocampus and cerebellum [78]. This transporter is known to interact with a broad range of drugs including antibiotics (penicillins, benzylpenicillin and carbenicillin), antineoplastics (methotrexate) and even cholesterol lowering drugs including the statins and fibrates such as fluvastatin, pravastatin, and bezafibrate, respectively [78]. OAT2, on the other hand, is predominantly expressed in the liver and very little is found in the kidney and brain. The expression level of this transporter in a particular tissue can be influenced by a variety of factors; including gender and species differences [79]. For example, in the adult male rat, the mRNA for OAT2 expression is greater in the liver than the kidney, and the opposite is true for the adult female rat where the mRNA level in the kidney is greater than in the liver [79]. However, this phenomenon has not been observed in humans. Furthermore, the expression level of OAT2 is also influenced by hepatocyte nuclear factors and endogenous gas molecules including nitric oxide [80,81]. Given the similar molecular structure to OAT1, OAT2 also mediates the transport of a broad range of solutes including cholesterol lowering drugs (i.e. statins), antibiotics such as cephalosporins, and antineoplastic drugs like 5-fluorouracil [78].

From a CNS perspective, OAT3 appears to have the greatest expression levels in the brain [78]. Within the CNS, OAT3 is primarily localized in the brain capillaries and in epithelial cells of the choroid plexus, specifically on the basolateral side of the plasma membrane of the cells [82]. The predominantly basolateral localization of OAT3 in the BBB and BCSFB implies that the primary function of OAT3 is to aid in the removal of compounds from the brain. Endogenous products of neurotransmitter and hormone metabolism are potential candidates for OAT3-mediated removal. Potential therapeutic agents that may be transported out of the brain through OAT3-dependent processes at the BBB and BCSFB include the various statins, diuretics, antibiotics and antivirals [78]. As OAT3 interacts with a large number of therapeutic agents, drug-drug interactions may be of potential concern in the BBB, although specific examples are at present not known.

6.3. Glucose Transporters (GLUT)

Glucose is the major source of energy for most mammalian cells, particularly in the brain. Despite the high dependence of the brain on glycolysis, the source of glucose comes entirely from the blood and is dependent on passage through the BBB. The entry of glucose into the brain is mediated by facilitative glucose transporter proteins. There are currently seven known isoforms, with the designation of GLUT1-7 [83]. The main isoforms found within the CNS are GLUT1 and GLUT3 that bring glucose into the cell through sodium independent transport mechanisms. A summary of the various GLUTs and their distribution within the CNS is shown in Figure 4. GLUT1 within the CNS exists as two distinct forms, which differ only by the extent of glycosylation [84]. A glycosylated, 55 KDa GLUT1 is found primarily in the endothelial cells of the BBB while the non-vascular, non-glycosylated 45 KDa form is mainly found in neural cells as well as the basolateral plasma of epithelial cells isolated from the choroid plexus [83]. Aside from the prominent expression found in the microvessels and choroid plexus, GLUT1 has also been detected in small cells with dark stained nuclei characteristic of glia cells [85].

Immunohistochemistry staining also showed a positive detection of GLUT1 in astrocytes that are in direct contact with the cerebral microvessels of rat brain slices. Electron microscopy also revealed dense distribution of GLUT1 within the astrocyte foot processes surrounding the microvessels of the gray matter and synaptic contacts [86].

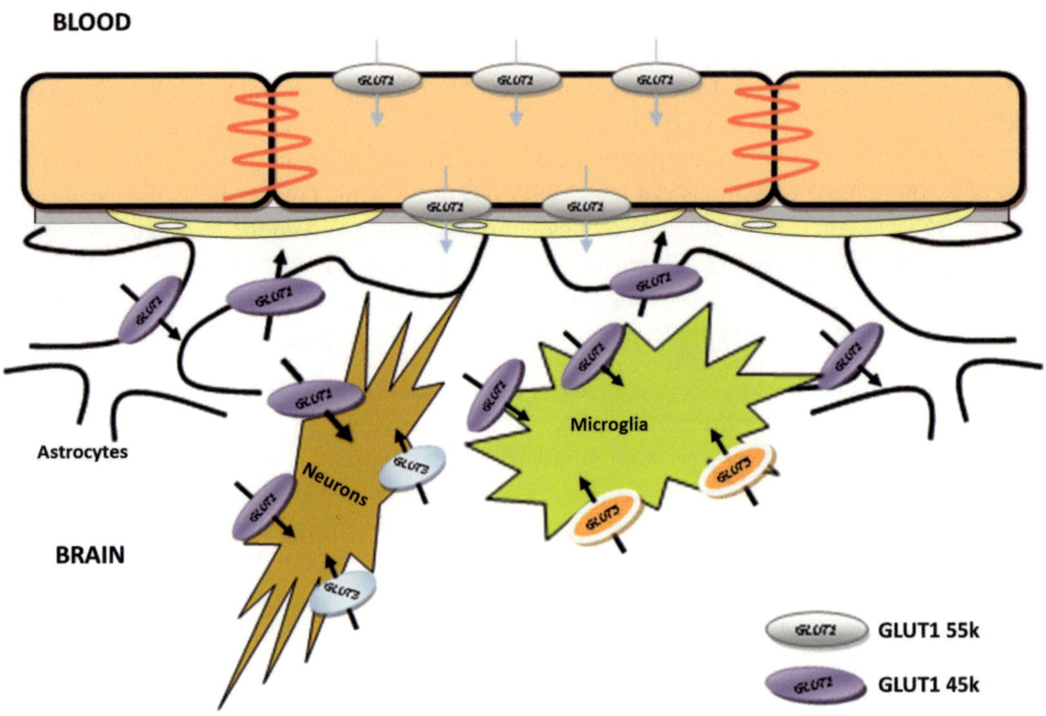

Figure 4. Cellular localization of different isoforms of glucose transporter in the CNS.

The main glucose transporter in the BBB is GLUT1. This same transporter is also highly expressed in the blood-retinal barrier, the placental barrier, and blood-CSF barrier (BCSFB) [87-89] highlighting its importance in regulation of glucose levels in these tissues. The transport of glucose through GLUT1 in the BBB is the rate-limiting step for glucose utilization in the brain and is highly responsive to metabolic changes within the brain. For example, GLUT1 expression in the BBB at both the mRNA and protein level can increase or decrease depending on the ambient concentration of hexose. High concentration of hexose decreases the expression of GLUT1 while low hexose concentration causes an up-regulation of both GLUT1 mRNA and protein levels [90]. Following brain injury such as a stroke and brain tumors, both mRNA and protein levels of GLUT1 are significantly increased [83,85,91].

The endothelial cells forming the BBB also express sodium glucose cotransporter (SGLT) [92]. Unlike GLUT1, glucose transport through SGLT is sodium-dependent. A functional role for SGLT in glucose homeostasis in the brain has not been established; however, it has been speculated that SGLT may help maintain intracellular glucose levels in the brain under stressful conditions such as hypoglycemia [92].

6.4. Monocarboxylate Transporter (MCT)

Monocarboxylic acids, including lactate, pyruvate, and ketones play an important role in energy metabolism within the body. Monocarboxylates such as pyruvate, lactate, and ketone bodies (i.e acetoacetate and β-hydroxybutyarate) can be utilized by neurons, in the absence of glucose, to generate a substantial amount of energy for the brain [93]. Under pathological and physiological conditions including diabetes, prolonged starvation, hypoglycemia, or even intense exercise, the build-up of lactate provides an energy source, which can be utilized by the brain [3,94,95]. In addition, monocarboxylates including lactic acid are a metabolic by-product produced and released within the CNS by neurons [96,97], astrocytes [96] and oligodendrocytes [98]. As monocarboxylates are hydrophilic compounds that cannot readily diffuse cross the BBB, specific transporter systems are required to maintain proper levels of these endogenous metabolic products in the brain [93].

Sequence homology indicates that the monocarboxylate transporter family (previous known as SLC16 gene family) consists of 14 members identified as MCT1-9, MCT11-14 and T-type amino acid transporter 1 (TAT1) [99]. MCT1-4 is a symporter mediating the co-transport of monocarboxylate and proton in a one to one stoichiometry ratio. MCT1-4 is present in almost all tissues including the muscles, liver, kidney, heart, testes, and brain [93,99]. While MCT1 and MCT2 are found in the muscles, liver, kidney, heart and CNS, [93], MCT3 is exclusively expressed on the basolateral side of the retinal pigment epithelium and MCT4 is highly expressed in the skeletal muscles and also in the brain. Within the BBB, MCT1 was the first monocarboxylic acid transporter identified in the brain microvessel endothelial cells and in the ependycytes lining the ventricles [100]. Both electron microscopy and immunohistochemistry revealed a small amount of MCT1 in astrocytic end-feet surrounding the capillaries [100,101]. The presence of MCT1 was found in the cytoplasm of astrocyte and also associated with the plasma membrane [93]. In contrast, MCT2 is found in endothelial cells forming the BBB, but absent in astrocytes [93,100]. MCT4, on the other hand, was exclusively expressed in the astrocytes and glial cells of rodent brain. Furthermore, when the hippocampus and the corpus callosum were labeled, the expression of MCT4 was restricted to astrocytes [93]. MCT8 was recently recognized as thyroid hormone transporter as opposed to monocarboxylate [102].

6.5. ATP-Binding Cassette Transporters (ABC)

The ATP-binding cassette (ABC) superfamily of transporter proteins are responsible for the active transport of a wide variety of compounds including phospholipids, ions, peptides, steroids, polysaccharides, amino acids, organic anions, bile acids, drugs and other xenobiotic compounds across cellular membranes. There are roughly 48 genes encoding the various human ABC transporters, each is organized into seven subfamilies designated ABCA to ABCG [103]. Over-expression of ABC transporters are major contributors to the development of multidrug resistance (MDR) in cancer cells. For instance, when the MDR gene that codes for an efflux transporter is being transfected into drug sensitive cells, the transfectant cells become resistant to the drugs that are substrates for the transporters resulting in a decrease in the intracellular concentration of the drugs, thereby conferring multidrug resistance [104]. MDR in tumor cell lines is often linked to an ATP-dependent decrease in cellular accumulation of drugs namely through p-glycoprotein (p-gp encoded by ABCB1), multidrug resistance proteins (MRP encoded by ABCC), and breast cancer resistance protein (BCRP encoded by ABCG2) drug efflux transporters [105]. In addition to their function as multidrug resistance proteins, these transporters are also expressed in normal tissue such as intestines, liver, kidney and the BBB and BCSFB, suggesting that they also have a protective function in limiting accumulation and distribution and speeding the elimination of xenobiotic compounds which could result in tissue toxicity [106].

6.6. Multidrug Resistance Protein (MRP)

The multidrug resistance-associated proteins (MRPs) are a subfamily of ABC transporters. There are currently 12 members of this subfamily designated as ABCC1-12. Of the 12, 9 have demonstrated drug efflux transporter function and play an important role in absorption, distribution and elimination of various drugs and metabolites. While all MRPs have the capability to transport amphiphatic organic anions, transport substrates are not limited to anionic species. Examples of this include the transport of nucleotide based analogs by MRP4 and MRP5, efflux of prostaglandins by MRP1, co-transport of neutral or cationic solutes as well as glucoronide drug conjugates by MRP1 and MRP2 [107]. Within the MRPs and other ABC transport proteins there tends to be substantial substrate affinity overlap. This is a fascinating feature considering most members are structurally and functionally distinct from other ABC binding cassette transporters. For example, there is only approximately 15% amino acid sequence homology between MRPs and P-gp [108]. In addition, when comparing amino acid sequence between different members within the MRP subfamily to MRP1, amino acid sequence homology ranges between 33% for MRP8 and 58% for MRP3 [109].

The brain endothelial cells that form the BBB express several different MRP. Collectively the MRP efflux transporters function to restrict the uptake and aid in the elimination of drugs, xenobiotics and endogenous compounds from the brain. Currently, members of the MRP family that have been reported in the BBB include MRP1, 2,4-9. The evidence for the localization and function of each of the MRPs within the BBB are discussed below.

6.6.1. MRP1

MRP1 is expressed in primary cultured bovine, murine [110], rat [111] and porcine [112] brain microvessel endothelial cells. While studies by Seetharaman and coworkers [113] suggested up-regulation of MRP1 expression in human culture brain microvessel endothelial cells compared to freshly isolated human brain capillaries, more recent studies support robust expression of MRP1 within the brain capillaries isolated from human brain tissue [114]. Two independent studies reported that MRP1 is localized primarily to the apical (luminal) plasma membrane in brain microvessel endothelial cells [114,115]. This is in contrast to studies by Roberts et al. [116] suggesting MRP1 has a basolateral (abluminal) plasma membrane localization in rat brain microvessels. As MRP1 shows high transporter activity for conjugated

http://dx.doi.org/10.5772/57604

compounds such as estradiol 17β glucuronides [117], it is interesting to note that Sugiyama and colleagues [118] demonstrated a reduction in elimination of estradiol 17β glucuronide from the brain of *Mrp1* knockout mice compared to that observed in the wild-type controls with functional MRP1. These functional studies support the luminal expression of MRP1 and suggest a role in limiting brain exposure to drugs and endogenous solutes.

6.6.2. MRP2

The expression and localization of MRP2 within the BBB is the subject of much debate. Studies by Miller et al. [119] indicated MRP2 was expressed in the luminal plasma membrane of isolated rat brain capillaries. These initial findings were supported by reports of MRP2 expression in both human brain capillaries as well as zebrafish [120,121]. In contrast, no detectable expression of MRP2 was found, at either the mRNA or protein level, in bovine brain microvessel endothelial cells [122,123] or mouse brain microvessel endothelial cells [110,118]. Furthermore, studies examining MRP2 protein expression in isolated human brain capillaries were below detection limits [114,124]. Interestingly, expression of MRP2 in rat brain endothelial cells was inducible by activation of either pregnane X receptor (PXR) or constitutive androstane receptor (CAR) pathways [125,126].

Functionally, MRP2 mediates the transport of glucuronide and GSH conjugates to a lesser extent than MRP1 [127]. It also actively transports chemotherapeutics such as methotrexate, vinca alkaloids, anthracyclins, antiepileptics such as phenytoin and endogenous agents like leukotriene C4 [107,109,128,129]. Thus if MRP2 is expressed in the BBB, it could have a profound effect on the brain distribution of many therapeutic agents. However, there are few studies showing a significant impact of MRP2 on the BBB permeability. One such study demonstrated an increased accumulation of phenytoin in the brain of Mrp2 deficient rats compared to controls [129]. There is also evidence for MRP2-mediated changes in brain penetration of drugs in epileptic animals. Based on available information, most evidence indicates that MRP2 expression in the BBB is low or below detectable limits and as such has negligible effects on solute and macromolecule distribution into the brain. However, as MRP2 expression appears highly inducible, there is a possibility that MRP2 activity in the BBB could be of importance during pathological events within the CNS.

6.6.3. MRP3

Studies by Zhang et al. [122] identified low and variable expression of MRP3 in bovine brain microvessel endothelial cells. Subsequent proteomics based studies of both mouse [130] and human [131] BBB indicated that MRP3 expression was below detection limits.

6.6.4. MRP4

Evidence supporting a significant functional role for MRP4 in the BBB is perhaps the strongest of all the MRPs. The first evidence of MRP4 expression in the BBB was the studies by Zhang et al. [122] in bovine brain microvessel endothelial cells. Follow-up studies examining the localization of MRP4 suggested both luminal and abluminal presence of the transporter [115]. The expression of MRP4 has since been reported in human, mouse and rat BBB [114,116,132]. Comparison of MRP4 expression in the brains of wild-type and *Mrp4* knockout mice confirmed BBB localization as well as expression in the choroid plexus epithelial cells forming the BCSFB [132].

Functionally, MRP4 can transport a wide variety of substrates and is important in the efflux of many nucleotide analog based chemotherapeutics. As with MRP1 and MRP2, MRP4 transports the endogenous substrate leukotriene C4 [133,134]. However, in addition, MRP4 can also transport endogenous nucleotides such as cAMP and cGMP [135]. Common chemotherapeutic purine nucleotide anion analogs that are effluxed by this transporter include bis(pivaloyloxymethyl)-9-[2-(phosphonomethoxy)ethyl]-adenine (PMEA), and active metabolites of 6-mercaptopurine and 6-thioguanine [72,107,136]. Using *Mrp4* -/- knockout mice significant increases in topotecan [132] and PMEA [137] accumulation in the brain was observed.

6.6.5. MRP5 and MRP6

Within the BBB, MRP5 is highly expressed, whereas MRP6 is expressed to a lesser extent [122]. Presently their locations within the BBB remain unclear. Previous studies by Zhang et al. [115] found MRP5 protein expression to be primarily in the apical membrane fraction of brain microvessel endothelial cells. These findings were supported by Nies et al. [114]. In contrast, Roberts et al. [116] found low levels of abluminal MRP5 expression when staining in rat brain microvessel endothelial cells. Currently, the location of MRP6 remains to be seen because no specific MRP6 antibody is available at this time [115].

MRP5 can transport purine nucleotide analogs [127] and is the primary active transporter of cGMP and cAMP [138]. Therefore MRP5 and -4 may work in concert to regulate cGMP and cAMP levels [127] in the brain. MRP6 can transport anionic organic ions but cannot transport glucuronide or GSH [127] and has been shown to transport leukotrinene C4 [139].

6.6.6. MRP7, -8 and -9

Currently, little is known about these transporters with regards to the BBB. MRP7, -8 and -9 have been found to be expressed in brain [140]. MRP7 can transport glucuronide E2 17betaG and exhibits high levels of resistance to taxane docetaxel, approximately 9 to 13 fold [140]. MRP8 is able to transport nucleotide analogues such as PMEA, glutathione conjugates and methotrexate [140]. No substrates for MRP9 have been identified at this time [109].

When looking at drug resistant efflux transport in the literature, major focus has been put on P-gp and BCRP and limited research has been focused on members within the MRP subfamily as it relates to the BBB. As has been demonstrated here, many of these MRP transporters can transport substrates that are important both physiologically and in the clinic. Particularly within the CNS, it is important to decipher any discrepancies in location and expression of MRP members within the BBB because they can have relevant impact on CNS drug concentrations reaching therapeutic levels within the brain and thus can affect our ability to treat important brain pathologies.

http://dx.doi.org/10.5772/57604

6.7. Breast Cancer Resistance Protein (BCRP)

BCRP was originally discovered in the MCF-7 AdrVp breast cancer cell line after observing that the cells are resistant to chemotherapeutic drugs including mitoxantrone, doxorubicin, and daunorubicin [141]. The gene sequence of the protein was isolated shortly after and was classified as the group G subfamily of ABC transporters. There are at least 5 members of ABCG subfamily identified in humans (ABCG1, ABCG2, ABCG4, ABCG5, and ABCG8). However, the primary form that plays a crucial role in the transport of substances between the blood and the CNS is ABCG2 [141]. At the protein level, ABCG2 is approximately 72-kDa with 665 amino acids and is considered as a half-transporter as shown in Figure 5. Other ABC transporters have two sets of membrane spanning regions (6 transmembrane α-helices) and two nucleotide binding domains (NBD); the G subfamily of protein consists of only one set of membrane spanning domain 6 transmembrane α-helices and only one NBD [141]. In order to function, it is believed that these half-transporters form homodimers [142].

The specific localization of ABCG2 within the CNS is primarily confined to the luminal plasma membrane of the brain microvessel endothelial cells. Given the localization within the BBB and the compounds that are transported by ABCG2, it has been suggested that ABCG2 most likely protects the brain from xenobiotics and toxins similar to other ABC transporters [141]. Furthermore, ABCG2 also plays a role in the accumulation and disposition of various endogenous substrates including sulfate and glucuronide conjugates of estrone and dehydroepiandrosterone [143,144]. In addition to endogenous substrates, ABCG2 also binds and recognizes a broad range of structurally-unrelated drugs and xenobiotics [141]. Many of these transport substrates also interact with other ABC transporters including ABCB1 and the ABCC subfamily; thus, the accumulation and distribution of drugs can be significantly altered.

6.8. P-glycoprotein (P-gp)

P-glycoprotein (P-gp) was the first ABC transporter to be characterized. First identified by Juliano and Ling [145] in 1976 using Chinese hamster ovary cells with selected resistance to colchicine, they discovered that the drug resistance properties of the mutated cells were consistently correlated with a high molecular weight component found in the plasma membrane with an approximate weight of 170,000 Da [145]. They also observed that the component was likely a glycoprotein associated with the plasma membrane of the mutated cells and was consistently absent or expressed at a lower level in the wild-type cells. Furthermore, they also noticed that the mutant cells with high levels of glycoprotein displayed an alter drug permeability; thus, they designated it as "P-glycoprotein" [145]. P-gp is also expressed in numerous tissues, including adrenal glands, kidneys, liver, colon, small intestine, heart, testes, peripheral nerves, and the brain. At the BBB, it is the most extensively studied ABC transporter being expressed in the luminal plasma membrane of brain endothelial cells [104]. Under normal conditions, the presence of P-gp in the BBB limits a broad range of substances from penetrating the brain tissue. Some notable drug classes with reduced brain penetration due to P-gp efflux at the BBB include anti-epileptics, anti-cancer drugs, anti-histamines and HIV protease inhibitors [103]. Numerous studies using drugs such as cyclosporine, digoxin, domperidone, etoposide, loperamide, ondansetron, taxol and vinblastine have shown the important role of

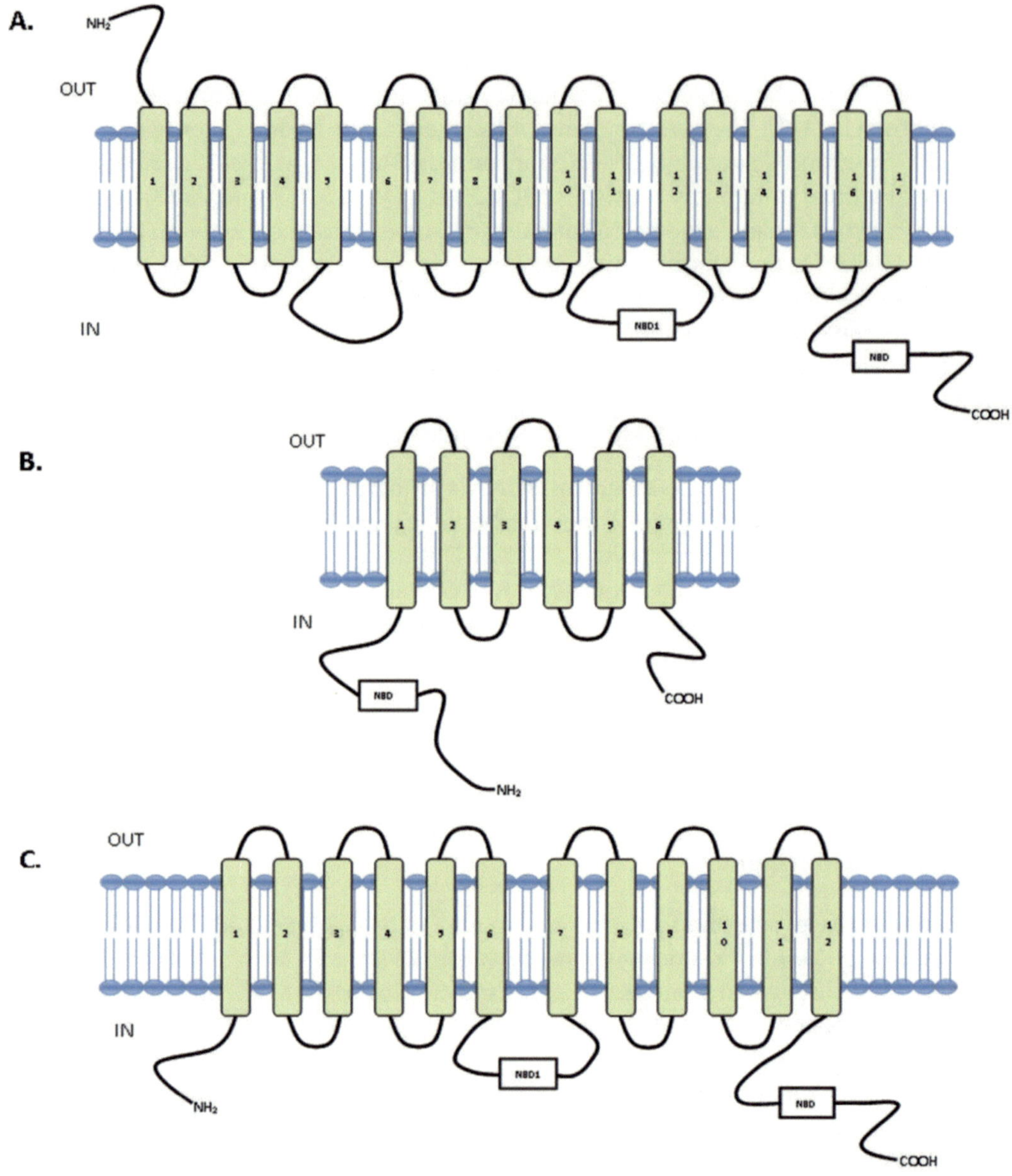

Figure 5. Structures of (A) MRP transporter, (B) BCRP transporter, and (C) P-glycoprotein transporter.

P-gp in the pharmacokinetics of P-gp substrates in multiple parts of the body. Table 1 shows some of the drugs that are known substrates for P-gp.

Similar to other ABC transporters, P-gp is a transmembrane protein with a molecular weight of 170 KDa formed by two homologous subunits that function as an efflux pump in an ATP-dependent manner (shown in Figure 5). The protein is assembled in two halves connected by a 75 amino acid linker region. Each half contains 6 transmembrane segments, an intracellular nucleotide binding domain, and both intracellular N and C terminal regions. The exact localization of P-gp had been a subject of some debate with evidence supporting both luminal and abluminal expression of the protein. Luminal P-gp expression had been observed in rat and mouse brain capillaries [115,146,147]. Furthermore, the luminal expression of P-gp has also been isolated in human brain microvessels [113,148]. In contrast, electron microscope techniques have shown an enhanced expression of P-gp on the abluminal side of the rat brain endothelial cells [149]. Nevertheless, recent studies using immunoreactivity support the localization of P-gp on the luminal side of the endothelial cells [116].

Cancer Drugs	Immuno-suppressive Drugs	Lipid Lowering Agent	Steroids	HIV Protease Inhibitors	Cardiac Drugs	Anti-Diarrheal Drugs	Anti-Gout Agent	Anti-Bacterial Agents	Anti-Helminthic Agent
Doxorubicin	Cyclosporin A	Lovastatin	Aldosterone	Amprenavir	Digoxin	Loperamide	Colchicine	Erythromyccin	Ivermectin
Daunourbicin	FK506		Cortisol	Indinavir	Quinidine	Antiemetics		Rifampin	Abamectin
Vinblastine	Tacrolimus		Corticosterone	Nelfinavir		Domperidone		Valinomycin	
Vincristine			Hydrocortisone	Ritonavir		Ondansetron		Gramicidin	
Vindesine			Dexamethaxone	Saquinavir				Grepafloxacin	
Vinorelbine			Triamcinolone	Lopinavir					
Paclitaxel									
Etoposide									
Teniposide									
Epirubicin									
Irinotecan									
Tamoxifen									
Methotrexate									
Amsacrine									
Imatinib									

Table 1 Representative compounds that are known to be P-glycoprotein substrates. (Adapted from [156])

Numerous studies have attempted to identify and characterize P-gp substrates. Unlike conventional transporters, which recognize specific substrates, P-gp recognizes a broad range of compounds and has the capacity to extract its substrates directly from the plasma membrane [150]. Some of the most common features of P-gp substrates include their lipophilic nature that enables them to cross the lipid bilayer of the cell membrane. Furthermore, many P-gp substrates commonly consist of two aromatic rings and a basic nitrogen atom. These molecules can be uncharged or basic in nature, although some acidic compounds including methotrexate and phenytoin can also bind to P-gp but at a lower rate. Molecules with molecular weight ranges from 300 to 2000 Da are capable of binding to the protein and being transported [151]. Peptide substrates consisting of 3 to 15 amino acids with molecular weight ranges from 380 to

1880 Da can also interact with P-gp [151]. Most recently, beta amyloid protein, the component found in amyloid plaques in Alzheimer's disease was reported to be a transport substrate of both P-gp but not BCRP [152,153].

One method for overcoming the limited permeability of P-gp transport substrates is to pharmacologically inhibit Pgp. P-glycoprotein inhibitors are themselves non-cytotoxic agents that can be used in combination with P-gp substrates to maintain the intracellular drug concentration. An inhibitor binds to P-gp and prevents the transport of P-gp substrates. There are at least three generations of P-gp inhibitors. The first generation compounds are less potent and non-selective with undesirable side effects at inhibitory concentrations. Examples of first generation inhibitors include the calcium channel blocker, verapamil, and the immunosuppressive agent cyclosporin A. First generation P-gp inhibitors act as competitive inhibitors of P-gp transport [154].

The second-generation compounds including dexverapamil or dexniguldipine were developed to reduce the toxicity associated with P-gp inhibition. They eliminate the undesirable side effects while retaining the ability to inhibit P-gp. The third generation inhibitors including tariquidar and elacridar are much more specific and more potent than earlier compounds. Unlike the first and second generation of P-gp inhibitors, the third generation of drugs acts as non-competitive inhibitors of P-gp, and the compounds themselves are not transported by P-gp [155]. Table 2 summarizes representative P-gp inhibitors [104].

Cyclopropylibenzosuberane	Immunosupp-ressant	Calcuim channel blocker	Progesterone antagonist	Antiarrhythmic agent	Antifungal agent	Acridonecarboxamide derivative	Topoisomerase
LY335979	Cyclosporin A Valspodar (PSC833)	Verapamil	Mefiprostone (RU486)	Quinidine	Ketoconazole	GG918 (GF120918)	Xenova (XR 5944)

Table 2 Representative compounds that are known to be P-glycoprotein inhibitors. (Adapted from [156])

The ability of P-gp to extrude xenobiotics provides protection and detoxification of cells under normal conditions. For example, knockout mice (MDR1a$^{-/-}$) have been shown to be more sensitive to ivermectin and are susceptible to serious neurotoxicity compared to wild type control mice [156]. Considering the broad range of P-gp substrates and the expression of P-gp in tissues responsible for absorption, distribution and elimination of drugs, it is no surprise that this particular drug efflux transporter can significantly affect the absorption and distribution of drugs. This is especially true for cancer therapies used in the treatment of brain tumors. The tight junctions of the BBB restrict paracellular diffusion of chemotherapeutic agents into the CNS, while the presence of the various drug efflux transporters, such as P-gp, within the endothelial cells of the BBB reduces transcellular passage of chemotherapeutic agents into the brain and tumor sites.

http://dx.doi.org/10.5772/57604

7. Conclusion

The brain capillaries are structurally and functionally different from capillaries formed in the other organs. The selectiveness and permissiveness of the endothelial cell monolayer within the CNS is dependent on the tight junctions as wells as the numerous transporter systems located on the luminal and the abluminal surface of the endothelial cells forming the BBB. The restrictive nature of the tight junctions along with transporter systems expressed in the BBB can significantly altered the accumulation and distribution of fatty acids and drugs in the CNS under pathological conditions. Improved delivery to the brain can be achieved by reversibly disrupting the physical tight junctions and/or inhibiting the activity of efflux transporter systems.

Author details

Siddhartha Dalvi[1], Ngoc On[1], Hieu Nguyen[1], Michael Pogorzelec[1], Donald W. Miller[1] and Grant M. Hatch[1,2]

*Address all correspondence to: ghatch@mich.ca

1 Departments of Pharmacology & Therapeutics, Center for Research and Treatment of Atherosclerosis, University of Manitoba, DREAM Manitoba Institute of Child Health, Canada

2 Biochemistry and Medical Genetics, Center for Research and Treatment of Atherosclerosis, University of Manitoba, DREAM Manitoba Institute of Child Health, Canada

References

[1] Rubin LL, Hall DE, Porter S, Barbu K, Cannon C, Horner HC, et al. A cell culture model of the blood-brain barrier. J Cell Biol 1991 Dec;115(6):1725-1735.

[2] Gloor SM, Wachtel M, Bolliger MF, Ishihara H, Landmann R, Frei K. Molecular and cellular permeability control at the blood-brain barrier. Brain Res Brain Res Rev 2001 Oct;36(2-3):258-264.

[3] Hawkins BT, Davis TP. The blood-brain barrier/neurovascular unit in health and disease. Pharmacol Rev 2005 Jun;57(2):173-185.

[4] Kniesel U, Wolburg H. Tight junctions of the blood-brain barrier. Cell Mol Neurobiol 2000 Feb;20(1):57-76.

[5] Mitchell RW, Edmundson CL, Miller DW, Hatch GM. On the mechanism of oleate transport across human brain microvessel endothelial cells. J Neurochem 2009 Aug; 110(3):1049-1057.

[6] Mitchell RW, On NH, Del Bigio MR, Miller DW, Hatch GM. Fatty acid transport protein expression in human brain and potential role in fatty acid transport across human brain microvessel endothelial cells. J Neurochem 2011 May;117(4):735-746.

[7] Urich E, Lazic SE, Molnos J, Wells I, Freskgård P. Transcriptional Profiling of Human Brain Endothelial Cells Reveals Key Properties Crucial for Predictive In Vitro Blood-Brain Barrier Models. PloS one 2012;7(5).

[8] Huber JD, Egleton RD, Davis TP. Molecular physiology and pathophysiology of tight junctions in the blood-brain barrier. Trends Neurosci 2001 Dec;24(12):719-725.

[9] Zlokovic BV. The blood-brain barrier in health and chronic neurodegenerative disorders. Neuron 2008 Jan 24;57(2):178-201.

[10] Abbott NJ, Ronnback L, Hansson E. Astrocyte-endothelial interactions at the blood-brain barrier. Nat Rev Neurosci 2006 Jan;7(1):41-53.

[11] Haseloff RF, Blasig IE, Bauer HC, Bauer H. In search of the astrocytic factor(s) modulating blood-brain barrier functions in brain capillary endothelial cells in vitro. Cell Mol Neurobiol 2005 Feb;25(1):25-39.

[12] Janzer RC, Raff MC. Astrocytes induce blood-brain barrier properties in endothelial cells. Nature 1987 Jan 15-21;325(6101):253-257.

[13] Balabanov R, Dore-Duffy P. Role of the CNS microvascular pericyte in the blood-brain barrier. J Neurosci Res 1998 Sep 15;53(6):637-644.

[14] Lai CH, Kuo KH. The critical component to establish in vitro BBB model: Pericyte. Brain Res Brain Res Rev 2005 Dec 15;50(2):258-265.

[15] Ballabh P, Braun A, Nedergaard M. The blood-brain barrier: an overview: structure, regulation, and clinical implications. Neurobiol Dis 2004 Jun;16(1):1-13.

[16] Matter K, Balda MS. Signalling to and from tight junctions. Nat Rev Mol Cell Biol 2003 Mar;4(3):225-236.

[17] Morita K, Sasaki H, Furuse M, Tsukita S. Endothelial claudin: claudin-5/TMVCF constitutes tight junction strands in endothelial cells. J Cell Biol 1999 Oct 4;147(1): 185-194.

[18] Sonoda N, Furuse M, Sasaki H, Yonemura S, Katahira J, Horiguchi Y, et al. Clostridium perfringens enterotoxin fragment removes specific claudins from tight junction strands: Evidence for direct involvement of claudins in tight junction barrier. J Cell Biol 1999 Oct 4;147(1):195-204.

[19] Krause G, Winkler L, Mueller SL, Haseloff RF, Piontek J, Blasig IE. Structure and function of claudins. Biochim Biophys Acta 2008 Mar;1778(3):631-645.

[20] Furuse M, Fujita K, Hiiragi T, Fujimoto K, Tsukita S. Claudin-1 and -2: novel integral membrane proteins localizing at tight junctions with no sequence similarity to occludin. J Cell Biol 1998 Jun 29;141(7):1539-1550.

[21] Liebner S, Fischmann A, Rascher G, Duffner F, Grote EH, Kalbacher H, et al. Claudin-1 and claudin-5 expression and tight junction morphology are altered in blood vessels of human glioblastoma multiforme. Acta Neuropathol 2000 Sep;100(3): 323-331.

[22] Hirase T, Staddon JM, Saitou M, Ando-Akatsuka Y, Itoh M, Furuse M, et al. Occludin as a possible determinant of tight junction permeability in endothelial cells. J Cell Sci 1997 Jul;110 (Pt 14)(Pt 14):1603-1613.

[23] Feldman GJ, Mullin JM, Ryan MP. Occludin: structure, function and regulation. Adv Drug Deliv Rev 2005 Apr 25;57(6):883-917.

[24] Aurrand-Lions M, Johnson-Leger C, Wong C, Du Pasquier L, Imhof BA. Heterogeneity of endothelial junctions is reflected by differential expression and specific subcellular localization of the three JAM family members. Blood 2001 Dec 15;98(13): 3699-3707.

[25] Mandell KJ, Parkos CA. The JAM family of proteins. Adv Drug Deliv Rev 2005 Apr 25;57(6):857-867.

[26] Lippoldt A, Kniesel U, Liebner S, Kalbacher H, Kirsch T, Wolburg H, et al. Structural alterations of tight junctions are associated with loss of polarity in stroke-prone spontaneously hypertensive rat blood-brain barrier endothelial cells. Brain Res 2000 Dec 8;885(2):251-261.

[27] Gumbleton M, Audus KL. Progress and limitations in the use of in vitro cell cultures to serve as a permeability screen for the blood-brain barrier. J Pharm Sci 2001 Nov; 90(11):1681-1698.

[28] Miller D.W., Audus K.L. and Borchardt R.T. Application of cultured endothelial cells of the brain microvasculature in the study of the blood-brain barrier. J. Tiss. Cult. Meth 1992;14:217-224.

[29] Trickler WJ, Mayhan WG, Miller DW. Brain microvessel endothelial cell responses to tumor necrosis factor-alpha involve a nuclear factor kappa B (NF-kappaB) signal transduction pathway. Brain Res 2005 Jun 28;1048(1-2):24-31.

[30] de Vries HE, Blom-Roosemalen MC, de Boer AG, van Berkel TJ, Breimer DD, Kuiper J. Effect of endotoxin on permeability of bovine cerebral endothelial cell layers in vitro. J Pharmacol Exp Ther 1996 Jun;277(3):1418-1423.

[31] Cecchelli R, Dehouck B, Descamps L, Fenart L, Buee-Scherrer VV, Duhem C, et al. In vitro model for evaluating drug transport across the blood-brain barrier. Adv Drug Deliv Rev 1999 Apr 5;36(2-3):165-178.

[32] Abumrad N, Coburn C, Ibrahimi A. Membrane proteins implicated in long-chain fatty acid uptake by mammalian cells: CD36, FATP and FABPm. Biochim Biophys Acta 1999 Oct 18;1441(1):4-13.

[33] Schaffer JE. Fatty acid transport: the roads taken. Am J Physiol Endocrinol Metab 2002 Feb;282(2):E239-46.

[34] Brouns F, van der Vusse GJ. Utilization of lipids during exercise in human subjects: metabolic and dietary constraints. Br J Nutr 1998 Feb;79(2):117-128.

[35] Pohl J, Ring A, Ehehalt R, Schulze-Bergkamen H, Schad A, Verkade P, et al. Long-chain fatty acid uptake into adipocytes depends on lipid raft function. Biochemistry 2004 Apr 13;43(14):4179-4187.

[36] Drewes LR. What is the blood-brain barrier? A molecular perspective. Cerebral vascular biology. Adv Exp Med Biol 1999;474:111-122.

[37] Kamp F, Hamilton JA, Kamp F, Westerhoff HV, Hamilton JA. Movement of fatty acids, fatty acid analogues, and bile acids across phospholipid bilayers. Biochemistry 1993 Oct 19;32(41):11074-11086.

[38] Watkins PA, Hamilton JA, Leaf A, Spector AA, Moore SA, Anderson RE, et al. Brain uptake and utilization of fatty acids: applications to peroxisomal biogenesis diseases. J Mol Neurosci 2001 Apr-Jun;16(2-3):87-92; discussion 151-7.

[39] Hamilton JA, Johnson RA, Corkey B, Kamp F. Fatty acid transport: the diffusion mechanism in model and biological membranes. J Mol Neurosci 2001 Apr-Jun; 16(2-3):99-108; discussion 151-7.

[40] Hamilton JA, Guo W, Kamp F. Mechanism of cellular uptake of long-chain fatty acids: Do we need cellular proteins? Mol Cell Biochem 2002 Oct;239(1-2):17-23.

[41] Abumrad N, Harmon C, Ibrahimi A. Membrane transport of long-chain fatty acids: evidence for a facilitated process. J Lipid Res 1998 Dec;39(12):2309-2318.

[42] Schwenk RW, Holloway GP, Luiken JJ, Bonen A, Glatz JF. Fatty acid transport across the cell membrane: regulation by fatty acid transporters. Prostaglandins Leukot Essent Fatty Acids 2010 Apr-Jun;82(4-6):149-154.

[43] Hamilton JA. Transport of fatty acids across membranes by the diffusion mechanism. Prostaglandins Leukot Essent Fatty Acids 1999 May-Jun;60(5-6):291-297.

[44] Hamilton JA. Fatty acid transport: difficult or easy? J Lipid Res 1998 Mar;39(3): 467-481.

[45] Frohnert BI, Bernlohr DA. Regulation of fatty acid transporters in mammalian cells. Prog Lipid Res 2000 Jan;39(1):83-107.

[46] Hui TY, Bernlohr DA. Fatty acid transporters in animal cells. Front Biosci 1997 May 15;2:d222-31.

[47] Storch J, Corsico B. The emerging functions and mechanisms of mammalian fatty acid-binding proteins. Annu Rev Nutr 2008;28:73-95.

[48] Rapoport SI, Chang MC, Spector AA. Delivery and turnover of plasma-derived essential PUFAs in mammalian brain. J Lipid Res 2001 May;42(5):678-685.

[49] Duncan RE, Bazinet RP. Brain arachidonic acid uptake and turnover: implications for signaling and bipolar disorder. Curr Opin Clin Nutr Metab Care 2010 Mar;13(2): 130-138.

[50] Katsuki H, Okuda S. Arachidonic acid as a neurotoxic and neurotrophic substance. Prog Neurobiol 1995 Aug;46(6):607-636.

[51] Chan PH, Fishman RA, Caronna J, Schmidley JW, Prioleau G, Lee J. Induction of brain edema following intracerebral injection of arachidonic acid. Ann Neurol 1983 Jun;13(6):625-632.

[52] Chan PH, Fishman RA, Longar S, Chen S, Yu A. Cellular and molecular effects of polyunsaturated fatty acids in brain ischemia and injury. Prog Brain Res 1985;63:227-235.

[53] Jaworowicz DJ,Jr, Korytko PJ, Singh Lakhman S, Boje KM. Nitric oxide and prostaglandin E2 formation parallels blood-brain barrier disruption in an experimental rat model of bacterial meningitis. Brain Res Bull 1998 Aug;46(6):541-546.

[54] Stanimirovic D, Satoh K. Inflammatory mediators of cerebral endothelium: a role in ischemic brain inflammation. Brain Pathol 2000 Jan;10(1):113-126.

[55] Deli MA, Abraham CS, Kataoka Y, Niwa M. Permeability studies on in vitro blood-brain barrier models: physiology, pathology, and pharmacology. Cell Mol Neurobiol 2005 Feb;25(1):59-127.

[56] Mark KS, Trickler WJ, Miller DW. Tumor necrosis factor-alpha induces cyclooxygenase-2 expression and prostaglandin release in brain microvessel endothelial cells. J Pharmacol Exp Ther 2001 Jun;297(3):1051-1058.

[57] Jiang J, Quan Y, Ganesh T, Pouliot WA, Dudek FE, Dingledine R. Inhibition of the prostaglandin receptor EP2 following status epilepticus reduces delayed mortality and brain inflammation. Proc Natl Acad Sci U S A 2013 Feb 26;110(9):3591-3596.

[58] Easton AS, Fraser PA. Arachidonic acid increases cerebral microvascular permeability by free radicals in single pial microvessels of the anaesthetized rat. J Physiol 1998 Mar 1;507 (Pt 2)(Pt 2):541-547.

[59] Othman A, Ahmad S, Megyerdi S, Mussell R, Choksi K, Maddipati KR, et al. 12/15-Lipoxygenase-derived lipid metabolites induce retinal endothelial cell barrier dysfunction: contribution of NADPH oxidase. PLoS One 2013;8(2):e57254.

[60] Stuhlmeier KM, Tarn C, Csizmadia V, Bach FH. Selective suppression of endothelial cell activation by arachidonic acid. Eur J Immunol 1996 Jul;26(7):1417-1423.

[61] Farmer PJ, Bernier SG, Lepage A, Guillemette G, Regoli D, Sirois P. Permeability of endothelial monolayers to albumin is increased by bradykinin and inhibited by prostaglandins. Am J Physiol Lung Cell Mol Physiol 2001 Apr;280(4):L732-8.

[62] Esaki Y, Li Y, Sakata D, Yao C, Segi-Nishida E, Matsuoka T, et al. Dual roles of PGE2-EP4 signaling in mouse experimental autoimmune encephalomyelitis. Proc Natl Acad Sci U S A 2010 Jul 6;107(27):12233-12238.

[63] Ahmad M, Saleem S, Shah Z, Maruyama T, Narumiya S, Dore S. The PGE2 EP2 receptor and its selective activation are beneficial against ischemic stroke. Exp Transl Stroke Med 2010 Jul 8;2(1):12-7378-2-12.

[64] Denning GM, Figard PH, Spector AA. Effect of fatty acid modification on prostaglandin production by cultured 3T3 cells. J Lipid Res 1982 May;23(4):584-596.

[65] Eldor A, Vlodavsky I, Hy-Am E, Atzmon R, Weksler BB, Raz A, et al. Cultured endothelial cells increase their capacity to synthesize prostacyclin following the formation of a contact inhibited cell monolayer. J Cell Physiol 1983 Feb;114(2):179-183.

[66] Gerritsen ME, Nganele DM, Rodrigues AM. Calcium ionophore (A23187)- and arachidonic acid-stimulated prostaglandin release from microvascular endothelial cells: effects of calcium antagonists and calmodulin inhibitors. J Pharmacol Exp Ther 1987 Mar;240(3):837-846.

[67] Baker PN, Davidge ST, Barankiewicz J, Roberts JM. Plasma of preeclamptic women stimulates and then inhibits endothelial prostacyclin. Hypertension 1996 Jan;27(1): 56-61.

[68] Li X, Hong S, Li PL, Zhang Y. Docosahexanoic acid-induced coronary arterial dilation: actions of 17S-hydroxy docosahexanoic acid on K+ channel activity. J Pharmacol Exp Ther 2011 Mar;336(3):891-899.

[69] Hong S, Gronert K, Devchand PR, Moussignac RL, Serhan CN. Novel docosatrienes and 17S-resolvins generated from docosahexaenoic acid in murine brain, human blood, and glial cells. Autacoids in anti-inflammation. J Biol Chem 2003 Apr 25;278(17):14677-14687.

[70] Adkins Y, Kelley DS. Mechanisms underlying the cardioprotective effects of omega-3 polyunsaturated fatty acids. J Nutr Biochem 2010 Sep;21(9):781-792.

[71] Hermann DM, Bassetti CL. Implications of ATP-binding cassette transporters for brain pharmacotherapies. Trends Pharmacol Sci 2007 Mar;28(3):128-134.

[72] Urquhart BL, Kim RB. Blood-brain barrier transporters and response to CNS-active drugs. Eur J Clin Pharmacol 2009 Nov;65(11):1063-1070.

[73] Meier-Abt F, Mokrab Y, Mizuguchi K. Organic anion transporting polypeptides of the OATP/SLCO superfamily: identification of new members in nonmammalian species, comparative modeling and a potential transport mode. J Membr Biol 2005 Dec; 208(3):213-227.

[74] Gao B, Stieger B, Noe B, Fritschy JM, Meier PJ. Localization of the organic anion transporting polypeptide 2 (Oatp2) in capillary endothelium and choroid plexus epithelium of rat brain. J Histochem Cytochem 1999 Oct;47(10):1255-1264.

[75] Hagenbuch B, Meier PJ. Organic anion transporting polypeptides of the OATP/ SLC21 family: phylogenetic classification as OATP/ SLCO superfamily, new nomenclature and molecular/functional properties. Pflugers Arch 2004 Feb;447(5):653-665.

[76] Kalliokoski A, Niemi M. Impact of OATP transporters on pharmacokinetics. Br J Pharmacol 2009 Oct;158(3):693-705.

[77] Ose A, Kusuhara H, Endo C, Tohyama K, Miyajima M, Kitamura S, et al. Functional characterization of mouse organic anion transporting peptide 1a4 in the uptake and efflux of drugs across the blood-brain barrier. Drug Metab Dispos 2010 Jan;38(1): 168-176.

[78] Burckhardt G, Burckhardt BC. In vitro and in vivo evidence of the importance of organic anion transporters (OATs) in drug therapy. Handb Exp Pharmacol 2011;(201): 29-104. doi(201):29-104.

[79] Buist SC, Cherrington NJ, Choudhuri S, Hartley DP, Klaassen CD. Gender-specific and developmental influences on the expression of rat organic anion transporters. J Pharmacol Exp Ther 2002 Apr;301(1):145-151.

[80] Aoki K, Saso N, Kato S, Sugiyama Y, Sato H. Nitric oxide and peroxynitrite regulate transporter transcription in rat liver slices. Biol Pharm Bull 2008 Oct;31(10):1882-1887.

[81] Popowski K, Eloranta JJ, Saborowski M, Fried M, Meier PJ, Kullak-Ublick GA. The human organic anion transporter 2 gene is transactivated by hepatocyte nuclear factor-4 alpha and suppressed by bile acids. Mol Pharmacol 2005 May;67(5):1629-1638.

[82] Kikuchi R, Kusuhara H, Sugiyama D, Sugiyama Y. Contribution of organic anion transporter 3 (Slc22a8) to the elimination of p-aminohippuric acid and benzylpenicillin across the blood-brain barrier. J Pharmacol Exp Ther 2003 Jul;306(1):51-58.

[83] Vannucci SJ, Maher F, Simpson IA. Glucose transporter proteins in brain: delivery of glucose to neurons and glia. Glia 1997 Sep;21(1):2-21.

[84] Birnbaum MJ, Haspel HC, Rosen OM. Cloning and characterization of a cDNA encoding the rat brain glucose-transporter protein. Proc Natl Acad Sci U S A 1986 Aug; 83(16):5784-5788.

[85] Bondy CA, Lee WH, Zhou J. Ontogeny and cellular distribution of brain glucose transporter gene expression. Mol Cell Neurosci 1992 Aug;3(4):305-314.

[86] Morgello S, Uson RR, Schwartz EJ, Haber RS. The human blood-brain barrier glucose transporter (GLUT1) is a glucose transporter of gray matter astrocytes. Glia 1995 May;14(1):43-54.

[87] Pardridge WM. Blood-brain barrier biology and methodology. J Neurovirol 1999 Dec;5(6):556-569.

[88] Pardridge WM, Boado RJ, Farrell CR. Brain-type glucose transporter (GLUT-1) is selectively localized to the blood-brain barrier. Studies with quantitative western blotting and in situ hybridization. J Biol Chem 1990 Oct 15;265(29):18035-18040.

[89] Farrell CL, Yang J, Pardridge WM. GLUT-1 glucose transporter is present within apical and basolateral membranes of brain epithelial interfaces and in microvascular endothelia with and without tight junctions. J Histochem Cytochem 1992 Feb;40(2):193-199.

[90] Klip A, Tsakiridis T, Marette A, Ortiz PA. Regulation of expression of glucose transporters by glucose: a review of studies in vivo and in cell cultures. FASEB J 1994 Jan;8(1):43-53.

[91] Au KK, Liong E, Li JY, Li PS, Liew CC, Kwok TT, et al. Increases in mRNA levels of glucose transporters types 1 and 3 in Ehrlich ascites tumor cells during tumor development. J Cell Biochem 1997 Oct 1;67(1):131-135.

[92] Vemula S, Roder KE, Yang T, Bhat GJ, Thekkumkara TJ, Abbruscato TJ. A functional role for sodium-dependent glucose transport across the blood-brain barrier during oxygen glucose deprivation. J Pharmacol Exp Ther 2009 Feb;328(2):487-495.

[93] Pierre K, Pellerin L. Monocarboxylate transporters in the central nervous system: distribution, regulation and function. J Neurochem 2005 Jul;94(1):1-14.

[94] Nybo L, Secher NH. Cerebral perturbations provoked by prolonged exercise. Prog Neurobiol 2004 Mar;72(4):223-261.

[95] Gjedde A, Crone C. Induction processes in blood-brain transfer of ketone bodies during starvation. Am J Physiol 1975 Nov;229(5):1165-1169.

[96] Bouzier-Sore AK, Merle M, Magistretti PJ, Pellerin L. Feeding active neurons: (re)emergence of a nursing role for astrocytes. J Physiol Paris 2002 Apr-Jun;96(3-4):273-282.

[97] Pellerin L. Lactate as a pivotal element in neuron-glia metabolic cooperation. Neurochem Int 2003 Sep-Oct;43(4-5):331-338.

[98] Waniewski RA, Martin DL. Astrocytes and synaptosomes transport and metabolize lactate and acetate differently. Neurochem Res 2004 Jan;29(1):209-217.

[99] Simpson IA, Carruthers A, Vannucci SJ. Supply and demand in cerebral energy metabolism: the role of nutrient transporters. J Cereb Blood Flow Metab 2007 Nov; 27(11):1766-1791.

[100] Pierre K, Pellerin L, Debernardi R, Riederer BM, Magistretti PJ. Cell-specific localization of monocarboxylate transporters, MCT1 and MCT2, in the adult mouse brain revealed by double immunohistochemical labeling and confocal microscopy. Neuroscience 2000;100(3):617-627.

[101] Leino RL, Gerhart DZ, Drewes LR. Monocarboxylate transporter (MCT1) abundance in brains of suckling and adult rats: a quantitative electron microscopic immunogold study. Brain Res Dev Brain Res 1999 Mar 12;113(1-2):47-54.

[102] Friesema EC, Ganguly S, Abdalla A, Manning Fox JE, Halestrap AP, Visser TJ. Identification of monocarboxylate transporter 8 as a specific thyroid hormone transporter. J Biol Chem 2003 Oct 10;278(41):40128-40135.

[103] Tai LM, Reddy PS, Lopez-Ramirez MA, Davies HA, Male DK, Loughlin AJ, et al. Polarized P-glycoprotein expression by the immortalised human brain endothelial cell line, hCMEC/D3, restricts apical-to-basolateral permeability to rhodamine 123. Brain Res 2009 Oct 6;1292:14-24.

[104] Dantzig AH, de Alwis DP, Burgess M. Considerations in the design and development of transport inhibitors as adjuncts to drug therapy. Adv Drug Deliv Rev 2003 Jan 21;55(1):133-150.

[105] Potschka H. Targeting regulation of ABC efflux transporters in brain diseases: a novel therapeutic approach. Pharmacol Ther 2010 Jan;125(1):118-127.

[106] Loscher W, Potschka H. Role of drug efflux transporters in the brain for drug disposition and treatment of brain diseases. Prog Neurobiol 2005 May;76(1):22-76.

[107] Kruh GD, Belinsky MG. The MRP family of drug efflux pumps. Oncogene 2003 Oct 20;22(47):7537-7552.

[108] Su W, Pasternak GW. The role of multidrug resistance-associated protein in the blood-brain barrier and opioid analgesia. Synapse 2013 Sep;67(9):609-619.

[109] Keppler D. Multidrug resistance proteins (MRPs, ABCCs): importance for pathophysiology and drug therapy. Handb Exp Pharmacol 2011;(201):299-323. doi(201): 299-323.

[110] Kusuhara H, Suzuki H, Naito M, Tsuruo T, Sugiyama Y. Characterization of efflux transport of organic anions in a mouse brain capillary endothelial cell line. J Pharmacol Exp Ther 1998 Jun;285(3):1260-1265.

[111] Regina A, Koman A, Piciotti M, El Hafny B, Center MS, Bergmann R, et al. Mrp1 multidrug resistance-associated protein and P-glycoprotein expression in rat brain microvessel endothelial cells. J Neurochem 1998 Aug;71(2):705-715.

[112] Gutmann H, Torok M, Fricker G, Huwyler J, Beglinger C, Drewe J. Modulation of multidrug resistance protein expression in porcine brain capillary endothelial cells in vitro. Drug Metab Dispos 1999 Aug;27(8):937-941.

[113] Seetharaman S, Barrand MA, Maskell L, Scheper RJ. Multidrug resistance-related transport proteins in isolated human brain microvessels and in cells cultured from these isolates. J Neurochem 1998 Mar;70(3):1151-1159.

[114] Nies AT, Jedlitschky G, Konig J, Herold-Mende C, Steiner HH, Schmitt HP, et al. Expression and immunolocalization of the multidrug resistance proteins, MRP1-MRP6 (ABCC1-ABCC6), in human brain. Neuroscience 2004;129(2):349-360.

[115] Zhang Y, Schuetz JD, Elmquist WF, Miller DW. Plasma membrane localization of multidrug resistance-associated protein homologs in brain capillary endothelial cells. J Pharmacol Exp Ther 2004 Nov;311(2):449-455.

[116] Roberts LM, Black DS, Raman C, Woodford K, Zhou M, Haggerty JE, et al. Subcellular localization of transporters along the rat blood-brain barrier and blood-cerebral-spinal fluid barrier by in vivo biotinylation. Neuroscience 2008 Aug 13;155(2): 423-438.

[117] Stanley LA, Horsburgh BC, Ross J, Scheer N, Wolf CR. Drug transporters: gatekeepers controlling access of xenobiotics to the cellular interior. Drug Metab Rev 2009;41(1):27-65.

[118] Sugiyama D, Kusuhara H, Lee YJ, Sugiyama Y. Involvement of multidrug resistance associated protein 1 (Mrp1) in the efflux transport of 17beta estradiol-D-17beta-glucuronide (E217betaG) across the blood-brain barrier. Pharm Res 2003 Sep;20(9): 1394-1400.

[119] Miller DS, Nobmann SN, Gutmann H, Toeroek M, Drewe J, Fricker G. Xenobiotic transport across isolated brain microvessels studied by confocal microscopy. Mol Pharmacol 2000 Dec;58(6):1357-1367.

[120] Dombrowski SM, Desai SY, Marroni M, Cucullo L, Goodrich K, Bingaman W, et al. Overexpression of multiple drug resistance genes in endothelial cells from patients with refractory epilepsy. Epilepsia 2001 Dec;42(12):1501-1506.

[121] Miller DS, Graeff C, Droulle L, Fricker S, Fricker G. Xenobiotic efflux pumps in isolated fish brain capillaries. Am J Physiol Regul Integr Comp Physiol 2002 Jan; 282(1):R191-8.

[122] Zhang Y, Han H, Elmquist WF, Miller DW. Expression of various multidrug resistance-associated protein (MRP) homologues in brain microvessel endothelial cells. Brain Res 2000 Sep 8;876(1-2):148-153.

[123] Berezowski V, Landry C, Dehouck MP, Cecchelli R, Fenart L. Contribution of glial cells and pericytes to the mRNA profiles of P-glycoprotein and multidrug resistance-

associated proteins in an in vitro model of the blood-brain barrier. Brain Res 2004 Aug 20;1018(1):1-9.

[124] Ma JJ, Chen BL, Xin XY. Inhibition of multi-drug resistance of ovarian carcinoma by small interfering RNA targeting to MRP2 gene. Arch Gynecol Obstet 2009 Feb;279(2): 149-157.

[125] Bauer B, Hartz AM, Lucking JR, Yang X, Pollack GM, Miller DS. Coordinated nuclear receptor regulation of the efflux transporter, Mrp2, and the phase-II metabolizing enzyme, GSTpi, at the blood-brain barrier. J Cereb Blood Flow Metab 2008 Jun;28(6): 1222-1234.

[126] Lombardo L, Pellitteri R, Balazy M, Cardile V. Induction of nuclear receptors and drug resistance in the brain microvascular endothelial cells treated with antiepileptic drugs. Curr Neurovasc Res 2008 May;5(2):82-92.

[127] Kruh GD, Zeng H, Rea PA, Liu G, Chen ZS, Lee K, et al. MRP subfamily transporters and resistance to anticancer agents. J Bioenerg Biomembr 2001 Dec;33(6):493-501.

[128] Bakos E, Evers R, Sinko E, Varadi A, Borst P, Sarkadi B. Interactions of the human multidrug resistance proteins MRP1 and MRP2 with organic anions. Mol Pharmacol 2000 Apr;57(4):760-768.

[129] Potschka H, Fedrowitz M, Loscher W. Multidrug resistance protein MRP2 contributes to blood-brain barrier function and restricts antiepileptic drug activity. J Pharmacol Exp Ther 2003 Jul;306(1):124-131.

[130] Agarwal S, Elmquist WF. Insight into the cooperation of P-glycoprotein (ABCB1) and breast cancer resistance protein (ABCG2) at the blood-brain barrier: a case study examining sorafenib efflux clearance. Mol Pharm 2012 Mar 5;9(3):678-684.

[131] Uchida Y, Ohtsuki S, Katsukura Y, Ikeda C, Suzuki T, Kamiie J, et al. Quantitative targeted absolute proteomics of human blood-brain barrier transporters and receptors. J Neurochem 2011 Apr;117(2):333-345.

[132] Leggas M, Adachi M, Scheffer GL, Sun D, Wielinga P, Du G, et al. Mrp4 confers resistance to topotecan and protects the brain from chemotherapy. Mol Cell Biol 2004 Sep;24(17):7612-7621.

[133] Chen ZS, Lee K, Kruh GD. Transport of cyclic nucleotides and estradiol 17-beta-D-glucuronide by multidrug resistance protein 4. Resistance to 6-mercaptopurine and 6-thioguanine. J Biol Chem 2001 Sep 7;276(36):33747-33754.

[134] Lai L, Tan TM. Role of glutathione in the multidrug resistance protein 4 (MRP4/ABCC4)-mediated efflux of cAMP and resistance to purine analogues. Biochem J 2002 Feb 1;361(Pt 3):497-503.

[135] van Aubel RA, Smeets PH, Peters JG, Bindels RJ, Russel FG. The MRP4/ABCC4 gene encodes a novel apical organic anion transporter in human kidney proximal tubules:

putative efflux pump for urinary cAMP and cGMP. J Am Soc Nephrol 2002 Mar; 13(3):595-603.

[136] Sampath J, Adachi M, Hatse S, Naesens L, Balzarini J, Flatley RM, et al. Role of MRP4 and MRP5 in biology and chemotherapy. AAPS PharmSci 2002;4(3):E14.

[137] Belinsky MG, Guo P, Lee K, Zhou F, Kotova E, Grinberg A, et al. Multidrug resistance protein 4 protects bone marrow, thymus, spleen, and intestine from nucleotide analogue-induced damage. Cancer Res 2007 Jan 1;67(1):262-268.

[138] Jedlitschky G, Burchell B, Keppler D. The multidrug resistance protein 5 functions as an ATP-dependent export pump for cyclic nucleotides. J Biol Chem 2000 Sep 29;275(39):30069-30074.

[139] Belinsky MG, Chen ZS, Shchaveleva I, Zeng H, Kruh GD. Characterization of the drug resistance and transport properties of multidrug resistance protein 6 (MRP6, ABCC6). Cancer Res 2002 Nov 1;62(21):6172-6177.

[140] Kruh GD, Guo Y, Hopper-Borge E, Belinsky MG, Chen ZS. ABCC10, ABCC11, and ABCC12. Pflugers Arch 2007 Feb;453(5):675-684.

[141] Nicolazzo JA, Katneni K. Drug transport across the blood-brain barrier and the impact of breast cancer resistance protein (ABCG2). Curr Top Med Chem 2009;9(2): 130-147.

[142] Ozvegy C, Litman T, Szakacs G, Nagy Z, Bates S, Varadi A, et al. Functional characterization of the human multidrug transporter, ABCG2, expressed in insect cells. Biochem Biophys Res Commun 2001 Jul 6;285(1):111-117.

[143] Imai Y, Asada S, Tsukahara S, Ishikawa E, Tsuruo T, Sugimoto Y. Breast cancer resistance protein exports sulfated estrogens but not free estrogens. Mol Pharmacol 2003 Sep;64(3):610-618.

[144] Suzuki M, Suzuki H, Sugimoto Y, Sugiyama Y. ABCG2 transports sulfated conjugates of steroids and xenobiotics. J Biol Chem 2003 Jun 20;278(25):22644-22649.

[145] Juliano RL, Ling V. A surface glycoprotein modulating drug permeability in Chinese hamster ovary cell mutants. Biochim Biophys Acta 1976 Nov 11;455(1):152-162.

[146] Beaulieu E, Demeule M, Ghitescu L, Beliveau R. P-glycoprotein is strongly expressed in the luminal membranes of the endothelium of blood vessels in the brain. Biochem J 1997 Sep 1;326 (Pt 2)(Pt 2):539-544.

[147] Tatsuta T, Naito M, Oh-hara T, Sugawara I, Tsuruo T. Functional involvement of P-glycoprotein in blood-brain barrier. J Biol Chem 1992 Oct 5;267(28):20383-20391.

[148] Virgintino D, Robertson D, Errede M, Benagiano V, Girolamo F, Maiorano E, et al. Expression of P-glycoprotein in human cerebral cortex microvessels. J Histochem Cytochem 2002 Dec;50(12):1671-1676.

[149] Bendayan R, Ronaldson PT, Gingras D, Bendayan M. In situ localization of P-glycoprotein (ABCB1) in human and rat brain. J Histochem Cytochem 2006 Oct;54(10): 1159-1167.

[150] Seelig A, Landwojtowicz E. Structure-activity relationship of P-glycoprotein substrates and modifiers. Eur J Pharm Sci 2000 Nov;12(1):31-40.

[151] Ueda K, Taguchi Y, Morishima M. How does P-glycoprotein recognize its substrates? Semin Cancer Biol 1997 Jun;8(3):151-159.

[152] Wijesuriya HC, Bullock JY, Faull RL, Hladky SB, Barrand MA. ABC efflux transporters in brain vasculature of Alzheimer's subjects. Brain Res 2010 Oct 28;1358:228-238.

[153] Kania KD, Wijesuriya HC, Hladky SB, Barrand MA. Beta amyloid effects on expression of multidrug efflux transporters in brain endothelial cells. Brain Res 2011 Oct 18;1418:1-11.

[154] Hollo Z, Homolya L, Hegedus T, Sarkadi B. Transport properties of the multidrug resistance-associated protein (MRP) in human tumour cells. FEBS Lett 1996 Mar 25;383(1-2):99-104.

[155] Bauer F, Kuntner C, Bankstahl JP, Wanek T, Bankstahl M, Stanek J, et al. Synthesis and in vivo evaluation of [11C]tariquidar, a positron emission tomography radiotracer based on a third-generation P-glycoprotein inhibitor. Bioorg Med Chem 2010 Aug 1;18(15):5489-5497.

[156] Balayssac D, Authier N, Cayre A, Coudore F. Does inhibition of P-glycoprotein lead to drug-drug interactions? Toxicol Lett 2005 Apr 28;156(3):319-329.

Chapter 2

TRP Channels in Neuronal and Glial Signal Transduction

Christian Harteneck and Kristina Leuner

Additional information is available at the end of the chapter

http://dx.doi.org/10.5772/58232

1. Introduction

Many physiological processes like muscle contraction, hormone secretion and intracellular signalling processes are triggered by calcium as intracellular signalling molecule. The signal transduction capacity of calcium depends on the 10,000-fold gradient across the plasma membrane with 2.5 mM extracellular and resting intracellular calcium ion concentration of approximately 100 nM. Low intracellular calcium concentrations are managed by the extrusion of calcium by ATPases and transporters [1, 2], whereas rapid and distinct increases in intracellular calcium up to micromolar concentrations are mediated by calcium-permeable ion channels of the plasma membrane as well intracellular calcium storage compartments. Calcium mediates its biological functions by protein structures capable to bind calcium. These calcium-binding domains are building blocks of the proteins modulated by calcium directly or part of calcium sensor proteins (calmodulin, calcium binding protein, calcineurin, S100, NCS etc) mediating calcium-dependent modulation by protein-protein interaction [3].

In excitable cells like neurons, heart or skeletal or smooth muscle cells, calcium currents first identified are mediated by voltage-gated calcium channels [4-6]. Later, additional calcium-permeable ion channels have been identified mediating hormone-induced calcium entry also in non-excitable cells like endothelial, epithelial, immune cells. The identity of these channels has been unravelled via analysis of phototransduction in flies [7]. Montell and Rubin cloned Transient Receptor Potential (TRP) from *Drosophila melanogaster* and described TRP as a phospholipase C-modulated, calcium-permeable ion channel [8]. Mammalian TRP-homologous channels have been identified by comparing the *Drosophila* TRP sequences with sequences resulting from the upcoming genome and expression profiling projects at that time. The first channel protein showing the highest degree of sequence similarities with *Drosophila* TRP were named classic TRP family (TRPC1) [9-11]. Additional TRP-homologous proteins establishing the melastatin-like and vanilloid-like TRP subfamilies, TRPM and TRPV, respectively, were identified by other approaches [12-14]. An additional fascinating feature of TRP channels became obvious with the identification of TRPV1 (vanilloid receptor 1, VR1) as molecular target of capsaicin [15]. Capsaicin is the active molecule of chilli peppers and an irritant that is responsible for providing a sensation of burning, e.g., on the tongue. TRPV1 characterization revealed that TRP channels are targets of many secondary plant compounds and are involved in sensory functions [16]. Last but not least, the TRP superfamily comprises the mucolipin [TRPML [17]] and the polycystin [TRPP [18]] calcium-permeable channel proteins sharing a comparable transmembrane topology and features like ion permeability [13, 14, 19]. TRP channels are integrated in many cellular signal transduction pathways and a variety of physiological processes as discussed below.

TRP channels have been identified and characterized by common biochemical, immunochemical and physiological methods. The function of TRP channels can be directly studied by patch clamp electrophysiology as well as imaging techniques. Patch clamp techniques enable to monitor currents across the plasma membrane mediated by TRP channels using small electrodes in small pipettes together with the ground electrode in the bath solution [20]. In this configuration, the electrical activity of ion channels in the plasma membrane can be monitored. Depending on configuration and access of the electrode within the patch pipette, different configurations can be discriminated (cell-attached, whole cell, inside-out or outside-out). On the other hand, a growing number of methods has been developed to monitor changes in ion concentrations in intact cells using small chemical compounds or artificial proteins constructs [21]. Fura-2 is one of the best known calcium dyes, a small chemical compound changing its fluorescence features depending on calcium concentration [22]. In the meantime a variety of new compounds have been developed characterized by changed ion selectivity, changes in Kd values or fluorescence intensities. The intracellular concentration of the indicator dyes depend on the activity and capability of organic solute carrier to export the dyes and thereby lowering intracellular dye concentrations. This disadvantage can be overcome by the use of the new protein-based probes. These artificial proteins are constructs of ion binding domains conjugated with fluorescence protein domains transcribed transiently from transfected plasmids or permanently from genomic localized expression cassettes [23, 24].

The following review will give an introduction in the broad field of TRP channel research related to their expression in the central nervous system (CNS), their physiological function in neurons as well as in glia cells, and their role in neurological and psychiatric CNS disorders. The involvement of TRP channels in the pathophysiology of glioma and the sensing of pain is not discussed here [for comprehensive reviews please refer to [25, 26]].

2. TRP channels in the brain

2.1. TRPC channels

The classic TRP channel family comprises seven different genes with proteins showing the highest sequence similarity to the prototypic *Drosophila* TRP [8, 12, 19]. The mammalian channel proteins are involved in receptor-regulated calcium entry [27]. Receptor activation by hormones, neurotransmitter and in *Drosophila* light results in the phospholipase C-mediated breakdown of phosphatidylinositides leading to the formation of inositol 1,4,5-trisphosphate and diacylglycerol (Figure 1). Inositol 1,4,5-trisphosphate induces calcium release from intracellular stores via the activation of inositol 1,4,5-trisphosphate receptors (IP3 receptor), whereas diacylglycerol directly activates mammalian classic transient receptor potential (TRPC) channels (TRPC2, TRPC3, TRPC6 and TRPC7) in a protein kinase C-independent manner [27, 28]. The prerequisite of phospholipase C stimulation has been shown for TRPC1, TRPC4 and TRPC5 currents, however the molecular mechanism is still unclear [27].

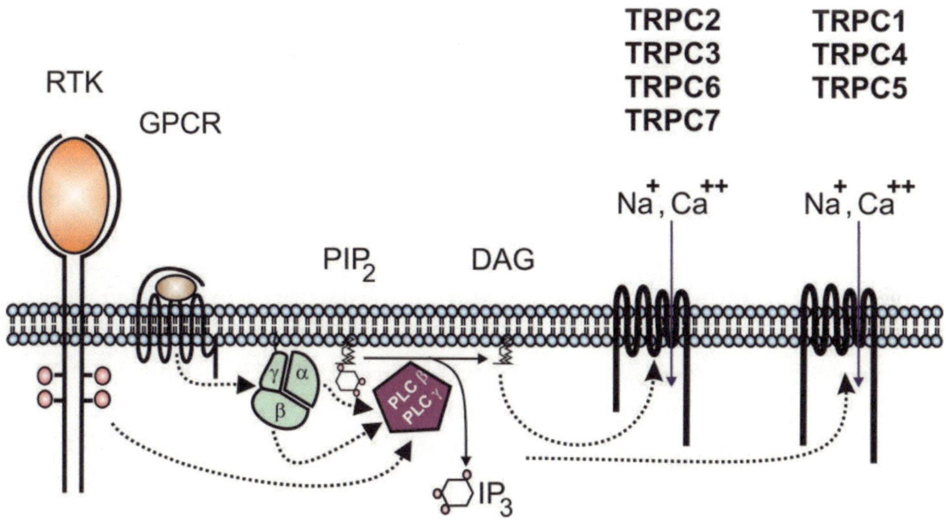

Figure 1. Receptor-induced activation mechanisms of TRP channels in mammals. RTK: receptor tyrosine kinase; GPCR: G protein-coupled receptor; PLC: phospholipase C; PIP2: phosphatidylinositol-4,5-bisphosphate; IP3: inositol-1,4,5-trisphosphate; DAG: diacylglycerol.

In the brain, TRPC1 expression was confirmed using a set of techniques ranging from RT-PCR, western blotting to confocal and electron microscopy. TRPC1 was detected in different brain regions of adult mice including the cerebellum, the hippocampus, the basal ganglia, the amygdala and the forebrain [29-31]. Strübing et al. showed that TRPC1 and TRPC5 channels are expressed in similar brain areas suggesting that they might form heteromers for example in the hippocampus [31]. However, empirical evidence for the existence of these heteromers is still lacking [32]. Only little is known about the distribution of TRPC channels in neurons. TRPC5 channels were suggested to be expressed mainly in distal dendrites and dendritic spines in lateral septal neurons. However, the expression pattern might differ in different brain areas and neurons [33]. Interestingly, TRPC1 protein was not only detected in neurons such as in the hippocampal CA1 or CA3 pyramidal cells [31], but also in astrocytes and oligodendrocyte progenitor cells [34-36]. Furthermore, mRNA for all TRPC channels including TRPC1 was found in the cortex of the mouse developing brain [37]. TRPC1, together with TRPC3 and TRPC5 were the main isoforms detected in this study. This expression pattern might be time dependent and species specific because TRPC4 and TRPC5 were the most prominent isoforms in the adult rat prefrontal cortex [38], whereas TRPC3 and TRPC6 channels are major TRPC mRNAs detected in adult mice [29]. TRPC2 being expressed in the rodent vomeronasal organ is clearly an exception [39]. In humans, TRPC2 is a pseudogene; the transcribed mRNA is functionless due to various stop codons [40]. In rodents, the transcription of the TRPC2 gene results in a functionally active protein involved in sensory responses to pheromones [39]. Genetic inactivation of TRPC2 in mice leads to loss of sex discrimination of male mice [41-43]. TRPC4 mRNA expression was observed in the adult mouse brain in the cortex, the hippocampus, the thalamus, the amygdala, the basal ganglia as well as the prefrontal cortex [29, 30, 38, 44]. TRPC4 protein expression was shown in the hippocampus, the cortex as well as the cerebellum [38, 44]. Using in situ hybridisation or immunocytochemistry, the expression of TRPC4 channels in different brain areas was specified. For example, TRPC4 was detected in cell layers of the prefrontal cortex [38] or in pyramidal CA1 and CA3 neurons of the hippocampus. In lateral septal neurons, TRPC4 channels were found on the cell surface of the soma and primary dendrites [33].

TRPC3 and TRPC6 mRNAs were demonstrated in the basal ganglia, the cerebellum, hippocampus as well as the forebrain [29]. TRPC3 protein expression in the brain especially in the prefrontal cortex and cerebellum was not only shown in rat and mouse tissues but also in human tissue obtained from subjects of different age groups [45]. TRPC3 channel expression was higher in the developing cortex compared to the adult cortex, whereas TRPC3 cerebral expression was not age-dependent. The protein expression of TRPC6 channels in the hippocampus is controversial. While several groups using pharmacological approaches or RT-PCR or western blot analyses describe TRPC6 channels being expressed in all hippocampal regions [46-51], Nagy and co-workers as well as Chung and colleagues show expression of TRPC6 channels selectively in the dentate gyrus and interneurons [52, 53]. Interestingly, in contrast to Tai et al. 2008, who described TRPC6 expression in hippocampal CA1 soma as well as in dendrites, Nagy's data suggest that TRPC6 channels are mainly expressed in dendrites of interneurons and neurons from the dentate gyrus [49, 53]. In the developing brain TRPC6 channels protein expression peaked between postnatal day 7 and 14, a period known to be important for maximal dendritic growth [49]. For TRPC7, only low mRNA expression levels were published [29, 30]. TRPC3 channels are also expressed in astrocytes [54].

2.2. TRPM channels

Melastatin, the founding member of the melastatin-like TRP family, was identified within a screen for proteins differentially regulated in melanocytes and melanoma cells [55]. Analysis of clinical data showed that the presence of melastatin expression in melanoma patients inversely correlates with the severity and survival [56-58]. Although melastatin is the first member of the TRPM family its activation mechanism and physiological role is still unclear. In line with the first description as protein involved in melanocyte physiology several reports confirmed this view. A completely unexpected function, the integration in retinal signal processing, has recently been discovered by the identification of TRPM1 expression in retinal ON bipolar cells [59]. The critical role of TRPM1 in mammalian phototransduction is also highlighted by several reports describing TRPM1 mutations in patients suffering from congenital stationary night blindness [60-63]. Only very little is known about TRPM1 function and expression in the CNS. Rather low mRNA TRPM1 expression was found in three studies in the brain [29, 64, 65].

From sequence similarity, TRPM3 is phylogenetically the closest neighbour to melastatin. TRPM3 is a polymodal ion channel activated by a variety of different stimuli like hypotonicity [66], sphingolipids [67], steroids [68, 69], nifedipine [69], and heat [70]. TRPM3 is activated by hypotonic extracellular solution and represents together with TRPV4, the volume-regulated TRP channels in the kidney [71, 72]. With the help of pharmacological tools, calcium entry induced by the application of hypotonic extracellular solutions can be assigned to TRPV4 and TRPM3 [71, 73-75]. While TRPV4 is activated by 4α-Isomers of phorbolesters and is blocked by ruthenium red, TRPM3 is activated by sphingosine and by pregnenolone-sulphate and blocked by gadolinium ions. TRPM3 is expressed in different areas of the CNS such as the hippocampus, the corpus callosum, the cortex or the hippocampus. These findings were reproduced in different studies using RT-PCR [29], northern blot [66, 76], as well as immunohistochemistry [77, 78]. TRPM3 channels are found in neurons (cerebral Purkinje neurons) as well as in oligodendrocytes [76-78]. Interestingly, neuronal expression of TRPM3 is present throughout development. However, it is almost lost in the adult brain [77]. In contrast, TRPM3 is highly expressed in oligodendrocytes in the adult brain.

The phylogenetically next neighbours to TRPM1 and TRPM3 are TRPM6 and TRPM7 [79]. The latter ones are involved in the body magnesium homeostasis [80]. While TRPM7 is ubiquitously expressed, TRPM6 is expressed in epithelial cells of the gut and the kidney and responsible for magnesium absorption and reabsorption. Loss-of-function mutations in TRPM6 are linked to autosomal-recessive hypomagnesemia with secondary hypocalcemia [81, 82]. TRPM6, TRPM7 and TRPM2 share a common structural feature. All three genes code for chimeric proteins combining a hexahelical transmembrane channel forming domain with a C-terminal enzymatic active domain [83]. In the case of TRPM6 and TRPM7, the pore-forming domains are fused to atypical alpha kinase-like structures. The functional role for the enzymatic domain is still under dispute. TRPM6 and TRPM7 are permeable for magnesium and for other essential divalent cations like Ca^{2+}, Zn^{2+}, Mn^{2+}, Co^{2+} as well as toxic cations like Ba^{2+}, Sr^{2+}, Ni^{2+}, Cd^{2+} [84, 85]. While TRPM6 mRNA was detected at low level in different brain areas [29], nothing is known about its role in the CNS. In contrast to TRPM6 channels, TRPM7 mRNA is highly expressed in the brain [29, 86]. In primary hippocampal neurons as well as in pyramidal hippocampal CA1 neurons in rat brain slices, TRPM7 was detected by different groups using immunocyto- and immunohistochemistry [87-89].

While divalent ions are the preferentially carried ion of TRPM6- and TRPM7-mediated currents, TRPM4 and TRPM5 form ion pores impermeable for divalent ions and allow selectively sodium to pass [90]. As sodium channels, TRPM4 and TRPM5 are paradoxically activated by increased intracellular calcium concentrations and represent calcium-activated sodium channels. TRPM4 is expressed in different brain regions including the thalamus, the hypothalamus, the medulla oblongata, the hippocampus and the spinal cord in mouse, rat as well as human brain (Lein et al., 2007; [29, 91]. In contrast to TRPM4, the expression of TRPM5 is restricted to a few cell types. TRPM5 is expressed in taste buds of the tongue and involved in the sensation of bitter and sweet taste [92, 93].

The remaining two TRPM channels proteins, TRPM2 and TRPM8, can also be discussed in the light of sensory functions. As already mentioned, TRPM2 represents a chimeric protein integrating an ADP-ribose hydrolase domain C-terminal to the pore-forming transmembrane domains [83]. Simultaneously to the ADP-ribose hydrolysing activity of the C-terminal enzymatic domain, TRPM2 is activated by ADP-ribose and it has been shown that the C-terminal part is essential for the function of the pore forming channel protein [94, 95]. Increased intracellular ADP-ribose concentrations are linked to genotoxic and/or oxidative stress of cells leading to the activation of the poly(ADP-ribose) polymerase (PARP) modulating protein stability by the mono and poly ADP-ribosylation of proteins [96]. This process of protein stability regulation is additionally controlled by an enzyme called poly(ADP-ribose) glucohydrolase (PARG). PARG reduces the post-translational poly ADP-ribose modifications to mono ADP-ribosylation, thereby increasing the intracellular ADP-ribose concentration leading to the activation of TRPM2. In whole cell calcium imaging experiments, the extracellular application of hydrogen peroxide results in the activation of TRPM2 validating its function as redox sensor. TRPM2 channels are preferentially expressed in microglia cells, the host macrophages of the CNS [97, 98]. In addition, in several brain regions such as the hippocampus, the cortex and the substantia nigra TRPM2 channels were also detected in neurons using RT-PCR, western blotting as well as immunohistochemistry [99, 100]. It was suggested that TRPM2 and TRPM7 channels form heteromers because knock-down of TRPM7 with siRNA is accompanied by down-regulation of TRPM2 channels [101]. TRPM8, the cold sensor, is mainly expressed in sensory neurons. TRPM8 is activated at temperatures between 8 °C to 28 °C as well as the secondary plant compound menthol and synthetic cooling compounds. Together with TRPA1, TRPM8 represent the cold sensors in human. Noxious cold is mediated by TRPA1 [26, 102].

2.3. TRP channels in the brain - TRPV channels

Vanilloid structures, derivates of vanillin comprising eugenol, zingerone and capsaicin, are found in many spice plants and known for their individual characteristic flavour. Beside the use as spice, vanilloid containing plant extracts are used as remedy in the various traditions of folk medicines. Therapeutic and experimental use of capsaicin in pain treatment inspired research resulting in the unravelling of the molecular target of capsaicin. The molecular target, an ion channel related to *Drosophila* TRP, was named capsaicin or vanilloid receptor and became eponym of the subgroup or structurally related ion channels of the TRP channel superfamily [15]. The vanilloid-like TRP channels comprise six members, four proteins (TRPV1 to TRPV4) like TRPV1 are non selective ion channels involved in thermosensation [14, 73, 74, 102, 103], while two ion channels (TRPV5 and TRPV6) represent highly calcium-selective ion channels [75, 104].

The warm and heat sensors (TRPV1 to TRPV4) and the cold sensors (TRPM8 and TRPA1) represent the thermosensors of the human body and cover the complete temperature range necessary for human life. As warning sensors expressed in dorsal root ganglia, the thermo TRPs are also involved in sensation and modulation of pain and therefore interesting as molecular targets for new pain-treating drugs. Most studies dealing with the structural and functional properties of the TRPV channel family in the CNS are focused on TRPV1. However, TRPV2, TRPV3 and TRPV4 are also detected in the CNS. In contrast for TRPV5 and TRPV6, there is no evidence for their expression in the CNS.

Localization	Function	References
Hippocampus (interneurons, dentate gyrus)	involved in anxiety and fear	[132, 151]
	involved in LTD	[152, 153]
	involved in LTP	[152]
	involved in pathogenesis of epilepsy	[126, 127]
hypothalamus	central osmoregulation	[154, 155]
	central regulation of temperature	[108]
Locus coeruleus	potentiation of glutamate,	
	adrenaline or norepinephrine release	[151]
Cortex	involved in cortical excitability	[156]
	involved in pathogenesis of epilepsy	[126]
Striatum	facilitation of glutamatergic	[157]
	postsynaptic neurotransmission	[158]
	glutamate release	[159]

Table 1 Localization and putative function of TRPV1 channels

TRPV1 expression in the CNS was investigated using a variety of methods ranging from pharmacological characterization and immunohistochemistry [105] to RT-PCR [106], western blotting to radio ligand binding [107]. Beside the great variety of methods and studies the expression of TRPV1 in the brain remains controversial. Several studies showed a wide spread TRPV1 expression in the CNS suggesting an expression of TRPV1 in pyramidal neurons of the CA1, CA3 area of the hippocampus, the dentate gyrus, the locus coeruleus, the hypothalamus, the substantia nigra, the cerebellum, the cortex and other limbic structures [108]. Other studies reported TRPV1 expression which was highly restricted to primary sensory ganglia with minimal expression in few brain regions which are adjacent to the caudal hypothalamus [107] (expression profiles and methods are summarized in Table 1). However several groups used TRPV1 agonists or antagonists as well as TRPV1 knock-out mice to define the role of TRPV1 channels in the CNS and reported versatile functions in different brain regions such as the hippocampus, the substantia nigra, the cortex or the hypothalamus. TRPV1 channels are not only activated by capsaicin but also by the CB1 agonist anandamide [109], other endovanilloids such as N-acyldopamines or the endogenous lipoxygenase derivates HPETE which are released for example in the hippocampus after mGluR1 activation [108]. Importantly, colocalization of TRPV1 and CB1 receptors was found in different mouse brain regions including the pyramidal cells of the hippocampus and basal glia [110, 111]. Regarding its cellular localisation, TRPV1 channels were detected in neuronal cell bodies, presynaptic terminals as well as in dendrites on postsynaptic spines [105, 106, 112, 113]. Furthermore, these channels are also present in pericytes and at the feet of astrocytes surrounding small vessels [105, 114].

TRPV2 channels are widely distributed in the brain compromising the colocalisation with TRPV1 in the cortex [19, 112, 115, 116]. TRPV3 mRNA was detected throughout the cortex, hippocampus, thalamus, striatum and cerebellum [117, 118]. TRPV4 mRNA is present in the hypothalamus, the cerebellum, basal ganglia, as well as in pyramidal neurons of the hippocampus [29, 119, 120]. Importantly, TRPV1-4 were also found in astrocytes [121, 122].

3. TRP channels in CNS diseases

3.1. Developmental disorders — Rett syndrome

Rett syndrome (RTT) is severe X-linked neurodevelopmental disorder which is unique among genetic, chromosomal and other developmental disorders because of its extreme female gender bias, early normal development, and subsequent developmental regression with loss of motor and language skills. RTT is caused by heterozygosity for mutations in the X-linked gene *MECP2*, which encodes methyl-CpG binding protein 2. Rett syndrome patients suffer from stereotypic wringing hand movements, social withdrawal, communication dysfunction, cognitive impairment, respiratory dysfunction as well as failing locomotion [123]. MeCP2 regulates expression of multiple genes, including BDNF. BDNF signaling was strongly altered in Mecp2 mutant mice [48].

Importantly, TRPC3 and TRPC6 channel expression and function was significantly lower in the hippocampus and several other brain regions of Mecp2 mutant mice revealing a cellular phenotype certainly contributing to hippocampal dysfunction in Mecp2 mutant mice as well as Rett syndrome etiology. These results suggest that compounds which enhance BDNF release or boost TRPC3/TRPC6 channel function might be an interesting new preclinical concept which needs to be evaluated in Rett mouse models [124, 125].

3.2. Epilepsy

Recent data suggests that TRPV1 channels might contribute to the pathophysiology of epilepsy. In the cortex and hippocampus from patients suffering from mesial temporal lobe epilepsy, the most common form of chronic and intractable epilepsy, TRPV1 mRNA and protein expression was significantly increased compared to healthy controls [126]. In a mouse model of temperal lobe epilepsy, these findings were supported [127]. The expression of TRPV1 in the dentate gyrus was significantly enhanced. Furthermore, capsaicin and anandamide significantly enhanced glutamate release in a TRPV1-dependent manner in mice with temperal lobe epilepsy [128, 129]. In contrast, the TRPV1 antagonist capsazepine reduced 4-aminopyridine-induced seizure-like activity in mice [128].

Beside TRPV1 channels, data from knockout mice point to a role of TRPC1/4/5 as well as for TRPC3/6 channels in the pathophysiology of epilepsy. Phelan et al. described a major role of TRPC1 and TRPC4 channels in the plateau potential of lateral septal neurons which show a high vulnerability to seizure-induced neuronal death as well as direct excitotoxicity by the application of group I mGluR receptor agonists [33]. *In vivo* results using the pilocarpine-induced status epileptics in TRPC1/TRPC4 double knockout animals showed surprising results. Cell death was significantly reduced in the lateral septum but also in the CA1 region of the hippocampus after severe seizures. However, the severity of the seizures *per se* was not altered. The authors concluded that this conundrum might be explained by the hypothesis that TRPC5 channels might be important for epileptiform burst in other limbic brain areas. This hypothesis was recently supported using TRPC5 knockout mice [32]. They exhibit significantly reduced seizures and minimal seizure-induced cell death in the CA1 region of the hippocampus. Importantly, spatial learning was not affected making TRPC5 channels an attractive novel target for the treatment of epilepsy.

TRPC3 channels are also discussed to play a "toxic" role in status epilepticus [46, 130]. After pilocarpine-induced status epilepticus in rats, TRPC3 expression was significantly enhanced in CA1, CA3 pyramidal neurons as well as dentate granule cells, whereas TRPC6 channel expression was reduced in these areas. Using two pharmacological approaches, first the inhibition of TRPC3 with the selective antagonist Pyr3 and second activation of TRPC6 channels with the TRPC6 activator hyperforin protected against neuronal damages following the status epilepticus [46].

3.3. Migraine

TRP channels might be involved in several processes relevant for the pathophysiology of migraine such as altered central calcium homeostasis, multimodal sensory and pain perception, or central or peripheral sensitization. Therefore, a recent study investigated single nucleotide polymorphisms (SNPs) in TRP genes in 1040 patients and 1037 healthy controls in Spain. For TRPV1, a nominal association was found for TRPV1 rs 222741 in the overall migraine group, for TRPV3 a correlation with TRPV3 rs7217270 was detected in the migraine group with aura [131].

3.4. Mood disorders – anxiety, unipolar and bipolar depression

TRPV1 and TRPV3 channels might be involved in fear and anxiety [107, 132]. TRPV1 knockout mice showed decreased anxiety-related behavior in several behavior paradigms such as the elevated plus maze test or the light dark test [107, 132]. Furthermore, fear and stress reaction were also reduced in TRPV1 knockout mice [107]. Therefore, TRPV1 antagonists such as capsazepine were investigated when they were applied directly into the ventral hippocampus or the periaqueductal grey. In both studies capsazepine showed anxiolytic effects. Recent studies investigated if compounds which act on both TRPV1 as well as CB1 receptors might be more effective than selective TRPV1 blocker [133]. N-arachidonoyl-serotonin which blocks TRPV1 channels and indirectly activates CB1 receptors and Arachidonyl-2-chloroethylamide (ACEA) which activates both TRPV1 as well as CB1 receptors were investigated. N-arachidonyl-serotonin was more effective than arachidonyl-2-chloroethylamide in behavioral paradigms for anxiety [134, 135]. The TRPV1/CB1 agonist ACEA showed anxiolytic effects in a bell shaped dose dependency in a mouse model using electrical stimulation of a brain area, the medial dorsal periaqueductal gray, which has an important role in orchestrating anxiety- and panic-related responses [133, 136]. The panicolytic effects are dependent on CB1 receptors. Importantly, in higher concentrations ACEA loses its anxiolytic effect probably via TRPC1 activation. This assumption is supported by the finding that ACEA effects in higher concentrations can be unmasked by the addition of the TRPV1 antagonist capsazepine. TRPV1 blockade per se also showed panicolytic effects suggesting opposite functions for TRPV1 and CB_1 receptors in the modulation of panic-like responses [136].

The evidence for the role of TRPC6 channels in depression comes from the active antidepressant constituent of St. Johns wort, hyperforin. Hyperforin resembles in its effects several classical antidepressants and neurotrophic factors such brain derived neurotrophic factor (BDNF) or nerve growth factor (NGF) [137-140]. Hyperforin inhibits neurotransmitter reuptake and improves synaptic plasticity ranging from increased neuritic outgrowth in PC12 cells to altered spine morphology in CA1 and CA3 neurons of the hippocampus via the activation of TRPC6 channels [137-139]. Recently, we showed that several signal cascades are involved in the alteration of synaptic plasticity such as Ras/MEK/ERK, PI3K/Akt as well as CAMKIV which finally result in CREB phorsphorylation [137]. In addition, enhanced CREB phosphorylation and TRPC6 channel expression was detected in the cortex but not the hippocampus after chronic hyperforin treatment for 4 weeks in adult mice [141]. However, hippocampal neurogenesis remained unchanged. Bouron et al. suggests that not only the hyperforin-mediated calcium influx but also its effects on intracellular zinc might be important for its antidepressant activity [142, 143]

Oxidative stress, mitochondrial dysfunction, and disrupted intracellular Ca^{2+} homeostasis are discussed to play a role in bipolar disorder (BD). TRPM2 channels, as a regulator and connector between reactive oxygen species (ROS) and intracellular Ca^{2+}, seem to be implicated in bipolar disorder. In B-lymphocytes from patients, TRPM2 channel expression is elevated associated with enhanced intracellular Ca^{2+} levels [144]. In addition, several groups reported genetic association between several intronic and extronic single nucleotide polymorphisms in TRPM2 and BD [145-149]. In a recent study using B-lymphocytes from small group of patients (n = 6) suffering from bipolar disorder, no change in TRPM2 expression could be detected. However, they were more susceptible to oxidative stress when stimulated with H_2O_2 [150].

3.5. Multiple sclerosis

Multiple sclerosis is a neurodegenerative disease caused by chronic inflammation of the CNS. Schattling et al. recently demonstrated that TRPM4 channels are involved in the pathogenesis of multiple sclerosis by using TRPM4 knockout mice and inducing an experimental autoimmune encephalomyelitis (EAE) in these animals [91]. TRPM4 channels are located in hippocampal neurons from mice and humans as well as in the spinal cord and cortex. TRPM4 deficiency reduced overall disease severity. Importantly, deficiency or pharmacological inhibition of TRPM4 resulted in reduced axonal and neuronal degeneration without altering

EAE relevant immune function. In addition, axonal TRPM4 expression in axons was significantly elevated in demyelinating white matter brain lesions of patients with multiple sclerosis in comparison to healthy controls. The authors further demonstrate that TRPV4 channels are involved in toxic effects of high glutamate levels which are a major contributor to neurodegeneration in multiple sclerosis.

4. Conclusion

Transient receptor potential (TRP) channels comprise a large family of non selective, calcium-permeable channel proteins which are activated and regulated by different mechanisms. TRP channels respond to secondary plant compounds as well as intracellular stimuli such as calcium, metabolites of the arachidonic acid or phosphatidylinositol signal transduction pathways. TRP channels sense environmental stimuli such as changes in temperature, osmolarity and pH and represent the molecular target of pheromones, taste and secondary plant compounds. The broad function of TRP channels in CNS physiology becomes apparent through their involvement in several psychiatric and neurological CNS disorders. This makes them an interesting topic for further research and drug development. The diversity of the chemical structures and the selectivity of the naturally occurring compounds modulating TRP channels show the possibility for pharmacological modulation of TRP channels and inspire the development of new synthetic structures for TRP channel interference at bench and bedside.

Author details

Christian Harteneck[1] and Kristina Leuner[2]

1 Institute of Pharmacology and Toxicology & Interfaculty Centre for Pharmacogenomics and Drug Research, Eberhard-Karls-University, Tübingen, Germany

2 Molecular und Clinical Pharmacy, Friedrich-Alexander-University Erlangen/Nürnberg, Germany

References

[1] Berridge, M.J., M.D. Bootman, and H.L. Roderick, *Calcium signalling: dynamics, homeostasis and remodelling.* Nat Rev Mol Cell Biol, 2003. 4: p. 517-29.

[2] Berridge, M.J., P. Lipp, and M.D. Bootman, *The versatility and universality of calcium signalling.* Nat Rev Mol Cell Biol, 2000. 1: p. 11-21.

[3] Yanez, M., J. Gil-Longo, and M. Campos-Toimil, *Calcium binding proteins.* Adv Exp Med Biol, 2012. 740: p. 461-82.

[4] Atlas, D., *The voltage-gated calcium channel functions as the molecular switch of synaptic transmission.* Annu Rev Biochem, 2013. 82: p. 607-35.

[5] Catterall, W.A., *Voltage-gated calcium channels.* Cold Spring Harb Perspect Biol, 2011. 3: p. a003947.

[6] Dolphin, A.C., *Calcium channel diversity: multiple roles of calcium channel subunits.* Curr Opin Neurobiol, 2009. 19: p. 237-44.

[7] Montell, C., *Drosophila visual transduction.* Trends Neurosci, 2012. 35: p. 356-63.

[8] Montell, C. and G.M. Rubin, *Molecular characterization of the Drosophila trp locus: a putative integral membrane protein required for phototransduction.* Neuron, 1989. 2: p. 1313-23.

[9] Wes, P.D., et al., *TRPC1, a human homolog of a Drosophila store-operated channel.* Proc Natl Acad Sci U S A, 1995. 92: p. 9652-6.

[10] Zhu, X., et al., *Molecular cloning of a widely expressed human homologue for the Drosophila trp gene.* FEBS Lett, 1995. 373: p. 193-8.

[11] Zitt, C., et al., *Cloning and functional expression of a human Ca^{2+}-permeable cation channel activated by calcium store depletion.* Neuron, 1996. 16: p. 1189-96.

[12] Harteneck, C., T.D. Plant, and G. Schultz, *From worm to man: three subfamilies of TRP channels.* Trends Neurosci, 2000. 23: p. 159-66.

[13] Montell, C., et al., *A unified nomenclature for the superfamily of TRP cation channels.* Mol Cell, 2002. 9: p. 229-31.

[14] Wu, L.J., T.B. Sweet, and D.E. Clapham, *International Union of Basic and Clinical Pharmacology. LXXVI. Current progress in the mammalian TRP ion channel family.* Pharmacol Rev, 2010. 62: p. 381-404.

[15] Caterina, M.J., et al., *The capsaicin receptor: a heat-activated ion channel in the pain pathway.* Nature, 1997. 389: p. 816-24.

[16] Voets, T., et al., *Sensing with TRP channels.* Nat Chem Biol, 2005. 1: p. 85-92.

[17] Puertollano, R. and K. Kiselyov, *TRPMLs: in sickness and in health.* Am J Physiol Renal Physiol, 2009. 296: p. F1245-54.

[18] Hofherr, A. and M. Kottgen, *TRPP channels and polycystins.* Adv Exp Med Biol, 2011. 704: p. 287-313.

[19] Venkatachalam, K. and C. Montell, *TRP channels.* Annu Rev Biochem, 2007. 76: p. 387-417.

[20] Talavera, K. and B. Nilius, *Electrophysiological Methods for the Study of TRP Channels*, in *TRP Channels*, M.X. Zhu, Editor. 2011: Boca Raton (FL).

[21] Yang, F. and J. Zheng, *Fluorescence Microscopy in ThermoTRP Channel Research*, in *TRP Channels*, M.X. Zhu, Editor. 2011: Boca Raton (FL).

[22] Grynkiewicz, G., M. Poenie, and R.Y. Tsien, *A new generation of Ca^{2+} indicators with greatly improved fluorescence properties.* J Biol Chem, 1985. 260: p. 3440-50.

[23] Shaner, N.C., P.A. Steinbach, and R.Y. Tsien, *A guide to choosing fluorescent proteins.* Nat Methods, 2005. 2: p. 905-9.

[24] Wallace, D.J., et al., *Single-spike detection in vitro and in vivo with a genetic Ca^{2+} sensor.* Nat Methods, 2008. 5: p. 797-804.

[25] Chung, M.K., S.J. Jung, and S.B. Oh, *Role of TRP channels in pain sensation.* Adv Exp Med Biol, 2011. 704: p. 615-36.

[26] Vay, L., C. Gu, and P.A. McNaughton, *The thermo-TRP ion channel family: properties and therapeutic implications.* Br J Pharmacol, 2012. 165: p. 787-801.

[27] Birnbaumer, L., *The TRPC class of ion channels: a critical review of their roles in slow, sustained increases in intracellular Ca^{2+} concentrations.* Annu Rev Pharmacol Toxicol, 2009. 49: p. 395-426.

[28] Dietrich, A., et al., *Functional characterization and physiological relevance of the TRPC3/6/7 subfamily of cation channels.* Naunyn Schmiedebergs Arch Pharmacol, 2005. 371: p. 257-65.

[29] Kunert-Keil, C., et al., *Tissue-specific expression of TRP channel genes in the mouse and its variation in three different mouse strains.* BMC Genomics, 2006. 7: p. 159.

[30] Riccio, A., et al., *mRNA distribution analysis of human TRPC family in CNS and peripheral tissues.* Brain Res Mol Brain Res, 2002. 109: p. 95-104.

[31] Strübing, C., et al., *TRPC1 and TRPC5 form a novel cation channel in mammalian brain.* Neuron, 2001. 29: p. 645-55.

[32] Phelan, K.D., et al., *Canonical transient receptor channel 5 (TRPC5) and TRPC1/4 contribute to seizure and excitotoxicity by distinct cellular mechanisms.* Mol Pharmacol, 2013. 83: p. 429-38.

[33] Phelan, K.D., et al., *Heteromeric canonical transient receptor potential 1 and 4 channels play a critical role in epileptiform burst firing and seizure-induced neurodegeneration.* Mol Pharmacol, 2012. 81: p. 384-92.

[34] Li, B., et al., *Effects of chronic treatment with fluoxetine on receptor-stimulated increase of $[Ca^{2+}]_i$ in astrocytes mimic those of acute inhibition of TRPC1 channel activity.* Cell Calcium, 2011. 50: p. 42-53.

[35] Malarkey, E.B., Y. Ni, and V. Parpura, *Ca^{2+} entry through TRPC1 channels contributes to intracellular Ca^{2+} dynamics and consequent glutamate release from rat astrocytes.* Glia, 2008. 56: p. 821-35.

[36] Paez, P.M., et al., *Modulation of canonical transient receptor potential channel 1 in the proliferation of oligodendrocyte precursor cells by the golli products of the myelin basic protein gene.* J Neurosci, 2011. 31: p. 3625-37.

[37] Boisseau, S., et al., *Heterogeneous distribution of TRPC proteins in the embryonic cortex.* Histochem Cell Biol, 2009. 131: p. 355-63.

[38] Fowler, M.A., et al., *Corticolimbic expression of TRPC4 and TRPC5 channels in the rodent brain.* PLoS One, 2007. 2: p. e573.

[39] Liman, E.R., D.P. Corey, and C. Dulac, *TRP2: a candidate transduction channel for mammalian pheromone sensory signaling.* Proc Natl Acad Sci U S A, 1999. 96: p. 5791-6.

[40] Vannier, B., et al., *Mouse trp2, the homologue of the human trpc2 pseudogene, encodes mTrp2, a store depletion-activated capacitative Ca^{2+} entry channel.* Proc Natl Acad Sci U S A, 1999. 96: p. 2060-4.

[41] Leypold, B.G., et al., *Altered sexual and social behaviors in trp2 mutant mice.* Proc Natl Acad Sci U S A, 2002. 99: p. 6376-81.

[42] Lucas, P., et al., *A diacylglycerol-gated cation channel in vomeronasal neuron dendrites is impaired in TRPC2 mutant mice: mechanism of pheromone transduction.* Neuron, 2003. 40: p. 551-61.

[43] Stowers, L., et al., *Loss of sex discrimination and male-male aggression in mice deficient for TRP2.* Science, 2002. 295: p. 1493-500.

[44] Zechel, S., S. Werner, and O. von Bohlen Und Halbach, *Distribution of TRPC4 in developing and adult murine brain.* Cell Tissue Res, 2007. 328: p. 651-6.

[45] Roedding, A.S., et al., *TRPC3 protein is expressed across the lifespan in human prefrontal cortex and cerebellum.* Brain Res, 2009. 1260: p. 1-6.

[46] Kim, D.S., et al., *The reverse roles of transient receptor potential canonical channel-3 and -6 in neuronal death following pilocarpine-induced status epilepticus.* Cell Mol Neurobiol, 2013. 33: p. 99-109.

[47] Li, H., et al., *TRPC6 inhibited NMDA receptor activities and protected neurons from ischemic excitotoxicity.* J Neurochem, 2012. 123: p. 1010-8.

[48] Li, W., et al., *Activity-dependent BDNF release and TRPC signaling is impaired in hippocampal neurons of Mecp2 mutant mice.* Proc Natl Acad Sci U S A, 2012. 109: p. 17087-92.

[49] Tai, Y., et al., *TRPC6 channels promote dendritic growth via the CaMKIV-CREB pathway.* J Cell Sci, 2008. 121: p. 2301-7.

[50] Xu, P., et al., *Expression of TRPC6 in renal cortex and hippocampus of mouse during post-natal development.* PLoS One, 2012. 7: p. e38503.

[51] Zhou, J., et al., *Critical role of TRPC6 channels in the formation of excitatory synapses.* Nat Neurosci, 2008. 11: p. 741-3.

[52] Chung, Y.H., et al., *Immunohistochemical study on the distribution of TRPC channels in the rat hippocampus.* Brain Res, 2006. 1085: p. 132-7.

[53] Nagy, G.A., et al., *DAG-sensitive and Ca^{2+} permeable TRPC6 channels are expressed in dentate granule cells and interneurons in the hippocampal formation.* Hippocampus, 2013. 23: p. 221-32.

[54] Shirakawa, H., et al., *Transient receptor potential canonical 3 (TRPC3) mediates thrombin-induced astrocyte activation and upregulates its own expression in cortical astrocytes.* J Neurosci, 2010. 30: p. 13116-29.

[55] Hunter, J.J., et al., *Chromosomal localization and genomic characterization of the mouse melastatin gene (Mlsn1).* Genomics, 1998. 54: p. 116-23.

[56] Deeds, J., F. Cronin, and L.M. Duncan, *Patterns of melastatin mRNA expression in melanocytic tumors.* Hum Pathol, 2000. 31: p. 1346-56.

[57] Duncan, L.M., et al., *Down-regulation of the novel gene melastatin correlates with potential for melanoma metastasis.* Cancer Res, 1998. 58: p. 1515-20.

[58] Fang, D. and V. Setaluri, *Expression and Up-regulation of alternatively spliced transcripts of melastatin, a melanoma metastasis-related gene, in human melanoma cells.* Biochem Biophys Res Commun, 2000. 279: p. 53-61.

[59] Shen, Y., et al., *A transient receptor potential-like channel mediates synaptic transmission in rod bipolar cells.* J Neurosci, 2009. 29: p. 6088-93.

[60] Audo, I., et al., *TRPM1 is mutated in patients with autosomal-recessive complete congenital stationary night blindness.* Am J Hum Genet, 2009. 85: p. 720-9.

[61] Li, Z., et al., *Recessive mutations of the gene TRPM1 abrogate ON bipolar cell function and cause complete congenital stationary night blindness in humans.* Am J Hum Genet, 2009. 85: p. 711-9.

[62] Nakamura, M., et al., *TRPM1 mutations are associated with the complete form of congenital stationary night blindness.* Mol Vis, 2010. 16: p. 425-37.

[63] van Genderen, M.M., et al., *Mutations in TRPM1 are a common cause of complete congenital stationary night blindness.* Am J Hum Genet, 2009. 85: p. 730-6.

[64] Dong, H.W., et al., *Expression of transient receptor potential (TRP) channel mRNAs in the mouse olfactory bulb.* Neurosci Lett, 2012. 524: p. 49-54.

[65] Yang, J., et al., *Receptor for activated C kinase 1 (RACK1) inhibits function of transient receptor potential (TRP)-type channel Pkd2L1 through physical interaction.* J Biol Chem, 2012. 287: p. 6551-61.

[66] Grimm, C., et al., *Molecular and functional characterization of the melastatin-related cation channel TRPM3.* J Biol Chem, 2003. 278: p. 21493-501.

[67] Grimm, C., et al., *Activation of the melastatin-related cation channel TRPM3 by D-erythro-sphingosine [corrected].* Mol Pharmacol, 2005. 67: p. 798-805.

[68] Majeed, Y., et al., *Cis-isomerism and other chemical requirements of steroidal agonists and partial agonists acting at TRPM3 channels.* Br J Pharmacol, 2010. 161: p. 430-41.

[69] Wagner, T.F., et al., *Transient receptor potential M3 channels are ionotropic steroid receptors in pancreatic beta cells.* Nat Cell Biol, 2008. 10: p. 1421-30.

[70] Vriens, J., et al., *TRPM3 is a nociceptor channel involved in the detection of noxious heat.* Neuron, 2011. 70: p. 482-94.

[71] Harteneck, C. and B. Reiter, *TRP channels activated by extracellular hypo-osmoticity in epithelia.* Biochem Soc Trans, 2007. 35: p. 91-5.

[72] Harteneck, C. and G. Schultz, *TRPV4 and TRPM3 as Volume-Regulated Cation Channels,* in *TRP Ion Channel Function in Sensory Transduction and Cellular Signaling Cascades,* W.B. Liedtke and S. Heller, Editors. 2007: Boca Raton (FL).

[73] Liedtke, W., *Role of TRPV ion channels in sensory transduction of osmotic stimuli in mammals.* Exp Physiol, 2007. 92: p. 507-12.

[74] Vriens, J., G. Appendino, and B. Nilius, *Pharmacology of vanilloid transient receptor potential cation channels.* Mol Pharmacol, 2009. 75: p. 1262-79.

[75] Woudenberg-Vrenken, T.E., R.J. Bindels, and J.G. Hoenderop, *The role of transient receptor potential channels in kidney disease.* Nat Rev Nephrol, 2009. 5: p. 441-9.

[76] Oberwinkler, J., et al., *Alternative splicing switches the divalent cation selectivity of TRPM3 channels.* J Biol Chem, 2005. 280: p. 22540-8.

[77] Hoffmann, A., et al., *TRPM3 is expressed in sphingosine-responsive myelinating oligodendrocytes.* J Neurochem, 2010. 114: p. 654-65.

[78] Zamudio-Bulcock, P.A., et al., *Activation of steroid-sensitive TRPM3 channels potentiates glutamatergic transmission at cerebellar Purkinje neurons from developing rats.* J Neurochem, 2011. 119: p. 474-85.

[79] Runnels, L.W., *TRPM6 and TRPM7: A Mul-TRP-PLIK-cation of channel functions.* Curr Pharm Biotechnol, 2011. 12: p. 42-53.

[80] Ferre, S., J.G. Hoenderop, and R.J. Bindels, *Insight into renal Mg^{2+} transporters.* Curr Opin Nephrol Hypertens, 2011. 20: p. 169-76.

[81] Schlingmann, K.P., et al., *Hypomagnesemia with secondary hypocalcemia is caused by mutations in TRPM6, a new member of the TRPM gene family.* Nat Genet, 2002. 31: p. 166-70.

[82] Walder, R.Y., et al., *Mutation of TRPM6 causes familial hypomagnesemia with secondary hypocalcemia.* Nat Genet, 2002. 31: p. 171-4.

[83] Harteneck, C., *Function and pharmacology of TRPM cation channels.* Naunyn Schmiedebergs Arch Pharmacol, 2005. 371: p. 307-14.

[84] Gwanyanya, A., et al., *Magnesium-inhibited, TRPM6/7-like channel in cardiac myocytes: permeation of divalent cations and pH-mediated regulation.* J Physiol, 2004. 559: p. 761-76.

[85] Kerschbaum, H.H., J.A. Kozak, and M.D. Cahalan, *Polyvalent cations as permeant probes of MIC and TRPM7 pores.* Biophys J, 2003. 84: p. 2293-305.

[86] Fonfria, E., et al., *Tissue distribution profiles of the human TRPM cation channel family.* J Recept Signal Transduct Res, 2006. 26: p. 159-78.

[87] Sun, H.S., et al., *Suppression of hippocampal TRPM7 protein prevents delayed neuronal death in brain ischemia.* Nat Neurosci, 2009. 12: p. 1300-7.

[88] Wei, W.L., et al., *TRPM7 channels in hippocampal neurons detect levels of extracellular divalent cations.* Proc Natl Acad Sci U S A, 2007. 104: p. 16323-8.

[89] Zhang, J., et al., *Hypoxia induces an increase in intracellular magnesium via transient receptor potential melastatin 7 (TRPM7) channels in rat hippocampal neurons in vitro.* J Biol Chem, 2011. 286: p. 20194-207.

[90] Guinamard, R., L. Salle, and C. Simard, *The non-selective monovalent cationic channels TRPM4 and TRPM5.* Adv Exp Med Biol, 2011. 704: p. 147-71.

[91] Schattling, B., et al., *TRPM4 cation channel mediates axonal and neuronal degeneration in experimental autoimmune encephalomyelitis and multiple sclerosis.* Nat Med, 2012. 18: p. 1805-11.

[92] Perez, C.A., et al., *A transient receptor potential channel expressed in taste receptor cells.* Nat Neurosci, 2002. 5: p. 1169-76.

[93] Zhang, Y., et al., *Coding of sweet, bitter, and umami tastes: different receptor cells sharing similar signaling pathways.* Cell, 2003. 112: p. 293-301.

[94] Perraud, A.L., et al., *ADP-ribose gating of the calcium-permeable LTRPC2 channel revealed by Nudix motif homology.* Nature, 2001. 411: p. 595-9.

[95] Sano, Y., et al., *Immunocyte* Ca^{2+} *influx system mediated by LTRPC2.* Science, 2001. 293: p. 1327-30.

[96] Eisfeld, J. and A. Lückhoff, *Trpm2.* Handb Exp Pharmacol, 2007: p. 237-52.

[97] Kraft, R., et al., *Hydrogen peroxide and ADP-ribose induce TRPM2-mediated calcium influx and cation currents in microglia.* Am J Physiol Cell Physiol, 2004. 286: p. C129-37.

[98] Naziroglu, M., *TRPM2 cation channels, oxidative stress and neurological diseases: where are we now?* Neurochem Res, 2011. 36: p. 355-66.

[99] Jia, J., et al., *Sex differences in neuroprotection provided by inhibition of TRPM2 channels following experimental stroke.* J Cereb Blood Flow Metab, 2011. 31: p. 2160-8.

[100] Roedding, A.S., et al., *Chronic oxidative stress modulates TRPC3 and TRPM2 channel expression and function in rat primary cortical neurons: relevance to the pathophysiology of bipolar disorder.* Brain Res, 2013. 1517: p. 16-27.

[101] Aarts, M., et al., *A key role for TRPM7 channels in anoxic neuronal death.* Cell, 2003. 115: p. 863-77.

[102] Talavera, K., B. Nilius, and T. Voets, *Neuronal TRP channels: thermometers, pathfinders and life-savers.* Trends Neurosci, 2008. 31: p. 287-95.

[103] Basbaum, A.I., et al., *Cellular and molecular mechanisms of pain.* Cell, 2009. 139: p. 267-84.

[104] Hoenderop, J.G. and R.J. Bindels, *Calciotropic and magnesiotropic TRP channels.* Physiology (Bethesda), 2008. 23: p. 32-40.

[105] Toth, A., et al., *Expression and distribution of vanilloid receptor 1 (TRPV1) in the adult rat brain.* Brain Res Mol Brain Res, 2005. 135: p. 162-8.

[106] Mezey, E., et al., *Distribution of mRNA for vanilloid receptor subtype 1 (VR1), and VR1-like immunoreactivity, in the central nervous system of the rat and human.* Proc Natl Acad Sci U S A, 2000. 97: p. 3655-60.

[107] Marsch, R., et al., *Reduced anxiety, conditioned fear, and hippocampal long-term potentiation in transient receptor potential vanilloid type 1 receptor-deficient mice.* J Neurosci, 2007. 27: p. 832-9.

[108] Kauer, J.A. and H.E. Gibson, *Hot flash: TRPV channels in the brain.* Trends Neurosci, 2009. 32: p. 215-24.

[109] Ross, R.A., *Anandamide and vanilloid TRPV1 receptors.* Br J Pharmacol, 2003. 140: p. 790-801.

[110] Hajos, N. and T.F. Freund, *Pharmacological separation of cannabinoid sensitive receptors on hippocampal excitatory and inhibitory fibers.* Neuropharmacology, 2002. 43: p. 503-10.

[111] Rouach, N. and R.A. Nicoll, *Endocannabinoids contribute to short-term but not long-term mGluR-induced depression in the hippocampus.* Eur J Neurosci, 2003. 18: p. 1017-20.

[112] Liapi, A. and J.N. Wood, *Extensive co-localization and heteromultimer formation of the vanilloid receptor-like protein TRPV2 and the capsaicin receptor TRPV1 in the adult rat cerebral cortex.* Eur J Neurosci, 2005. 22: p. 825-34.

[113] Roberts, J.C., J.B. Davis, and C.D. Benham, *[$_3$H]Resiniferatoxin autoradiography in the CNS of wild-type and TRPV1 null mice defines TRPV1 (VR-1) protein distribution.* Brain Res, 2004. 995: p. 176-83.

[114] Mannari, T., et al., *Astrocytic TRPV1 ion channels detect blood-borne signals in the sensory circumventricular organs of adult mouse brains.* Glia, 2013. 61: p. 957-71.

[115] Lewinter, R.D., G. Scherrer, and A.I. Basbaum, *Dense transient receptor potential cation channel, vanilloid family, type 2 (TRPV2) immunoreactivity defines a subset of motoneurons in the dorsal lateral nucleus of the spinal cord, the nucleus ambiguus and the trigeminal motor nucleus in rat.* Neuroscience, 2008. 151: p. 164-73.

[116] Wainwright, A., et al., *Discrete expression of TRPV2 within the hypothalamo-neurohypophysial system: Implications for regulatory activity within the hypothalamic-pituitary-adrenal axis.* J Comp Neurol, 2004. 474: p. 24-42.

[117] Smith, G.D., et al., *TRPV3 is a temperature-sensitive vanilloid receptor-like protein.* Nature, 2002. 418: p. 186-90.

[118] Xu, H., et al., *TRPV3 is a calcium-permeable temperature-sensitive cation channel.* Nature, 2002. 418: p. 181-6.

[119] Mutai, H. and S. Heller, *Vertebrate and invertebrate TRPV-like mechanoreceptors.* Cell Calcium, 2003. 33: p. 471-8.

[120] Vriens, J., et al., *Cell swelling, heat, and chemical agonists use distinct pathways for the activation of the cation channel TRPV4.* Proc Natl Acad Sci U S A, 2004. 101: p. 396-401.

[121] Benfenati, V., et al., *Expression and functional characterization of transient receptor potential vanilloid-related channel 4 (TRPV4) in rat cortical astrocytes.* Neuroscience, 2007. 148: p. 876-92.

[122] Benfenati, V., et al., *An aquaporin-4/transient receptor potential vanilloid 4 (AQP4/TRPV4) complex is essential for cell-volume control in astrocytes.* Proc Natl Acad Sci U S A, 2011. 108: p. 2563-8.

[123] Briggs, A., *Primary care of a child with Rett syndrome.* J Am Assoc Nurse Pract, 2013.

[124] Chapleau, C.A., et al., *Evaluation of current pharmacological treatment options in the management of Rett syndrome: from the present to future therapeutic alternatives.* Curr Clin Pharmacol, 2013. 8: p. 358-69.

[125] Li, W. and L. Pozzo-Miller, *BDNF deregulation in Rett syndrome.* Neuropharmacology, 2014. 76 Pt C: p. 737-46.

[126] Sun, F.J., et al., *Increased expression of TRPV1 in the cortex and hippocampus from patients with mesial temporal lobe epilepsy.* J Mol Neurosci, 2013. 49: p. 182-93.

[127] Bhaskaran, M.D. and B.N. Smith, *Effects of TRPV1 activation on synaptic excitation in the dentate gyrus of a mouse model of temporal lobe epilepsy.* Exp Neurol, 2010. 223: p. 529-36.

[128] Gonzalez-Reyes, L.E., et al., *TRPV1 antagonist capsazepine suppresses 4-AP-induced epileptiform activity in vitro and electrographic seizures in vivo.* Exp Neurol, 2013. 250: p. 321-32.

[129] Manna, S.S. and S.N. Umathe, *Involvement of transient receptor potential vanilloid type 1 channels in the pro-convulsant effect of anandamide in pentylenetetrazole-induced seizures.* Epilepsy Res, 2012. 100: p. 113-24.

[130] Ryu, H.J., et al., *Endothelial transient receptor potential conical channel (TRPC)-3 activation induces vasogenic edema formation in the rat piriform cortex following status epilepticus.* Cell Mol Neurobiol, 2013. 33: p. 575-85.

[131] Carreno, O., et al., *SNP variants within the vanilloid TRPV1 and TRPV3 receptor genes are associated with migraine in the Spanish population.* Am J Med Genet B Neuropsychiatr Genet, 2012. 159B: p. 94-103.

[132] You, I.J., et al., *Alterations in the emotional and memory behavioral phenotypes of transient receptor potential vanilloid type 1-deficient mice are mediated by changes in expression of 5-HT$_{1A}$, GABA$_{A}$, and NMDA receptors.* Neuropharmacology, 2012. 62: p. 1034-43.

[133] Fogaca, M.V., et al., *The endocannabinoid and endovanilloid systems interact in the rat prelimbic medial prefrontal cortex to control anxiety-like behavior.* Neuropharmacology, 2012. 63: p. 202-10.

[134] John, C.S. and P.J. Currie, *N-arachidonoyl-serotonin in the basolateral amygdala increases anxiolytic behavior in the elevated plus maze.* Behav Brain Res, 2012. 233: p. 382-8.

[135] Micale, V., et al., *Anxiolytic effects in mice of a dual blocker of fatty acid amide hydrolase and transient receptor potential vanilloid type-1 channels.* Neuropsychopharmacology, 2009. 34: p. 593-606.

[136] Casarotto, P.C., et al., *Opposing roles for cannabinoid receptor type-1 (CB$_1$) and transient receptor potential vanilloid type-1 channel (TRPV1) on the modulation of panic-like responses in rats.* Neuropsychopharmacology, 2012. 37: p. 478-86.

[137] Heiser, J.H., et al., *TRPC6 channel-mediated neurite outgrowth in PC12 cells and hippocampal neurons involves activation of RAS/MEK/ERK, PI3K, and CAMKIV signaling.* J Neurochem, 2013. 127: p. 303-13.

[138] Leuner, K., et al., *Hyperforin--a key constituent of St. John's wort specifically activates TRPC6 channels.* FASEB J, 2007. 21: p. 4101-11.

[139] Leuner, K., et al., *Hyperforin modulates dendritic spine morphology in hippocampal pyramidal neurons by activating Ca^{2+}-permeable TRPC6 channels.* Hippocampus, 2013. 23: p. 40-52.

[140] Tu, P., et al., *Diacylglycerol analogues activate second messenger-operated calcium channels exhibiting TRPC-like properties in cortical neurons.* J Neurochem, 2009. 108: p. 126-38.

[141] Gibon, J., et al., *The antidepressant hyperforin increases the phosphorylation of CREB and the expression of TrkB in a tissue-specific manner.* Int J Neuropsychopharmacol, 2013. 16: p. 189-98.

[142] Gibon, J., P. Richaud, and A. Bouron, *Hyperforin changes the zinc-storage capacities of brain cells.* Neuropharmacology, 2011. 61: p. 1321-6.

[143] Gibon, J., et al., *The over-expression of TRPC6 channels in HEK-293 cells favours the intracellular accumulation of zinc.* Biochim Biophys Acta, 2011. 1808: p. 2807-18.

[144] Yoon, I.S., et al., *Altered TRPC7 gene expression in bipolar-I disorder.* Biol Psychiatry, 2001. 50: p. 620-6.

[145] McQuillin, A., et al., *Fine mapping of a susceptibility locus for bipolar and genetically related unipolar affective disorders, to a region containing the C21ORF29 and TRPM2 genes on chromosome 21q22.3.* Mol Psychiatry, 2006. 11: p. 134-42.

[146] Perova, T., et al., *Hyperactive intracellular calcium dynamics in B lymphoblasts from patients with bipolar I disorder.* Int J Neuropsychopharmacol, 2008. 11: p. 185-96.

[147] Xu, C., et al., *TRPM2 variants and bipolar disorder risk: confirmation in a family-based association study.* Bipolar Disord, 2009. 11: p. 1-10.

[148] Xu, C., et al., *Association of the putative susceptibility gene, transient receptor potential protein melastatin type 2, with bipolar disorder.* Am J Med Genet B Neuropsychiatr Genet, 2006. 141B: p. 36-43.

[149] Xu, C., et al., *Association of the iPLA$_2$beta gene with bipolar disorder and assessment of its interaction with TRPM2 gene polymorphisms.* Psychiatr Genet, 2013. 23: p. 86-9.

[150] Roedding, A.S., et al., *Effect of oxidative stress on TRPM2 and TRPC3 channels in B lymphoblast cells in bipolar disorder.* Bipolar Disord, 2012. 14: p. 151-61.

[151] Marinelli, S., et al., *Capsaicin activation of glutamatergic synaptic transmission in the rat locus coeruleus in vitro.* J Physiol, 2002. 543: p. 531-40.

[152] Brown, T.E., et al., *Loss of interneuron LTD and attenuated pyramidal cell LTP in Trpv1 and Trpv3 KO mice.* Hippocampus, 2013. 23: p. 662-71.

[153] Gibson, H.E., et al., *TRPV1 channels mediate long-term depression at synapses on hippocampal interneurons.* Neuron, 2008. 57: p. 746-59.

[154] Ciura, S., W. Liedtke, and C.W. Bourque, *Hypertonicity sensing in organum vasculosum lamina terminalis neurons: a mechanical process involving TRPV1 but not TRPV4.* J Neurosci, 2011. 31: p. 14669-76.

[155] Sinke, A.P. and P.M. Deen, *The physiological implication of novel proteins in systemic osmoregulation.* FASEB J, 2011. 25: p. 3279-89.

[156] Mori, F., et al., *TRPV1 channels regulate cortical excitability in humans.* J Neurosci, 2012. 32: p. 873-9.

[157] Musella, A., et al., *TRPV1 channels facilitate glutamate transmission in the striatum.* Mol Cell Neurosci, 2009. 40: p. 89-97.

[158] Marinelli, S., et al., *Activation of TRPV1 in the VTA excites dopaminergic neurons and increases chemical- and noxious-induced dopamine release in the nucleus accumbens.* Neuropsychopharmacology, 2005. 30: p. 864-70.

[159] Marinelli, S., et al., *Presynaptic facilitation of glutamatergic synapses to dopaminergic neurons of the rat substantia nigra by endogenous stimulation of vanilloid receptors.* J Neurosci, 2003. 23: p. 3136-44.

Chapter 3

Cytosolic Calcium Homeostasis in Neurons — Control Systems, Modulation by Reactive Oxygen and Nitrogen Species, and Space and Time Fluctuations

Carlos Gutierrez-Merino, Dorinda Marques-da-Silva,
Sofia Fortalezas and Alejandro K. Samhan-Arias

Additional information is available at the end of the chapter

http://dx.doi.org/10.5772/57576

1. Introduction

Cytosolic calcium plays a major and central role in neuronal activity and functions both in brain and in peripheral nervous systems, and its sustained alteration is a critical event that leads to neuronal death. On these grounds, it is not surprising that a sustained alteration of intracellular calcium homeostasis in neurons is a point of convergence of the cellular mechanisms underlying many neurodegenerative processes in the brain. Indeed, this has been shown to be the case for the brain's neurodegenerative diseases of higher incidence to humans, like Alzheimer's and Parkinson's, or in the acute neurodegeneration observed in amyotrophic lateral sclerosis, and also for major brain insults, such as excitotoxicity in trauma and ischemia-reperfusion, inflammation and neurotoxicity by drugs and environmental chemicals.

Sustained deregulation of cytosolic calcium concentration have been reported in neuronal apoptosis and necrosis, the two major cellular death pathways involved in brain neurodegeneration. It has been experimentally demonstrated and confirmed by many investigations using cell cultures that a sustained rise of cytosolic calcium concentration in the neuronal soma within the range 0.5-1 μM elicits a rapid necrotic neuronal death, mediated by calcium-dependent proteases activation, like calpains. On the other hand, long-term sustained cytosolic calcium concentrations below 60-70 nM in the neuronal soma promote the slow development of apoptotic neuronal death of neurons in culture [1,2]. Since the central role of calcium in neurotransmitter secretion and neuronal plasticity is also well known, the basal steady state cytosolic calcium concentration in the neuronal soma can be considered as a bioenergetics marker of neuronal activity and survival. We shall then present the major calcium transport systems that control the cytosolic calcium homeostasis in the wider space within neurons, i.e. in the neuronal soma. Owing to the large subcellular regionalization of neuronal processes essential for the normal activity of neurons and especially in neuronal signal transduction pathways, we shall also place a particular emphasis in the subcellular compartmentation of these calcium transport systems.

Noteworthy, neurodegenerative processes in the brain also share another common metabolic deviation, namely, that neurons are also exposed to an enhanced oxidative stress in the brain. Using different types of neuronal cultures, many investigators have shown during the last 15 years that the cellular oxidative stress produced by reactive oxygen species (ROS) and reactive nitrogen species (RNS) and a sustained alteration of the intracellular calcium homeostasis are metabolic deregulations usually observed during the early stages of the development of the process of neuronal death and before the cell viability loss induced entry in the irreversible steps characterized by the activation of proteases. In addition, it has been proposed that alterations of the intracellular calcium homeostasis of glial cells can also contribute to inflammation and damage in the brain in neurodegenerative processes [3]. Therefore, a better knowledge of the major molecular pathways contributing to induce the oxidative stress in the brain and the deregulation of intracellular calcium homeostasis in neurons should be expected to lead to the development of novel and more efficient therapies against brain neurodegeneration.

The fact that the most relevant calcium transport systems for the fine tuning of cytosolic calcium homeostasis in neurons have been shown to be molecular targets for ROS/RNS generated in neurodegenerative insults and diseases will be analyzed next in this context. As most of neurotoxic ROS/RNS species react with many intracellular molecules and these species are short-lived within the cells, the extent of chemical modification of each calcium transport system by ROS/RNS is strongly dependent on its relative proximity to the ROS/RNS source. In functional terms, it has been shown by many studies that ROS/RNS can elicit estimulation or inhibition of key proteins of calcium signalling pathways in neurons, and that these effects are strongly dependent on the specific protein, on the ROS/RNS concentration in the micro-environment and on the accummulated dose of ROS/RNS (time of exposure). Therefore, clustering of these systems within subcellular microdomains plays a major role in cross-modulation between calcium and ROS/RNS intracellular signalling, and this point will be specifically addressed thereafter in this chapter.

Furthermore, the accummulated experimental evidences pointing out that there is an intimate cross-talk between calcium and ROS/RNS intracellular signalling pathways are now ovel-whelming, including the modulation of ROS/RNS sources by calcium in neurons and the redox modulation of calcium transport systems. Both, calcium and ROS/RNS intracellular signalling show a clear pattern of local and focalized transients of intracellular concentration (peaks). Therefore, clustering of calcium transport systems responsible of the rise of cytosolic calcium and ROS/RNS sources within the same subcellular microcompartments will generate over-lapping focalized points of high concentration of calcium and ROS/RNS. In addition, this clustering will produce transient and highly focalized cytosolic calcium concentration peaks near the calcium entry points and associated calcium concentration waves owing to the rapid diffusion coefficient of calcium ions. Thus, we shall discuss the space and time fluctuations of cytosolic calcium concentrations that are known to be produced by the activity of calcium transport systems more relevant for the control of cytosolic calcium homeostasis in the neuronal soma. Finally, the last section of this chapter is focussed in the most relevant calcium buffering systems expressed in neurons and their modulation by oxidative stress, since calcium buffering systems of the neuronal cytosol play a major role to attenuate the local gradients of calcium concentration.

2. Neuronal cytosolic calcium homeostasis is attained by functional coupling between different types of calcium transport systems

A highly efficient spatial and temporal coupling between the activity of transport systems producing calcium entry to the cytosol and those extruding calcium out of the cytosol is a basic bioenergetics need for brain neurons, as they establish many functional synapses and have to maintain and rapidly restore cytosolic calcium in the neuronal soma within the narrow concentration window that allows for neuron survival. Extensive experimental studies carried out during last thirty years have settled the major molecular actors that allow neurons to achieve this goal, see for example the reviews [4-7], and these are schematically presented in the diagram of the Figure 1. Thus, the control of cytosolic calcium homeostasis in neurons is primarily the result of the activity of transport systems at the plasma membrane acting in concert, with the help of calcium transport systems located in intracellular stores, mainly in the endoplasmic reticulum and mitochondria. The concentration gradient of calcium ions across the neuronal plasma membrane in the brain is by far larger than the concentration gradients of other ions involved in the control of neuronal excitability, like potassium, sodium and chloride. In addition, cytosolic calcium binding proteins provide the neurons with buffering capacity to attenuate the peak height of free cytosolic calcium concentration spikes after focal neuronal stimulation by some neurotransmitters or after high frequency repetitive neuronal stimulation [8].

In primary cultures of cerebellar granule neurons, calcium entry through L-type voltage-operated calcium channel (L-VOCC) accounts for more than 75% of the increase of the steady-state cytosolic calcium in the neuronal soma after partial depolarization of the plasma membrane upon raising the extracellular potassium concentration from 5 to 25 mM [9]. The particular relevance of this observation for neuronal survival is highlighted by the fact that the apoptosis of these neurons induced by low potassium (5 mM) in the extracellular medium can be blocked simply by raising the extracellular potassium concentration up to 25 mM [1,10].

Many other experimental data accumulated along the last two decades point out that the transport systems more potent to elicit a fast and sustained increase of cytosolic calcium in neurons are located at the plasma membrane, i.e. ionotropic receptors and VOCC. These calcium transport systems are activated by extracellular stimuli, neurotransmitters or neuro-modulators, either directly or indirectly through plasma membrane depolarization. Let us recall here, for example, that high frequency stimulation of neurons by application of electrical

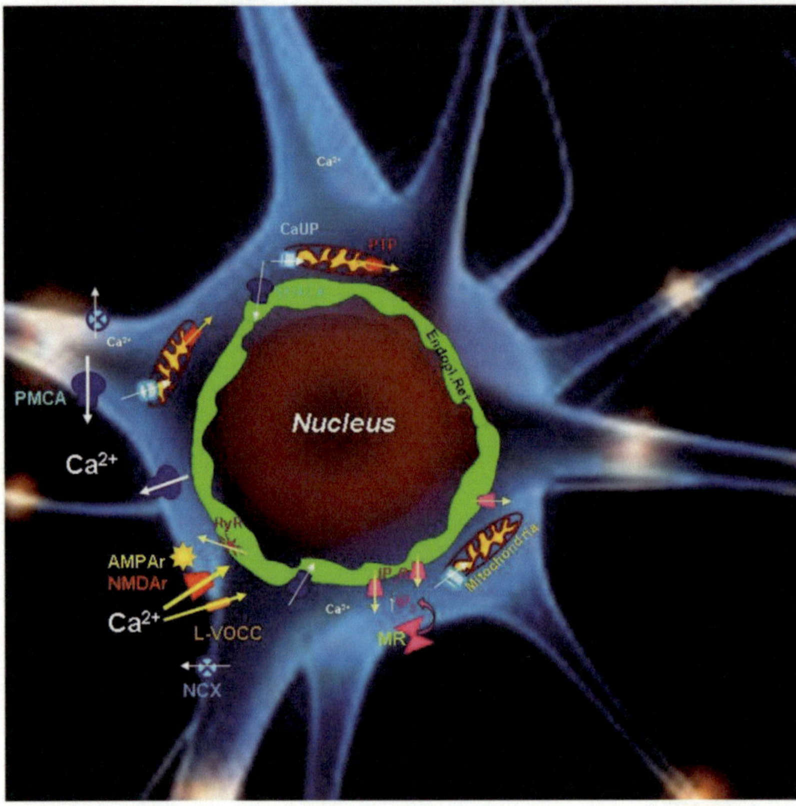

Figure 1. Diagrammatic image illustrating the major calcium transport systems controlling the concentration of cytosolic calcium in the neuronal soma. Yellow and white arrows indicate cytosolic calcium entry and extrusion transport systems, respectively. The thickness of the arrow indicates the relative relevance. Abbreviations: Endopl.Ret., endoplasmic reticulum (green space); NMDAr, NMDA receptor; AMPAr, AMPA receptor; L-VOCC, L-type voltage- operated calcium channel; PMCA, plasma membrane calcium pump; NCX, sodium-calcium exchanger; MR, metabotropic receptor; RyR, ryanodine receptor; IP_3R, IP_3 receptor; SERCA, endoplasmic reticulum calcium pump; PTP, mitochondrial permeability transition pore; CaUP, mitochondrial calcium uniporter.

depolarizing pulses or of the appropriate neurotransmitter (chemical stimulation) can lead to neuronal tetanic activity. Because of their focalized distribution pattern in the neurons and also because of the large differences in the intensity of calcium currents across activated ionotropic receptors and VOCC, significant calcium concentration gradients between different cytosolic regions of the neuron during normal neuronal activity are expected to develop at least transiently. In contrast, the rise of IP_3 following activation of phospholipase C after stimulation of members of the large family of G-coupled neurotransmitter receptors [5], also located at the plasma membrane, promoted calcium release from intracellular stores displaying calcium spikes of smaller intensity and a more widespread increase of calcium concentration within the cytosol.

Taking into consideration the large number of different chemical molecules that promote neuronal stimulation within the brain and the high frequency of the stimulation events, it is wonderful for its simplicity that the concerted action of only a few calcium transport systems can maintain neurons functional and alive for so many years during human lifetime. Why such a simple design? As the evolution selects the living structures and organisms that optimize the use of metabolic energy [11] and the bioenergetics costs for building a complex structural design is always higher than the costs for building simpler structures, probably the answer is: to optimize the use of the metabolic energy in neurons. Let us recall here that the large needs of metabolic energy to continuously restore the electric potential of the plasma membrane of active brain neurons, which is essential for their proper biological functions, would not allow them to develop a safe system for the control of cytosolic calcium homeostasis of a high-bioenergetics cost of maintenance and repair. Noteworthy, maximal energy optimization within the cells can be attained when the coupling between molecules involved in energy transduction makes use of the information or entropic energy stored in subcellular structures, i.e. minimizing stochastic collisional events that dissipate a large amount of energy, and this seems to be the case. For example, the subcellular distribution of the calcium transport systems in neurons enables them to use cytosolic calcium for highly polarized, rapid and specific synaptic responses, and also for more slowly developing adaptative responses, like long term post-synaptic potentiation or depression [4,5]. Furthermore, the different levels of expression of ionotropic and metabotropic receptors in distinct types of neurons allows for differential selectivity and sensitivity in calcium modulation of neuronal threshold excitability, thereby linking regionalization of neuronal responses within the brain structures with the major neurotransmitter pathways.

2.1. The calcium entry systems of the neuronal plasma membrane

All neurons express different types of functional VOCC. On the basis of their unitary conductance, on their rate of inactivation and their subcellular location the most relevant for neuronal calcium homeostasis are the L-VOCC. The L-VOCC unitary conductance has been reported to be in the range of 20-25 pS, while reported unitary conductances for N-, P/Q- and R-type range between 10 and 20 pS, and L-VOCC inactivation kinetics is slower than that of the other VOCC types [12-17]. In addition, L-VOCC are polarised in the neuronal soma and at the conical neck leading to neurite extensions [18], whereas N-, P/Q and R-types of VOCC are largely enriched in the presynaptic plasma membranes and its activation serves largely to elicit neurotransmitter release at the synapses [14,19-21]. On these grounds, taking also into consideration the rate of kinetics inactivation of the P/Q-VOCC, these channels should afford a contribution to the cytosolic calcium homeostasis of the neuronal soma much lower than that of L-VOCC but higher than that of N-, R- and T-types of VOCC. Indeed, using specific channels blockers we have experimentally assessed that the sum of the contributions of non-L-VOCC calcium channels to the cytosolic calcium homeostasis of the neuronal soma of primary cultures of cerebellar granule neurons in a standard Locke's medium with 25 mM K^+ is lower than 20%, while the L-VOCC contribution is 80% or higher (*unpublished results*).

L-VOCC, which are expressed in all neurons, are by far the most relevant calcium channels not only for the tuning of steady-state cytosolic calcium homeostasis in neurons (see above), but also for the overall threshold neuronal excitability, see [22-24]. The L-VOCC family, also known as Ca_V1, has four subtypes: $Ca_V1.1$, $Ca_V1.2$, $Ca_V1.3$ and $Ca_V1.4$ [25]. $Ca_V1.2$ and $Ca_V1.3$ are expressed in neurons, cardiac and endocrine cells, while $Ca_V1.1$ and $Ca_V1.4$ are specific of skeletal muscle and retina, respectively [26]. In brain, near 80% of L-VOCC belongs to the $Ca_V1.2$ subtype and 10-25% to the subtype $Ca_V1.3$ [27]. It has been reported that inactivation of the gene encoding for $Ca_V1.2$ in the hippocampus and neocortex of mouse ($Ca_V1.2$HKO) leads to a selective loss of N-methyl-D-aspartate (NMDA) receptors-independent long-term potentiation [28]. The activity of these calcium channels is modulated not only by the plasma membrane potential but it is also dependent upon their phosphorylation by protein kinases. Meanwhile the activation of different isoforms of protein kinase C (PKC) has been reported to produce stimulation or inhibition of L-VOCC activity in different cellular types [29], the activation of protein kinase A (PKA) and of calcium/calmodulin-dependent protein kinase II (CaMKII) have been shown to increase the activity of L-VOCC. Moreover, both PKA and CaMKII have been shown to form complexes with L-VOCC subunits. In brain, PKA associates with L-VOCC subunit α1c [30]. L-VOCC subunits α1c and β2 are phosphorylated by PKA [31-34], and this produces an increase of L-VOCC activity. It has been demonstrated that this increase of L-VOCC activity is mediated by phosphorylation of Ser478 and Ser479 of the β-subunit and also by phosphorylation of Ser1928 of the α1c-subunit, as their mutations led to complete elimination of the PKA-induced increase of calcium currents catalyzed by L-VOCC [29,35]. Regarding CaMKII, the amino acids sequence near Thr498 of the L-VOCC subunit β2a shows a high homology with the self-inhibitory domain of the CaMKII and with the binding domain of this kinase in the NR2B subunit of NMDA receptors [36]. Indeed, it has been shown the co-localization within neurons of the L-VOCC ($Ca_V1.2$ type) and CaMKII [37] and also of the L-VOCC subunit β2a with CaMKII, and this has led to the suggestion that the L-VOCC subunit β2a can act as an associated protein of CaMKII *in vivo* [36]. Phosphorylation of L-VOCC by CaMKII takes place not only in Thr498 of the β2a subunit but also in Ser1512 and Ser1570 of the α1 subunit and leads to an increase of the intensity of calcium currents through these channels [36, 38-40]. It has been proposed that the modulation of L-VOCC by CaMKII can be relevant to potentiate the raise of cytosolic calcium concentration in response to hormones and growth factors [41,42]. In contrast, the excessive activation of the L-VOCC ($Ca_V1.3$ type) by CaMKII over-stimulation has been correlated with the loss of dendritic spines in the striatum observed after dopamine depletion in animal models of parkinsonism [43].

The most potent calcium ionotropic receptors present in the neurons of the mammalian brain are L-glutamate receptors of the NMDA and α-amino-3-hydroxy-5-methylisoxazole-4-propionic acid (AMPA) subtypes, except those AMPA receptors formed only with GluR2 subunits [44,45], and P_{2X}-purinergic receptors [46]. NMDA and AMPA receptors are present in most fast excitatory synapses in the brain, allowing for neuronal responses in the milliseconds time scale range, and P_{2X}-purinergic receptors display also a widespread distribution in the brain. The more limited distribution in brain of L-glutamate receptors of the kainate subtype, its low ionic selectivity for calcium and the slight calcium currents generated upon its activation compared to those observed upon activation of AMPA and NMDA receptors [47], suggest that they can play at most a secondary role in the tuning of cytosolic calcium homeostasis of a very limited number of brain neurons.

The L-glutamate receptors are expressed in the vast majority of glutamatergic neurons, and they are present in the major structures of mammalian brain (neocortex, striatum, hippocampus and cerebellum). NMDA, AMPA and kainate receptors are oligomeric integral membrane proteins, being their calcium channel structure predominantly formed by a combination of different, though highly homologous, subunits [48]. Among these receptors, NMDA receptors play an outstanding role in neurosciences, as supported by many experimental evidences in studies of brain development [49], long term post-synaptic potentiation [4] or brain damage after ischemia-reperfusion [44,45]. Three major reasons allows to explain the dominant role of NMDA receptors over AMPA and kainate receptors in the brain: (1) the NMDA single channel conductance is higher than AMPA single channel conductance, 40-50 pS versus ~20 pS [16,50]; (2) their higher affinity for the endogenous agonist L-glutamate, e.g. the EC_{50} for L-glutamate is ~10 μM for NMDA receptors and ~200 μM for AMPA receptors, and (3) the slower desensitization rate of NMDA receptors, e.g. several hundreds of milliseconds for NMDA receptors while it is ~10 milliseconds for AMPA receptors [48]. Nevertheless, the maximal activation of NMDA receptors not only requires the presence of L-glutamate but also co-stimulation by glycine or D-serine in the brain and relief of Mg^{2+} inhibition [48,51]. Both, AMPA and P_{2x} receptors can potentiate NMDA receptor activation in the brain. AMPA receptors co-localization with NMDA receptors allows that plasma membrane depolarization induced by activation of AMPA receptors elicits the relief of Mg^{2+} inhibition of NMDA receptors. Phosphorylation by PKC and CaMKII promotes synaptic incorporation of AMPA receptors during long-term post-synaptic potentiation (LTP), and the latter kinase also enhances the channel conductance of this receptor [52-54]. On the other hand, it has been shown that facilitation of L-glutamate release by P_{2x} activation can lead to a stronger NMDA receptor activation. The calcium channel in the NMDA-receptor structure can be formed by different combinations of subunit 1 (NR1) and one of the isoforms of subunit 2 (NR2A, NR2B, NR2C and NR2D) [55]. The expression of functional NMDA receptors is a relatively slow process during the maturation of neurons [56]. Therefore, in molecular terms there are different isoforms of functional NMDA receptors whose level of expression varies from one type of neurons to another, and also during neuronal maturation. In addition, NMDA receptors are found in synaptic and in extra-synaptic locations [56-58]. As activation of extra-synaptic NMDA receptors can lead to a less focalized increase of cytosolic calcium, the extra-synaptic NMDA receptors are likely to play a role more relevant than synaptic NMDA receptors in the control of cytosolic calcium homeostasis in the neuronal soma. Phosphorylation of NMDA receptors *in vitro* by PKA and by some PKC isoforms increases their activity [59]. The co-stimulation of PKA and PKC elicits the phosphorylation of Ser896 and Ser897 leading to activation of NMDA receptors, while phosphorylation of Ser890 by only PKC leads to a subcellular re-localization of the NR1 subunit of NMDA receptors, which is reverted upon dephosphorylation [60].

2.2. Transport systems that release calcium from intracellular stores

The long-term control of neuronal calcium homeostasis also involves several major calcium transport systems of the subcellular organelles that behave as relevant neuronal intracellular stores, namely, endoplasmic reticulum and mitochondria.

The endoplasmic reticulum Ca^{2+}-ATPase (SERCA) helps to pump calcium out from the cytosol to the endoplasmic reticulum internal space [5], while calcium release from the endoplasmic reticulum involves the activation of IP_3 receptors and/or ryanodine receptors in different neuronal responses and in synaptic plasticity [5,61-63]. Although the neuronal endoplasmic reticulum can accumulate much lower amounts of calcium than the sarcoplasmic reticulum of muscle cells, it is still significant for hippocampal neurons as shown in several studies, see e.g. [4,64]. In these cases, calcium release from the endoplasmic reticulum can sustain a moderate increase of cytosolic calcium, which has been shown to play a significant role in the process of LTP in hippocampal neurons [4,64]. By itself, calcium filling of the endoplasmic reticulum is relevant for neuronal survival to ensure the correct protein folding of many proteins, particularly proteins of the plasma membrane or to be secreted to the extracellular space, as the activity of several endoplasmic reticulum protein-chaperones is dependent on the calcium concentration in the internal space of the endoplasmic reticulum [65]. Depletion of calcium in the endoplasmic reticulum has been shown to elicit the opening of specific calcium channels of the plasma membrane, the store-operated calcium entry (SOCE) [5,66-67]. The presence of SOCE in neurons has been documented during last years [4,68], and its opening elicits a transient increase of cytosolic calcium under neuronal stress conditions to restore the calcium levels of intracellular stores. The inhibition of SERCA by selective inhibitors, thapsigargin or cyclopiazonic acid, is needed to induce the large calcium depletion in the endoplasmic reticulum required for SOCE in experiments with cells in culture. Thus, this process can be seen as a 'rescue call' at the cellular level and operates under conditions of severe energetic depletion of the neurons. Indeed, it is to be recalled here that these channels and in particular the isoforms TRPC-3 and -6 have been also involved in neuronal survival of CGN [69]. More recently, Selvaraj *et al.* [70] have demonstrated that in a mouse neurotoxin-based model of Parkinson's disease, reduced Ca^{2+} influx through transient receptor potential C1 (TRPC1) channels in the plasma membrane of dopaminergic neurons triggers a cell death-inducing endoplasmic reticulum-stress response. These latter results highlighted for the first time the relevance of calcium homeostasis in Parkinson's disease.

In contrast, the large population of neuronal mitochondria can store relatively large amounts of calcium, high enough to elicit a large increase of cytosolic calcium as shown by several studies, see e.g. [71,72]. Nevertheless, the rate of calcium fluxes across the mitochondrial membrane transporters in normal cells is much slower than that measured for the major endoplasmic reticulum calcium transport systems listed above. However, calcium release from mitochondria high enough to promote a large and sustained rise of cytosolic calcium in neurons has been observed only during the development of neuronal cell death, as a consequence of the steady opening of the high permeability mitochondrial transition pore [73]. On these grounds, large calcium release from mitochondria has been proposed to be part of the molecular mechanism that triggers irreversible events in neuronal cell death through calpains activation. On the other hand, the uptake of calcium by mitochondria takes place through a calcium uniporter [71,73], with a rate of uptake in the submicromolar calcium range much lower than the major cytosolic calcium extrusion pathways, namely, PMCA and SERCA in neurons [4,6].

2.3. The transport systems involved in calcium extrusion from the cytosol

The major plasma membrane calcium extrusion systems, PMCA and Na^+/Ca^{2+}-exchanger (NCX) are expressed in all neuronal types. PMCA provides the major extrusion pathway operating in neurons for the maintenance of cytosolic calcium concentrations below the neurotoxic calcium range, i.e. <0.4 μM cytosolic calcium [6,74,75]. As PMCA is active at cytosolic calcium concentrations below 0.4 μM [6,74], neurons must spend a significant amount of metabolic energy (ATP) to maintain cytosolic calcium within the short concentration range which is required for neuronal survival. Therefore, the cytosolic calcium concentration can be considered a key bioenergetics marker of neuronal activity and survival. In contrast, NCX is more potent than the PMCA at cytosolic calcium concentrations ≥0.5 μM [6,76]. On these grounds, NCX can be seen as a safety system to minimise neuronal damage associated with cytosolic calcium ≥0.4 μM, as its activation when cytosolic calcium reaches this range allows neurons to rapidly reset cytosolic calcium to the concentration window that allows neuronal survival, see above. The expression levels of different neuronal isoforms of PMCA undergo significant changes during neuronal maturation [77], and a similar observation has been reported for NCX isoforms [78]. This has been seen as a neuronal adaptative response to the fine set of free cytosolic calcium concentration and control of cytosolic calcium homeostasis, since it has been demonstrated that different PMCA isoforms show different affinity for calcium [79]. On the other hand, although both PMCA and NCX are found in the plasma membrane of the neuronal soma and neuronal dendrites, recent data cast doubt on the current assumption that both PMCA and NCX are homogeneously distributed in the plasma membrane. For example, regulatory effects of actin cytoskeleton have been recently reported on the NCX activity [80], and actin filaments are components of caveolin-rich structures associated with 'lipid rafts' [81].

SERCA, which catalyzes the ATP-dependent calcium uptake by this subcellular organelle, plays only a secondary role as a system for calcium extrusion from the cytosol because in neurons PMCA is a calcium pump more potent than SERCA [4]. The calcium uptake by mitochondria is performed mainly via the Ca^{2+} uniporter driven by the large mitochondrial inner membrane potential [73], although the contribution of an alternate transport system yet ill-defined in molecular terms cannot be excluded under conditions of high frequency of cytosolic calcium peaks [82]. Nevertheless, in neurons the rate of calcium uptake by mitochondria is much slower than the rate of calcium extrusion from the cytosol via the plasma membrane systems, i.e. the PMCA and NCX, and via the SERCA.

3. Compartmentation of calcium transport systems relevant for the control of cytosolic calcium homeostasis in nanodomains of the neuronal plasma membrane and functional implications

Many recent experimental evidences have demonstrated that the calcium transport systems of the neuronal plasma membrane more relevant for the control of cytosolic calcium homeostasis are clustered within focalized nanodomains of a diameter size lower or equal to few hundreds of nanometers. Lipid rafts of the plasma membrane are dynamic nanodomains of a dimension between 10 and 200 nm [83], which define cellular sub-microdomains of the plasma membrane anchoring caveolins, see e.g. [81], and it has been suggested that caveolin-rich nanodomains associated with neuronal plasma membrane lacking the morphological appearance of "caveola invaginations" can serve to focalize signal transduction in neurons [84]. Indeed, the putative implication of lipid rafts in the regulation of intracellular calcium homeostasis and calcium signalling pathways was already suggested in the 1970's [85,86], but only during the last decade this hypothesis has been experimentally demonstrated, see [87,88].

Lipid rafts are enriched in cholesterol and sphingolipids [83], including a lipid family particularly enriched in the plasma membrane of neurons: the gangliosides [89], and define nanodomains of the plasma membrane for the anchoring of caveolins, flotillin, actin microfilaments and also an increasingly higher number of palmitoylated or farnesylated proteins, see [81]. The isoform caveolin-1 binds to cholesterol and sphingolipids [90-92], and also promotes the transport of cholesterol from the endoplasmic reticulum to the plasma membrane [93]. These nanodomains are merging as unique platforms for intracellular signalling in neurons, as pointed out in [84,94,95], and their stability is currently rationalized in terms of specific protein/protein or protein/lipid interactions. Noteworthy, as caveolins can act as scaffolding proteins in protein/protein interactions within these nanodomains [96,97], these interactions also bear functional relevance for the protein partners and, therefore, these nanodomains cannot be solely seen as structural elements of the plasma membrane. In this regard, it has been reported that cholesterol depletion with methyl-β-cyclodextrin, a chemical widely used to solubilise lipid rafts, alters the basal current of L-VOCC in foetal mouse skeletal muscle cells and cardiomyocytes [98,99]. Also the calcium-dependent exocytosis in synaptosomes is sensible to the cholesterol content of the plasma membrane [100], and probably one of the best documented functions of caveolins is their implication in the maintenance of intracellular cholesterol homeostasis [101].

Noteworthy, using hippocampal neurons in culture it has been demonstrated the regulation of caveolins expression by L-glutamate [102], and an increased level of caveolins expression has been reported in Alzheimer's disease which has been correlated with the increased level of cellular cholesterol observed in these patients [103]. On the other hand, knockout mice in caveolin-1 have impaired nitric oxide and calcium signalling pathways, displaying severe vascular and pulmonary anomalies and uncontrolled cellular proliferation [104], and caveolins mutations has been associated with muscle disorders and cancer [96]. Moreover, lipid rafts alterations have been reported in a significant number of pathologies [105,106].

The association of the muscle type of L-VOCC with lipid rafts sub-microdomains in cardiomyocytes was established nearly 10 years ago [81,107]. Later, we have demonstrated L-VOCC association with lipid rafts nanodomains in mature primary cultures of cerebellar granule neurons using FRET microscopy imaging [108]. This association of L-VOCC with lipid rafts nanodomains has a major functional relevance for the regulation by protein kinases of the calcium influx through these channels in neurons. First, as noted previously in this chapter within the brain the α1c subunit of L-VOCC forms a complex with PKA [30] and Razani *et al.* [109] have demonstrated the co-localization and direct interaction between the scaffolding domain of caveolin-1 and the catalytic subunit of PKA *in vivo* and *in vitro*, respectively. Second, some experimental data have suggested the possibility of direct association of CaMKII with lipid rafts [110], which is consistent with the reported co-localization of $Ca_V1.2$, the predominant L-VOCC subtype in the brain, and CaMKII [37]. Functional regulation of L-VOCC by lipid rafts is also supported by the modulation of the level of phosphorylation of L-VOCC by cholesterol depletion in cardiomyocytes [99].

Since the two major subtypes of L-VOCC present in the brain, namely $Ca_V1.2$ and $Ca_V1.3$, directly interact with many proteins having the PDZ binding domain [111,112], proteins that also bind to the NMDA receptor [113], the association of these receptors with lipid rafts nanodomains is not an unexpected finding. The presence of NMDA receptors in isolated lipid rafts has been shown by different investigators [114-117], and using fluorescence resonance energy transfer (FRET) microscopy imaging their association with lipid rafts nanodomains in mature primary cultures of cerebellar granule neurons has been demonstrated in a recent work of our laboratory [117]. The critical role of proteins with PDZ domains in the association of NMDA receptors with neuronal lipid rafts has been experimentally demonstrated using genetically modified mice, as mutations in the NR2A and NR2B subunits which impair their interaction with PDZ domains led to a reduction of NMDA receptors association with lipid rafts [118]. It has been suggested that the clustering of NMDA receptors in lipid rafts-associated sub-microdomains can potentiate the activation of these receptors, thereby serving as a molecular mechanism for potentiation of the synaptic efficiency in neuronal connections [116,117]. Because AMPA receptor clustering near NMDA receptors plays a key role for NMDA receptor activation and LTP induction, it is of special neurophysiological relevance to note here that the association of AMPA receptors with molecular components of the lipid rafts of neuronal plasma membranes has also been experimentally demonstrated [114,119,120].

The association with lipid rafts of the major systems of the neuronal plasma membrane for extrusion of calcium from the cytosol, PMCA and NCX, has also been experimentally assessed, although to the best of our knowledge only in the case of PMCA this has been reported with neuronal plasma membranes at the time this chapter was written. PMCA association with lipid rafts has been shown using preparations of synaptic plasma membranes [121] and also in primary cultures of rat cortical and hippocampal neurons [122]. Earlier, it was shown that the C-terminal domain of the PMCA interacts with proteins with PDZ domains [123]. Moreover, Jiang *et al.* [122] showed that disruption of lipid rafts domains by chronic depletion of cholesterol elicited a marked decrease of PMCA activity, suggesting that PMCA associated with lipid rafts is more active than PMCA bound to non-raft domains. NCX has been shown to be associated with lipid rafts in the smooth muscle of coronary arteries [124], it has also been shown to be present in membrane fractions of vascular endothelial cells enriched in the lipid rafts markers caveolin-1 and e-NOS [125] and the direct interaction of cardiac NCX with caveolin-3 has been demonstrated by co-precipitation [126].

On these grounds, lipid rafts nanodomains of the neuronal plasma membrane can be seen as microchip-like structures for the fine coupling and control of systems playing a major role in the maintenance of a cytosolic calcium homeostasis within the range that allows for survival and normal functionality of neurons. Because of the relevance of oxidative stress in neurodegeneration it is of utmost importance to note that two enzymatic sources of ROS/RNS have been shown to be also associated with these lipid rafts nanodomains in the neuronal plasma membrane, namely, neuronal nitric oxide synthase (nNOS) and cytochrome b_5 reductase (Cb_5R). Sato *et al.* [127] showed that two domains of the nNOS, the oxygenase and the reductase domains, interact with the scaffolding domain of caveolin-1. More recently, using FRET microscopy imaging our group has shown that nNOS is associated with lipid rafts nanodomains enriched in NMDA receptors and L-VOCC in mature cultures of primary cerebellar granule neurons [117]. Since nitric oxide play a very important role in neuromodulation, this association bears a special relevance as protein/protein interactions regulate the enzyme activity of nNOS as well as define anchoring points for the subcellular location of this protein [127,128]. Indeed, it has been shown that the interaction of nNOS with caveolin-3 in skeletal muscle modulates the catalytic activity of NOS [128]. In addition, previous works of our laboratory have shown that the Cb_5R, whose deregulation at the onset of neuronal apoptosis generates a burst of superoxide anion that stimulates the entry in the irreversible phase characterized by caspases activation [10,129-131], is also associated with lipid rafts nanodomains enriched in L-VOCC and NMDA receptors in mature cultures of primary cerebellar granule neurons [108,130,131]. Moreover, the association with these lipid rafts nanodomains of a source of nitric oxide (nNOS) and of a source of superoxide anion (Cb_5R) point out that these nanodomains may play also a major role in the focalized generation of the harmful oxidant peroxynitrite in the plasma membrane when the neurons are exposed to sustained cellular stress conditions. Let us recall here also that some mitochondria, a widely accepted major ROS-producing subcellular compartment, are also close to the plasma membrane in many neuronal types, because the cell nucleus occupies a large volume of the neuronal soma.

This protein clustering associated with lipid rafts nanodomains of the neuronal plasma membrane is summarized in the Table 1, where proteins of the cytoskeleton typically associated with lipid rafts are also included. Noteworthy, ROS significantly alter the actin polymerisation/depolymerisation dynamics, reviewed in [132]. Because actin microfilaments are part of the structural protein network of proteins associated with lipid rafts nanodomains, ROS are expected to produce a significant distortion of this protein network, like nNOS which has been shown to associate with the neuronal cytoskeleton in synaptic terminals [133]. Indeed, regulatory effects of actin cytoskeleton have been reported on NMDA receptors activation [134], on the distribution of L-type calcium channels in myocytes [135], and on the activity of NCX [80].

Structural elements	Calcium transport systems	ROS/RNS sources	Regulatory kinases
Cholesterol, Caveolins,	L-VOCC,	nNOS and Cb_5R	PKA and CaMKII
Sphingolipids, Flotillin,	NMDA and AMPA receptors,		
Actin microfilaments,	PMCA and NCX		
PDZ-binding proteins			

Table 1 Molecules associated with lipid rafts in the neuronal plasma membrane of special relevance for cytosolic calcium homeostasis and ROS/RNS-calcium signalling cross-modulation.

In spite of the well known relevance of L-glutamate AMPA and NMDA receptors clustering in LTP, the regulation of incorporation and dissociation of proteins in nanodomains or sub-microdomains associated with lipid rafts is still poorly understood and, thus, it is a pending issue. It is to be noted also that knowledge of the time scale range of the clustering dynamics of proteins within these nanodomains is a basic need to properly understand their formation and plasticity, and this is particularly relevant to reach firm conclusions regarding their role as structural or adaptive elements in rapid and slow neuronal responses.

In conclusion, a close spatial location of these calcium transport proteins in the neuronal plasma membrane can also afford a fast and fine tuning of cytosolic calcium concentrations. Moreover, as major redox centers producing ROS are also tighly associated with lipid rafts nanodomains, this compartmentation allows also to rationalize on simple grounds the intimate cross-talk between ROS and calcium signalling in neurons, as well as between oxidative stress and sustained cytosolic calcium deregulation, reviewed in [136,137].

4. Sustained alteration of cytosolic calcium homeostasis in neuronal death

Neuronal survival is extremely dependent of the fine tuning of cytosolic calcium homeostasis, because cytosolic calcium concentration has to be maintained within a relatively narrow window for neuronal survival [1], for example, between 70 and 200 nM for cerebellar granule neurons in culture [9,138]. An overwhelming amount of experimental data reported by many investigators from different countries show that sustained deviations of cytosolic calcium concentration out of this narrow window lead to neuronal cell death. Besides rapid necrotic neuronal death induced by sustained cytosolic calcium concentration higher than 0.4 μM for periods in the minutes time scale range [1,9,44,45,138,139], it has also been shown that apoptotic neuronal death can be induced when cytosolic calcium concentration remains very low for longer periods of time, in the hours time scale range [1,2]. As the extracellular free calcium concentration is approximately 1 mM, this implies that neurons need to sustain a large calcium gradient across their plasma membranes. Owing to the large number of synaptic connections established by neurons in the brain, these cells need to spend a large amount of metabolic energy to maintain their cytosolic calcium homeostasis, because during synaptic activity calcium entry is activated through VOCC and some ionotropic receptors, mainly NMDA receptors. In addition, many neuronal processes are extremely dependent upon cytosolic calcium concentration, such as neurotransmitter secretion and synaptic plasticity [140], neurite growth and sprouting [141] and signalling pathways which mediate the metabolic neuronal responses to a large number of relevant extracellular stimuli [4,5]. Therefore, the cytosolic calcium concentration should be considered a major bioenergetic marker for neuronal activity and survival.

The increase of oxidative stress in brain is a biochemical marker associated with neurodegenerative insults, like ischemia-reperfusion or inflammation, or neurodegenerative diseases of high prevalence and relevance to humans, for example, Alzheimer's, Parkinson's, amyotrophic lateral sclerosis and Huntington's diseases. Many studies have shown that cellular oxidative stress is caused by an imbalance between endogenous antioxidant defences and ROS production in favour of the latter, which results in an excessive exposure of cells to harmful ROS/RNS. On the other hand, it is well established now that the calcium transport systems most relevant for the cytosolic calcium homeostasis in neurons are molecular targets for ROS/RNS and that their chemical modification by these reactive species lead to their functional impairment. Indeed, oxidative chemical modifications of these calcium transport systems have been reported to take place *in vivo*. Moreover, many experimental studies reported during last 10 years led to the conclusion that ROS produce a sustained deregulation of cytosolic calcium homeostasis in neurons. For example, neuronal death mediated by calpains activation can be taken as a biological marker of a sustained rise of cytosolic calcium concentration [142-144]. Another examples are provided by the central role of L-VOCC and ROS in the apoptosis induced by low extracellular potassium concentration [2,9,10,129,131,145], and also by L-glutamate excitoxicity-induced neuronal death [44,45,146]. Thus, sustained alterations of neuronal cytosolic calcium are expected to be a convergent cellular mechanism in brain neurodegeneration. Consistent with this hypothesis, alterations of neuronal calcium homeostasis and brain oxidative stress have been reported in the case for the brain neurodegenerative diseases of higher incidence to humans, like Alzheimer's [147,148] and Parkinson's [149,150], or in the acute neurodegeneration observed in amyotrophic lateral sclerosis [146,151], and also for major brain insults, such as excitotoxicity in trauma and ischemia-reperfusion [44,45], inflammation [152,153] and neurotoxicity by drugs and environmental chemicals [139,154].

Most ROS/RNS that are produced in cellular oxidative stress in mammalian tissues have been demonstrated to be strongly neurotoxic to neurons *in vitro*. This is a relatively large list of ROS/RNS, and we shall concentrate in this chapter in those most studied as agents in brain neurodegeneration, namely, superoxide anion, H_2O_2, hydroxyl radicals, lipid hydroperoxides, and nitric oxide-derived ROS, mainly peroxynitrite and nitrogen dioxide. Because of the calcium dependence of the activity of nNOS, the main enzymatic system responsible for the production of nitric oxide in neurons [133], RNS should be expected to play a particularly relevant role as intracellular biomarkers of the level of coordination or deregulation of calcium and ROS signalling pathways in neurons. However, it is still a matter of debate whether *in vivo* all of these ROS/RNS can reach concentrations high enough to act as causal agents or merely as agents that potentiate or accelerate the rate of an ongoing neuronal death process in the brain. Moreover, the analysis and dissection of the chemical reaction pathways of each one of this ROS/RNS is further complicated by the fact that *in vivo* they generate radicalic chain chemical reactions. Therefore, it is critical to identify the major subcellular primary sources of these ROS/RNS in different neurons and in different degenerative processes in the brain, and this is an issue yet to be settled in many cases, as during lasts years the experimental evidences have pointed out that the relative relevance of different ROS/RNS seems to be largely dependent on the neurodegenerative disease or brain insult.

5. Modulation by ROS/RNS of calcium transport systems relevant for the control of neuronal cytosolic calcium homeostasis

ROS and RNS producing oxidative stress to neurons can be generated by neuronal and also by non-neuronal cells, like microglia or endothelial cells of the brain blood vessels. It is to be noted that oxidative stress-induced brain degeneration is a relatively slow process, in most neurodegenerative diseases developing in periods of time of years and in acute brain ischemia-reperfusion in a time range from minutes to several days, depending upon the intensity of the oxidative stress insult. Thus, in a brain suffering oxidative stress neurons are exposed for relatively large time periods to either extracellularly and/or intracellularly generated ROS/RNS. Because the extracellular liquid bathing the brain and stem neurons is poorer in antioxidants than the blood, due to the low permeability and high selectivity of the blood-brain barrier, the extracellular antioxidant protection in the brain is notably lower than that of other organs and tissues in mammals. Under these environmental conditions the plasma membrane of neurons, where major calcium transport systems controlling the cytosolic calcium homeostais are located, is particularly sensitive to the oxidative stress generated in the brain by vicinal neuronal and non-neuronal cells. The major ROS/RNS reported to play a significant role in the enhanced brain oxidative stress associated with neurodegenerative diseases and insults like ischemia-reperfusion and inflammation can be split into three major groups: (i) primary biochemical ROS/RNS, i.e. chemical species directly generated by some enzymes or proteins during brain activity in normal or pathophysiological conditions, (ii) secondary biochemical ROS/RNS, chemical species derived by rapid reaction between the primary biochemical ROS/RNS or by systems involved in their detoxification, and (iii) radicalic chain ROS/RNS, chemical radicals involved in the initiation of radical reaction chains or that are largely generated within radical reaction chains.

Superoxide anion is a primary biochemical ROS that plays a key role in the generation of many of the more harmful ROS and RNS detected in the oxidative stress-induced degeneration of the brain. Superoxide anion can be produced by neuronal and non-neuronal cells within the brain. Because of the relatively low permeability to superoxide anion of lipid bilayers [155], extracellular superoxide anion must be largely generated by redox centres of the plasma membrane of neuronal and non-neuronal cells. In glial, macrophages and endothelial cells there are NADPH oxidases of the NOX family, which are under the control of transcriptional antioxidant-responsive elements (ARE), reviewed in [156]. In contrast, we found that in the plasma membrane of neurons the NADH-dependent production of superoxide anion associated with their NADH oxidase activity was nearly ten-fold higher than their NADPH activity [157,158]. Indeed, an overshot of superoxide anion production at the plasma membrane is an early event in the apoptosis of cerebellar granule neurons induced by extracellular K^+ deprivation [10,131], an overshot that we have found to be largely catalyzed by deregulation of cytochrome b_5 reductase associated with plasma membrane lipid rafts sub-microdomains [130,131]. Mitochondria is now widely accepted as the major source of intracellular superoxide anion in oxidative stress-induced neuronal death in cultures *in vitro*, particularly by complexes I and III of the mitochondrial respiratory chain [159]. In addition, non-mitochondrial enzymes that use oxygen as substrate can also become a source of intracellular superoxide anion in neurons, such as the conversion of xanthine dehydrogenase into xanthine oxidase either by direct oxidation and/or by proteolytic activation during oxidative stress-induced neuronal death [160].

Nitric oxide is the major primary biochemical RNS produced in oxidative stress-induced brain degeneration, and although not harmful by itself, its reaction with superoxide anion yields peroxynitrite (a secondary biochemical ROS/RNS), probably the most neurotoxic ROS/RNS generated during oxidative stress-mediated brain neurodegeneration, see e.g. [161,162]. The reaction between nitric oxide and superoxide anion is very fast, such that it is considered a diffusion-controlled chemical reaction due to the very high value of the bimolecular rate constant, (4-7) 10^9 M^{-1} s^{-1} [163]. Peroxynitrite, in spite of its short lifetime within the cells [162], has been shown to be a very harmful ROS/RNS involved in the brain damage produced by ischemia-reperfusion [161], by inflammation and spinal cord injury [164,165] and also in neurodegenerative diseases and aging [166,167]. Peroxynitrite can elicit functional damage of biomolecules and subcellular structures acting either as a potent oxidant ($E^{0'}$ = 1.2-1.4 V) or through the generation of harmful radicals such as hydroxyl and nitrogen dioxide free radicals, reviewed in [162,168]. Due to this, peroxynitrite can produce oxidation of protein cysteines to disulfide bonds, sulfenic and sulfinic acids eventually leading to sulfonic acids, oxidation of protein methionines, nitration of protein tyrosines and lipids, lipid peroxidation, coenzyme Q oxidation, and DNA and RNA oxidation. Because the activation of neuronal nitric oxide synthase requires an increase of cytosolic calcium, peroxynitrite is one of the more harmful ROS/RNS produced in the oxidative stress accompanied by sustained alterations of the neuronal cytosolic calcium homeostasis. Indeed, this has been shown to be the case for the excitotoxic neuronal death elicited by L-glutamate through activation of NMDA receptors [166,169].

ROS/RNS initiating lipid oxidation and peroxidation, i.e. self-accelerating chemical radical chains, are the other group of ROS/RNS playing a major role in brain damage by oxidative stress. Among them, H_2O_2 has required a large attention because is one of the major products generated under conditions that elicit over-production of superoxide anion, as it is a product of superoxide dismutase activity. In addition, intracellular traces of metal ions such as Fe^{3+} or Cu^{2+} can catalyse Fenton-like reactions in neurons, generating hydroxyl radical from superoxide and H_2O_2 [170]. Hydroxyl radical is one of the most potent cytotoxic oxygen radicals, which can attack a large variety of important biomolecules, from small biomolecules such as coenzyme Q or α-tocopherol [171] up to large biomolecules like proteins, RNA and DNA [170,172]. Since hydroxyl radical can be also generated from peroxynitrite decomposition (see above), it turns out that it is a converging point between the oxidative stress pathways involving ROS and RNS derived from nitric oxide. The involvement of hydroxyl radical in oxidative stress-induced neuronal damage has been suggested, for example, in the pathophysiological case of spinal cord trauma [173], amyotrophic lateral sclerosis [174] and Parkinson's disease [170,175].

Lipid ROS are a family of harmful ROS detected in oxidative stress-mediated brain degeneration that also catalyze chemical radical reaction chains. They can be produced as primary biochemical ROS by cyclooxygenases (COX) and lipoxygenases in some brain oxidative stress insults, such as ischemia-reperfusion [176], or Parkinson's disease [177]. Indeed, inhibitors of the neuronal COX-2 isoform have been reported to attenuate brain damage after ischemia-reperfusion [176]. Moreover, the oxidation of dopamine by the microglial COX-1 isoform and also by COX-2 isoform in the dopaminergic neurons of the substantia nigra has been involved in the pathogenesis of Parkinson's disease [177]. It is to be noted though that lipid ROS are also generated during hydroxyl radical- and hydrogen peroxide-induced lipid oxidation and peroxidation, respectively [170]. In addition, lipid oxidation and peroxidation also release the aldehydes malondialdehyde and 4-hydroxynonenal, which have been shown to be highly neurotoxic compounds [178,179]. Because of the self-propagating properties of lipid radical chains once they are initiated, and also due to the high toxicity for neurons of lipid breakdown compounds released, the possibility of cell rescue after the threshold antioxidant barrier against lipid oxidation/peroxidation is surpassed can be considered negligible. The extent of lipid oxidation marking the 'point of no return' for neurons survival has not been firmly established yet, but it is likely to be at most only a few per cent of the total lipids [180]. On these grounds, an enhanced lipid oxidation should be expected to be a late and largely irreversible step in neuronal death. This view is consistent with the many reports showing that largely damaged brain areas after an ischemia-reperfusion insult display a marked increase of lipid peroxidation.

5.1. Modulation by ROS/RNS of the major calcium entry systems of the neuronal plasma membrane

5.1.1. Voltage-operated calcium channels

As indicated above in the section 2 of this chapter, the L-type are the most relevant VOCC in the fine tuning of the steady state level of cytosolic calcium concentration in the neuronal soma and, thus, in the fine tuning of threshold neuronal excitability [22-24]. L-type VOCC as a primary target for ROS in brain is also supported by the hypoxic up-regulation of these channels, which is mediated by Alzheimer's amyloid peptides [181]. L-VOCC contain two vicinal cysteines at positions 271 and 272 which are involved in their interaction with syntaxin 1A, thereby playing a major role in their regional localization in plasma membrane microdomains [182]. In addition, three cysteines are located in the calcium-pore region (Cys^{330}, Cys^{1383} and Cys^{1396}) [183]. Therefore, L-VOCC contains redox centres that have been shown to react with ROS/RNS in other proteins, for example, in NMDA-receptors (see below).

Studies with neurons in culture have provided ample experimental evidences of direct modulation of L-VOCC by the major ROS/RNS involved in brain ischemia-reperfusion, inflammation and/or neurodegeneration. The L-VOCC antagonist nifedipine has been reported to protect CNS neurons against hydrogen peroxide-induced death, which is mediated by a sustained increase of cytosolic calcium, pointing out activation of L-type VOCC by H_2O_2 [184]. H_2O_2 was shown later to activate recombinant calcium channel α_{1C} subunit stably expressed in HEK 293 cells [185]. In addition, nitric oxide has been reported to induce activation of L-VOCC in hippocampal neurons by plasma membrane depolarization [186] or to inhibit calcium channel gating via activation of cGMP-dependent protein kinases [187]. In contrast, exposure to peroxynitrite has been reported to produce decrease of calcium influx through L-VOCC at low submicromolar doses in rat cerebellar granule neurons in culture and increase of calcium influx through L-VOCC at higher micromolar doses in rat cerebellar granule neurons in culture [9] and in mouse cerebral cortical neurons [188]. Hydroxyl radicals, a radical produced during the decomposition of peroxynitrite, have been reported to suppress the calcium influx through L-VOCC in mouse cortical neurons [189]. Consistent with these results, dihydropyridine L-VOCC blockers afford protection against neuronal death induced by exposure of neurons *in vitro* to the peroxynitrite-releasing agent SIN-1 [9,190]. Because of the short lifetime and high reactivity of these radicals this is likely to be due to direct chemical modification of L-VOCC, although it is to be noted that this chemical modification is yet unknown. In addition, it has been reported that eicosanoids and ROS generated during arachidonic acid oxidative metabolism also activate L-VOCC [191], and that the lipid peroxidation product 4-hydroxynonenal causes opening of the L-VOCC, resulting in an increase of cytosolic calcium and neuronal death which is prevented by the L-VOCC blocker nimodipine [192]. Direct redox modulation of L-VOCC is further supported by its activation by hydrogen sulphide [138]. Further studies are needed to reach firm conclusions regarding the molecular mechanisms of modulation of different neuronal L-VOCC subtypes by ROS.

Only very scarce experimental studies have been done on the putative modulation of N-, P/Q- and R-type VOCC by ROS/RNS, despite the fact that N- and R-type of calcium channels are blocked by heavy metals such as Pb^{2+} and Hg^{2+} that are likely to interact with thiols [193]. $Ca_V2.2$ (N-type) channel gating is inhibited by nitric oxide via cGMP-dependent protein kinase, as it is also the Ca_V1 (L-type) channel [187]. Also, the lipid peroxidation product 4-hydroxynonenal increased the calcium influx through L-type and other ill-defined types of VOCC [178].

5.1.2. NMDA and other ionotropic receptors with calcium channel activity

It is well known the relevant role of NMDA-receptor mediated excitotoxic neuronal death in ischemia-reperfusion brain injury, see [44,45], in multiple chemical sensitivity in brain [194], in neuronal glutathione depletion [195] and in hydrogen sulfide-induced neuronal death [138,196]. Therefore, it is not surprising that the redox modulation of the NMDA-receptor is by far the most studied within the group of ionotropic receptors. The redox modulatory site of the NMDA-receptor consists of thiols groups that are vicinal in the three-dimensional structure and may form disulfide bonds under the cellular oxidative stress conditions induced by ROS [197], and it acts as a gain control for current flux through the NMDA-receptor [197,198]. Moreover, a significant number of NMDA-receptor cysteines are in the domains of this receptor facing the extracellular space, including at least one pair of vicinal thiols [199]. Thus, this receptor can also play a major role in the rapid neuronal adaptation to changes of the redox potential in the extracellular fluids within the brain, and the different types of NMDA-receptors display a redox response that is dependent on the type of NR2 forming the channels [55]. The differential redox-sensitivity of NMDA receptors isoforms led to the discovery of two redox modulatory centres within the NMDA-receptor structure, one formed by Cys744 and Cys798 on the subunit NR1 and a second one on the subunit NR2A [200,201]. Whereas the redox centre of the subunit NR1 plays a major role in the redox modulation of NR1/NR2C- and NR1/NR2B-containing receptors, the redox centre of subunit NR2A is sufficient for the expression of redox sensitivity in NR1/NR2A-containing receptors [201]. Redox active compounds modulate NMDA-receptors such that reduction of NMDA-receptor increases NMDA-receptor activity and their oxidation leads to a decrease of NMDA-receptor activity [202].

Because of the high physiological relevance of nitric oxide and of NMDA receptors in the brain, the modulation of NMDA receptors by nitric oxide is of particular relevance. Nitric oxide inhibition of NMDA-receptor response in cortical neurons in culture has been rationalized in terms of NO-induced disulfide bonds between vicinal thiols of the NMDA-receptor, and was proposed to afford neuronal protection against L-glutamate excitotoxicity [203]. Indeed, it has also been reported that thiol-reducing agents such as dithiothreitol increase the open dwell-time and opening frequency of NR1/NR2A channels [55,201]. Consistent with these findings, it has been reported that the novel neuromodulator hydrogen sulphide potentiates NMDA-receptor response in hippocampal neurons [204] and in cerebellar granule neurons [138], and that over-stimulation of NMDA-receptors by hydrogen sulphide can lead to excitotoxic neuronal death [138,196]. Glutamate-induced excitotoxic neuronal death has been shown to mediate brain injury after a transient focal cerebral ischemia episode [44,45]. Inhibitors of the H_2S-producing enzymes cystathionine β-synthase and cystathionine γ-lyase reduced the infarct volume in a dose-dependent manner, while administration of sodium hydrosulfide significantly increased the infarct volume after a transient focal cerebral ischemia insult [205]. Exposure of neurons to peroxynitrite also leads to activation of calcium entry through NMDA-receptors [166,169]. This effect of peroxynitrite has been rationalized in terms of the rise of L-glutamate concentration within the synaptic cleft, either due to potentiation by nitric oxide and/or peroxynitrite of L-glutamate secretion in synaptic terminals [194,206] or of inhibition of L-glutamate transporters catalyzing its re-uptake [207].

Besides the major role of NMDA-receptors on the neuronal damage elicited by ROS and/or oxidative stress, AMPA receptors have been also involved in the neurotoxicity of ROS. It has been reported that the increase of cytosolic calcium associated with the influx of Ca^{2+} through the ionotropic AMPA-receptors can stimulate nNOS leading to an enhanced production of nitric oxide within L-glutamatergic neurons [208]. Moreover, antagonists of AMPA/kainate-receptors have been reported to prevent the loss of cell viability induced by the peroxynitrite-releasing agent SIN-1 in mixed cortical cell cultures containing both neurons and astrocytes [209]. AMPA-receptors contain a disulfide bond between cysteines 260 and 315 in the ligand binding domain of receptor subunit GluRD, which has been proposed to act as a redox centre implicated in direct redox modulation of these receptors [210]. Nevertheless, the redox modulation of AMPA-receptors is a topic that will require further studies to develop an integrative view of its modulation by the different ROS that has been implicated in brain damage.

Finally, the response of the purinergic ionotropic P2X-receptors has been shown to be altered by acute hypoxia, an effect that has been proposed to be mediated by ROS because H_2O_2 attenuated the effect of hypoxia on homomeric P2X2 whole-cell currents, which are reversibly reduced to 38% of control by H_2O_2 [211]. Yet, studies regarding the putative modulation of P2X-receptors by other ROS are a pending issue.

5.2. Modulation by ROS/RNS of the transport systems that release calcium from intracellular stores

5.2.1. Endoplasmic reticulum

ROS/RNS have been shown to elicit a potent stimulation of calcium release from the endoplasmic reticulum, through activation of IP_3 and ryanodine receptors.

Superoxide anion and H_2O_2 have been reported to induce calcium release from the endoplasmic reticulum of neurons through activation of IP_3 receptors [212,213]. Oxidized glutathione and the alkyl mercury compound thimerosal, a thiol specific agent, increase the affinity of IP_3 receptors for IP_3, thereby sensitizing this receptor to basal IP_3 level in the cell and promoting calcium release from the endoplasmic reticulum to the cytosol [214,215]. Cysteine clusters highly reactive against ROS have been recently identified in the IP_3 receptors [216]. IP_3 receptors are inhibited by interaction with luminal endoplasmic reticulum proteins through luminal-facing domains of the receptor containing reduced cysteines, and oxidation of these cysteines weakens these interactions leading to IP_3 receptor activation [63,217]. Moreover, nitric oxide-induced increase of IP_3 binding to the IP_3 receptor in hypoxic brain has been proposed to mediate IP_3 receptors activation in calcium-dependent neuronal apoptotic death induced by hypoxia [218].

Although all ryanodine receptor isoforms are expressed in the brain, the isoform 2 is the most heavily expressed [219, 220]. Many studies have addressed the redox modulation of the ryanodine receptors in myocytes and in neurons, reviewed in [62,64,221]. Nitric oxide activates the skeletal and cardiac ryanodine receptors [222,223]. The activation of the ryanodine receptor by nitric oxide has been shown to be due to the presence of highly reactive cysteines of the receptor, which are S-nitrosylated upon exposure to nitric oxide [222-224]. The cysteines that are S-nitrosylated upon *in vitro* exposure to nitric oxide have been identified [225]. However, *in vivo* the extent of S-nitrosylation of ryanodine receptor cysteines is highly modulated by the physiological oxygen tension, leading to the concept that ryanodine receptors can operate as a coupled redox sensor for oxygen and nitric oxide [226,227]. *In vitro* studies have shown that these cysteines of the ryanodine receptor are highly sensitive to oxidative stress and are likely to mediate the redox ryanodine receptor response to another ROS, as they are also prone to reversible S-glutathionylation or oxidation to disulfide bonds [225]. The ryanodine receptors are also activated by hydroxyl radical, H_2O_2, the disulfide bond-forming agent diamide and also by oxidized glutathione [221,224,228]. Overall, oxidizing conditions favor the opening of the ryanodine receptor calcium channel, and on these grounds it has been proposed that activation of these calcium channels are also involved in the pathology of brain ischemia-reperfusion [229] and Alzheimer's disease [230]. Noteworthy, a moderate and sustained stimulation of the ryanodine receptors in the hippocampus has been involved in the sustained increase of cytosolic calcium needed for the induction of the long-term postsynaptic potentiation associated with memory formation [231,232].

Calcium accumulation within the luminal space of the endoplasmic reticulum is performed by Ca^{2+}-ATPases (SERCA), whose activity is inhibited by exposure to H_2O_2, superoxide anion and peroxynitrite [233-236], the major ROS produced in brain insults such as ischemia-reperfusion or inflammation and in neurodegeneration. Despite that the isoforms of SERCA most sensitive to ROS, i.e. SERCA2 isoforms, are expressed in brain, the relevance of the impairment of their activity to alterations of neuronal cytosolic calcium homeostasis has yet to be conclusively demonstrated, probably because in neurons the PMCA is a calcium pump more potent than SERCA for calcium extrusion from the cytosol.

The apparently higher susceptibility to ROS/RNS of the calcium release systems of the endoplasmic reticulum, ryanodine and IP_3 receptors, should lead under oxidative stress conditions to at least a partial depletion of the calcium concentration within the luminal space of this subcellular compartment, see for example [237]. It should be noted, though, that in neurons the amount of calcium stored in the endoplasmic reticulum is small compared with the amount of calcium entering through plasma membrane calcium channels and ionotropic receptors. However, in most severe cases the depletion of calcium can elicit the opening of plasma membrane SOCE, see section 2.2 of this chapter. Thus, the relevance of calcium release from the endoplasmic reticulum or of inhibition of the SERCA to the observed alterations by ROS/RNS of cytosolic calcium homeostasis will strongly depend on the differential expression of SOCE isoforms in different type of neurons. On the other hand, the depletion of calcium of the endoplasmic reticulum may lead to a dysfunctional endoplasmic reticulum by itself, because of the relevance of the endoplasmic calcium concentration for the correct folding and processing of membrane and secretory proteins [65, 238]. On these grounds, these authors have proposed that ROS/RNS-induced endoplasmic reticulum dysfunction can be a mechanism underlying slow-developing cell injury in ischemia-reperfusion, epileptic seizures and degenerative diseases of the brain like Alzheimer's and Parkinson's diseases. In addition, it has been recently shown that mutations in presenilin-1 and -2 observed in nearly 40% of familial Alzheimer's disease lead to calcium release from the endoplasmic reticulum [239]. Moreover, presenilins by themselves can form calcium leak channels in the endoplasmic reticulum whose properties are altered in mutant presenilins linked to Alzheimer's disease [240].

5.2.2. Mitochondria

A key role has been proposed for mitochondrial dysfunctions in the onset or development of neuronal death in the brain mediated by the enhanced oxidative stress observed in relevant neurodegenerative disorders, such as Alzheimer's and Parkinson's diseases, amyotrophic lateral sclerosis and Friedreich's ataxia, and in harmful brain insults like ischemia-reperfusion and glutamate excitotoxicity, reviewed in [166,241,242]. Mitochondrial calcium overload is observed in excitotoxic conditions that produce a sustained increase of neuronal cytosolic calcium or high frequency repetitive cytosolic calcium peaks [73]. ROS/RNS have been shown to promote opening of the permeability transition pore of mitochondria and this effect of ROS/RNS is enhanced by mitochondrial calcium overload [71,73,166]. Opening of the permeability transition pore leads to a significant calcium release from mitochondria which contributes to foster excitotoxic neuronal death [71, 243], and also is an important factor in necrotic cell death following ischemia-reperfusion [73] or in neurons exposed to transient hypoglycemia [244]. Consistently, calcium-dependent mitochondrial dysfunction by peroxynitrite has been demonstrated to elicit necrotic cell death via activation of calpains [245]. In addition, opening of this pore has also been shown to mediate the neuronal apoptosis elicited by 3-nitropropionic acid, an agent which has been used to mimic in model rodents the brain neurodegeneration observed in Huntington's disease [246]. Despite that most of studies concerning ROS-stimulated release of calcium from mitochondria point out a major role of the permeability transition pore, it should be recalled that the inner membrane Na^+/Ca^{2+}-exchanger, i.e. the other major mitochondrial calcium release system [71], is also sensitive to oxidative stress. It has been reported that oxidative stress mediated by H_2O_2 modulates this exchanger and can lead to activation of caspase 3-dependent apoptosis due to mitochondrial Na^+ overload [247].

The permeability transition pore opening induced by ROS/RNS is mediated by oxidation of critical thiols of proteins forming the pore, as it can be elicited by a relatively large number of oxidizing agents such as diamide, dithiopyridine, singlet oxygen, diazoxide, nitric oxide, S-nitrosothiols and selenium [221]. The adenine nucleotide transporter of the inner mitochondrial membrane and the voltage-dependent anion channel of the outer mitochondrial membrane have been proposed to be part of the molecular structure of the permeability transition pore, and both proteins have shown to be modulated by oxidative stress and exposure of mitochondria to chemically defined ROS, such that oxidation of thiols of the adenine nucleotide transporter facing to the mitochondrial matrix have been shown to elicit the opening of the permeability transition pore, reviewed in [73].

5.3. Modulation by ROS/RNS of the transport systems involved in calcium extrusion from the cytosol

Much of the interest on modulation of PMCA and Na^+/Ca^{2+}-exchanger of neurons by ROS is based on the reported decrease of these activities in synaptic plasma membranes in aging, and the possibility that this could lead to a sustained increase of the steady state cytosolic calcium in aged animals with respect to young animals [248,249].

5.3.1. PMCA

It has been shown that incubation of brain synaptic plasma membranes with Fe^{2+}/EDTA, H_2O_2, peroxyl radicals generated by azo-initiators and peroxynitrite resulted in a significant loss of PMCA activity [250-253]. Inhibition of purified PMCA by H_2O_2 has been proposed to be due to oxidation of two cysteines of this protein [253]. Also, lipid peroxidation and the lipid peroxidation product 4-hydroxynonenal have been shown to inhibit the PMCA actvity [254]. In the case of incubation with peroxynitrite, the loss of Ca^{2+}-ATPase activity was paralleled by decrease of ATP-dependent calcium uptake activity and by a significant increase of tyrosine nitration of the PMCA [252]. However, it is to be noted that all these studies were carried out *in vitro* with purified plasma membranes in an altered environment with respect to the normal redox cytosolic environment in living neurons, and this has to be taken into account since endogenous antioxidant levels of reduced glutathione has been shown to largely attenuate the inhibition of PMCA by peroxynitrite [252]. In addition, the concentrations of H_2O_2 and peroxynitrite producing approximately 50% inhibition of the PMCA in these studies, higher than 100 μM in both cases, were much higher than those reported to be attained in brain after transient focal ischemia or inflammation. For the case of neuronal exposure to peroxynitrite fluxes mimicking those attained in inflammation or ischemia-reperfusion, in a previous work of our laboratory it was shown that in cerebellar granule neurons in culture the PMCA is significantly inhibited in less than 2 hours exposure to micromolar concentrations of peroxynitrite, although it was also noted that the PMCA has nearly ten-fold lower sensitivity to peroxynitrite than L-VOCC [9].

$Na^+/Ca^{2+}-exchanger\ (NCX)$

The NCX has been reported to be less sensitive to inhibition by the peroxyl radical azo initiator 2,2'- azobis (2-amidinopropane) dihydrochloride (AAPH) and peroxynitrite than the PMCA [251], and also to be insensitive to inhibition by up to 700 μM of H_2O_2 [255]. The Na^+/Ca^{2+}-exchanger activity of synaptic brain plasma membranes and in transfected CHO-K1 cells has been reported to be inhibited by exposure to AAPH and also to peroxynitrite [255], although it must be noted that peroxynitrite only afforded a partial inhibition of the exchanger caused by decrease of its affinity for calcium without a significant change of the V_{max}. The inhibition induced by both oxidants correlated with the formation of higher molecular weight aggregates of the Na^+/Ca^{2+}-exchanger, and in addition AAPH also caused fragmentation of the exchanger protein.

In contrast, in cardiac muscle myocytes, hypoxia inhibits the Na^+/Ca^{2+}-exchanger and ROS are required for its rapid reactivation upon reoxygenation [256]. This is consistent with the earlier demonstration in ventricular myocytes of stimulation of the Na^+/Ca^{2+}-exchanger by H_2O_2 and superoxide anion [257]. Owing to the different pattern of Na^+/Ca^{2+}-exchanger isoforms expression in brain cells and cardiac myocytes, more experimental studies are needed to reach solid conclusions regarding the effects of oxidative stress on the activity of this exchanger in different neuronal types and also in the glial cells of the brain.

6. Space and time fluctuations of cytosolic calcium in the neuronal soma

As indicated previously in this chapter, protein compartmentation within microdomains allows for a more efficient and rapid functional coupling between influx and efflux calcium transport systems, and this is particularly relevant for neuronal activity, as neurons have to deliver fast responses to many repetitive and simultaneous extracellular stimuli coming from different neighbour cells. Studies on calcium signalling in neurons have played a pioneer role to demonstrate the outstanding role of subcellular compartmentation in the control of neuronal activity, see for example [5]. As analyzed in more detail in the section 3 of this chapter more recently reported experimental data point out that the calcium transport systems of the plasma membrane more relevant for the control of cytosolic calcium homeostasis in neurons are associated with lipid rafts sub-microdomains or nanodomains. This is an emerging scenario that opens new perspectives for the rationalization of the modulation of cytosolic calcium peaks amplitude and also of the rate of attenuation of calcium local gradients in neurons, as both parameters are strongly dependent on the spatial proximity between systems controlling calcium entry and extrusion from the cytosol. For example, the rationalization of the transient calcium gradients observed between different regions of the neuronal cytosol can be done on simple grounds taking into account a polarised or focalized distribution of the major calcium transport systems of the neuronal plasma membrane. Note that, as indicated before in this chapter, sustained cytosolic calcium concentrations higher than 0.4 μM are strongly cytotoxic to neurons, but it is a need for neurons to reach these concentrations in the environment of cytosolic proteins and enzymes having EC_{50} values for calcium between 0.4 and 1 μM. Indeed, some of these proteins play a key role in neuronal plasticity and functional responses critical for proper brain development and function, like calmodulin, nNOS, GAP-43 and CaMK, to cite only a few of well-established examples.

The calcium concentration reaches values in the micromolar range upon activation of L-VOCC and NMDA receptors in small volume elements close to the cytosolic side of their calcium channel structures [258], see also the Figure 2a. This generates a calcium concentration wave that diffuses within the cytosolic space, because the protein cytosolic buffering systems are not fast enough to trap all incoming calcium ions through these calcium channels [259, 260]. Due to the rapid diffusion of calcium ions in the aqueous space of the cytoplasm, ~300 $\mu m^2 s^{-1}$, the calcium entry through the high conductance L-VOCC and NMDA receptors channels will rapidly raise the calcium concentration to the micromolar range within the associated lipid rafts nanodomains. As these nanodomains have sizes lower than 200 nm, it can be derived that in less than 1 microsecond the incoming calcium ions will diffuse within the whole space of the nanodomain, i.e. in the time scale range characteristic for fast conformational relaxation in proteins. Thus, this clustering serves to built up a very efficient molecular switch for signal transduction in calcium signalling pathways within neurons, with a time response as fast as the rapid conformational relaxations elicited by regulatory direct protein/protein interactions. However, nanodomains can be seen as multi-port exit molecular devices that can serve to many uni-port exit molecular devices, through regulatory direct protein/protein interactions. Therefore, the localized calcium rise within these nanodomains not only serves to guarantee the maximal possible activation of proteins or enzymes with EC_{50} values ≥0.4 micromolar, such as those listed above, but also to elicit rapid integrative cellular responses. We shall next briefly analyze several integrative responses of relevance for the rapid and fine control of cytosolic calcium homeostasis in neurons elicited by the localized calcium rise within the nanodomains associated with lipid rafts.

The association of CaMKII with L-VOCC subunit β2a and with NMDA receptors subunit NR2B, mentioned in the section 2.1 of this chapter, implies that this protein is present in neuronal nanodomains associated with lipid rafts. A direct consequence of the steep calcium concentration gradient generated by calcium entry through L-VOCC and NMDA receptors is the stronger selective activation of the pool of CaMKII that lies in their vicinity over other CaMKII pools present in neurons. Thus, this will selectively potentiate phosphorylation of CaMKII substrates present in lipid rafts associated nanodomains. Regarding the cytosolic calcium homeostasis in neurons, the more relevant effect is the activation of L-VOCC upon phosphorylation by CaMKII, as this potentiates the increase of the local gradient of calcium concentration within these nanodomains, leading to a longer lasting increase of the concentration of cytosolic calcium with the concomitant increase in neuronal secretory activity and excitability (Figure 2b). Indeed, it has been shown that L-VOCC plays a relevant physiological role in NMDA receptors-independent long-term potentiation [28]. The activation and synaptic clustering of AMPA receptors upon phosphorylation by CaMKII has been shown to potentiate NMDA receptors activation in the induction of LTP [53]. Noteworthy, L-VOCC blockers like nifedipine and nimodipine and AMPA antagonists/inhibitors have been shown to have anti-epileptic therapeutic effects, pointing out that overstimulation of L-VOCC and/or AMPA underlies, at least, some types of epileptic seizures.

The high concentration of calcium attained within the nanodomains associated with lipid rafts allows for a stronger and faster selective stimulation of the pool of nNOS localized therein. Because of the rapid diffusion coefficient of nitric oxide, these nanodomains can be seen as the most relevant plasma membrane points for focalized nitric oxide generation in neurons and, therefore, define the sub-microcompartments of neurons where higher transient concentrations of nitric oxide are attained upon nNOS stimulation. This fact and the vicinal location of nNOS and NMDA receptors within these nanodomains, i.e. separated by a distance lower than 40 nm [117], makes of NMDA receptors a major cellular target for the chemical reactivity of released nitric oxide. As the calcium currents through NMDA receptors are inhibited by exposure of these receptors to nitric oxide, see the section 5.1 of this chapter, the co-localization of nNOS and NMDA receptors within these nanodomains serves to potentiate a feedback retroinhibition mechanism for the attenuation of excessive NMDA receptors activity which would lead to neuronal excitotoxicity [117], i.e. these nanodomains can be also seen as a molecular microchip-like structure designed for neuronal protection against the harmful consequences of overstimulation by L-glutamate (Figure 2c). On these grounds, the reported stimulation of L-VOCC by nitric oxide, see the section 5.1 of this chapter, can be rationalized as a molecular compensatory mechanism for the fine tuning of NMDA receptor activity, as it will lead to an increase of L-glutamate secretion near these nanodomains and this should avoid excessive depression of NMDA receptor activity in the neuron.

The latter point already highlights a major role of the nanodomains associated with lipid rafts in the intimate cross-talk between calcium and nitric oxide signalling for the normal physiological activity of neurons, but also points out that excessive calcium entry through L-VOCC or NMDA receptors should rapidly lead to unusually large peaks of nitric oxide generation in these nanodomains. As indicated above in this chapter, it is well established now that the sustained rise of intracellular calcium and/or nitric oxide can induce neuronal death and are common features in brain degeneration. Many experimental evidences accumulated up to date reveal that in some cases the induction of oxidative stress in brain neurodegeneration takes place before a sustained cytosolic calcium homeostasis deregulation can be observed. For example, in the case of inflammation of a brain area induced either by a traumatic shock injury or cerebral stroke the neurons are exposed to a ROS/RNS overshot largely generated by vicinal glial and vascular endothelial cells. The major sources for the overshot of ROS/RNS observed in this inflammation episode are the increase of iNOS expression, which produces a nitric oxide overshot, and activation of plasma membrane NADPH oxidases, which produces a superoxide anion overshot. Therefore, within the brain area affected by inflammation neurons suffer a long-lasting exposure to an extracellular microenvironment where the simultaneous presence

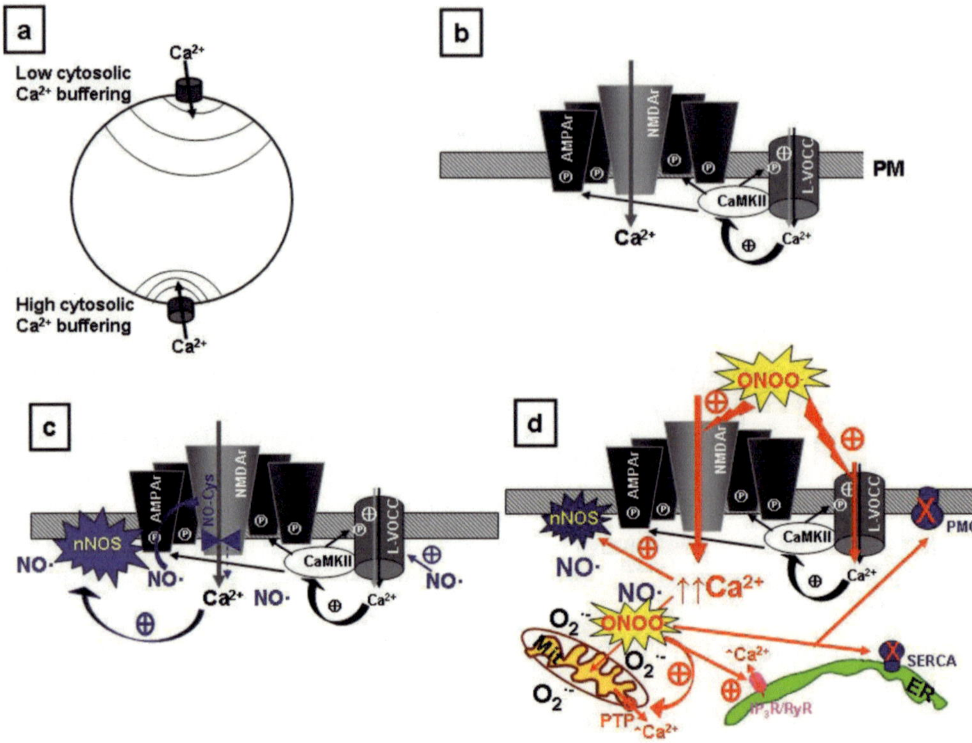

Figure 2. Functional implications of the association of calcium transport systems and ROS/RNS-sources in the neuronal plasma membrane. (a) Generation of transients of micromolar calcium concentrations within nano- or sub-micro-volume elements. The size attained by these volume elements is strongly dependent on the intensity of the total calcium inward current through the calcium transport systems clusters within lipid rafts-associated nanodomains and on the cytosolic calcium buffering capacity (see the text). (b) Faster and long-lasting potentiation of NMDA receptors (NMDAr). Calcium entry through L-VOCC triggers the activation of associated CaMKII, which elicits (i) a feedback activation of L-VOCC potentiating calcium entry and (ii) a recruitment of activated AMPA receptors (AMPAr). (c) Potentiation of NO -mediated protection against L-glutamate excitotoxicity. The co-localization of nNOS allows to reach higher NO concentrations near NMDA receptors and L-VOCC potentiating its effects on these calcium transport systems. (d) Peroxynitrite-induced sustained cytosolic calcium deregulation. A dramatic consequence of an unbalanced overstimulation of calcium transport systems that raise the cytosolic calcium concentration. Other abbreviations used in this figure: PM, plasma membrane; Mit, mitochondria; ER, endoplasmic reticulum; $ONOO^-$, peroxynitrite;, protein phosphorylation; ⊕, stimulation; ⋈ and X, inhibition or blockade.

of high nitric oxide and superoxide anion concentrations generate significant amounts of peroxynitrite, see e.g. [162,169]. In this oxidative scenario, the calcium-entry transport systems more relevant for the control of neuronal cytosolic calcium homeostasis associated with lipid rafts nanodomains, NMDA and AMPA receptors and L-VOCC, are strongly activated by peroxynitrite, see the section 5.1 of this chapter. This produces a large peak of calcium concentration within these nanodomains, large enough to elicit a large increase of cytosolic calcium and a strong stimulation of nNOS, leading to an intracellular burst of nitric oxide, and stimulation of the neuronal metabolic activity and associated intracellular superoxide anion generation, oxidative conditions that generate intracellular peroxynitrite. In turn, these intracellular oxidative conditions produce the release of calcium from endoplasmic reticulum and mitochondria (see the section 5.2 of this chapter), contributing to a further and more widespread rise of cytosolic calcium concentration, and partial inactivation of the extrusion systems of the neuronal plasma membrane, PMCA and NCX (see the section 5.3 of this chapter). These latter effects lead to impairment of the ability of neurons to restore the low cytosolic calcium concentration needed for their normal function, and as a result lead to a long-lasting rise of cytosolic calcium concentration which can eventually reach the level that elicits a rapid necrotic death. Thus, impairment of the calcium transport systems of nanodomains associated with lipid rafts results in generation of an intracellular ROS/RNS oxidative stress that amplifies the oxidative stress suffered by exposure of neurons to a combined ROS/RNS extracellular oxidative stress (Figure 2d). Indeed, many experimental studies have shown that pharmacological compounds that inhibit the calcium currents through NMDA and AMPA receptors and L-VOCC behave as protection agents against neuronal death in inflammatory brain insults.

Experimental evidences have pointed out that there is a large mesh/network of lipid rafts-associated nanodomains in the plasma membrane of the soma of primary cultures of cerebellar granule neurons, where they are particularly enriched in neuron/neuron contact areas [130], and microscopy images have also shown a distribution map that closely overlap with the distribution map of flavoproteins bound to the plasma membrane [130,261], consistent with the association of the flavoproteins nNOS and cytochrome b_5 reductase with these nanodomains. Because of the strong impairment of the activity of calcium transport systems present in these nanodomains by many ROS/RNS that can be generated in the neuronal cytoplasm under a variety of cellular stress conditions, it should be expected that even exposure of neurons to a relatively mild oxidative stress should elicit a partial failure of the control of calcium homeostasis within these neurons. Owing to the large intracellular space occupied by nuclei in these neurons, partial failure in the control of cytosolic calcium homeostasis should elicit significant fluctuations of the cytosolic calcium concentration even in the absence of neuronal stimulation. The occurrence of basal endogenous oscillations of the cytosolic calcium concentration have been reported in *in vitro* cultures of different types of neurons, see for example [186,262-264]. We have recorded synchronized fluctuations of the cytosolic calcium concentration in primary cultures of rat cerebellar granule neurons, of an average amplitude of ±0.15 units of the ratio 340/380 in cells loaded with fura-2, by simply increasing the intensity of UV-irradiation in the epifluorescence microscope [Marques-da-Silva D and Gutierrez-Merino C, *unpublished results*], conditions that promote an increase of H_2O_2 production by cellular flavoproteins. The implication of nanodomains associated with lipid rafts in the generation of these cytosolic calcium fluctuations is unravelled by their attenuation by specific inhibitors or blockers of the calcium transport systems associated with these nanodomains. In this particular case the calcium entry through L-VOCC plays a major role in the modulation of the amplitude of the UV-induced fluctuations of cytosolic calcium concentrations. However, it is to be noted that other calcium transport systems associated with lipid rafts can also play a major role under different experimental conditions, as it has been shown that NCX interactions with another proteins bound to lipid rafts can elicit cytosolic calcium oscillations in oocytes [265].

6.1. The role and relevance of cytosolic calcium buffering systems

The activation of a channel with a typical conductance of 2.6 pS, like that of some calcium channels, can generate a calcium diffusion sub-microcompartment where the calcium concentration is higher than 1 μM, but the effective dimensions of this volume element is largely dependent upon the calcium buffering capacity of the microenvironment, increasing from only several nanometers with a millimolar calcium buffering capacity up to 82 nm in presence of a calcium buffering capacity equal to that afforded by 0.1 mM fura-2 [258]. The higher the conductance of the calcium channel, the higher the effective dimension of this sub-microcompartment. Using the equations derived in [260], for channels with unitary calcium conductances in the range of 20 to 40 pS, i.e. that of L-VOCC and NMDA receptors (section 2.1 of this chapter), effective dimensions of a sub-microcompartment with calcium concentrations higher than 1 μM can extend to several hundreds of nanometers taking into account that only micromolar concentrations of calcium buffering systems are present in the neuronal cytosol (Figure 2a). Because of the high neurotoxicity of cytosolic calcium concentrations in the micromolar range, a decrease of the calcium buffering capacity of the cytosol shall increase the propensity for rapid degeneration of neurons.

On these grounds, it can be easily understood that the role of the cytosolic calcium buffering in neurons has attracted considerable interest, not only because of the abundance of calcium-binding proteins in the nervous system but also because of the specificity of their regional distribution in the brain. It is also relevant herein to note that an altered expression of the major calcium-binding proteins has been noticed in damaged brain regions of patients suffering from acute insults, such as stroke or epileptic seizures, and from chronic human neurodegenerative disorders which develop with an enhanced oxidative stress in the brain, such as Alzheimer's, Huntington's, Parkinson's and Pick's diseases [266]. Several of the major calcium-buffering proteins present in the brain have been reported to show altered expression levels in degenerating brain regions, namely, parvalbumin, calbindin-D28K and S100, all of them members of the EF-hand calcium binding proteins like the calcium-binding protein calmodulin ubiquitously expressed in all mammalian cells. Furthermore, it has been proposed that the lack of calcium buffering proteins parvalbumin and calbindin-D28K may be considered one of the factors that render human motor neurons particularly vulnerable to calcium toxicity following glutamate receptor activation in amyotrophic lateral sclerosis [267]. Consistently, it has been reported that parvalbumin overexpression delays disease onset in a transgenic model of familial amyotrophic lateral sclerosis [268], a devastating and oxidative stress-mediated neurodegenerative disease of the brain.

Because of the high relevance of calmodulin as a multifunctional modulator of cellular calcium homeostasis and also of cellular calcium signalling pathways [4-6], this is the calcium binding protein of the EF-hand family whose functional and structural alterations by ROS have been more extensively studied [269]. In this regard, calmodulin-dependent proteins particularly relevant for the control of calcium homeostasis in neurons are the calcium transport systems

PMCA and IP_3-receptors, see above. In addition, calmodulin modulates signalling pathways controlling neuronal activity and synaptic plasticity like the protein phosphatase calcineurin, CaMK and IQ motif-containing proteins, such as myosins, Ras exchange proteins and GAP-43 among others [141,270,271]. Noteworthy, the activity of calcineurin has been reported to be decreased in sporadic and familial amyotrophic lateral sclerosis [272]. Calmodulin has been shown to become more oxidized in aged animals [269], pointing out that the physiological oxidative stress developed in the tissues is enough to lead to a sustained chemical modification of this protein. *In vitro* calmodulin suffers chemical oxidative modifications upon exposure to either H_2O_2 or peroxynitrite, for a review on this topic see [269]. Two vicinal methionine residues close to the carboxyl-terminus of calmodulin, Met-144 and Met145, are oxidized to methionine sulfoxide in aged tissues and also by H_2O_2 and more efficiently by peroxynitrite. Calmodulin oxidation leads to inhibition of the target proteins by non-productive association and stabilization of their inactive state. This has been experimentally demonstrated for the PMCA [273-275]. The oxidation of these methionines is reversible *in vivo*, as methionine sulfoxide reductases can efficiently reduce them back to methionine, restoring normal calmodulin function [269]. The fact that in aged tissues this oxidation is not fully reverted indicates a functional loss of this recycling process during aging. Thus, oxidation of calmodulin leads to a transient inactivation of neuronal PMCA. On these grounds, the fact that high levels of expression of calcium binding proteins are observed in neurons expressing nNOS [276-279] can be seen as a protective mechanism to attenuate long-lasting calcium transients in these neurons, which could eventually elicit cell death through calpains activation.

The widespread expression of calmodulin in the brain, its high level of expression in neurons relative to other cell types and its pleiotropic cellular functions confer a high relevance to the oxidative modifications of this protein by ROS/RNS. Regarding specifically the calcium transport systems associated with lipid rafts nanodomains, a loss of functional calmodulin leads to a marked decrease of the CaMK activity and this, in turn, leads to a decrease of the activity of the calcium entry systems L-VOCC and AMPA and NMDA receptors. As a result, the calcium concentration within these sub-microcompartments will be lowered up to levels closer to those found in the overall cytosol. Although the PMCA will also be inhibited, this inhibition by itself cannot compensate a large decrease of the inward calcium currents for two major reasons: (i) in neurons PMCA is also stimulated by phosphatidylserine and in these cells calmodulin stimulation is weak relative to other cell types [280], and (ii) the higher potency for transport across the open calcium channels of L-VOCC and NMDA receptors with respect to that of PMCA. Therefore, these nanodomains can eventually enter in a latent state regarding calcium and nitric oxide signalling in neurons. A simple and rational hypothesis merges from this conclusion, namely, that this could be a molecular mechanism underlying the observed loss of neuronal threshold excitability in aging and brain neurodegeneration. Owing to its putative relevance for the search of new therapeutic drugs and treatments for slow-developing neurodegenerative processes, this hypothesis deserve to be experimentally assessed in future studies.

7. Concluding remarks

The organization of the major calcium transport systems controlling the cytosolic calcium homeostasis within nanodomains of the neuronal plasma membrane associated with lipid rafts is opening new perspectives for regulation and deregulation of calcium signalling in neurons. In addition to the relevance of this fact for the efficient neuronal function in brain associative structures, like the concerted activity in neuronal circuits and LTP, the co-localization of ROS/RNS enzyme sources within these nanodomains is of particular relevance for neurodegenerative insults and diseases. The basic reason for this conclusion is that the calcium transport systems playing a major role in cytosolic calcium homeostasis and calcium-mediated neuronal activity are highly sensitive to modulation by ROS/RNS, and that oxidative stress is a common feature observed during the development of brain damage elicited in the most frequent brain insults and neurodegenerative diseases of high prevalence in humans. Yet, the actual knowledge of the molecular structure and plasticity of these nanodomains is still very limited, both in terms of their molecular composition in different types of neurons and of the factors controlling its formation and structural organization. Moreover, the molecular mechanisms leading to deregulation of the ROS/RNS enzyme sources associated with these nanodomains remain to be established, as well as the structural changes induced in these nanodomains by exposure to the different ROS/RNS that are generated in neurodegenerative insults and diseases. Because of the central role of cytosolic calcium in the control of neuronal activity, plasticity and survival it can be foreseen that these nanodomains will become a relevant pharmacological target in the search for alternate and novel therapies aiming to prevent or slowdown neurodegenerative processes in the brain.

Abbreviations used in the text

AAPH, 2,2'- azobis (2-amidinopropane) dihydrochloride; AMPA, α-amino-3-hydroxy-5-methylisoxazole-4-propionic acid; CaMKII, calcium/calmodulin-dependent protein kinase, isoform II; Cb_5R, cytochrome b_5 reductase; cGMP, 3′,5′-cyclic guanosine monophosphate; CNS, central nervous system; COX, cyclooxygenase; EDTA, ethylenediamine-tetraacetic acid; FRET, fluorescence resonance energy transfer; LTP, long-term post-synaptic potentiation; NCX, sodium-calcium exchanger; NMDA, N-methyl-D-aspartate; nNOS, neuronal nitric oxide synthase; NOX, ROS-generating NADPH oxidases; PKA, protein kinase A; PKC, protein kinase C; PMCA, plasma membrane calcium pump; ROS, reactive oxygen species; RNS, reactive nitrogen species; SIN-1, 3-morpholinosydnonimine; SOCE, store-operated calcium entry; UV, ultraviolet; VOCC, voltage-operated caclium channels (L-VOCC, L-type VOCC; N-VOCC, N-type VOCC; etc).

Acknowledgements

This work has been supported by Grant BFU2011-30178 of the Spanish Plan Nacional de I+D +I and by Grant GR10092 of the Gobierno de Extremadura to the Research Group "Estrés oxidativo y bioenergética en neuronas y cerebro", both with co-financing by the European Funds for Structural Development (FEDER). DMS and SF have been supported by predoctoral fellowships of the Spanish Ministerio de Ciencia y Tecnología and of the Portuguese Fundação para a Ciência e a Tecnologia (FCT), respectively, and AKSA by a post-doctoral fellowship of the Gobierno de Extremadura with FEDER co-financing (reference number RE000008).

Author details

Carlos Gutierrez-Merino, Dorinda Marques-da-Silva, Sofia Fortalezas and Alejandro K. Samhan-Arias

*Address all correspondence to: carlosgm@unex.es

Dept. Biochemistry and Molecular Biology, School of Sciences, University of Extremadura, Badajoz, Spain

References

[1] Franklin JL, Johnson EMJr. Suppression of programmed neuronal death by sustained elevation of cytoplasmic calcium. Trends Neurosci 1992;15: 501-508.

[2] Franklin JL, Johnson EMJr. Block of neuronal apoptosis by a sustained increase of steady-state free Ca2+ concentration. Philos Trans R Soc Lond B Biol Sci 1994;345: 251-256.

[3] Mattson MP, Chan SL. Neuronal and glial calcium signaling in Alzheimer's disease. Cell Calcium 2003;34: 385-397.

[4] Berridge MJ. Neuronal calcium signaling. Neuron 1998;21: 13-26.

[5] Berridge MJ, Lipp P, Bootman MD. The versatility and universality of calcium signalling. Nat Rev Mol Cell Biol 2000; 1: 11-21.

[6] Carafoli E, Santella L, Branca D, Brini M. Generation, control, and processing of cellular calcium signals. Crit Rev Biochem Mol Biol 2001;36: 107-260.

[7] Carafoli E. Calcium signaling: a tale for all seasons. Proc Natl Acad Sci USA 2002;99: 1115-1122.

[8] Baimbridge KG, Celio MR, Rogers JH. Calcium-binding proteins in the nervous system. Trends Neurosci 1992;15: 303-308.

[9] Gutierrez-Martin Y, Martin-Romero FJ, Henao F, Gutierrez-Merino C. Alteration of cytosolic free calcium homeostasis by SIN-1: high sensitivity of L-type Ca2+ channels

to extracellular oxidative/nitrosative stress in cerebellar granule cells. J Neurochem 2005;92: 973-989.

[10] Martin-Romero FJ, Garcia-Martin E, Gutierrez-Merino C. Inhibition of the oxidative stress produced by plasma membrane NADH oxidase delays low-potassium induced apoptosis of cerebellar granule cells. J Neurochem 2002;82: 705–715.

[11] Harold FM. The Vital Force: A Study of Bioenergetics. New York: WH Freeman and Co; 1986.

[12] Tsien RW, Lipscombe D, Madison DV, Bley KR, Fox AP. Multiple types of neuronal calcium channels and their selective modulation. Trends Neurosci 1988;11: 431-438.

[13] Forti L, Tottene A, Moretti A, Pietrobon D. Three novel types of voltage-dependent calcium channels in rat cerebellar neurons. J Neurosci 1994;14: 5243-5256.

[14] Olivera BM, Miljanich GP, Ramachandran J, Adams ME. Calcium channel diversity and neurotransmitter release: the omega-conotoxins and omega-agatoxins. Annu Rev Biochem 1994;63: 823-867.

[15] Catterall WA. Structure and function of voltage-gated ion channels. Annu Rev Biochem 1995;64: 493-531.

[16] Hammond C., editor. Cellular and Molecular Neurobiology. San Diego: Academic Press; 1996.

[17] Tottene A, Moretti A, Pietrobon D. Functional diversity of P-type and R-type calcium channels in rat cerebellar neurons. J Neurosci 1996;16: 6353-6363.

[18] Schild D, Geiling H, Bischofberger J. Imaging of L-type Ca2+ channels in olfactory bulb neurones using fluorescent dihydropyridine and a styryl dye. J Neurosci Methods 1995;59: 183-190.

[19] Cohen R, Atlas D. R-type voltage-gated Ca(2+) channel interacts with synaptic proteins and recruits synaptotagmin to the plasma membrane of Xenopus oocytes. Neuroscience 2004;128: 831-841.

[20] Khanna R, Sun L, Li Q, Guo L, Stanley EF. Long splice variant N type calcium channels are clustered at presynaptic transmitter release sites without modular adaptor proteins. Neuroscience 2006;138: 1115-1125.

[21] Tai C, Kuzmiski JB, MacVicar BA. Muscarinic enhancement of R-type calcium currents in hippocampal CA1 pyramidal neurons. J Neurosci 2006;26: 6249-6258.

[22] Marchetti C, Usai C. High affinity block by nimodipine of the internal calcium elevation in chronically depolarized rat cerebellar granule neurons. Neurosci Lett 1996;207: 77-80.

[23] Maric D, Maric I, Barker JL. Developmental changes in cell calcium homeostasis during neurogenesis of the embryonic rat cerebral cortex. Cereb Cortex 2000;10: 561-573.

[24] Arakawa Y, Nishijima C, Shimizu N, Urushidani T. Survival-promoting activity of nimodipine and nifedipine in rat motoneurons: implications of an intrinsic calcium toxicity in motoneurons. J Neurochem 2002;83: 150-156.

[25] Ertel EA, Campbell KP, Harpold MM, Hofmann F, Mori Y, Perez-Reyes E, Schwartz A, Snutch TP, Tanabe T, Birnbaumer L, Tsien RW, Catterall WA. Nomenclature of voltage-gated calcium channels. Neuron 2000;25: 533–535.

[26] Catterall WA. Structure and regulation of voltage-gated Ca2+ Channels. Annu Rev Cell Dev Biol 2000;16: 521–555.

[27] Clark NC, Nagano N, Kuenzi FM, Jarolimek W, Huber I, Walter D, Wietzorrek G, Boyce S, Kullmann DM, Striessnig J, Seabrook GR. Neurological phenotypeand synaptic function in mice lacking the CaV1.3 alpha subunit of neuronal L-type voltage-dependent Ca2+ channels. Neuroscience 2003;120: 435 – 442.

[28] Moosmang S, Haider N, Klugbauer N, Adelsberger H, Langwieser N, Müller J, Stiess M, Marais E, Schulla V, Lacinova L, Goebbels S, Nave KA, Storm DR, Hofmann F, Kleppisch T. Role of hippocampal Cav1.2 Ca2+ channels in NMDA receptor-independent synaptic plasticity and spatial memory. J Neurosci 2005;25: 9883 – 9892.

[29] Kamp TJ, Hell JW. Regulation of Cardiac L-Type Calcium Channels by Protein Kinase A and Protein Kinase C. Circ Res 2000;87: 1095-1102.

[30] Davare MA, Dong F, Rubin CS, Hell JW. The A-kinase anchor protein MAP2B and cAMP-dependent protein kinase are associated with class C L-type calcium channels in neurons. J Biol Chem 1999;274: 30280–30287.

[31] De Jongh KS, Murphy BJ, Colvin AA, Hell JW, Takahashi M, Catterall WA. Specific phosphorylation of a site in the full-length form of the alpha 1 subunit of the cardiac L-type calcium channel by adenosine 3',5'-cyclic monophosphate-dependent protein kinase. Biochemistry 1996;35: 10392–10340.

[32] Mitterdorfer J, Froschmayr M, Grabner M, Moebius FF, Glossmann H, Striessnig J. Identification of PK-A phosphorylation sites in the carboxyl terminus of L-type calcium channel alpha 1 subunits. Biochemistry 1996;35: 9400–9406.

[33] Gao T, Yatani A, Dell'Acqua ML, Sako H, Green SA, Dascal N, Scott JD, Hosey MM. cAMP-dependent regulation of cardiac L-type Ca2+ channels requires membrane targeting of PKA and phosphorylation of channel subunits. Neuron 1997;19: 185–196.

[34] Puri TS, Gerhardstein BL, Zhao XL, Ladner MB, Hosey MM. Differential effects of subunit interactions on protein kinase A- and C-mediated phosphorylation of L-type calcium channels. Biochemistry 1997;36: 9605–9615.

[35] Bünemann M, Gerhardstein BL, Gao T, Hosey MM. Functional Regulation of L-type Calcium Channels via Protein Kinase A-mediated Phosphorylation of the β2 Subunit. J Biol Chem 1999;274: 33851–33854.

[36] Grueter CE, Abiria SA, Dzhura I, Wu Y, Ham AJL, Mohler PJ, Anderson ME, Colbran RJ. L-Type Ca2+ Channel Facilitation Mediated by Phosphorylation of the β Subunit by CaMKII. Mol Cell 2006;23: 641–650.

[37] Pinard CR, Mascagni F, McDonald AJ. Neuronal localization of Cav1.2 L-type calcium channels in the rat basolateral amygdala. Brain Res 2005;1064: 52 – 55.

[38] Hudmon A, Schulman H, Kim J, Maltez JM, Tsien RW, Pitt GS. CaMKII tethers to L-type Ca2+ channels, establishing a local and dedicated integrator of Ca2+ signals for facilitation. J Cell Biol 2005;171: 537–547.

[39] Lee TS, Karl R, Moosmang S, Lenhardt P, Klugbauer N, Hofmann F, Kleppisch T, Welling A. Calmodulin kinase II is involved in voltage-dependent facilitation of the L-type Cav1.2 calcium channel: Identification of the phosphorylation sites. J Biol Chem 2006;281: 25560–25567.

[40] Grueter CE, Abiria SA, Wu Y, Anderson ME, Colbran RJ. Differential regulated interactions of calcium/calmodulin-dependent protein kinase II with isoforms of voltage-gated calcium channel beta subunits. Biochemistry 2008;47: 1760-1767.

[41] O-Uchi J, Komukai K, Kusakari Y, Obata T, Hongo K, Sasaki H, Kurihara S. Alpha1-adrenoceptor stimulation potentiates L-type Ca2+ current through Ca2+/calmodulin-dependent PK II (CaMKII) activation in rat ventricular myocytes. Proc Natl Acad Sci USA 2005;102: 9400–9405.

[42] Gao L, Blair LA, Salinas GD, Needleman LA, Marshall J. Insulin-like growth factor-1 modulation of CaV1.3 calcium channels depends on Ca2+ release from IP3-sensitive stores and calcium/calmodulin kinase II phosphorylation of the alpha1 subunit EF hand. J Neurosci 2006;26: 6259–6268.

[43] Brown AM, Deutch AY, Colbran RJ. Dopamine depletion alters phosphorylation of striatal proteins in a model of Parkinsonism. Eur J Neurosci 2005;22: 247–256.

[44] Choi DW, Rothman SM. The role of glutamate neurotoxicity in hypoxic-ischemic neuronal death. Annu Rev Neurosci 1990;13: 171-182.

[45] Choi DW. Glutamate neurotoxicity and diseases of the nervous system. Neuron 1998;1: 623–634.

[46] Robertson SJ, Ennion SJ, Evans RJ, Edwards FA. Synaptic P2X receptors. Curr Opin Neurobiol 2001;11: 378-386.

[47] Huettner JE. Kainate receptors and synaptic transmission. Prog Neurobiol 2003;70: 387-407.

[48] Dingledine R., McBain C.J. Glutamate and aspartate. In: Siegel G.J., Agranoff B.W., Albers R.W., Fisher S.K., Uhler M.D. (eds.). Basic Neurochemistry. Molecular, Cellular and Medical Aspects (6th ed.). Philadelphia: Lippincott Williams & Wilkins; 1998. p. 315-333.

[49] Contestabile A. Roles of NMDA receptor activity and nitric oxide production in brain development. Brain Res Brain Res Rev 2000;32: 476-509.

[50] Smith TC, Wang L-Y, Howe JR. Heterogeneous conductance levels of native AMPA receptors. J Neurosci 2000;20: 2073-2085.

[51] Mothet JP, Parent AT, Wolosker H, Brady ROJr, Linden DJ, Ferris CD, Rogawski MA, Snyder SH. D-serine is an endogenous ligand for the glycine site of the N-methyl-D-aspartate receptor. Proc Natl Acad Sci USA 2000;97: 4926-4931.

[52] Derkach V, Barria A, Soderling TR. Ca2+/calmodulin-kinase II enhances channel conductance of alpha-amino-3-hydroxy-5-methyl-4-isoxazolepropionate type glutamate receptors. Proc Natl Acad Sci USA 1999;96: 3269–3274.

[53] Hayashi Y, Shi SH, Esteban JA, Piccini A, Poncer JC, Malinow R. Driving AMPA receptors into synapses by LTP and CaMKII: requirement for GluR1 and PDZ domain interaction.Science 2000;287: 2262–2267.

[54] Boehm J, Kang MG, Johnson RC, Esteban J, Huganir RL, Malinow R. Synaptic incorporation of AMPA receptors during LTP is controlled by a PKC phosphorylation site on GluR1. Neuron 2006;51: 213–225.

[55] Kohr G, Eckardt S, Luddens H, Monyer H, Seeburg PH. NMDA receptor channels: subunit-specific potentiation by reducing agents. Neuron 1994;12: 1031-1040.

[56] Rumbaugh G, Vicini S. Distinct synaptic and extrasynaptic NMDA receptors in developing cerebellar granule neurons. J Neurosci 1999;19: 10603-10610.

[57] Petralia RS, Wang YX, Hua F, Yi Z, Zhou A, Ge L, Stephenson FA, Wenthold RJ. Organization of NMDA receptors at extrasynaptic locations. Neuroscience 2010;167:68-87.

[58] Li ST, Ju JG. Functional roles of synaptic and extrasynaptic NMDA receptors in physiological and pathological neuronal activities. Curr Drug Targets 2012;13: 207-221.

[59] Leonard AS, Hell JW. Cyclic AMP-dependent Protein Kinase and Protein Kinase C Phosphorylate N-Methyl-D-aspartate Receptors at Different Sites. J Biol Chem 1997;272: 12107–12115.

[60] Tingley WG, Ehlers MD, Kameyama K, Doherty C, Ptak JB, Riley CT, Huganir RL. Characterization of Protein Kinase A and Protein Kinase C Phosphorylation of the N-Methyl-D-aspartate Receptor NR1 Subunit Using Phosphorylation Site-specific Antibodies. J Biol Chem 1997;272: 5157–5166.

[61] Fill M, Copello JA. Ryanodine receptor calcium release channels. Physiol Rev 2002;82: 893-922.

[62] Hamilton SL. Ryanodine receptors. Cell Calcium 2005;38: 253-260.

[63] Mikoshiba K. Inositol 1,4,5-trisphosphate IP(3) receptors and their role in neuronal cell function. J Neurochem 2006;97: 1627-1633.

[64] Hidalgo C. Cross talk between Ca2+ and redox signalling cascades in muscle and neurons through the combined activation of ryanodine receptors/Ca2+ release channels. Philos Trans R Soc Lond B Biol Sci 2005;360: 2237-2246.

[65] Paschen W, Frandsen A. Endoplasmic reticulum dysfunction-a common denominator for cell injury in acute and degenerative diseases of the brain? J Neurochem 2001;79: 719-725.

[66] Montero M, Alvarez J, Garcia-Sancho J. Agonist-induced Ca2+ influx in human neutrophils is secondary to the emptying of intracellular calcium stores. Biochem J 1991;277: 73-79.

[67] Parekh AB, Putney JWJr. Store-operated calcium channels. Physiol Rev 2005;85: 757-810.

[68] Arakawa N, Sakaue M, Yokoyama I, Hashimoto H, Koyama Y, Baba A, Matsuda T. KB-R7943 inhibits store-operated Ca(2+) entry in cultured neurons and astrocytes. Biochem Biophys Res Commun 2000;279: 354-357.

[69] Jia Y, Zhou J, Tai Y, Wang Y. TRPC channels promote cerebellar granule neuron survival. Nat Neurosci 2007 ;10 : 559-567.

[70] Selvaraj S, Sun Y, Watt JA, Wang S, Lei S, Birnbaumer L, Singh BB. Neurotoxin-induced ER stress in mouse dopaminergic neurons involves downregulation of TRPC1 and inhibition of AKT/mTOR signaling. J Clin Invest 2012;122: 1354-1367.

[71] Smaili SS, Hsu YT, Youle RJ, Russell JT. Mitochondria in Ca2+ signaling and apoptosis. J Bioenerg Biomembr 2000;32: 35-46.

[72] Simpson PB. The local control of cytosolic Ca2+ as a propagator of CNS communication-integration of mitochondrial transport mechanisms and cellular responses. J Bioenerg Biomembr 2000;32: 5-13.

[73] Crompton M. The mitochondrial permeability transition pore and its role in cell death. Biochem J. 1999;341: 233-249.

[74] Garcia-Martin E, Gutierrez-Merino C. Rate of Na+/Ca2+ exchange across the plasma membrane of synaptosomes measured using the fluorescence of chlorotetracycline. Implications to calcium homeostasis in synaptic terminals. Biochim Biophys Acta 1996;1280: 257-264.

[75] Garcia ML, Strehler EE. Plasma membrane calcium ATPases as critical regulators of calcium homeostasis during neuronal cell function. Front Biosci 1999;4: D869–D882.

[76] Gill DL, Chueh SH, Whitlow LC. Functional importance of the synaptic plasma membrane calcium pump and sodium-calcium exchanger. J Biol Chem 1984;259: 10807-10813.

[77] Guerini D, García-Martín E, Gerber A, Volbracht C, Leist M, Gutierrez-Merino C, Carafoli E. The expression of plasma membrane Ca2+ pump isoforms in cerebellar granule neurons is modulated by cytosolic free Ca2+. J Biol Chem 1999;274: 1667-1676.

[78] Kip SN, Gray NW, Burette A, Canbay A, Weinberg RJ, Strehler EE. Changes in the expression of plasma membrane calcium extrusion systems during the maturation of hippocampal neurons. Hippocampus 2006;16: 20-34.

[79] Hilfiker H, Guerini D, Carafoli E. Cloning and expression of isoform 2 of the human plasma membrane Ca2+ ATPase. Functional properties of the enzyme and its splicing products. J Biol Chem 1994;269: 26178-26183.

[80] Condrescu M, Reeves JP. Actin-dependent regulation of the cardiac Na+/Ca2+ exchanger. Am J Physiol Cell Physiol 2006;290: C691-C701.

[81] O′ Connell KMM, Martens JR, Tamkun MM. Localization of ion channels to lipid raft domains within the cardiovascular system. Trends Cardiovasc Med 2004;14: 37–42.

[82] Gunter TE, Yule DI, Gunter KK, Eliseev RA, Salter JD. Calcium and mitochondria. FEBS Lett 2004;567: 96-102.

[83] Pike LJ. Rafts defined: a report on the keystone symposium on lipid rafts and cell function. J Lipid Res 2006;47: 1597–1598.

[84] Head BP, Insel PA. Do caveolins regulate cells by actions outside of caveolae? Trends Cell Biol 2007;17: 51–57.

[85] Gabella G. Caveolae intracellulares and sarcoplasmic reticulum in smooth muscle. J Cell Sci 1971;8: 601–609.

[86] Popescu LM, Diculescu I, Zelck U, Ionescu N. Ultrastructural distribution of calcium in smooth muscle cells of guinea-pig taenia coli. A correlated electron microscopic and quantitative study. Cell Tissue Res 1974;154: 357–378.

[87] Brazer SC, Singh BB, Liu X, Swaim W, Ambudkar IS. Caveolin-1 contributes to assembly of store-operated Ca2+ influx channels by regulating plasma membrane localization of TRPC1. J Biol Chem 2003;278: 27208–27215.

[88] Murata T, Lin MI, Stan RV, Bauer PM, Yu J, Sessa WC. Genetic evidence supporting caveolae microdomain regulation of calcium entry in endothelial cells. J Biol Chem 2007;282: 16631–16643.

[89] Anderson RG. The caveolae membrane system. Annu Rev Biochem 1998;67: 199–225.

[90] Fra AM, Masserini M, Palestini P, Sonnino S, Simons K. A photo-reactive derivative of ganglioside GM1 specifically cross-links VIP21-caveolin on the cell surface. FEBS Lett 1995;375: 11-14.

[91] Murata M, Peranen J, Schreiner R, Weiland F, Kurzchalia T, Simons K. VIP21/caveolin is a cholesterol-binding protein. Proc Natl Acad Sci USA 1995;92: 10339–10343.

[92] Thiele C, Hannah MJ, Fahrenholz F, Huttner WB. Cholesterol binds to synaptophysin and is required for biogenesis of synaptic vesicles. Nat Cell Biol 2000;2: 42-49.

[93] Smart EJ, Ying Y-S, Donzell WC, Anderson RGW. A Role for Caveolin in Transport of Cholesterol from Endoplasmic Reticulum to Plasma Membrane. J Biol Chem 1996;271: 29427–29435.

[94] Toselli M, Biella G, Taglietti V, Cazzaniga E, Parenti M. Caveolin-1 expression and membrane cholesterol content modulate N-type calcium channel activity in NG108-15 cells. Biophys J 2005;89: 2443–2457.

[95] Head BP, Patel HH, Tsutsumi YM, Hu Y, Mejia T, Mora RC, Insel PA, Roth DM, Drummond JC, Patel PM. Caveolin-1 expression is essential for N-methyl-D-aspartate receptor-mediated Src and extracellular signal-regulated kinase 1/2 activation and protection of primary neurons from ischemic cell death. FASEB J 2008;22: 828–840.

[96] Razani B, Woodman SE, Lisanti MP. Caveolae: From Cell Biology to Animal Physiology. Pharmacol Rev 2002;54: 431–467.

[97] van Deurs B, Roepstorff K, Hommelgaard AM, Sandvig K. Caveolae: anchored, multifunctional platforms in the lipid ocean. Trends Cell Biol 2003;13: 92-100.

[98] Pouvreau S, Berthier C, Blaineau S, Amsellem J, Coronado R, Strube C. Membrane cholesterol modulates dihydropyridine receptor function in mice fetal skeletal muscle cells. J Physiol 2004;555: 365-381.

[99] Tsujikawa H, Song Y, Watanabe M, Masumiya H, Gupte SA, Ochi R, Okada T. Cholesterol depletion modulates basal L-type Ca2+ current and abolishes its β-adrenergic enhancement in ventricular myocytes. Am J Physiol Heart Circ Physiol 2008;294: H285–H292.

[100] Waseem TV, Kolos VA, Lapatsina LP, Fedorovich SV. Influence of cholesterol depletion in plasma membrane of rat brain synaptosomes on calcium-dependent and calcium-independent exocytosis. Neurosci Lett 2006;405: 106–110.

[101] Fielding CJ, Fielding PE. Intracellular cholesterol transport. J Lipid Res 1997;38: 1503–1521.

[102] Bu J, Bruckner SR, Sengoku T, Geddes JW, Estus S. Glutamate regulates caveolin expression in rat hippocampal neurons. J Neurosci Res 2003;72: 185-190.

[103] Gaudreault SB, Dea D, Poirier J. Increased caveolin-1 expression in Alzheimer's disease brain. Neurobiol Aging 2004;25: 753-759.

[104] Drab M, Verkade P, Elger M, Kasper M, Lohn M, Lauterbach B, Menne J, Lindschau C, Mende F, Luft FC, Schedl A, Haller H, Kurzxhalia TV. Loss of caveolae, vascular

dysfunction, and pulmonary defects in caveolin-1 gene disrupted mice. Science 2001;293: 2449-2452.

[105] Simons K, Ehehalt R. Cholesterol lipid rafts, and disease. J Clin Invest 2002;110: 597-603.

[106] Cohen AW, Hnasko R, Schubert W, Lisanti P. Role of caveolae and caveolins in health and disease. Physiol Rev 2004;84: 1341-1379.

[107] Balijepalli RC, Foell JD, Hall DD, Hell JW, Kamp TJ. Localization of cardiac L-type Ca2+ channels to a caveolar macromolecular signaling complex is required for b2-adrenergic regulation. Proc Natl Acad Sci USA 2006;103: 7500–7505.

[108] Marques-da-Silva D, Samhan-Arias AK, Tiago T, Gutierrez-Merino C. L-type calcium channels and cytochrome b5 reductase are components of protein complexes tightly associated with lipid rafts microdomains of the neuronal plasma membrane. J Proteomics 2010;73: 1502-1510.

[109] Razani B, Rubin CS, Lisanti MP. Regulation of cAMP-mediated Signal Transduction via Interaction of Caveolins with the Catalytic Subunit of Protein Kinase A. J Biol Chem 1999;274: 26353–26360.

[110] Suzuki T, Du F, Tian Q-B, Zhang J, Endo S. Ca2+/calmodulin-dependent protein kinase IIα clusters are associated with stable lipid rafts and their formation traps PSD-95. J Neurochem 2008;104: 596–610.

[111] Weick JP, Groth RD, Isaksen AL, Mermelstein PG. Interactions with PDZ proteins are required for L-type calcium channels to activate cAMP response element-binding protein-dependent gene expression. J Neurosci 2003;23: 3446–3456.

[112] Zhang H, Maximov A, Fu Y, Xu F, Tang TS, Tkatch T, Surmeier DJ, Bezprozvanny I. Association of CaV1.3 L-type calcium channels with Shank. J Neurosci 2005;25: 1037-1049.

[113] Prybylowski K, Chang K, Sans N, Kan L, Vicini S, Wenthold RJ. The synaptic localization of NR2B-containing NMDA receptors is controlled by interactions with PDZ proteins and AP-2. Neuron 2005;47: 845-857.

[114] Hering H, Lin C-C, Sheng M. Lipid Rafts in the Maintenance of Synapses, Dendritic Spines, and Surface AMPA Receptor Stability. J Neurosci 2003;23: 3262–3271.

[115] Besshoh S, Chen S, Brown IR, Gurd JW. Developmental Changes in the Association of NMDA Receptors With Lipid Rafts. J Neurosci Res 2007;85:1876–1883.

[116] Delínte-Ramirez I, Salcedo-Tello P, Bermudez-Rattoni F. Spatial memory formation induces recruitment of NMDA receptor and PSD-95 to synaptic lípid rafts. J Neurochem 2008;106: 1658–1668.

[117] Marques-da-Silva D, Gutierrez-Merino C. L-type voltage-operated calcium channels, N-methyl-D-aspartate receptors and neuronal nitric-oxide synthase form a calcium/

redox nano-transducer within lipid rafts. Biochem Biophys Res Commun 2012;420: 257-262.

[118] Delinte-Ramirez I, Fernández E, Bayés A, Kicsi E, Komiyama NH, Grant SGN. In Vivo Composition of NMDA Receptor Signaling Complexes Differs between Membrane Subdomains and Is Modulated by PSD-95 and PSD-93. J Neurosci 2010;30: 8162– 8170.

[119] Hou Q, Huang Y, Amato S, Snyder SH, Huganir RL, Man HY. Regulation of AMPA receptor localization in lipid rafts. Mol Cell Neurosci 2008;38: 213-223.

[120] Keith DJ, Sanderson JL, Gibson ES, Woolfrey KM, Robertson HR, Olszewski K, Kang R, El-Husseini A, Dell'acqua ML. Palmitoylation of A-kinase anchoring protein 79/150 regulates dendritic endosomal targeting and synaptic plasticity mechanisms. J Neurosci 2012;32: 7119-7136.

[121] Sepúlveda MR, Berrocal-Carrillo M, Gasset M, Mata AM. The plasma membrane Ca2+-ATPase isoform 4 is localized in lipid rafts of cerebellum synaptic plasma membranes. J Biol Chem 2006;281: 447-453.

[122] Jiang L, Fernandes D, Mehta N, Bean JL, Michaelis ML, Zaidi A. Partitioning of the plasma membrane Ca2+-ATPase into lipid rafts in primary neurons: effects of cholesterol depletion. J Neurochem 2007;102: 378–388.

[123] Vorherr T, Kessler T, Hofmann F, Carafoli E. The calmodulin-binding domain mediates the self-association of the plasma membrane Ca2+ pump. J Biol Chem 1991;266: 22–27.

[124] Kuszczak I, Samson SE, Pande J, Shen DQ, Grover AK. Sodium–calcium exchanger and lipid rafts in pig coronary artery smooth muscle. Biochim Biophys Acta 2011;1808: 589–596.

[125] Teubl M, Groschner K, Kohlwein SD, Mayer B, Schmidt K. Na+/Ca2+ exchange facilitates Ca2+-dependent activation of endothelial nitric-oxide synthase. J Biol Chem 1999;274: 29529-29535.

[126] Bossuyt J, Taylor BE, James-Kracke M, Hale CC. Evidence for cardiac sodium-calcium exchanger association with caveolin-3. FEBS Lett 2002;511: 113-117.

[127] Sato Y, Sagami I, Shimizu T. Identification of Caveolin-1-interacting Sites in Neuronal Nitric-oxide Synthase. J Biol Chem 2004;279: 8827–8836.

[128] Venema VJ, Ju H, Zou R, Venema RC. Interaction of neuronal nitric-oxide synthase with caveolin-3 in skeletal muscle. Identification of a novel caveolin scaffolding/ inhibitory domain. J Biol Chem 1997;272: 28187–28190.

[129] Samhan-Arias AK, Martin-Romero FJ, Gutierrez-Merino C. Kaempferol blocks oxidative stress in cerebellar granule cells and reveals a key role for the plasma membrane

NADH oxidase activity in the commitment of apoptosis. Free Radic Biol Med 2004;37: 48-61.

[130] Samhan-Arias AK, Garcia-Bereguiain MA, Martin-Romero FJ, Gutierrez-Merino C. Clustering of plasma membrane-bound cytochrome b5 reductase within 'lipid rafts' microdomains of the neuronal plasma membrane. Mol Cell Neurosci 2009;40: 14–26.

[131] Samhan-Arias AK, Marques-da-Silva D, Yanamala N, Gutierrez-Merino C. Stimulation and clustering of cytochrome b(5) reductase in caveolin-rich lipid microdomains is an early event in oxidative stress-mediated apoptosis of cerebellar granule neurons. J Proteomics 2012;75: 2934-2949.

[132] Tiago T, Aureliano M, Gutierrez-Merino C. Effects of reactive oxygen and nitrogen species on actomyosin and their implications for muscle contractility. In: Gutierrez-Merino C., Leeuwenburgh C. (eds.) Free Radicals in Biology and Medicine. Kerala: Research Signpost; 2008. p. 131-149.

[133] Brenman JE, Bredt DS. Synaptic signalling by nitric-oxide. Curr Opin Neurobiol 1997;7: 374–378.

[134] Bonfoco E, Leist M, Zhivotovsky B, Orrenius S, Lipton SA, Nicotera P. Cytoskeletal breakdown and apoptosis elicited by NO donors in cerebellar granule cells require NMDA receptor activation. J Neurochem 1996;67: 2484–2493.

[135] Leach RN, Desai JC, Orchard CH. Effect of cytoskeleton disruptors on L-type Ca channel distribution in rat ventricular myocytes. Cell Calcium 2005;38: 515-526.

[136] Gutierrez-Merino C. Redox modulation of neuronal calcium homeostasis and its deregulation by reactive oxygen species. In: Gutierrez-Merino C., Leeuwenburgh C. (eds.) Free Radicals in Biology and Medicine. Kerala: Research Signpost; 2008. p. 67-101.

[137] Hidalgo C, Donoso P. Crosstalk between calcium and redox signalling: from molecular mechanisms to health implications. Antioxid Redox Signal 2008;10: 1275-1312.

[138] Garcia-Bereguiain MA, Samhan-Arias AK, Martin-Romero FJ, Gutierrez-Merino C. Hydrogen sulfide raises cytosolic calcium in neurons through activation of L-type Ca2+ channels. Antioxid Redox Signal 2008;10: 31-42.

[139] Orrenius S, McConkey DJ, Bellomo G, Nicotera P. Role of Ca2+ in toxic cell killing. Trends Pharmacol Sci 1989;10: 281-285.

[140] Triffaró JM, Vitale ML. Cytoskeleton dynamics during neurotransmitter release. Trends Neurosci 1993;16: 466-472.

[141] Benowitz LI, Routtenberg A. GAP-43: an intrinsic determinant of neuronal development and plasticity. Trends Neurosci 1997;20: 84-91.

[142] Bizat N, Hermel J-M, Boyer F, Jacquard C, Créminon C, Ouary S, Escartin C, Hantraye P, Krajewski S, Brouillet E. Calpain Is a Major Cell Death Effector in Selective

Striatal Degeneration Induced In Vivo by 3-Nitropropionate: Implications for Huntington's Disease. J Neurosci 2003;23: 5020-5030.

[143] Volbracht C, Chua BT, Ng CP, Bahr BA, Hong W, Li P. The critical role of calpain versus caspase activation in excitotoxic injury induced by nitric oxide. J Neurochem 2005;93: 1280-1292.

[144] Lagoa R, Lopez-Sanchez C, Samhan-Arias AK, Gañan CM, Garcia-Martinez V, Gutierrez-Merino C. Kaempferol protects against rat striatal degeneration induced by 3-nitropropionic acid. J Neurochem 2009;111: 473-487.

[145] Valencia A, Morán J. Role of oxidative stress in the apoptotic cell death of cultured cerebellar granule cells. J Neurosci Res 2001;64: 284–297.

[146] van Damme P, Dewil M, Robberecht W, van den Bosch L. Excitotoxicity and amyotrophic lateral sclerosis. Neurodegener Dis 2005;2: 147-159.

[147] Thibault O, Gant JC, Landfield PW. Expansion of the calcium hypothesis of brain aging and Alzheimer's disease: minding the store. Aging Cell 2007;6: 307-317.

[148] Marx J. Alzheimer's disease. Fresh evidence points to an old suspect: calcium. Science 2007;318: 384-385.

[149] Mattson MP. Calcium and neurodegeneration. Aging Cell2007; 6: 337-350.

[150] Surmeier DJ. Calcium, ageing, and neuronal vulnerability in Parkinson's disease. Lancet Neurol 2007;6: 933-938.

[151] Ionov ID. Survey of ALS-associated factors potentially promoting Ca2+ overload of motor neurons. Amyotroph Lateral Scler 2007;8: 260-265.

[152] Craft JM, Watterson DM, Marks A, Van Eldik LJ. Enhanced susceptibility of S-100B transgenic mice to neuroinflammation and neuronal dysfunction induced by intracerebroventricular infusion of human beta-amyloid. Glia 2005;51: 209-216.

[153] Vesce S, Rossi D, Brambilla L, Volterra A. Glutamate release from astrocytes in physiological conditions and in neurodegenerative disorders characterized by neuroinflammation. Int Rev Neurobiol 2007;82: 57-71.

[154] Farber JL. The role of calcium ions in toxic cell injury. Environ Health Perspect 1990;84: 107-111.

[155] Mao GD, Poznansky MJ. Electron spin resonance study on the permeability of superoxide radicals in lipid bilayers and biological membranes. FEBS Lett 1992;305: 233-236.

[156] Bedard K, Krause KH. The NOX family of ROS-generating NADPH oxidases: physiology and pathophysiology. Physiol Rev 2007;87: 245-313.

[157] Martin-Romero FJ, Gutierrez-Martin Y, Henao F, Gutierrez-Merino C. The NADH oxidase activity of the plasma membrane of synaptosomes is a major source of superoxide anion and is inhibited by peroxynitrite. J Neurochem 2002;82: 604–614.

[158] Samhan-Arias AK, Duarte RO, Martin-Romero FJ, Moura JJG, Gutierrez-Merino C. Reduction of ascorbate free radical by the plasma membrane of synaptic terminals from rat brain. Arch Biochem Biophys 2008;469: 243–254.

[159] Herrero A, Barja G. Localization of the site of oxygen radical generation inside the complex I of heart and nonsynaptic brain mammalian mitochondria. J Bioenerg Biomembr 2000;32: 609-615.

[160] Zimmerman BJ, Granger DN. Mechanisms of reperfusion injury. Am J Med Sci 1994;307: 284-292.

[161] Iadecola C. Bright and dark sides of nitric oxide in ischemic brain injury. Trends Neurosci 1997;20: 132-139.

[162] Szabo C, Ischiropoulos H, Radi R. Peroxynitrite: biochemistry, pathophysiology and development of therapeutics. Nat Rev Drug Discov 2007;6: 662-680.

[163] Huie RE, Padmaja S. The reaction of NO with superoxide. Free Radic Res Commun 1993;18: 195-199.

[164] van der Veen RC, Hinton DR, Incardonna F, Hofman FM. Extensive peroxynitrite activity during progressive stages of central nervous system inflammation. J Neuroimmunol 1997;77: 1-7.

[165] Liu D, Ling X, Wen J, Liu J. The role of reactive nitrogen species in secondary spinal cord injury: formation of nitric oxide, peroxynitrite, and nitrated protein. J Neurochem 2000;75: 2144-2154.

[166] Beal MF. Energetics in the pathogenesis of neurodegenerative diseases. Trends Neurosci. 2000;23: 298–304.

[167] Beal MF. Oxidatively modified proteins in aging and disease. Free Radic Biol Med 2002;32: 797-803.

[168] Murphy MP, Packer MA, Scarlett JL, Martin SW. Peroxynitrite: a biologically significant oxidant. General Pharmacology 1998;31: 179–186.

[169] Bolaños JP, Almeida A, Stewart V, Peuchen S, Land JM, Clark JB, Heales SJ. Nitric oxide-mediated mitochondrial damage in the brain: mechanisms and implications for neurodegenerative diseases. J Neurochem 1997;68: 2227-2240.

[170] Olanow CW. A radical hypothesis for neurodegeneration. Trends Neurosci 1993;16: 439-444.

[171] Espinosa-Garcia J, Gutierrez-Merino C. The Trapping of the OH Radical by Coenzyme Q. A Theoretical and Experimental Study. J Phys Chem A 2003;107: 9712-9723.

[172] Spencer JP, Jenner A, Aruoma OI, Cross CE, Wu R, Halliwell B. Oxidative DNA damage in human respiratory tract epithelial cells. Time course in relation to DNA strand breakage. Biochem Biophys Res Commun 1996;224: 17-22.

[173] Bao F, Liu D. Hydroxyl radicals generated in the rat spinal cord at the level produced by impact injury induce cell death by necrosis and apoptosis: protection by a metalloporphyrin. Neuroscience 2004:126: 285-295.

[174] Andrus PK, Fleck TJ, Gurney ME, Hall ED. Protein oxidative damage in a transgenic mouse model of familial amyotrophic lateral sclerosis. J Neurochem 1998;71: 2041-2048.

[175] Li SW, Lin TS, Minteer S, Burke WJ. 3,4-Dihydroxyphenylacetaldehyde and hydrogen peroxide generate a hydroxyl radical: possible role in Parkinson's disease pathogenesis. Brain Res Mol Brain Res 2001;93: 1-7.

[176] Sugimoto K, Iadecola C. Delayed effect of administration of COX-2 inhibitor in mice with acute cerebral ischemia. Brain Res 2003;960: 273-276.

[177] Teismann P, Tieu K, Choi DK, Wu DC, Naini A, Hunot S, Vila M, Jackson-Lewis V, Przedborski S. Cyclooxygenase-2 is instrumental in Parkinson's disease neurodegeneration. Proc Natl Acad Sci U S A 2003;100: 5473-5478.

[178] Mattson MP. Modification of ion homeostasis by lipid peroxidation: roles in neuronal degeneration and adaptive plasticity. Trends Neurosci 1998;21: 53-57.

[179] Sharma SS, Kaundal RK. Neuroprotective effects of 6-hydroxy-2,5,7,8-tetramethylchroman-2-carboxylic acid (Trolox), an antioxidant in middle cerebral artery occlusion induced focal cerebral ischemia in rats. Neurol Res 2007;29: 304-309.

[180] Bazan NG. Synaptic signaling by lipids in the life and death of neurons. Mol Neurobiol 2005;31: 219-230.

[181] Scragg JL, Fearon IM, Boyle JP, Ball SG, Varadi G, Peers C. Alzheimer's amyloid peptides mediate hypoxic up-regulation of L-type Ca2+ channels. FASEB J 2005;19: 150-152.

[182] Arien H, Wiser O, Arkin IT, Leonov H, Atlas D. Syntaxin 1A modulates the voltage-gated L-type calcium channel (Ca(v)1.2) in a cooperative manner. J Biol Chem 2003;278: 29231-29239.

[183] Koch SE, Bodi I, Schwartz A, Varadi G. Architecture of Ca(2+) channel pore-lining segments revealed by covalent modification of substituted cysteines. J Biol Chem 2000;275: 34493-34500.

[184] Nakajima M, Miura M, Aosaki T, Shirasawa T. Deficiency of presenilin-1 increases calcium-dependent vulnerability of neurons to oxidative stress in vitro. J Neurochem 2001;78: 807-814.

[185] Hudasek K, Brown ST, Fearon IM. H2O2 regulates recombinant Ca2+ channel alpha1C subunits but does not mediate their sensitivity to acute hypoxia. Biochem Biophys Res Commun 2004;318: 135-141.

[186] Willmott NJ, Wong K, Strong AJ. Intercellular Ca(2+) waves in rat hippocampal slice and dissociated glial-neuron cultures mediated by nitric oxide. FEBS Lett 2000;487: 239-247.

[187] Grassi C, D'Ascenzo M, Azzena GB. Modulation of Ca(v)1 and Ca(v)2.2 channels induced by nitric oxide via cGMP-dependent protein kinase. Neurochem Int 2004;45: 885-893.

[188] Ohkuma S, Katsura M, Higo A, Shirotani K, Hara A, Tarumi C, Ohgi T. Peroxynitrite affects Ca2+ influx through voltage-dependent calcium channels. J Neurochem 2001;76: 341-350.

[189] Shirotani K, Katsura M, Higo A, Takesue M, Mohri Y, Shuto K, Tarumi C, Ohkuma S. Suppression of Ca2+ influx through L-type voltage-dependent calcium channels by hydroxyl radical in mouse cerebral cortical neurons. Mol Brain Res 2001;92: 12-18.

[190] Mak IT, Zhang J, Weglicki WB. Protective effects of dihydropyridine Ca-blockers against endothelial cell oxidative injury due to combined nitric oxide and superoxide. Pharmacological Res 2002;45: 27-33.

[191] Yagami T, Ueda K, Asakura K, Nakazato H, Hata S, Kuroda T, Sakaeda T, Sakaguchi G, Itoh N, Hashimoto Y, Hori Y. Human group IIA secretory phospholipase A2 potentiates Ca2+ influx through L-type voltage-sensitive Ca2+ channels in cultured rat cortical neurons. J Neurochem 2003;85: 749-758.

[192] Lu C, Chan SL, Fu W, Mattson MP. The lipid peroxidation product 4-hydroxynonenal facilitates opening of voltage-dependent Ca2+ channels in neurons by increasing protein tyrosine phosphorylation. J Biol Chem 2002;277: 24368-24375.

[193] Peng S, Hajela RK, Atchison WD. Characteristics of block by Pb2+ of function of human neuronal L-, N- and R-type Ca2+ channels transiently expressed in human embryonic kidney 293 cells. Mol Pharmacol 2002;62: 1418-1430.

[194] Pall ML. NMDA sensitization and stimulation by peroxynitrite, nitric oxide, and organic solvents as the mechanism of chemical sensitivity in multiple chemical sensitivity. FASEB J 2002;16: 1407-1417.

[195] Fonnum F, Lock EA. The contributions of excitotoxicity, glutathione depletion and DNA repair in chemically induced injury to neurones: exemplified with toxic effects on cerebellar granule cells. J Neurochem 2004;88: 513-31.

[196] Cheung NS, Peng ZF, Chen MJ, Moore PK, Whiteman M. Hydrogen sulfide induced neuronal death occurs via glutamate receptor and is associated with calpain activation and lysosomal rupture in mouse primary cortical neurons. Neuropharmacology 2007;53: 505-514.

[197] Aizenman E, Lipton SA, Loring RH. Selective modulation of NMDA responses by reduction and oxidation. Neuron 1989;2: 1257-1263.

[198] Levy DI, Sucher NJ, Lipton SA. Redox modulation of NMDA receptor-mediated toxicity in mammalian central neurons. Neurosci Lett 1990;110: 291-296.

[199] Moriyoshi K, Masu M, Ishii T, Shigemoto R, Mizuno N, Nakanishi S. Molecular cloning and characterization of the rat NMDA receptor. Nature 1991;354: 31-37.

[200] Sullivan JM, Traynelis SF, Chen HS, Escobar W, Heinemann SF, Lipton SA. Identification of two cysteine residues that are required for redox modulation of the NMDA subtype of glutamate receptor. Neuron 1994;13: 929-936.

[201] Brimecombe JC, Potthoff WK, Aizenman E. A critical role of the N-methyl-D-aspartate (NMDA) receptor subunit (NR) 2A in the expression of redox sensitivity of NR1/NR2A recombinant NMDA receptors. J Pharmacol Exp Ther 1999;291: 785-792.

[202] Sanchez RM, Wang C, Gardner G, Orlando L, Tauck DL, Rosenberg PA, Aizenman E, Jensen FE. Novel role for the NMDA receptor redox modulatory site in the pathophysiology of seizures. J Neurosci 2000;20: 2409-2417.

[203] Lei SZ, Pan ZH, Aggarwal SK, Chen HS, Hartman J, Sucher NJ, Lipton SA. Effect of nitric oxide production on the redox modulatory site of the NMDA receptor-channel complex. Neuron 1992;8: 1087-1099.

[204] Moore PK, Bhatia M, Moochhala S. Hydrogen sulfide: from the smell of the past to the mediator of the future? Trends Pharmacol Sci 2003;24: 609-611.

[205] Qu K, Chen CP, Halliwell B, Moore PK, Wong PT. Hydrogen sulfide is a mediator of cerebral ischemic damage. Stroke 2006;37: 889-893.

[206] Di Stasi AMM, Mallozzi C, Macchia G, Maura G, Petrucci TC, Minetti M. Peroxynitrite affects exocytosis and SNARE complex formation and induces tyrosine nitration of synaptic proteins. J Neurochem 2002;82: 420-429.

[207] Trotti D, Rossi D, Gjesdal O, Levy LM, Racagni G, Danbolt NC, Volterra A. Peroxynitrite inhibits glutamate transporter subtypes. J Biol Chem 1996;271: 5976-5979.

[208] Lin LH, Talman WT. Colocalization of GluR1 and neuronal nitric oxide synthase in rat nucleus tractus solitarii neurons. Neuroscience 2001;106: 801-809.

[209] Trackey JL, Uliasz TF, Hewett SJ. SIN-1-induced cytotoxicity in mixed cortical cell culture: peroxynitrite-dependent and –independent induction of excitotoxic cell death. J Neurochem 2001;79: 445–455.

[210] Abele R, Lampinen M, Keinanen K, Madden DR. Disulfide bonding and cysteine accessibility in the alpha-amino-3-hydroxy-5-methylisoxazole-4-propionic acid receptor subunit GluRD. Implications for redox modulation of glutamate receptors. J Biol Chem 1998;273: 25132-25138.

[211] Mason HS, Bourke S, Kemp PJ. Selective modulation of ligand-gated P2X purinoceptor channels by acute hypoxia is mediated by reactive oxygen species. Mol Pharmacol 2004;66: 1525-1535.

[212] Sayers LG, Brown GR, Michell RH, Michelangeli F. The effects of thimerosal on calcium uptake and inositol 1,4,5-trisphosphate-induced calcium release in cerebellar microsomes. Biochem J 1993;289: 883-887.

[213] Takahashi A, Mikami M, Yang J. Hydrogen peroxide increases GABAergic mIPSC through presynaptic release of calcium from IP3 receptor-sensitive stores in spinal cord substantia gelatinosa neurons. Eur J Neurosci 2007;25: 705-716.

[214] Hilly M, Pietri-Rouxel F, Coquil JF, Guy M, Mauger JP. Thiol reagents increase the affinity of the inositol 1,4,5-trisphosphate receptor. J Biol Chem 1993;268: 16488-16494.

[215] Lopez-Colome AM, Lee I. Pharmacological characterization of inositol-1,4,5,-trisphosphate binding to membranes from retina and retinal cultures. J Neurosci Res 1996;44: 149-156.

[216] Joseph SK, Nakao SK, Sukumvanich S. Reactivity of free thiol groups in type-I inositol trisphosphate receptors. Biochem J 2006;393: 575-582.

[217] Higo T, Hattori M, Nakamura T, Natsume T, Michikawa T, Mikoshiba K. Subtype-specific and ER lumenal environment-dependent regulation of inositol 1,4,5-trisphosphate receptor type 1 by ERp44. Cell 2005;120: 85-98.

[218] Renard-Rooney DC, Joseph SK, Seitz MB, Thomas AP. Effect of oxidized glutathione and temperature on inositol 1,4,5-trisphosphate binding in permeabilized hepatocytes. Biochem J 1995;310: 185-192.

[219] Furuichi T, Furutama D, Hakamata Y, Nakai J, Takeshima H, Mikoshiba K. Multiple types of ryanodine receptor/Ca2+ release channels are differentially expressed in rabbit brain. J Neurosci 1994;14: 4794-4805.

[220] Mori F, Fukaya M, Abe H, Wakabayashi K, Watanabe M. Developmental changes in expression of the three ryanodine receptor mRNAs in the mouse brain. Neuroscience Lett 2000;285: 57-60.

[221] Waring P. Redox active calcium ion channels and cell death. Arch Biochem Biophys 2005;434: 33-42.

[222] Stoyanovsky D, Murphy T, Anno PR, Kim YM, Salama G. Nitric oxide activates skeletal and cardiac ryanodine receptors. Cell Calcium 1997;21: 19-29.

[223] Xu L, Eu JP, Meissner G, Stamler JS. Activation of the cardiac calcium release channel (ryanodine receptor) by poly-S-nitrosylation. Science 1998;279: 234-237.

[224] Anzai K, Ogawa K, Ozawa T, Yamamoto H. Oxidative modification of ion channel activity of ryanodine receptor. Antioxid Redox Signal 2000;2: 35-40.

[225] Aracena-Parks P, Goonasekera SA, Gilman CP, Dirksen RT, Hidalgo C, Hamilton SL. Identification of cysteines involved in S-nitrosylation, S-glutathionylation, and oxidation to disulfides in ryanodine receptor type 1. J Biol Chem 2006;281: 40354-40368.

[226] Eu JP, Sun J, Xu L, Stamler JS, Meissner G. The skeletal muscle calcium release channel: coupled O2 sensor and NO signaling functions. Cell 2000;102: 499-509.

[227] Sun J, Xin C, Eu JP, Stamler JS, Meissner G. Cysteine-3635 is responsible for skeletal muscle ryanodine receptor modulation by NO. Proc Natl Acad Sci USA 2001;98: 11158-11162.

[228] Favero TG, Zable AC, Abramson JJ. Hydrogen peroxide stimulates the Ca2+ release channel from skeletal muscle sarcoplasmic reticulum. J Biol Chem 1995;270: 25557-25563.

[229] Lehotsky J, Kaplan P, Matejovicova M, Murin R, Racay P, Raeymaekers L. Ion transport systems as targets of free radicals during ischemia reperfusion injury. Gen Physiol Biophys 2002;21: 31-37.

[230] Kelliher M, Fastbom J, Cowburn RF, Bonkale W, Ohm TG, Ravid R, Sorrentino V, O'Neill C. Alterations in the ryanodine receptor calcium release channel correlate with Alzheimer's disease neurofibrillary and beta-amyloid pathologies. Neuroscience 1999;92: 499-513.

[231] Lu YF, Hawkins RD. Ryanodine receptors contribute to cGMP-induced late-phase LTP and CREB phosphorylation in the hippocampus. J Neurophysiol 2002;88: 1270-1278.

[232] Kemmerling U, Munoz P, Muller M, Sanchez G, Aylwin ML, Klann E, Carrasco MA, Hidalgo C. Calcium release by ryanodine receptors mediates hydrogen peroxide-induced activation of ERK and CREB phosphorylation in N2a cells and hippocampal neurons. Cell Calcium 2007;41: 491-502.

[233] Grover AK, Samson SE, Misquitta CM. Sarco(endo)plasmic reticulum Ca2+ pump isoform SERCA3 is more resistant than SERCA2b to peroxide. Am J Physiol 1997;273: C420-C425.

[234] Barnes KA, Samson SE, Grover AK. Sarco/endoplasmic reticulum Ca2+-pump isoform SERCA3a is more resistant to superoxide damage than SERCA2b. Mol Cell Biochem 2000;203: 17-21.

[235] Grover AK, Kwan CY, Samson SE. Effects of peroxynitrite on sarco/endoplasmic reticulum Ca2+ pump isoforms SERCA2b and SERCA3a. Am J Physiol Cell Physiol 2003;285: C1537-C1543.

[236] Viner RI, Ferrington DA, Williams TD, Bigelow DJ, Schoneich C. Protein modification during biological aging: selective tyrosine nitration of the SERCA2a isoform of the sarcoplasmic reticulum Ca2+-ATPase in skeletal muscle. Biochem J 1999;340: 657-669.

[237] Doutheil J, Althausen S, Treiman M, Paschen W. Effect of nitric oxide on endoplasmic reticulum calcium homeostasis, protein synthesis and energy metabolism. Cell Calcium 2000;27: 107-115.

[238] Zhang K, Kaufman RJ. The unfolded protein response: a stress signaling pathway critical for health and disease. Neurology 2006;66: S102-S109.

[239] Zatti G, Burgo A, Giacomello M, Barbiero L, Ghidoni R, Sinigaglia G, Florean C, Bagnoli S, Binetti G, Sorbi S, Pizzo P, Fasolato C. Presenilin mutations linked to familial Alzheimer's disease reduce endoplasmic reticulum and Golgi apparatus calcium levels. Cell Calcium 2006;39: 539-550.

[240] Tu H, Nelson O, Bezprozvanny A, Wang Z, Lee SF, Hao YH, Serneels L, De Strooper B, Yu G, Bezprozvanny I. Presenilins form ER Ca2+ leak channels, a function disrupted by familial Alzheimer's disease-linked mutations. Cell 2006;126: 981-93.

[241] Cassarino DS, Bennett JPJr. An evaluation of the role of mitochondria in neurodegenerative diseases: mitochondrial mutations and oxidative pathology, protective nuclear responses, and cell death in neurodegeneration. Brain Res Rev 1999;29: 1-25.

[242] Fiskum G. Mitochondrial participation in ischemic and traumatic neural cell death. J Neurotrauma 2000;17: 843-855.

[243] Stout AK, Raphael HM, Kanterewicz BI, Klann E, Reynolds IJ. Glutamate-induced neuron death requires mitochondrial calcium uptake. Nature Neurosci 1998;1: 366-373.

[244] Ferrand-Drake M, Zhu C, Gido G, Hansen AJ, Karlsson JO, Bahr BA, Zamzami N, Kroemer G, Chan PH, Wieloch T, Blomgren K. Cyclosporin A prevents calpain activation despite increased intracellular calcium concentrations, as well as translocation of apoptosis-inducing factor, cytochrome c and caspase-3 activation in neurons exposed to transient hypoglycemia. J Neurochem 2003;85: 1431-1442.

[245] Whiteman M, Armstrong JS, Cheung NS, Siau JL, Rose P, Schantz JT, Jones DP, Halliwell B. Peroxynitrite mediates calcium-dependent mitochondrial dysfunction and cell death via activation of calpains. FASEB J 2004;18: 1395-1397.

[246] Rosenstock TR, Carvalho AC, Jurkiewicz A, Frussa-Filho R, Smaili SS. Mitochondrial calcium, oxidative stress and apoptosis in a neurodegenerative disease model induced by 3-nitropropionic acid. J Neurochem 2004;88: 1220-1228.

[247] Yang KT, Pan SF, Chien CL, Hsu SM, Tseng YZ, Wang SM, Wu ML. Mitochondrial Na+ overload is caused by oxidative stress and leads to activation of the caspase 3-dependent apoptotic machinery. FASEB J 2004;18: 1442-1444.

[248] Michaelis ML, Foster CT, Jayawickreme C. Regulation of calcium levels in brain tissue from adult and aged rats. Mech Ageing Dev 1992;62: 291-306.

[249] Zaidi A, Gao J, Squier TC, Michaelis ML. Age-related decrease in brain synaptic membrane Ca2+-ATPase in F344/BNF1 rats. Neurobiol Aging 1998;19: 487-495.

[250] Rohn TT, Hinds TR, Vincenzi FF. Inhibition of Ca2+-pump ATPase and the Na+/K+-pump ATPase by iron-generated free radicals. Protection by 6,7-dimethyl-2,4-DI-1-pyrrolidinyl-7H-pyrrolo[2,3-d] pyrimidine sulfate (U-89843D), a potent, novel, antioxidant/free radical scavenger. Biochem Pharmacol 1996;51: 471-476.

[251] Zaidi A, Michaelis ML. Effects of reactive oxygen species on brain synaptic plasma membrane Ca2+-ATPase. Free Radic Biol Med 1999;27: 810-821.

[252] Gutierrez-Martin Y, Martin-Romero FJ, Henao F, Gutierrez-Merino C. Synaptosomal plasma membrane Ca2+ pump activity inhibition by repetitive micromolar ONOO-pulses. Free Radic Biol Med 2002;32: 46-55.

[253] Zaidi A, Barron L, Sharov VS, Schoneich C, Michaelis EK, Michaelis ML. Oxidative inactivation of purified plasma membrane Ca2+-ATPase by hydrogen peroxide and protection by calmodulin. Biochemistry 2003;42: 12001-12010.

[254] Mark RJ, Hensley K, Butterfield DA, Mattson MP. Amyloid beta-peptide impairs ion-motive ATPase activities: evidence for a role in loss of neuronal Ca2+ homeostasis and cell death. J. Neurosci 1995;15: 6239-6249.

[255] Huschenbett J, Zaidi A, Michaelis ML. Sensitivity of the synaptic membrane Na+/Ca2+ exchanger and the expressed NCX1 isoform to reactive oxygen species. Biochim Biophys Acta 1998;1374: 34-46.

[256] Eigel BN, Gursahani H, Hadley RW. ROS are required for rapid reactivation of Na+/Ca2+ exchanger in hypoxic reoxygenated guinea pig ventricular myocytes. Am J Physiol Heart Circ Physiol 2004;286: H955-H963.

[257] Goldhaber JI. Free radicals enhance Na+/Ca2+ exchange in ventricular myocytes. Am J Physiol 1996;271: H823-H833.

[258] Parekh AB. Ca2+ microdomains near plasma membrane Ca2+ channels: impact on cell function. J Physiol 2008;586: 3043–3054.

[259] Neher E. Vesicle pools and Ca2+ microdomains: new tools for understanding their roles in neurotransmitter release. Neuron 1998;20: 389–399.

[260] Neher E. Usefulness and limitations of linear approximations to the understanding of Ca2+ signals. Cell Calcium 1998;24: 345–357.

[261] Samhan-Arias AK, Garcia-Bereguiain MA, Martin-Romero FJ, Gutierrez-Merino C. Regionalization of plasma membrane-bound flavoproteins of cerebellar granule neurons in culture by fluorescence energy transfer imaging. J Fluorescence 2006;16: 393–401.

[262] Nunez L, Sanchez A, Fonteriz RI, Garcia-Sancho J. Mechanisms for synchronous calcium oscillations in cultured rat cerebellar neurons. Eur J Neurosci 1996;8: 192–201.

[263] Wang X, Gruenstein EI. Mechanism of synchronized Ca2+ oscillations in cortical neurons. Brain Res 1997;767:239-249.

[264] Huang L, Liu Y, Zhang P, Kang R, Liu Y, Li X, Bo L, Dong Z. In vitro dose-dependent inhibition of the intracellular spontaneous calcium oscillations in developing hippocampal neurons by ketamine. PLoS One 2013;8(3): e59804.

[265] Yi Y-H, Ho P-Y, Chen T-W, Lin W-J, Gukassyan V, Tsai T-H, Wang D-W, Lew T-S, Tang C-Y, Lo SL, Chen T-Y, Kao F-J, Lin C-H. Membrane Targeting and Coupling of NHE1-IntegrinαIIbβ3-NCX1 by Lipid Rafts following Integrin-Ligand Interactions Trigger Ca2+ Oscillations. J Biol Chem 2009;284: 3855–3864.

[266] Heizmann CW, Braun K. Changes in Ca(2+)-binding proteins in human neurodegenerative disorders. Trends in Neurosci 1992;15: 259-264.

[267] Shaw PJ, Eggett CJ. Molecular factors underlying selective vulnerability of motor neurons to neurodegeneration in amyotrophic lateral sclerosis. J. Neurol 2000;247: I17-I27.

[268] Beers DR, Ho BK, Siklos L, Alexianu ME, Mosier DR, Mohamed AH, Otsuka Y, Kozovska ME, McAlhany RE, Smith RG, Appel SH. Parvalbumin overexpression alters immune-mediated increases in intracellular calcium, and delays disease onset in a transgenic model of familial amyotrophic lateral sclerosis. J. Neurochem 2001;79: 499-509.

[269] Bigelow DJ, Squier TC. Redox modulation of cellular signaling and metabolism through reversible oxidation of methionine sensors in calcium regulatory proteins. Biochem Biophys Acta 2005;1703: 121-134.

[270] Bahler M, Rhoads A. Calmodulin signaling via the IQ motif. FEBS Lett 2002;513: 107-113.

[271] Xia Z, Storm DR. The role of calmodulin as a signal integrator for synaptic plasticity. Nat Rev Neurosci 2005;6: 267-276.

[272] Ferri A, Nencini M, Battistini S, Giannini F, Siciliano G, Casali C, Damiano MG, Ceroni M, Chio A, Rotilio G, Carri MT. Activity of protein phosphatase calcineurin is decreased in sporadic and familial amyotrophic lateral sclerosispatients. J Neurochem 2004;90: 1237-1242.

[273] Yao Y, Yin D, Jas GS, Kuczer K, Williams TD, Schoneich C, Squier TC. Oxidative modification of a carboxyl-terminal vicinal methionine in calmodulin by hydrogen peroxide inhibits calmodulin-dependent activation of the plasma membrane Ca-ATPase. Biochemistry 1996;35: 2767-2787.

[274] Gao J, Yin D, Yao Y, Williams TD, Squier TC. Progressive decline in the ability of calmodulin isolated from aged brain to activate the plasma membrane Ca-ATPase. Biochemistry 1998;37: 9536-9548.

[275] Bartlett RK, Bieber Urbauer RJ, Anbanandam A, Smallwood HS, Urbauer JL, Squier TC. Oxidation of Met144 and Met145 in calmodulin blocks calmodulin dependent activation of the plasma membrane Ca-ATPase. Biochemistry 2003;42: 3231-3238.

[276] Gonzalez-Albo MC, Elston GN, DeFelipe J. The human temporal cortex: characterization of neurons expressing nitric oxide synthase, neuropeptides and calcium-binding proteins, and their glutamate receptor subunit profiles. Cereb Cortex 2001;11: 1170-1181.

[277] Jinno S, Kosaka T. Patterns of expression of calcium binding proteins and neuronal nitric oxide synthase in different populations of hippocampal GABAergic neurons in mice. J Comp Neurol 2002;449: 1-25.

[278] Kowianski P, Morys JM, Wojcik S, Dziewiatkowski J, Luczynska A, Spodnik E, Timmermans JP, Morys J. Neuropeptide-containing neurons in the endopiriform region of the rat: morphology and colocalization with calcium-binding proteins and nitric oxide synthase. Brain Res 2004;996: 97-110.

[279] Lee JE, Jeon CJ. Immunocytochemical localization of nitric oxide synthase-containing neurons in mouse and rabbit visual cortex and co-localization with calcium-binding proteins. Mol Cells 2005;19: 408-417.

[280] Di Leva F, Domi T, Fedrizzi L, Lim D, Carafoli E. The plasma membrane Ca2+ ATPase of animal cells: structure, function and regulation. Arch Biochem Biophys 2008;476:65-74.

Section 2

Neural Processing and Intercellular Signaling

Chapter 4

Peptide and Protein Neurotoxin Toolbox in Research on Nicotinic Acetylcholine Receptors

Victor Tsetlin and Igor Kasheverov

Additional information is available at the end of the chapter

http://dx.doi.org/10.5772/58240

1. Introduction

The chapter briefly covers the history of protein and peptide neurotoxins in research on nicotinic acetylcholine receptors (nAChR). It all started with a great help of α-bungarotoxin and other similar α-neurotoxins from snake venoms in isolation from the *Torpedo* ray electric organ of the muscle-type nAChR as a first individual membrane receptor. The next contribution of α-neurotoxins was the discovery with their aid of the first neuronal nAChR in the brain now known as homooligomeric α7 nAChR. An overview of various α-neurotoxins (so-called three-finger toxins) is presented below showing the structural differences between them, as well as the benefits of their current application for identification and quantification of different nAChR subtypes at normal state and at various pathologies such as Alzheimer's and Parkinson's diseases, psychiatric diseases and nicotine addiction. A special emphasis is placed on the work at our institute, starting with the first detection of nAChRs as targets for the so-called weak or "non-conventional" neurotoxins. Recently, in proteomic studies of snake venoms, novel structural types have been discovered, such as covalently connected dimeric α-cobratoxin or, on the contrary - azemiopsin, the first peptide from venoms which does not contain disulfide bonds but still blocks selectively the muscle-type nAChR.

A generous source for sophisticated tools in research on nAChRs is combinatorial peptide libraries from the venoms of *Conus* marine snails. In particular, they contain α-conotoxins which not only distinguish muscle nAChRs from neuronal ones, but some of them block specifically distinct neuronal nAChR subtypes. At present, combinations of snake and snail toxins are widely used in fundamental research and in pharmacological studies.

The chapter briefly summarizes information on the spatial organization and subunit composition of different nAChR subtypes, but considers in more detail important contributions of peptide and protein neurotoxins into elucidation of the topography of the nAChR binding sites. The information mainly came from the X-ray structures of their complexes with the acetylcholine-binding protein (AChBP), an excellent structural model of the ligand-binding domain of nAChRs. These complexes are considered as initial blocks for design of novel drugs.

2. Muscle-type, neuronal and "non-neuronal" nAChRs — Brief overview

Before considering in detail protein and peptide neurotoxins on which the Chapter is mostly focused, it is reasonable to give very shortly the information about various types of nAChR which will make easier later discussions of the specificity of one or another toxin to a particular nAChR subtype.

As mentioned in the Introduction, α-bungarotoxin made possible identification and isolation in a pure form of the nAChR from the *Torpedo* ray electric organ. Later it was found that this receptor is composed of 5 subunits arranged around the central axis along which an ion channel should be arranged (Figure 1, A). The subunits in the order of their increasing molecular masses (estimated from the SDS-gel electrophoresis) have been named α, β, γ and δ. The molecular mass of the receptor complex is around 250 kD and it should contain two α subunits and by one of the "non- α" subunits. When nucleotide sequences of the *Torpedo* nAChR subunits and of those from mammalian muscles were established it became clear that those receptors are highly homologous. In fact, the mammalian embryonic nAChR has the same subunit stoichiometry (2α, β, γ and δ), but in the mature form it has an ε subunit instead of γ. Although the relevant information at present is available in numerous biochemistry books and reviews [1-4], it should be mentioned here that nAChRs are ligand-gated ion channels: binding of a ligand (acetylcholine, nicotine or other specific agonists) will result in the channel opening and passing sodium or calcium ions will activate a variety of signaling cascades. On the other hand, binding at the same sites of competitive antagonists such as α-bungarotoxin will prevent both binding of agonists and subsequent channel opening; some so-called non-competitive antagonists, like phencyclidine, bind directly to the channel moiety but they are not discussed here.

Earlier it was thought that the ligand-binding sites of nAChRs lie within the α-subunits, hence there should be two binding sites on the muscle-type nAChRs. To-day we know that, indeed, the main contributions to binding of agonists or competitive antagonists are donated by the α-subunits. Moreover, even isolated α-subunit and its fragment in the amino-acid region 170-200 can bind α-bungarotoxin, although with lower affinity than the whole-size receptors [5,6]. However, now it is well established that the binding sites are situated at the interfaces of the α-subunits with their neighbors, and it is the variability of functional groups brought to the binding sites by less conservative "non-alpha" subunits which underlies the differences in specificity between individual nAChR subtypes [4].

What are the types and subtypes of nicotinic acetylcholine receptors? As mentioned above, binding of radioactive α-bungarotoxin to brain membranes finally brought to life the nAChR presently known as homopentameric α7 nAChR that is composed of five identical α7-subunits. Thus, we have an example of homooligomeric receptor belonging to the family of neuronal

http://dx.doi.org/10.5772/58240

nAChRs. Neuronal heteromeric nAChRs are composed of two types of subunits: α and β. At present there are 9 types of neuronal α-subunits (α2-α10) and three types of β subunits (β2-β4); α and β subunits in the muscle-type receptors presumed to be α1 and β1 ones. The characteristic feature of α-subunit is a vicinal disulfide between two neighboring Cys residues in the binding site (Cys192-Cys193 in the amino-acid sequence of the *Torpedo* α-subunit) which is not present in β or other "non-α" subunits. In recent years it became clear that diverse nAChRs are very much widespread and play different functional roles also outside the neuromuscular junctions or central nervous system. In fact, neuronal nAChR subunits were found on the immune system cells, skin, lung tissue and other. The respective receptors got the name of "non-neuronal" nAChRs thus making a third group of nicotinic acetylcholine receptors (see reviews [7,8]).

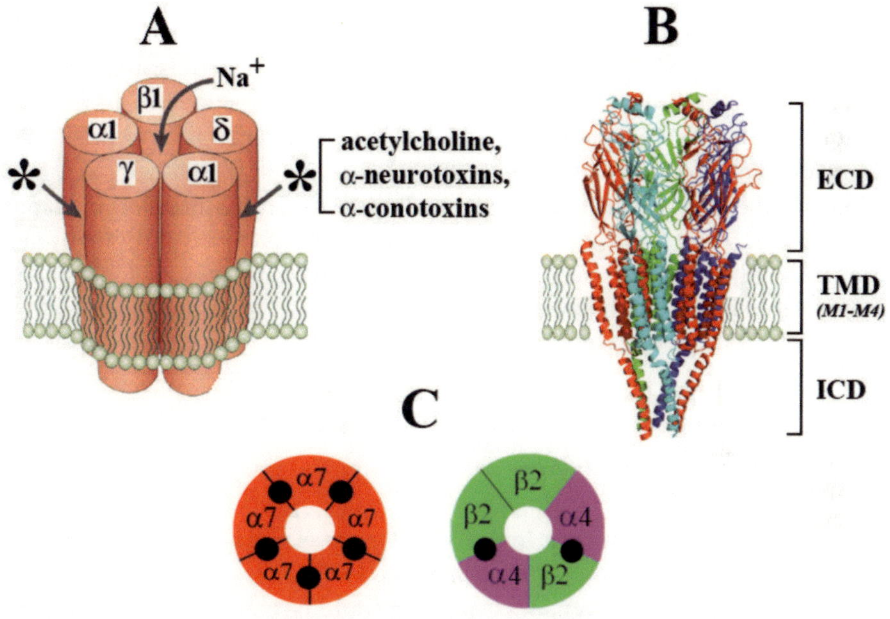

Figure 1. Spatial organization of nAChRs. A – Schematic presentation of *Torpedo* nAChR, consisting of 5 subunits with the ion channel along the central axis. Two binding sites of agonists (acetylcholine and others) and competitive antagonist (α-neurotoxins from snakes, α-conotoxins from *Conus* mollusks and others) are located at the interfaces of the α1/γ and α1/δ-subunits and marked with asterisks. B – Spatial organization of *Torpedo marmorata* nAChR derived from its cryo-electron microscopy structure. Subunits α1, β1, γ and δ are colored in red, green, cyanic and blue, respectively. Three main domains of the receptor – extracellular (ECD), transmembrane (TMD), consisting of 4 α-helical fragments (M1-M4), and intracellular (ICD) are shown. C – Schematic presentation of two representatives of neuronal nAChRs – homooligomeric and heterooligomeric ones. The probable binding sites of agonists and competitive antagonist are marked with black circles.

Structurally, the *Torpedo* nAChR is a prototype for all members of the nAChR family. First of all, it is a pentamer (composed of 5 subunits) as follows from the cryo-electron microscopy structure of the *Torpedo marmorata* receptor (see Figure 1, B). There are no structural data of this sort for any other nAChR, but their pentameric composition was presumed from computer modeling and from some indirect data like electrophysiology analysis. At present there are no doubts that all nAChRs are indeed either pentameric homooligomers (made exclusively of 5 α-type subunits, like $\alpha7$ nAChR, $\alpha9$ nAChR or $\alpha9/\alpha10$ nAChR) or pentameric heterooligomers (composed of α and other subunits) (Figure 1, C) – for example, one of the best presented in the brain is $\alpha4\beta2$ nAChR [9]. As already mentioned, all nAChRs should be built similarly to *Torpedo* nAChR: namely, four transmembrane fragments M1-M4 in each subunit, the most inner ones M2 fragments lining the channel, the N-terminal extracellular fragments of each subunit together forming the ligand-binding domain excellently imitated by the X-ray structure of the acetylcholine-binding protein (AChBP) (see below). The long intracellular loops between transmembrane fragments M3 and M4 of each subunit together form the cytoplasmic (intracellular) domain.

The first and the most direct structural evidence for a common three-dimensional organization of all nAChRs came from the crystal structure of AChBP [10]. Today even more convincing are the recently solved high-resolution X-ray structures of the whole-size prokaryotic membrane proteins belonging to the same superfamily of Cys-loop ligand-gated ion channels as nAChRs [11-13]. These proteins, each composed of 5 identical subunits, do not have large cytoplasmic domains (which apparently made their crystallization much more simple than of nAChRs or other mammalian Cys-loop receptors), but in the transmembrane and ligand-binding domains they are surprisingly similar to *Torpedo* nAChR. Moreover, the same type of structure was found for a Cys-loop receptor from *Caenorhabditis elegans* [14]. Now, after having these major facts about nicotinic acetylcholine receptors, we can open our toolbox and have a closer look on protein and peptide neurotoxins.

3. Snake venom neurotoxins utilized in research on nAChRs — Primary and three-dimensional structure

The word "toolbox" in the chapter title in the first place is related to the snake venom proteins, at least historically. It was the component of *Bungarus multicinctus* venom which was found to block very efficiently the muscle-type nAChRs and could be considered as a good marker of those receptors. The history of the discovery of such a tool, namely protein neurotoxin α-bungarotoxin, is presented in a recent review [15]. There Prof. Chang shares his memories about this discovery (exactly 50 years ago!) which played such a crucial role in understanding the structure and function of both snake neurotoxins and of one of their targets, namely nAChRs. Soon after the discovery of α-bungarotoxin, similar proteins were found in other snakes, in particular in cobra venoms and the whole family got the name of α-neurotoxins (see reviews [15-17]).

3.1. α-Neurotoxins

There are two structural types of α-neurotoxins: short-chain α-neurotoxins (60-62 amino acid residues, 4 disulfide bridges) and long-chain ones (66-75 amino acid residues, 5 disulfide bonds). The first X-ray structures have been determined for the short-chain α-neurotoxins,

http://dx.doi.org/10.5772/58240

namely for erabutoxins a and b [18,19] (see Figure 2, A). The molecule has three loops, with a predominant β-structure, fixed in the space by 4 disulfide bridges forming a sort of a knot. This folding gave the name of "three-finger proteins" to α-neurotoxins. Later spatial structures have been determined both by NMR and X-ray crystallography for different short- and long-chain α-neurotoxins, including α-bungarotoxin [20,21]. Long-chain α-neurotoxins have the same three -finger folding as the short ones, but contain a longer C-terminal tail and an additional 5th disulfide in the central loop II (Figure 2, B). In the structures of some long-chain α-neurotoxins (α-bungarotoxin, α-cobratoxin [22] or neurotoxin I from *Naja oxiana* [23]) a short α-helical fragment was found at the tip of the loop II (see Figure 2, B).

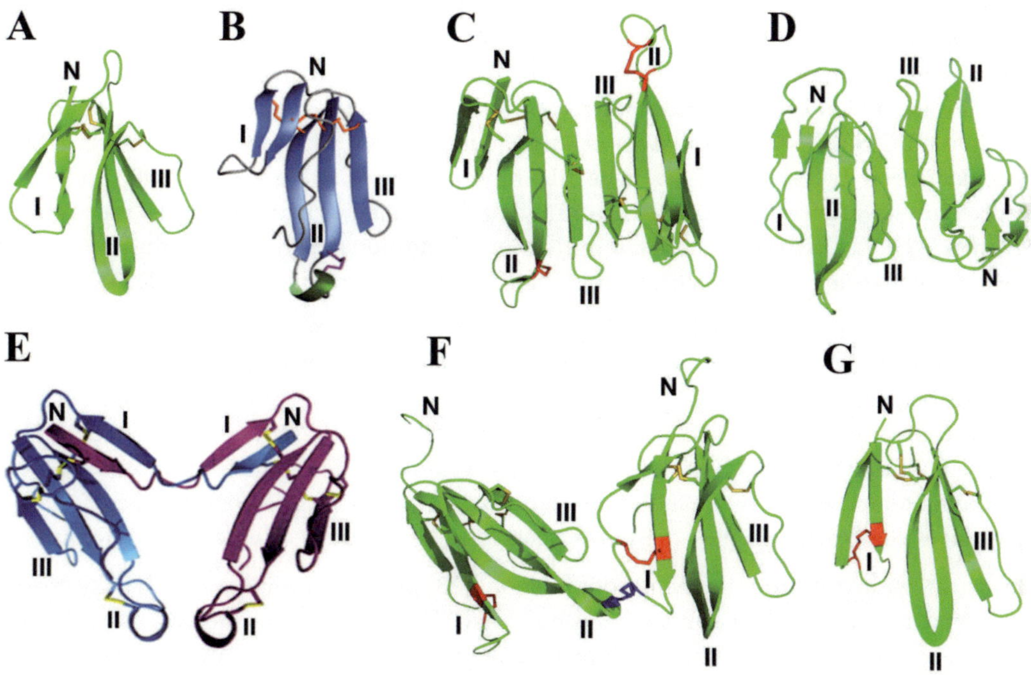

Figure 2. Spatial structures of snake 'three-finger' toxins interacting with nAChRs. The 'fingers' are marked with Roman numbers; N-termini are labeled as well. A - erabutoxin a (PDB ID: 5EBX). B – α-bungarotoxin (1KFH); the 5th disulfide bridge in loop II is colored in magenta (contrary to all other disulfides in orange) and α-helix at tip of this loop is colored intentionally in contrast green. C – κ-bungarotoxin (1KBA); 5th disulfide bridges in loops II are colored in red. D – haditoxin (3HH7). E – dimeric α-cobratoxin (4AEA), where disulfide bridges between Cys3 from one monomer and Cys20 from the second monomer stabilize the dimeric molecule; two monomers are shown in blue and magenta, respectively. F - irditoxin (2H7Z); 'non-conventional' disulfides in loops I are colored in red and disulfide bond between the monomers is shown in blue. G - candoxin (1JGK); disulfide in loop I is shown in red.

One of the characteristic features of α-neurotoxins is the stability of their three-dimensional structure fixed by 4 or 5 disulfide bridges. This conclusion is supported by high similarity of spatial structures determined by NMR at different conditions (varying pH and temperatures) and by X-ray crystallography. This may be one of the crucial factors explaining high efficiency of α-neurotoxin interactions with their targets, nicotinic acetylcholine receptors. As will be shown later, α-neurotoxins essentially preserve their conformation in complexes with the AChBP [24], with the ligand-binding domain of individual α1 subunit of nAChR [25] and with the chimera of AChBP and α7 nAChR extracellular domain [26].

3.2. Dimeric three-finger neurotoxins

First of all, we should mention here κ-bungarotoxins and several homologous neurotoxins which are dimers, but do not have covalent intermolecular bonds between monomers [27]. Each monomer is very similar to a typical long-chain α-neurotoxin: the same additional 5th disulfide at the tip of the central loop II, but a slightly shorter C-terminal tail (total number of amino acid residues 66 but not 75 as in α-bungarotoxin) (see Figure 2, C). The molecular targets of κ-bungarotoxins are neuronal nAChRs, but contrary to α-neurotoxins they have high affinity to neuronal α3β2 nAChR [28]. Interestingly, it was established about 20 years ago that there is one common property of α-neurotoxins and κ-neurotoxins, namely the additional disulfide in the loop II is essential for recognition of neuronal nAChRs. It was found that selective reduction of that disulfide and subsequent alkylation or removal of the respective cysteines in both types of toxins abolished their high affinity binding to α7 and α3β2 nAChRs, respectively (without decreasing the affinity of long-chain α-neurotoxins to muscle-type nAChRs [29,30]). On the other hand, introduction of additional disulfide into the central loop of short-chain α-neurotoxins considerably increased their affinity for α7 nAChR [31,32].

It is not yet absolutely clear why κ-bungarotoxins have preference for heteromeric nAChRs. There was a hypothesis that an important role in selectivity of κ-bungarotoxins towards α3β2 nAChRs belongs to the residue Lys26 [24]. However, its introduction to α-neurotoxin having a high affinity for α7 nAChRs only decreased considerably binding to this receptor but did not bring any affinity for α3β2 nAChRs [32]. Apparently, dimerization as such is important to force a protein, composed of two classical α-neurotoxins, to recognize a heteromeric neuronal nAChRs as can be seen on the example of other recently discovered dimeric neurotoxins.

One toxin, haditoxin from the King cobra venom [33] looks very similar to κ-bungarotoxin. Haditoxin is a non-covalent dimer composed of two short-chain α-neurotoxins, rather than of long-chain ones, and the monomers adopt a topological arrangement (Figure 2, D) reminiscent of that observed earlier for monomers in κ-bungarotoxin. Haditoxin can block not only muscle-type nAChRs, as typically observed for short-chain α-neurotoxins, but surprisingly it also blocks homooligomeric α7 and heterooligomeric α3β2 nAChRs. This finding appears to be in contradiction with the earlier found necessity of the additional disulfide in the central loop for recognition of neuronal nAChRs. However, it should be kept in mind that blocking of neuronal nAChRs by haditoxin was observed only at very high toxin concentrations [33]. It should be also mentioned that, strictly speaking, haditoxin cannot be assigned to classical short-chain α-neurotoxins because its homology to erabutoxin is only 50%, whereas it is 75-80% with the muscarinic toxin-like proteins (MTLP) having different targets [34].

Novel types of dimeric α-neurotoxins were recently discovered: contrary to κ-bungarotoxin or haditoxin, these are covalently bound where two molecules of α-cobratoxin are connected by two intermolecular disulfide bonds [35]. Before describing a biological activity of this new tool, it should be mentioned that such intermolecular disulfide is the first case of this posttranslational modification found for the whole huge family of three-finger toxins. Dimeric α-cobratoxin retained, although at a lower level, the capacity to block α7 and muscle-type nAChRs and in addition acquired the ability to block α3β2 nAChR - again, with lower potency than did κ-bungarotoxin [35]. Interestingly, selective reduction of the disulfides in the loop II of dimeric α-cobratoxin abolished its activity against α7 nAChR. It could be expected in view of earlier described similar modification of α-cobratoxin itself, but this chemical modification even increased the affinity for α3β2 nAChR [36]. Since dimeric α-cobratoxin is present in the *Naja kaouthia* cobra venom only in minute amounts (0.01% in crude venom, as compared to 10% for α-cobratoxin itself or to 0.1% for κ-bungarotoxin), unequivocal localization of intermolecular disulfides by chemical means could not be done. Fortunately, dimeric α-cobratoxin has been recently crystallized (Figure 2, E) and the high-resolution X-ray structure revealed the disposition of the intermolecular disulfide bridges: the disulfide Cys3-Cys20 or Cys3′-Cys20′ in each monomer is not formed, but Cys3 of one monomer finds Cys20′ of another monomer, while Cys3′ of the latter makes a disulfide with Cys20 of the former [36].

As will be shown later, the main contribution to binding of α-neurotoxins both to nAChRs and to their models comes from the tip of the central loop II of α-neurotoxins. In dimeric α-cobratoxin the two tips are in close proximity and computer modeling showed impossibility of docking such a structure to AChBP, suggesting that some conformational changes should occur in the dimeric α-cobratoxin to ensure its binding observed in radioligand and electrophysiology experiments [36].

The discovery of dimeric α-cobratoxin was followed by finding another three-fingered toxin where monomers are connected by a disulfide bridge [37]. It was irditoxin isolated from Colubrid snake *Boiga irregularis*. In contrast to dimeric α-cobratoxin present in venom in minor amounts, irditoxin is a main component of boiga venom. Again, strictly speaking, irditoxin is neither a short- nor a long-chain α-neurotoxin: the monomers forming this toxin belong to non-conventional toxin type (see below) and each monomer contains an extra cysteine residue forming one disulfide bridge between two monomers (or protomers). None of these cysteines is present in classical α-neurotoxins. In the first protomer, the additional cysteine is located in loop I whereas in the second protomer it is in loop II. The three-dimensional structure of irditoxin [37] (see Figure 2, F) shows that the central loops II of the two protomers are oriented in a similar way as the central loops of dimeric α-cobratoxin (Figure 2, E).

3.3. Weak (non-conventional) three-fingered neurotoxins

A characteristic feature of this group of three-fingered toxins is the presence of additional disulfide bridge not in the central loop II, as in long-chain α-neurotoxins or in κ-bungarotoxins, but in the N- terminal loop I. Some representatives of this group were known long ago, but many of them did not have a strong toxicity (that is why their name was "weak toxins") and their targets were unknown. At present this group of toxins, consisting of 62-68 amino acid residues, is quite well investigated and has a more general name "non-conventional neurotoxins" [38]. The toxicities for the most of group members are very low (5-80 mg/kg) in contrast to classical α-neurotoxin with toxicities in the range from 0.04 to 0.3 mg/kg. However, some very potent toxins (like γ-bungarotoxin with LD50 of 0.15 mg/kg) are also included in the group of non-conventional toxins. Since, as mentioned above, molecular targets of weak (non-conventional) toxins for a long time were unknown, an important step in this field was the work [39] where was discovered that weak toxin (WTX) from *Naja kaouthia* cobra venom interacted with micromolar affinity with the $\alpha7$ and muscle-type nAChRs, the binding being practically irreversible. Later it was found [40] that candoxin (Figure 2, G), another non-conventional toxin, interacted both with $\alpha7$ and muscle-type nAChR with high affinity. An interesting feature of candoxin is that its attachment to the muscle-type receptor was easily reversible. Even more impressing species specificity was reported for denmotoxin, a non-conventional toxin isolated from Colubrid snake *Boiga dendrophila*: it was able to interact irreversibly and with high affinity with chick muscle nAChR, but only with low affinity with mouse receptors [41].

3.4. Three-finger snake neurotoxins having other targets than nicotinic acetylcholine receptors

Before considering in detail the mechanisms of interactions between α-neurotoxins and nAChRs and describing their earlier and current roles of tools, it is appropriate to say a few words about the whole family of three-finger proteins from snake venoms (see reviews [16,17]). They all have the same "three-finger" fold but are decorated with quite different functionally active amino-acid residue and, as a result, attack distinct targets. For example, in the preceding paragraph we considered WTX from *Naja kaouthia* venom which blocked nicotinic acetylcholine receptors. Its very low toxicity allowed testing of its behavioural activity on rats which suggested action on muscarinic acetylcholine receptors [42]. Indeed, subsequent radioligand analyses revealed the WTX interaction with the different subtypes of muscarinic acetylcholine receptors [43]. It should be noted here that we have a dualism of action for this group of the three-finger proteins from snake venom: namely, blocking of one acetylcholine receptor (the nicotinic one) belonging to the family of ligand-gated ion channels and another acetylcholine receptor, the muscarinic one which is a member of the superfamily of G-protein-coupled receptors (GPCR).

Much more strong effects on muscarinic acetylcholine receptors exert so-called muscarinic neurotoxins isolated from the green mamba *Dendroaspis angusticeps* [44-46]. Structurally these proteins are of the same type as short-chain α-neurotoxins. Interestingly, they can distinguish different subtypes (M1-M7) of muscarinic acetylcholine receptors and on some of them exert not the inhibitory, but the potentiating effects. There is not yet much information about how muscarinic toxins recognize their targets. A large series of mutations was performed both on the muscarinic toxin MT7 and on the M1 muscarinic receptor and the results of this pair-wise mutagenesis, analyzed by computer modelling, indicated that all three loops I-III should be involved in the interaction and the main binding site for this allosteric modulator is located in the extracellular loops of the receptor [46].

There are also several three-finger proteins from snake venoms (calciceptin, FS2) blocking Ca^{2+} channels [47,48]. We should also mention here fasciculin, a three-finger protein with 4 disulfides, targeting the acetylcholinesterase. Interestingly, the X-ray structures of fasciculin in complex with acetylcholinesterases were the first examples presenting a three-finger toxin bound to its biological target [49,50].

One of the most well-represented groups in the snake venoms are so-called cytotoxins (some of them were earlier called cardiotoxins) which apparently do not have a single well-defined target but disrupt the cell membranes thus inducing a multitude of effects (see reviews [51,52]). As a result of proteomic studies new three-finger proteins are being found in the snake venoms, and one of the minor components in the *Naja kaouthia* cobra venom was identified as a glycosylated cytotoxin I [53]. This post-translational modification, for the first time discovered for the family of three-finger toxins, considerably decreased the cytotoxicity of this protein, whereas enzymatic deglycosylation restored it to the level of cytotoxin I activity [53]. Another really a minor component of that venom (less than 0.01% in the crude venom) was a dimer of cytotoxin and α-cobratoxin connected by two intermolecular disulfide bridges which revealed a weak activity against neuronal nicotinic acetylcholine receptors [35].

We also would like to mention here the recent discovery of three-finger neurotoxins which interact with another group of GPCR, namely with the adrenoreceptors [54,55]. These toxins are most similar to muscarinic toxins and were also isolated from the eastern green mamba *Dendroaspis angusticeps.* One such toxin (ϱ-Da1a) has a very high affinity (0.35 nM) for the α1 adrenoreceptor, while another one (ϱ-Da1b) has a lower affinity but is more selective towards α2 types [55]. Interestingly, these toxins are considered as possible drugs against prostate hypertrophy.

Although it is not the topic of the present review, it is appropriate to mention here that there are three-finger proteins in nervous and immune system of mammals and insects belonging to the Ly6 family and some of them bind to nicotinic acetylcholine receptors and regulate their functioning *in vivo* (see [56-59] and recent publications from our institute [60-63]).

3.5. Peptides from snake venoms acting on nicotinic acetylcholine receptors

Such peptides are not as numerous as α-neurotoxins or non-conventional toxins targeting different subtypes of nAChR. Until recently the only group was that of waglerins isolated from the venom of South Asian snake *Tropidolaemus wagleri* which consist of 22-24 amino acids and contain one disulfide bridge [64,65]. These toxins bind with high affinity to muscle-type nAChR [66]. Interestingly, waglerins can distinguish embryonic ($\alpha1_2\beta1\ \gamma\delta$) and "mature" ($\alpha1_2\beta1\varepsilon\delta$) muscle-type nAChR: waglerin-1 efficiently blocks the ε-containing form, but not the γ-form of this receptor [67]. While snake venom α-neurotoxins bind with practically equal efficiency to the two binding sites (formed by two α-subunits with their non-α neighbors) in the muscle-type nAChRs, waglerin-1 binds 2100-fold more tightly to the α-ε than to the α-δ binding site of the mouse nAChR [68]. Several amino acid residues in the nAChR subunits participating in waglerin binding were identified by site directed mutagenesis [69], namely Asp59 and Asp173 were shown to be important for waglerin binding at both sites. On the other hand, the disulfide in waglerin was found to be essential for its activity, as well as several residues in its N-terminal part of the amino acid sequence [70].

A new peptide was recently found in the snake venom possessing a capacity to block muscle-type nAChR [71]. It is azemiopsin, isolated from the *Azemiops feae* viper venom, which consists of 21 amino acid residues. By the chain length azemiopsin is similar to waglerins and, moreover, shares with them a homologous C-terminal fragment. However, it possesses a unique structural feature: contrary to all earlier known proteins and peptides from the venoms of snakes or poisonous *Conus* mollusks (see below), whose structure is fixed by one or several S–S-bonds, azemiopsin contains no disulfides. It dose-dependently blocked acetylcholine-induced currents in *Xenopus* oocytes heterologously expressing human muscle nAChR, and was more potent against the adult ($\alpha1_2\beta1\varepsilon\delta$) than the fetal ($\alpha1_2\beta1\gamma\delta$) form. Ala-scanning and analysis of competition with α-bungarotoxin for binding to *Torpedo* nAChR resulted in identification of the azemiopsin residues essential for its activity which in general were found to be different from those responsible for the waglerin activity [71].

4. α-Conotoxins, peptides from poisonous marine snails *Conus*, acting on nicotinic acetylcholine receptors

Historically, snake venom α-neurotoxins were the first extremely important tools which made possible "digging out" in a purified form the first representative of the nAChR family, namely the muscle-type receptor from the *Torpedo* ray electric organ. Then, in the early 80^s, the peptide toxins were discovered in the marine mollusk *Conus geographus* venom which caused postsynaptic inhibition at the neuromuscular junction in frog and got the name of conotoxins [72]. The following studies brought to life a tremendous number of so-called conotoxins or conopeptides from different species of *Conus* snails. The number of *Conus* species living in different seas and oceans is about 1000 and the available data show that the venom of each species should contain in excess of 1000 conopeptides. Thus, *Conus* mollusks provide researchers with huge combinatorial libraries of peptides. The main task of slowly moving *Conus* mollusks is to immobilize their preys (small fishes, worms etc.), that is why their venoms contain a variety of peptides paralyzing the nervous systems of their targets. Evolutionary each *Conus* species is adjusted to a particular area and a distinct food source, hence the individuality of each venom. There are several types of conotoxins differing in their targets: α-conotoxins block nAChRs, μ-conotoxins are acting on Na^+-channels, κ-conotoxins interact with K^+-channels, ω-conotoxins block specifically certain Ca^{2+}-channels and one of such ω-conotoxins became a very potent analgesic (trade name Ziconotide or Prialt; see more about these and many other conotoxins and conopeptides in recent reviews [73-75]). The number of discovered conotoxins is rapidly increasing because nowadays they appear not so much due to isolation from *Conus* venoms (usually available only in minute amounts) but due to deciphering mRNAs obtained from the venom glands.

Since this chapter is devoted to neurotoxic proteins and peptides interacting with nicotinic acetylcholine receptors, below we will consider only those conotoxins which target these receptors. The major group is α-conotoxins, competitive antagonists of nAChRs. They have 12-19 amino-acid residues, as a rule amidated C-terminus and two disulfide bonds between Cys residues C^1–C^3 and C^2–C^4 (see Table). There are also several other groups of conotoxins

http://dx.doi.org/10.5772/58240

acting on nAChRs (ψ-, αA-, αA_S-, αC-, αS- and αD), but they are not numerous, are not as widely used as α-conotoxins and will not be considered here.

Toxin	*Conus species*	Amino acid sequence [1]	Selectivity
3/5 α-conotoxins			
GI	*C. geographus*	ECCNPACGRHYSC*	α1β1γ/εδ
MI	*C. magus*	GRCCHPACGKNYSC*	α1β1γ/εδ
SIA	*C. striatus*	YCCHPACGKNFDC*	α1β1γ/εδ
4/3 α- conotoxins			
ImI	*C. imperialis*	GCCSDPRCAWRC*	α7, α9α10; α3β2; α3β4
RgIA	*C. regius*	GCCSDPRCRYRCR	α9α10
4/4 α- conotoxins			
BuIA	*C. bullatus*	GCCSTPPCAVLYC*	α3(α6)β2, α3(α6)β4
4/6 α- conotoxins			
AuIB	*C. aulicus*	GCCSYPPCFATNPDC*	α3β4
4/7 α- conotoxins			
PnIA	*C. pennaceus*	GCCSLPPCAANNPDYC*	α3β2
PnIB	*C. pennaceus*	GCCSLPPCALSNPDYC*	α7; α3β4
MII	*C. magus*	GCCSNPVCHLEHSNLC*	α3β2(β3); α6-containing
Vc1.1	*C. victoriae*	GCCSDPRCNYDHPEIC*	α9α10; α3β4, α3(α5)β2
TxIA	*C. textile*	GCCSRPPCIANNPDLC*	α3β2
ArIB	*C. arenatus*	DECCSNPACRVNNPHVCRRR	α7, α6α3β2β3, α3β2

[1] Scheme of disulfide closing for naturally-occurring α-conotoxins –

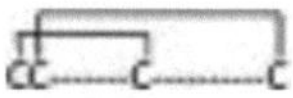

* indicates an amidated C-terminus; the names of α-conotoxins typed in italics mean that their structures were identified in cDNA libraries.

Table 1. Most studied members of naturally-occurring α-conotoxins.

α-Conotoxins are structurally subdivided into subgroups depending on the number of amino acid residues between the C^2–C^3 and C^3–C^4 cysteines (see Table) forming the first and second loops, respectively. This structural feature affects the α-conotoxin specificity to particular nAChR subtypes. All at present known 3/5 α-conotoxins are potent blockers of muscle type nAChRs (and conventionally can be called 'muscle' α-conotoxins). The members of other subgroups (4/3, 4/4, 4/6, 4/7) act on various neuronal nAChR subtypes (and can be called 'neuronal' α-conotoxins). It is very rare when naturally occurring neuronal α-conotoxin blocks specifically only one neuronal nAChR subtype, usually neuronal α-conotoxins interact with two or more nAChR subtypes (see Table).

Most of muscle 3/5 α-conotoxins can discriminate species-specifically two binding sites on muscle or *Torpedo* nAChRs. For example, α-conotoxins MI, GI or SIA have up to10000 times higher affinity for $\alpha1/\delta$- over $\alpha1/\gamma$ site in muscle nAChR [76,77]; in contrast to more effective binding of these peptides, although not with such a great difference, to $\alpha1/\gamma$ site in *Torpedo* receptor [78,79].

"Mutagenesis" studies of α-conotoxins (in fact not the mutagenesis as such, but substitutions of amino acid residues by solid-phase peptide synthesis) gave information about those residues which are the basis of the high affinity and selectivity to a particular receptor or receptor subgroup. For example, the crucial role of Arg9 in α-conotoxin GI, as well as of Pro6 and Tyr12 in α-conotoxin MI for discriminating the $\alpha1/\gamma$- and $\alpha1/\delta$-sites was revealed [80-82]. Interestingly, Arg9 proved important for a neuronal 4/3 α-conotoxin RgIA for its $\alpha9\alpha10$ nAChR specificity [83]. Similar "mutagenesis" studies resulting in revelation of residues crucial for activity were done also for many other α-conotoxins (ImI, PnIA, MII, GID, Vc1.1, AuIB) [84-89].

Like in the analysis of interactions between different nAChR types and snake venom neurotoxins, when much efforts has been spent by many laboratories to establish the topography of their binding, similar studies have been undertaken to elucidate the mechanism of nAChR recognition by α-conotoxins. Among them were above-mentioned multiple substitutions in the amino acid sequences of naturally occurring α-conotoxins, making their structures more rigid, syntheses of radioactive, fluorescent and photoactivatable derivatives. Combination with mutagenesis of the receptor subunits (pair-wise mutagenesis) gave information about possible contact points between α-neurotoxins and nAChRs, as well as between α-conotoxins and nAChRs. The relevant information can be found in numerous reviews (see, for example, [90-92]), but will not be considered in detail here, because this chapter contains a special section where crystal structures of α-neurotoxins and α-conotoxins in complexes with the relevant biological targets will be discussed.

5. Three-dimensional structures of peptide and protein neurotoxins in complexes with the nicotinic receptor models and fragments

It was already mentioned that the crystal structure of the acetylcholine-binding protein (AChBP) provided an impressing jump in the structural analysis of not only nicotinic acetylcholine receptors but of all other members of the Cys-loop receptor family. This water-soluble protein was found to modulated synaptic transmission in glia of *Lymnaea stagnalis* fresh-water mollusk and was purified using affinity chromatography on a column with the attached α-bungarotoxin [93]. Sufficient amounts of AChBP were obtained by heterologous expression and the crystal structure was determined at 2.7 Å resolution [10]. This structure clearly showed that AChBP is an excellent structural model of N-terminal ligand-binding domains of all nAChRs: crystal AChBP was in a pentameric state, similarly to the whole-size nAChRs. In spite of low homology with the amino-acid sequences of extracellular domains of nAChR subunits (not more than 25%), AChBP contains all those amino acid residues which earlier in receptor studies were found essential for interacting with the cholinergic agonists and antagonist. The

AChBP crystal structure revealed that such residues are all clustered in the middle of AChBP, at the interfaces between its subunits (or protomers). At present, the X-ray structures of several molluscan AChBPs are known (from *Lymnaea stagnalis, Aplysia californica, Bulinus truncatus*), as well of their complexes with a wide variety of agonists and antagonists which gave quite a detailed picture of the respective binding sites in these AChBPs and of their contacts with ligands. Biochemical data and computer modeling show convincingly that these structures shed light on the receptor binding sites *per se* and on the ligand disposition in the binding sites of muscle and neuronal nAChRs. The relevant information can be found in recent original papers [94-97] and reviews [98,99], and below we will consider in detail only the crystal structures of complexes with protein and peptide neurotoxins.

Interestingly, the first AChBP crystal structure in complex with a competitive antagonist was that of *Lymanaea stagnalis* AChBP with bound α-cobratoxin [24]. (In parentheses it may be mentioned that later more structures were solved for the *Aplysia californica* AChBP complexes, but *L. stagnalis* AChBP has a much higher affinity for α-neurotoxins than AChBPs from other species). First of all, X-ray analysis revealed 5 α-cobratoxin molecules attached at the interfaces between 5 identical subunits (or protomers) of AChBP (Figure 3, A). The major role in the organization of the binding site is played by aromatic residues (so-called "aromatic box") of AChBP. Long before crystallographic studies, protein chemistry and mutagenesis revealed that these aromatic residues were important for binding different agonists and antagonists to diverse muscle-type and neuronal nAChRs. It was proposed that the binding sites are formed by three fragments (A, B, C) of polypeptide chain of one subunit and by three fragments (D, E, F) of the polypeptide chain of the other one on which these aromatic residues are located (see review [100]). The first three fragments in real receptors are on the α-subunits and form the main (principal) binding surface, while the last three are on non-α-subunits and compose the complementary binding surface. In the case of homopentameric receptors like α7 ones, the A-C loops are on the "front surface" of one α7-subunit and D-F on the "back surface" of the neighboring identical subunit. In general, the X-ray structure of the AChBP complex with α-cobratoxin is in accord with the earlier ideas on the α-neurotoxin binding to nAChRs formulated on the basis of chemical modification of α-neurotoxins, their mutagenesis, photoaffinity labeling and mutagenesis of receptors (see reviews [101,102]). Indeed, there is a multipoint binding of α-cobratoxin and the major role, as earlier shown by "wet biochemistry" methods, is played by the toxin central loop II.

The comparison with the NMR and X-ray structures for α-neurotoxins revealed that α-cobratoxin did not need to change its conformation dramatically to be accommodated in the binding region of AChBP. On the contrary, the AChBP loop C containing the disulfide between the neighboring cysteines (which is also a characteristic feature of all nAChR α-subunits) had to move to periphery up to 10 Å from the position which it occupied in the AChBP containing no bound ligand. (This movement should be supplemented with essential changes in conformation of loop F from complementary AChBP protomer.) Moreover, the earlier solved structure of AChBP with such agonist as nicotine revealed that, when agonist comes to the binding site, loop C embraces it and moves closer to the central axis of the molecule [94]. At present there are many crystal structures of various AChBPs in complexes with versatile specific or nonselective agonists and antagonists of the muscle-type and neuronal nAChRs and it appears to be a general rule: antagonists versus agonists induce movements of the loop C in the opposite directions.

5.1. X-ray structure of the extracellular domain of muscle nAChR $\alpha 1$ subunit in complex with α-bungarotoxin

Until now we were considering the X-ray and Electron microscopy structures of closely related but independent objects of studies: acetylcholine binding proteins and *Torpedo* nAChR. It should be emphasized that the structures of bound cholinergic agonists and antagonists until recently were available only for their complexes with AChBPs. That is why when researchers wished to analyze in three-dimensions the interactions of agonists or antagonists with the muscle-type or neuronal nAChRs, they had to rely on computer modeling. Fortunately, one of the bridges between the AChBPs and nAChRs spatial structures has been recently open: the X-ray structure has been determined for the α-bungarotoxin complex with heterologously expressed ligand-binding domain of mouse muscle nAChR $\alpha 1$ subunit [25]. Many laboratories have earlier tried, with the aid of heterologous expression, to obtain ligand-binding domains of $\alpha 1$ or $\alpha 7$ subunits as individual proteins and to determine their three-dimensional structure. Although in certain cases those proteins could bind α-bungarotoxin with relatively high affinity (but not with the nanomolar constants as intact receptors) [103-106], in no case the proteins could be crystallized. In view of the above-said, the work [25] is clearly a breakthrough. Using random mutagenesis, the authors have chosen a protein with a low tendency to aggregation. In spite of its having the mutation of Trp149 (localized in loop B and known to be important for binding agonists and antagonists), the protein could bind α-bungarotoxin. It was namely the complex of α-bungarotoxin rather than the free domain which was successfully crystallized. (Thus, in addition to helping isolate the *Torpedo* nAChR and *L.stagnalis* AChBP, α-neurotoxins played again an important role, this time in crystallization of the nAChR subunit ligand-binding domain.) The structure of the complex has been solved at a very high resolution (1.94 Å) (see Figure 3, B).

Although this domain is a monomer, its spatial structure is very similar to an AChBP protomer in a pentameric complex. A molecule of bound α-bungarotoxin occupies the position similar to that of α-cobratoxin in complex with *L. stagnalis* AChBP (compare Figure 3, A and B). It should be emphasized that in the complex with $\alpha 1$ domain, α-bungarotoxin utilized for interaction only the principal side, while α-cobratoxin in complex with pentameric AChBP has contacts with both principal and complementary sides at the subunit interface. However, instead of this, α-bungarotoxin forms contacts with the sugar moiety present in the nAChR domain but absent in AChBPs.

5.2. X-ray structure of α-bungarotoxin with a chimera of L. stagnalis AChBP/ligand-binding domain of the human $\alpha 7$ subunit

This work can be considered as a further development of the recent breakthrough in the analysis of ligand binding domains of nAChRs when an important step was done in ascending from models to true receptors. The authors of [107] managed to substitute about

http://dx.doi.org/10.5772/58240

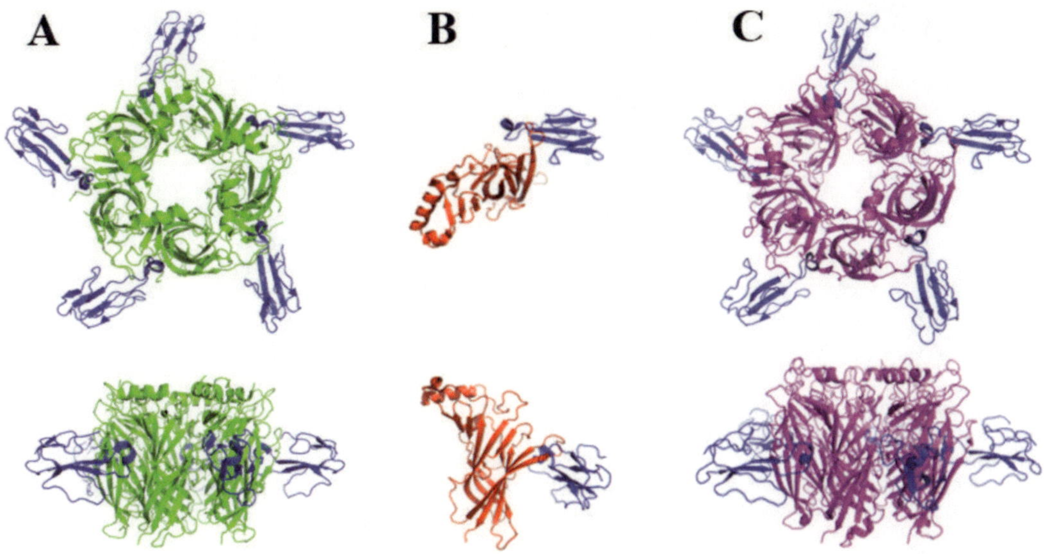

Figure 3. Crystal structures of the AChBP/nAChR domain-toxin complexes. Top and side views are in upper and lower lines, respectively. A - α-Cobratoxin bound to *L. stagnalis* AChBP (PDB ID: 1YI5); toxins and proteins are shown in blue and green. B – α-Bungarotoxin bound to the N-terminal domain of nAChR α1 subunit (2QC1); toxin and subunit are shown in blue and red; the sugar moiety presented in this complex were excluded for clarity. C - α-Bungarotoxin bound to the chimeric protein composed of N-terminal domain of nAChR α7 subunit and *L. stagnalis* AChBP (4HQP); toxins and chimeras are shown in blue and magenta.

70% of the amino-acid residues in *L. stagnalis*AChBP (not touching the less hydrophobic Cys-loop) for residues of the $\alpha 7$ subunit and crystallized this protein in free form and in complex with epibatidine, an potent but nonselective nAChR agonist[108]. The observed pentaoligomeric structure can be considered as the closest proximation to the 3D structure of the ligand-binding domain of the true $\alpha 7$ nAChR. Practically the same $\alpha 7$/AChBP chimera has been used to crystallize a complex with α-bungarotoxin [26]. Again, it was a pentaoligomer with 5 attached α-bungarotoxin molecules (see Figure 3, C). In general, disposition of α-bungarotoxin is very close to what was observed for α-bungarotoxin in complex with the $\alpha 1$ domain or for α-cobratoxin complex with the *L. stagnalis* AChBP (compare with Figure 3, B and A). Basing on the high-resolution structure of the $\alpha 7$/AChBP-α-bungarotoxin chimera, the authors designed a series of $\alpha 7$ nAChR mutants and from the analysis of their activities and efficiency of α-bungarotoxin binding collected a very detailed information about the intermolecular interactions which ensure the high affinity for α-bungarotoxin binding [26]. In particular, they not only confirmed the role of the "aromatic box", but also revealed the importance of amino-acid residues which in the amino acid sequence are direct neighbors of those aromatic residues.

5.3. X-ray structure structures of AChBP complexes with α-conotoxins

The first X-ray structure of the AChBP complex with α-conotoxin [109] has been solved soon after elucidation of the X-ray structure of the *L. stagnalis* AChBP complex with α-cobratoxin.

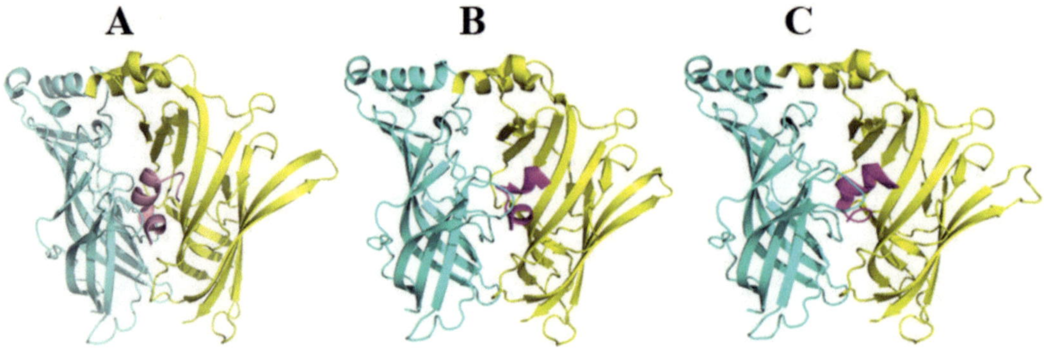

Figure 4. Spatial organization of complexes of α-conotoxins from different groups and *A. californica* AChBP derived from their crystal structures. Only two adjacent monomers of AChBP colored in cyan and yellow for clarity in side views are presented. All α-conotoxins are shown in magenta. A – complex with α-conotoxin PnIA[A10L, D14K] variant from 4/7 α-conotoxin group (PDB ID: 2BR8). B – complex with α-conotoxin ImI from 4/3 α-conotoxin group (2C9T). C - complex with α-conotoxin BuIA from 4/4 α-conotoxin group (4EZ1).

In this case it was another AChBP, namely the protein from the marine mollusk *Aplysia californica* [110]. First of all, contrary to the α-cobratoxin complex, it was a high-resolution (2.4 Å) structure and, secondly, it was the first X-ray structure for a representative of the huge conotoxin library in complex with a biological target. The crystals were raised for the complex of α-conotoxin PnIA analog having two substitutions ([A10L] and [D14K]) which had high affinity both for *L. stagnalis* and *A. californica* AChBPs and potently inhibited acetylcholine-induced currents in α7 nAChRs expressed in oocytes [109].

Hydrophobic contacts were found to play the major role in the interaction of α-conotoxin PnIA[A10L, D14K] with *A. californica* AChBP (Figure 4, A). As in other AChBP complexes with agonists or antagonists, at the principal side the contacts are formed mainly by highly conserved aromatic amino acid residues - Trp145, Tyr186, Tyr193. At the complementary side the contributions are from aliphatic residues (Val106, Met114, Ile116). It should be stressed again that loop C in the complex with α-conotoxin moves to the periphery of the AChBP molecule by more than 10 Å, as compared with its disposition in the "apo" form of *A. californica* AChBP. A similar shift was also observed, as mentioned above, for the α-cobratoxin complex [24], as well as for the majority of AChBP complexes with other antagonists (see reviews [98,111,112]). Thus, the conclusion that the most obvious distinction between the first steps in the binding modes of agonists versus antagonists is the induced movement of the loop C (to the central axis for the former and outwards for the latter) appears to be correct. However, there are some deviations from this trend: for example, strychnine is an antagonist both of the nAChRs and glycine receptors, but in the case of its complex with the *A. californica* AChBP, the loop C shift to the periphery was only very slight [113]. The changes in the disposition of the loop C were not pronounced also for AChBP complexes with partial agonists [96].

Another interesting feature of AChBP complexes was for the first time observed with partial agonists: in distinct binding sites within a pentameric AChBP molecule these compounds had different orientations [96]. Such multiplicity was first thought to be inherent only in partial agonists, but later altering dispositions in the 5 AChBP binding sites were observed for the complexes of such alkaloid antagonists as strychnine and d-tubocurarine [113]. Moreover, in several binding sites two alkaloid molecules managed to be accommodated simultaneously [113].

Variations of the ligand orientation in the binding sites of AChBPs and nAChRs are of undoubted interest. In the *A. californica* AChBP complex, all 5 bound α-conotoxin PnIA[A10L, D14K] molecules had the same conformation and orientation. This was also true for the later solved structures of α-conotoxin ImI complexes [114,115] (see Figure 4, B). These structures (very similar to those of α-conotoxin PnIA[A10L, D14K]) confirmed that, although bound α-conotoxin PnIA analog had two substitutions and was in this respect "unnatural α-conotoxin", the X-ray structure of its complex correctly revealed the structural principles of the α-conotoxin-AChBP recognition. Fine adjustments of such a recognition were brought to light by the structure of *A. californica* AChBP complex with the α-conotoxin TxIA[A10L] [116]. In general, the structure of this complex was very similar to those of α-conotoxin PnIA[A10L, D14K] or α-conotoxin ImI, but with a noticeable difference: this α-conotoxin derivative occupied exactly the same region as the two above-mentioned α-conotoxins, but it was turned around the central axis by about 20 degrees. The authors proposed that such rotation reflects certain differences in the selectivity of this particular α-conotoxin [116]. The latest published structure of the AChBP complex with α-conotoxin (November 2013) is announced by the Protein Data Bank (PDB) the structure with ID - 4EZ1. This is a complex of *A. californica* AChBP with α-conotoxin BuIA [117]. Despite the fact that α-conotoxin BuIA is a member of other subgroup of α-conotoxins (4/4) its position and orientation in the complex with AChBP (Figure 4, C) very close to that of both α-conotoxin PnIA analog (4/7 subgroup) and α-conotoxin ImI (4/3 subgroup) (compare Figure 4, A, B and C). In any case, from the four solved X-ray structures for AChBP complexes with α-conotoxins it followed that some variations in their attachment are possible. It might be expected that variations may be even more pronounced when α-conotoxins interact with true nAChRs, especially with heteroligomeric ones having different subunit interfaces.

Indeed, interpretation of the cross-linking of photoactivatable derivative of α-conotoxin GI to *Torpedo californica* nAChR in terms of the model built on the basis of the X-ray structure of the AChBP complex with α-conotoxin PnIA[A10L, D14K], suggested that for bound α-conotoxin two orientations are possible where the disposition of photoactivatable group differs by about 90 degrees [118]. Later a similar situation was demonstrated for an agonist, namely for the photoactivatable derivative of epibatidine [119]. This compound was shown to bind to only one site in the *T. californica* nAChR, but to 2 sites in the neuronal α4β2 nAChR which presumes two different dispositions of the bound ligand [119]. Naturally, cross-linking is not such a direct evidence as the X-ray structure, but the latter are available only for the AChBP complexes and the multiplicity of alkaloid antagonist orientations in the frames of one AChBP molecule [113] has been already mentioned.

6. Summary

In this chapter we tried to briefly present almost a 50-year history of using protein and peptide neurotoxins in fundamental and practical studies of nicotinic acetylcholine receptors (nAChRs). It was shown that the discovery of α-neurotoxins in the snake venoms was an extremely important step which made possible identification and isolation in individual form of the first nAChR from the *Torpedo* ray electric organ. Many laboratories comprehensively analyzed this receptor and it soon became clear that it is an appropriate model for nAChRs of all classes, namely muscle, neuronal and the so-called "non-neuronal" ones. Later, in addition to the three-finger α-neurotoxins, new shorter and smaller but not less efficient tools were found: namely, among a huge family of various peptides in the venoms of marine *Conus* mollusks, one particular group happened to be invaluable for research on nAChRs. Here we speak about α-conotoxins which not only discriminate the muscle-type from neuronal nAChRs, but some of them even are selective towards a particular neuronal nAChR subtype. One should not think that the discovery of α-conotoxins put the α-neurotoxins into archives. First of all, even to-day α-bungarotoxin and its radioactive and fluorescent derivatives are the most reliable tools for identification and measuring the levels of the functional α7 nAChRs. Secondly, α-neurotoxins played another leading role a decade ago helping to purify the acetylcholine-binding protein (AChBP). The discovery and the X-ray structure of this protein, an ideal model for the ligand-binding domains of all nAChRs, was the major breakthrough in elucidating the three-dimensional structure of nAChRs and especially of their ligand-binding site topography. Our chapter also presented the data on the crystal structures of AChBP complexes both with α-neurotoxins and α-conotoxins that gave information about the topography of their interactions with the key residues in the binding site, thus providing a basis for new drug design. The next step was the establishment of the crystal structures of α-neurotoxins with chimera of AChBP and α7 nAChR ligand-binding domain, which can be considered as a good mimic of the true α7 receptor, as well as the X-ray structure of the α-bungarotoxin complex with a mutated nAChR α1 subunit extracellular domain. In this chapter we were not discussing the bacterial pentameric ligand-gated ion channels (belonging to the same family as nAChRs), but at present not only high-resolution X-ray structures are available for them, but also for their complexes with different ligands. In particular, one of such receptors (ELIC) happened to be a close analog of the mammalian GABA-A receptors. We might hope that one day high resolution structures become available for nAChRs or their homologs in complexes with α-neurotoxins and/or α-conotoxins, to which the chapter is devoted. It will give new life to these still invaluable tools in fundamental research on nAChRs and in numerous practical applications.

Acknowledgements

The research was supported by RFBR grants and the grants of Presidium of RAS "Molecular and cellular biology" and "Fundamental principles of medicine".

Author details

Victor Tsetlin* and Igor Kasheverov

*Address all correspondence to: vits@mx.ibch.ru

Shemyakin-Ovchinnikov Institute of Bioorganic Chemistry, Russian Academy of Sciences, Moscow, Russian Federation

References

[1] Changeux JP. The nicotinic acetylcholine receptor: the founding father of the pentameric ligand-gated ion channel superfamily. Journal of Biological Chemistry 2012;287(48) 40207-40215.

[2] Kalamida D, Poulas K, Avramopoulou V, Fostieri E, Lagoumintzis G, Lazaridis K, Sideri A, Zouridakis M, Tzartos SJ. Muscle and neuronal nicotinic acetylcholine receptors. Structure, function and pathogenicity. FEBS Journal 2007;274(15) 3799-3845.

[3] Tsetlin V, Hucho F. Nicotinic acetylcholine receptors at atomic resolution. Current Opinion in Pharmacology 2009;9(3) 306-310.

[4] Sine SM, Engel AG. Recent advances in Cys-loop receptor structure and function. Nature 2006;440(7083) 448-455.

[5] Gershoni JM. Expression of the alpha-bungarotoxin binding site of the nicotinic acetylcholine receptor by Escherichia coli transformants. Proceedings of the National Academy of Sciences of the USA 1987;84(12) 4318-4321.

[6] Wilson PT, Hawrot E, Lentz TL. Distribution of alpha-bungarotoxin binding sites over residues 173-204 of the alpha subunit of the acetylcholine receptor. Molecular Pharmacology 1988;34(5) 643-650.

[7] Wessler I, Kirkpatrick CJ. Acetylcholine beyond neurons: the non-neuronal cholinergic system in humans. British Journal of Pharmacology 2008;154(8) 1558-1571.

[8] Fujii T, Takada-Takatori Y, Kawashima K. Basic and clinical aspects of non-neuronal acetylcholine: expression of an independent, non-neuronal cholinergic system in lymphocytes and its clinical significance in immunotherapy. Journal of Pharmacological Sciences 2008;106(2) 186-192.

[9] Picciotto MR, Kenny PJ. Molecular mechanisms underlying behaviors related to nicotine addiction. Cold Spring Harbor Perspectives in Medicine 2013;3(1) a012112. doi: 10.1101/cshperspect.a012112.

[10] Brejc K, van Dijk WJ, Klaassen RV, Schuurmans M, van Der Oost J, Smit AB, Sixma TK. Crystal structure of an ACh-binding protein reveals the ligand-binding domain of nicotinic receptors. Nature 2001;411(6835) 269-276.

[11] Hilf RJ, Dutzler R. X-ray structure of a prokaryotic pentameric ligand-gated ion channel. Nature 2008;452(7185) 375-379.

[12] Hilf RJ, Dutzler R. Structure of a potentially open state of a proton-activated pentameric ligand-gated ion channel. Nature 2009;457(7225) 115-118.

[13] Bocquet N, Nury H, Baaden M, Le Poupon C, Changeux JP, Delarue M, Corringer PJ. X-ray structure of a pentameric ligand-gated ion channel in an apparently open conformation. Nature 2009;457(7225) 111-114.

[14] Hibbs RE, Gouaux E. Principles of activation and permeation in an anion-selective Cys-loop receptor. Nature 2011;474(7349) 54-60.

[15] Chang CC. Looking back on the discovery of α-bungarotoxin. Journal of Biomedical Sciences 1999;6(6) 368-375.

[16] Tsetlin V. Snake venom α-neurotoxins and other 'three-finger' proteins. European Journal of Biochemistry 1999;264(2) 281-286.

[17] Kini RM, Doley R. Structure, function and evolution of three-finger toxins: mini proteins with multiple targets. Toxicon 2010;56(6) 855-867.

[18] Low BW, Preston HS, Sato A, Rosen LS, Searl JE, Rudko AD, Richardson JS. Three dimensional structure of erabutoxin b neurotoxic protein: inhibitor of acetylcholine receptor. Proceedings of the National Academy of Sciences of the USA 1976;73(9) 2991-2994.

[19] Tsernoglou D, Petsko GA. Three-dimensional structure of neurotoxin a from venom of the Philippines sea snake. Proceedings of the National Academy of Sciences of the USA 1977;74(3) 971-974.

[20] Love R, Stroud R. The crystal structure of α-bungarotoxin at 2.5 Å resolution: relation to solution structure and binding to acetylcholine receptor. Protein Engineering 1986;1(1) 37-46.

[21] Moise L, Piserchio A, Basus VJ, Hawrot E. NMR structural analysis of α-bungarotoxin and its complex with the principal α-neurotoxin-binding sequence on the α7 subunit of a neuronal nicotinic acetylcholine receptor. Journal of Biological Chemistry 2002;277(14) 12406-12417.

[22] Betzel C, Lange G, Pal GP, Wilson KS, Maelicke A, Saenger W. The refined crystal structure of alpha-cobratoxin from Naja naja siamensis at 2.4-Å resolution. Journal of Biological Chemistry 1991;266(32) 21530-21536.

[23] Nickitenko AV, Michailov AM, Betzel C, Wilson KS. Three-dimensional structure of neurotoxin-1 from Naja naja oxiana venom at 1.9 Å resolution. FEBS Letters 1993;320(2) 111-117.

[24] Bourne Y, Talley TT, Hansen SB, Taylor P, Marchot P.Crystal structure of a Cbtx-AChBP complex reveals essential interactions between snake alpha-neurotoxins and nicotinic receptors. EMBO Journal 2005;24(8) 1512-1522.

[25] Dellisanti CD, Yao Y, Stroud JC, Wang ZZ, Chen L. Crystal structure of the extracellular domain of nAChR alpha1 bound to alpha-bungarotoxin at 1.94 Å resolution. Nature Neuroscience 2007;10(8) 953-962.

[26] Huang S, Li SX, Bren N, Cheng K, Gomoto R, Chen L, Sine SM. Complex between α-bungarotoxin and an α7 nicotinic receptor ligand-binding domain chimaera. Biochemical Journal 2013;454(2) 303-310.

[27] Dewan JC, Grant GA, Sacchettini JC. Crystal structure of κ-bungarotoxin at 2.3-A resolution. Biochemistry 1994;33(44) 13147-13154.

[28] Chiappinelli VA, Weaver WR, McLane KE, Conti-Fine BM, Fiordalisi JJ, Grant GA. Binding of native κ-neurotoxins and site-directed mutants to nicotinic acetylcholine receptors. Toxicon 1996;34(11-12) 1243-1256.

[29] Servent D, Winckler-Dietrich V, Hu HY, Kessler P, Drevet P, Bertrand D, Ménez A. Only snake curaremimetic toxins with a fifth disulfide bond have high affinity for the neuronal α7 nicotinic receptor. Journal of Biological Chemistry 1997;272(39) 24279-24286.

[30] Grant GA, Luetje CW, Summers R, Xu XL. Differential roles for disulfide bonds in the structural integrity and biological activity of κ-bungarotoxin, a neuronal nicotinic acetylcholine receptor antagonist. Biochemistry 1998;37(35) 12166-12171.

[31] Mourier G, Servent D, Zinn-Justin S, Ménez A. Chemical engineering of a three-fingered toxin with anti-α7 neuronal acetylcholine receptor activity. Protein Engineering 2000;13(3) 217-225.

[32] Lyukmanova EN, Shenkarev ZO, Schulga AA, Ermolyuk YS, Mordvintsev DY, Utkin YN, Shoulepko MA, Hogg RC, Bertrand D, Dolgikh DA, Tsetlin VI, Kirpichnikov MP. Bacterial expression, NMR, and electrophysiology analysis of chimeric short/long-chain α-neurotoxins acting on neuronal nicotinic receptors. Journal of Biological Chemistry 2007;282(34) 24784-24791.

[33] Roy A, Zhou X, Chong MZ, D'hoedt D, Foo CS, Rajagopalan N, Nirthanan S, Bertrand D, Sivaraman J, Kini RM. Structural and functional characterization of a novel homodimeric three-finger neurotoxin from the venom of Ophiophagus hannah (king cobra). Journal of Biological Chemistry 2010;285(11) 8302-8315.

[34] Kukhtina VV, Weise C, Muranova TA, Starkov VG, Franke P, Hucho F, Wnendt S, Gillen C, Tsetlin VI, Utkin YN. Muscarinic toxin-like proteins from cobra venom. European Journal of Biochemistry 2000;267(23) 6784-6789.

[35] Osipov AV, Kasheverov IE, Makarova YV, Starkov VG, Vorontsova OV, Ziganshin RK, Andreeva TV, Serebryakova MV, Benoit A, Hogg RC, Bertrand D, Tsetlin VI, Utkin YN. Naturally occurring disulfide-bound dimers of three-fingered toxins: a paradigm for biological activity diversification. Journal of Biological Chemistry 2008;283(21) 14571-14580.

[36] Osipov AV, Rucktooa P, Kasheverov IE, Filkin SY, Starkov VG, Andreeva TV, Sixma TK, Bertrand D, Utkin YN, Tsetlin VI. Dimeric α-cobratoxin X-ray structure: localization of intermolecular disulfides and possible mode of binding to nicotinic acetylcholine receptors. Journal of Biological Chemistry 2012;287(9) 6725-6734.

[37] Pawlak J, Mackessy SP, Sixberry NM, Stura EA, Le Du MH, Ménez R, Foo CS, Ménez A, Nirthanan S, Kini RM. Irditoxin, a novel covalently linked heterodimeric three-finger toxin with high taxon-specific neurotoxicity. FASEB Journal 2009;23(2) 534-545.

[38] Nirthanan S, Gopalakrishnakone P, Gwee MC, Khoo HE, Kini RM. Non-conventional toxins from Elapid venoms. British Journal of Pharmacology 2003;139(4) 832-844.

[39] Utkin YN, Kukhtina VV, Kryukova EV, Chiodini F, Bertrand D, Methfessel C, Tsetlin VI. "Weak toxin" from Naja kaouthia is a nontoxic antagonist of α7 and muscle-type nicotinic acetylcholine receptors. Journal of Biological Chemistry 2001;276(19) 15810-15815.

[40] Nirthanan S, Charpantier E, Gopalakrishnakone P, Gwee MC, Khoo HE, Cheah LS, Bertrand D, Kini RM. Candoxin, a novel toxin from Bungarus candidus, is a reversible antagonist of muscle ($\alpha\beta\gamma\delta$) but a poorly reversible antagonist of neuronal α7 nicotinic acetylcholine receptors. Journal of Biological Chemistry 2002;277(20) 17811-17820.

[41] Pawlak J, Mackessy SP, Fry BG, Bhatia M, Mourier G, Fruchart-Gaillard C, Servent D, Ménez R, Stura E, Ménez A, Kini RM. Denmotoxin, a three-finger toxin from the colubrid snake Boiga dendrophila (Mangrove Catsnake) with bird-specific activity. Journal of Biological Chemistry 2006;281(39) 29030-29041.

[42] Mordvintsev DY, Rodionov DI, Makarova MV, Kamensky AA, Levitskaya NG, Ogay AY, Rzhevsky DI, Murashev AN, Tsetlin VI, Utkin YN. Behavioural effects in mice and intoxication symptomatology of weak neurotoxin from cobra Naja kaouthia. Basic and Clinical Pharmacology and Toxicology 2007;100(4) 273-278.

[43] Mordvintsev DY, Polyak YL, Rodionov DI, Jakubik J, Dolezal V, Karlsson E, Tsetlin VI, Utkin YN. Weak toxin WTX from Naja kaouthia cobra venom interacts with both nicotinic and muscarinic acetylcholine receptors. FEBS Journal 2009;276(18) 5065-5075.

[44] Ménez A. Functional architectures of animal toxins: a clue to drug design? Toxicon 1998;36(11) 1557-1572.

[45] Olianas MC, Adem A, Karlsson E, Onali P. Action of the muscarinic toxin MT7 on agonist-bound muscarinic M1 receptors. European Journal of Pharmacology 2004;487(1-3) 65-72.

[46] Marquer C, Fruchart-Gaillard C, Letellier G, Marcon E, Mourier G, Zinn-Justin S, Ménez A, Servent D, Gilquin B. Structural model of ligand-G protein-coupled receptor (GPCR) complex based on experimental double mutant cycle data: MT7 snake toxin bound to dimeric hM1 muscarinic receptor. Journal of Biological Chemistry 2011;286(36) 31661-31675.

[47] de Weille JR, Schweitz H, Maes P, Tartar A, Lazdunski M. Calciseptine, a peptide isolated from black mamba venom, is a specific blocker of the L-type calcium channel. Proceedings of the National Academy of Sciences of the USA 1991;88(6) 2437-2440.

[48] Albrand JP, Blackledge MJ, Pascaud F, Hollecker M, Marion D. NMR and restrained molecular dynamics study of the three-dimensional solution structure of toxin FS2, a specific blocker of the L-type calcium channel, isolated from black mamba venom. Biochemistry 1995;34(17) 5923-5937.

[49] Bourne Y, Taylor P, Marchot P. Acetylcholinesterase inhibition by fasciculin: crystal structure of the complex. Cell 1995;83(3) 503-512.

[50] Harel M, Kleywegt GJ, Ravelli RB, Silman I, Sussman JL. Crystal structure of an acetylcholinesterase-fasciculin complex: interaction of a three-fingered toxin from snake venom with its target. Structure 1995;3(12) 1355-1366.

[51] Kumar TK, Jayaraman G, Lee CS, Arunkumar AI, Sivaraman T, Samuel D, Yu C. Snake venom cardiotoxins-structure, dynamics, function and folding. Journal of Biomolecular Structure and Dynamics 1997;15(3) 431-463.

[52] Konshina AG, Dubovskii PV, Efremov RG. Structure and dynamics of cardiotoxins. Current Protein and Peptide Science 2012;13(6) 570-584.

[53] Osipov AV, Astapova MV, Tsetlin VI, Utkin YN. The first representative of glycosylated three-fingered toxins. Cytotoxin from the Naja kaouthia cobra venom. European Journal of Biochemistry 2004;271(10) 2018-2027.

[54] Quinton L, Girard E, Maiga A, Rekik M, Lluel P, Masuyer G, Larregola M, Marquer C, Ciolek J, Magnin T, Wagner R, Molgó J, Thai R, Fruchart-Gaillard C, Mourier G, Chamot-Rooke J, Ménez A, Palea S, Servent D, Gilles N. Isolation and pharmacological characterization of AdTx1, a natural peptide displaying specific insurmountable antagonism of the alpha1A-adrenoceptor. British Journal of Pharmacology 2010;159(2) 316-325.

[55] Maïga A, Mourier G, Quinton L, Rouget C, Gales C, Denis C, Lluel P, Sénard JM, Palea S, Servent D, Gilles N. G protein-coupled receptors, an unexploited animal toxin

targets: Exploration of green mamba venom for novel drug candidates active against adrenoceptors. Toxicon 2012;59(4) 487-496.

[56] Miwa JM, Ibanez-Tallon I, Crabtree GW, Sánchez R, Sali A, Role LW, Heintz N. Lynx1, an endogenous toxin-like modulator of nicotinic acetylcholine receptors in the mammalian CNS. Neuron 1999;23(1) 105-114.

[57] Adermann K, Wattler F, Wattler S, Heine G, Meyer M, Forssmann WG, Nehls M. Structural and phylogenetic characterization of human SLURP-1, the first secreted mammalian member of the Ly-6/uPAR protein superfamily. Protein Science 1999;8(4) 810-819.

[58] Miwa JM, Stevens TR, King SL, Caldarone BJ, Ibanez-Tallon I, Xiao C, Fitzsimonds RM, Pavlides C, Lester HA, Picciotto MR, Heintz N. The prototoxin lynx1 acts on nicotinic acetylcholine receptors to balance neuronal activity and survival in vivo. Neuron 2006;51(5) 587-600.

[59] Tekinay AB, Nong Y, Miwa JM, Lieberam I, Ibanez-Tallon I, Greengard P, Heintz N. A role for LYNX2 in anxiety-related behavior. Proc Natl Acad Sci U S A. 2009 Mar 17;106(11):4477-82.

[60] Lyukmanova EN, Shenkarev ZO, Shulepko MA, Mineev KS, D'Hoedt D, Kasheverov IE, Filkin SY, Krivolapova AP, Janickova H, Dolezal V, Dolgikh DA, Arseniev AS, Bertrand D, Tsetlin VI, Kirpichnikov MP. NMR structure and action on nicotinic acetylcholine receptors of water-soluble domain of human LYNX1. Journal of Biological Chemistry 2011;286(12) 10618-10627.

[61] Shulepko MA, Lyukmanova EN, Paramonov AS, Lobas AA, Shenkarev ZO, Kasheverov IE, Dolgikh DA, Tsetlin VI, Arseniev AS, Kirpichnikov MP. Human neuromodulator SLURP-1: bacterial expression, binding to muscle-type nicotinic acetylcholine receptor, secondary structure, and conformational heterogeneity in solution. Biochemistry (Moscow) 2013;78(2) 204-211.

[62] Lyukmanova EN, Shulepko MA, Buldakova SL, Kasheverov IE, Shenkarev ZO, Reshetnikov RV, Filkin SY, Kudryavtsev DS, Ojomoko LO, Kryukova EV, Dolgikh DA, Kirpichnikov MP, Bregestovski PD, Tsetlin VI. Water-soluble LYNX1 residues important for interaction with muscle-type and/or neuronal nicotinic receptors. Journal of Biological Chemistry 2013;288(22) 15888-15899.

[63] Thomsen MS, Cinar B, Jensen MM, Lyukmanova EN, Shulepko MA, Tsetlin V, Klein AB, Mikkelsen JD. Expression of the Ly-6 family proteins Lynx1 and Ly6H in the rat brain is compartmentalized, cell-type specific, and developmentally regulated. Brain Structure and Function 2013. doi 10.1007/s00429-013-0611-x.

[64] Weinstein SA, Schmidt JJ, Bernheimer AW, Smith LA. Characterization and amino acid sequences of two lethal peptides isolated from venom of Wagler's pit viper, Trimeresurus wagleri. Toxicon 1991;29(2) 227-236.

[65] Schmidt JJ, Weinstein SA, Smith LA. Molecular properties and structure-function relationships of lethal peptides from venom of Wagler's pit viper, Trimeresurus wagleri. Toxicon 1992;30(9) 1027-1036.

[66] Tsai MC, Hsieh WH, Smith LA, Lee CY. Effects of waglerin-I on neuromuscular transmission of mouse nerve-muscle preparations. Toxicon 1995;33(3) 363-371.

[67] McArdle JJ, Lentz TL, Witzemann V, Schwarz H, Weinstein SA, Schmidt JJ. Waglerin-1 selectively blocks the epsilon form of the muscle nicotinic acetylcholine receptor. Journal of Pharmacology and Experimental Therapeutics 1999;289(1) 543-550.

[68] Molles BE, Rezai P, Kline EF, McArdle JJ, Sine SM, Taylor P. Identification of residues at the α and ε subunit interfaces mediating species selectivity of Waglerin-1 for nicotinic acetylcholine receptors. Journal of Biological Chemistry 2002;277(7) 5433-5440.

[69] Molles BE, Tsigelny I, Nguyen PD, Gao SX, Sine SM, Taylor P. Residues in the ε subunit of the nicotinic acetylcholine receptor interact to confer selectivity of waglerin-1 for the α-ε subunit interface site. Biochemistry 2002;41(25) 7895-7906.

[70] Schmidt JJ, Weinstein SA. Structure-function studies of waglerin I, a lethal peptide from the venom of Wagler's pit viper, Trimeresurus wagleri. Toxicon 1995;33(8) 1043-1049.

[71] Utkin YN, Weise C, Kasheverov IE, Andreeva TV, Kryukova EV, Zhmak MN, Starkov VG, Hoang NA, Bertrand D, Ramerstorfer J, Sieghart W, Thompson AJ, Lummis SC, Tsetlin VI. Azemiopsin from Azemiops feae viper venom, a novel polypeptide ligand of nicotinic acetylcholine receptor. Journal of Biological Chemistry 2012;287(32) 27079-27086.

[72] Gray WR, Luque A, Olivera BM, Barrett J, Cruz LJ. Peptide toxins from Conus geographus venom. Journal of Biological Chemistry 1981;256(10) 4734-4740.

[73] Halai R, Craik DJ. Conotoxins: natural product drug leads. Natural Product Reports 2009;26(4) 526-536.

[74] Teichert RW, Olivera BM. Natural products and ion channel pharmacology. Future Medicinal Chemistry 2010;2(5) 731-444.

[75] Lewis RJ, Dutertre S, Vetter I, Christie MJ. Conus venom peptide pharmacology. Pharmacological Reviews 2012;64(2) 259-298.

[76] Kreienkamp HJ, Sine SM, Maeda RK, Taylor P. Glycosylation sites selectively interfere with α-toxin binding to the nicotinic acetylcholine receptor. Journal of Biological Chemistry 1994;269(11) 8108-8114.

[77] Groebe DR, Dumm JM, Levitan ES, Abramson SN. α-Conotoxins selectively inhibit one of the two acetylcholine binding sites of nicotinic receptors. Molecular Pharmacology 1995;48(1) 105-111.

[78] Utkin YN, Kobayashi Y, Hucho F, Tsetlin VI. Relationship between the binding sites for an α-conotoxin and snake venom neurotoxins in the nicotinic acetylcholine receptor from Torpedo californica. Toxicon 1994;32(9) 1153-1157.

[79] Hann RM, Pagán OR, Eterović VA. The α-conotoxins GI and MI distinguish between the nicotinic acetylcholine receptor agonist sites while SI does not. Biochemistry 1994;33(47) 14058-14063.

[80] Groebe DR, Gray WR, Abramson SN. Determinants involved in the affinity of α-conotoxins GI and SI for the muscle subtype of nicotinic acetylcholine receptors. Biochemistry 1997;36(21) 6469-6474.

[81] Hann RM, Pagan OR, Gregory LM, Jacome T, Eterovic VA. The 9-arginine residue of α-conotoxin GI is responsible for its selective high affinity for the $\alpha\gamma$ agonist site on the electric organ acetylcholine receptor. Biochemistry 1997;36(29) 9051-9056.

[82] Jacobsen RB, DelaCruz RG, Grose JH, McIntosh JM, Yoshikami D, Olivera BM. Critical residues influence the affinity and selectivity of α-conotoxin MI for nicotinic acetylcholine receptors. Biochemistry 1999;38(40) 13310-13315.

[83] Ellison M, Feng ZP, Park AJ, Zhang X, Olivera BM, McIntosh JM, Norton RS. α-RgIA, a novel conotoxin that blocks the $\alpha9\alpha10$ nAChR: structure and identification of key receptor-binding residues. Journal of Molecular Biology 2008;377(4) 1216-1227.

[84] Servent D, Thanh HL, Antil S, Bertrand D, Corringer PJ, Changeux JP, Ménez A. Functional determinants by which snake and cone snail toxins block the $\alpha7$ neuronal nicotinic acetylcholine receptors. Journal of Physiology-Paris 1998;92(2) 107-111.

[85] Hogg RC, Hopping G, Alewood PF, Adams DJ, Bertrand D. α-Conotoxins PnIA and [A10L]PnIA stabilize different states of the $\alpha7$-L247T nicotinic acetylcholine receptor. Journal of Biological Chemistry 2003;278(29) 26908-26914.

[86] Everhart D, Cartier GE, Malhotra A, Gomes AV, McIntosh JM, Luetje CW. Determinants of potency on α-conotoxin MII, a peptide antagonist of neuronal nicotinic receptors. Biochemistry 2004;43(10) 2732-2737.

[87] Millard EL, Nevin ST, Loughnan ML, Nicke A, Clark RJ, Alewood PF, Lewis RJ, Adams DJ, Craik DJ, Daly NL. Inhibition of neuronal nicotinic acetylcholine receptor subtypes by α-conotoxin GID and analogues. Journal of Biological Chemistry 2009;284(8) 4944-4951.

[88] Halai R, Clark RJ, Nevin ST, Jensen JE, Adams DJ, Craik DJ. Scanning mutagenesis of α-conotoxin Vc1.1 reveals residues crucial for activity at the $\alpha9\alpha10$ nicotinic acetylcholine receptor. Journal of Biological Chemistry 2009;284(30) 20275-20284.

[89] Grishin AA, Cuny H, Hung A, Clark RJ, Brust A, Akondi K, Alewood PF, Craik DJ, Adams DJ. Identifying key amino acid residues that affect α-conotoxin AuIB inhibition of $\alpha3\beta4$ nicotinic acetylcholine receptors. Journal of Biological Chemistry 2013. doi: 10.1074/jbc.M113.512582.

[90] Kasheverov IE, Utkin YN, Tsetlin VI. Naturally occurring and synthetic peptides acting on nicotinic acetylcholine receptors. Current Pharmaceutical Design 2009;15(21) 2430-2452.

[91] Armishaw CJ. Synthetic α-conotoxin mutants as probes for studying nicotinic acetylcholine receptors and in the development of novel drug leads. Toxins (Basel) 2010;2(6) 1471-1499.

[92] Muttenthaler M, Akondi KB, Alewood PF. Structure-activity studies on α-conotoxins. Current Pharmaceutical Design 2011;17(38) 4226-4241.

[93] Smit AB, Syed NI, Schaap D, van Minnen J, Klumperman J, Kits KS, Lodder H, van der Schors RC, van Elk R, Sorgedrager B, Brejc K, Sixma TK, Geraerts WP. A glia-derived acetylcholine-binding protein that modulates synaptic transmission. Nature 2001;411(6835) 261-268.

[94] Celie PH, van Rossum-Fikkert SE, van Dijk WJ, Brejc K, Smit AB, Sixma TK. Nicotine and carbamylcholine binding to nicotinic acetylcholine receptors as studied in AChBP crystal structures. Neuron 2004;41(6) 907-914.

[95] Ulens C, Akdemir A, Jongejan A, van Elk R, Bertrand S, Perrakis A, Leurs R, Smit AB, Sixma TK, Bertrand D, de Esch IJ. Use of acetylcholine binding protein in the search for novel α7 nicotinic receptor ligands. In silico docking, pharmacological screening, and X-ray analysis. Journal of Medicinal Chemistry 2009;52(8) 2372-2383.

[96] Hibbs RE, Sulzenbacher G, Shi J, Talley TT, Conrod S, Kem WR, Taylor P, Marchot P, Bourne Y. Structural determinants for interaction of partial agonists with acetylcholine binding protein and neuronal α7 nicotinic acetylcholine receptor. EMBO Journal 2009;28(19) 3040-3051.

[97] Akdemir A, Rucktooa P, Jongejan A, Elk Rv, Bertrand S, Sixma TK, Bertrand D, Smit AB, Leurs R, de Graaf C, de Esch IJ. Acetylcholine binding protein (AChBP) as template for hierarchical in silico screening procedures to identify structurally novel ligands for the nicotinic receptors. Bioorganic and Medicinal Chemistry 2011;19(20) 6107-6119.

[98] Rucktooa P, Smit AB, Sixma TK. Insight in nAChR subtype selectivity from AChBP crystal structures. Biochemical Pharmacology 2009;78(7) 777-787.

[99] Yakel JL. Gating of nicotinic ACh receptors: latest insights into ligand binding and function. Journal of Physiology 2010;588(Pt 4) 597-602.

[100] [100] Hucho F, Tsetlin VI, Machold J. The emerging three-dimensional structure of a receptor. The nicotinic acetylcholine receptor. European Journal of Biochemistry 1996;239(3) 539-557.

[101] Fruchart-Gaillard C, Gilquin B, Antil-Delbeke S, Le Novere N, Tamiya T, Corringer PJ, Changeux JP, Menez A, Servent D. Experimentally based model of a complex be-

tween a snake toxin and the $\alpha7$ nicotinic receptor. Proceedings of the National Academy of Sciences of the USA 2002;99(5) 3216-3221.

[102] Tsetlin VI, Hucho F. Snake and snail toxins acting on nicotinic acetylcholine receptors: fundamental aspects and medical applications. FEBS Letters 2004;557(1-3) 9-13.

[103] Gershoni JM, Hawrot E, Lentz TL. Binding of α-bungarotoxin to isolated α subunit of the acetylcholine receptor of Torpedo californica: quantitative analysis with protein blots. Proceedings of the National Academy of Sciences of the USA 1983;80(16) 4973-4977.

[104] Schrattenholz A, Pfeiffer S, Pejovic V, Rudolph R, Godovac-Zimmermann J, Maelicke A. Expression and renaturation of the N-terminal extracellular domain of Torpedo nicotinic acetylcholine receptor α-subunit. Journal of Biological Chemistry 1998;273(49) 32393-32399.

[105] Tsetlin VI, Dergousova NI, Azeeva EA, Kryukova EV, Kudelina IA, Shibanova ED, Kasheverov IE, Methfessel C. Refolding of the Escherichia coli expressed extracellular domain of $\alpha7$ nicotinic acetylcholine receptor (Cys116 mutation diminishes aggregation and stabilizes the β structure). European Journal of Biochemistry 2002;269(11) 2801-2809.

[106] Zouridakis M, Zisimopoulou P, Eliopoulos E, Poulas K, Tzartos SJ. Design and expression of human $\alpha7$ nicotinic acetylcholine receptor extracellular domain mutants with enhanced solubility and ligand-binding properties. Biochimica et Biophysica Acta 2009;1794(2) 355-366.

[107] Li SX, Huang S, Bren N, Noridomi K, Dellisanti CD, Sine SM, Chen L. Ligand-binding domain of an $\alpha7$-nicotinic receptor chimera and its complex with agonist. Nature Neuroscience 2011;14(10) 1253-1259.

[108] Dukat M, Glennon RA. Epibatidine: impact on nicotinic receptor research. Cellular and Molecular Neurobiology 2003;23(3) 365-378.

[109] Celie PH, Kasheverov IE, Mordvintsev DY, Hogg RC, van Nierop P, van Elk R, van Rossum-Fikkert SE, Zhmak MN, Bertrand D, Tsetlin V, Sixma TK, Smit AB. Crystal structure of nicotinic acetylcholine receptor homolog AChBP in complex with an α-conotoxin PnIA variant. Nature Structural and Molecular Biology 2005;12(7) 582-588.

[110] Hansen SB, Talley TT, Radic Z, Taylor P. Structural and ligand recognition characteristics of an acetylcholine-binding protein from Aplysia californica. Journal of Biological Chemistry 2004;279(23) 24197-24202.

[111] Dutertre S, Lewis RJ. Toxin insights into nicotinic acetylcholine receptors. Biochemical Pharmacology 2006;72(6) 661-670.

[112] Tsetlin V, Utkin Y, Kasheverov I. Polypeptide and peptide toxins, magnifying lenses for binding sites in nicotinic acetylcholine receptors. Biochemical Pharmacology 2009;78(7) 720-731.

[113] Brams M, Pandya A, Kuzmin D, van Elk R, Krijnen L, Yakel JL, Tsetlin V, Smit AB, Ulens C. A structural and mutagenic blueprint for molecular recognition of strychnine and d-tubocurarine by different cys-loop receptors. PLoS Biology 2011;9(3) e1001034.

[114] Hansen SB, Sulzenbacher G, Huxford T, Marchot P, Taylor P, Bourne Y. Structures of Aplysia AChBP complexes with nicotinic agonists and antagonists reveal distinctive binding interfaces and conformations. EMBO Journal 2005;24(20) 3635-46.

[115] Ulens C, Hogg RC, Celie PH, Bertrand D, Tsetlin V, Smit AB, Sixma TK. Structural determinants of selective α-conotoxin binding to a nicotinic acetylcholine receptor homolog AChBP. Proceedings of the National Academy of Sciences of the USA 2006;103(10) 3615-3620.

[116] Dutertre S, Ulens C, Büttner R, Fish A, van Elk R, Kendel Y, Hopping G, Alewood PF, Schroeder C, Nicke A, Smit AB, Sixma TK, Lewis RJ. AChBP-targeted α-conotoxin correlates distinct binding orientations with nAChR subtype selectivity. EMBO Journal 2007;26(16) 3858-3867.

[117] Talley TT, Reger AS, Kim C, Sankaran B, Ho K, Taylor P, McIntosh J.M. Crystal structure of acetylcholine binding protein (AChBP) from Aplysia Californica in complex with α-conotoxin BuIA. 2013. doi: 10.2210/pdb4ez1/pdb.

[118] Kasheverov IE, Chiara DC, Zhmak MN, Maslennikov IV, Pashkov VS, Arseniev AS, Utkin YN, Cohen JB, Tsetlin VI. α-Conotoxin GI benzoylphenylalanine derivatives. ^{1}H-NMR structures and photoaffinity labeling of the Torpedo californica nicotinic acetylcholine receptor. FEBS Journal 2006;273(7) 1373-1388.

[119] Srivastava S, Hamouda AK, Pandhare A, Duddempudi PK, Sanghvi M, Cohen JB, Blanton MP. [(3)H]Epibatidine photolabels non-equivalent amino acids in the agonist binding site of Torpedo and α4β2 nicotinic acetylcholine receptors. Journal of Biological Chemistry 2009;284(37) 24939-24947.

Synaptic Soluble and Membrane-Bound Choline Acetyltransferase as a Marker of Cholinergic Function In Vitro and In Vivo

E.I. Zakharova and A.M. Dudchenko

Additional information is available at the end of the chapter

http://dx.doi.org/10.5772/58307

1. Introduction

1.1. Synaptosomes — Definition, a bit of history

The synaptosome is the presynaptic part of the nerve ending with, as a rule, a postsynaptic membrane in the region of the junction of the pre- and postsynaptic membranes that remains with the presynapse during homogenization and centrifugation. The presynaptic part of the synaptosome is a membrane-bound structure with a preserved cytoplasm (synaptoplasm), synaptic vesicles, mitochondria and some other cellular components. The term *synaptosome* was adopted by V.P. Whittaker and coworkers [1]. Together, V.P. Whittaker and C.O. Hebb first isolated and identified nerve endings in nervous tissue [2].

Subcellular fractionation emerged in the 1930s and 1940s and has since established itself as a major technique in experimental biology. The first attempts at the fractionation of nervous tissue were made in the early 1950s. A few years later, the fraction of synaptosomes was successful, using discontinuous sucrose-density gradient centrifugation [2-4]. After this, researchers achieved the preparation of the synaptic components, including the synaptic membranes, synaptoplasm, synaptic vesicles [1, 5, 6] (Figure 1) and membrane junction complex [7, 8]. These studies were a powerful impetus for investigations into the biochemistry of synapses and in the development of new methods of synaptic fractionation. Synaptosomes, as nerve endings, are heterogeneous in density, size and mediator specificity. Therefore, a number of the methods were developed for separating the synaptosomal fraction into two fractions [4], as well as into many fractions using a continuous sucrose-density linear gradient [9-11]. Among the many publications at this time, two books stand out. In the first one, D.J. Jones recounts the story of subcellular fractionation techniques, and presents the entire set of modern synaptic and subsynaptic fractionation techniques and data about the ultrastructure of synaptosomes and synaptic components, their sedimentary characteristics and biomarkers [12]. In the second one, R.N. Glebov is focused on the achievements of that time in the field of the functional neurochemistry of synapses, their molecular structure as well as on the metabolism and biochemistry of "classic" neurotransmitters and on the concepts of mediator secretion [13].

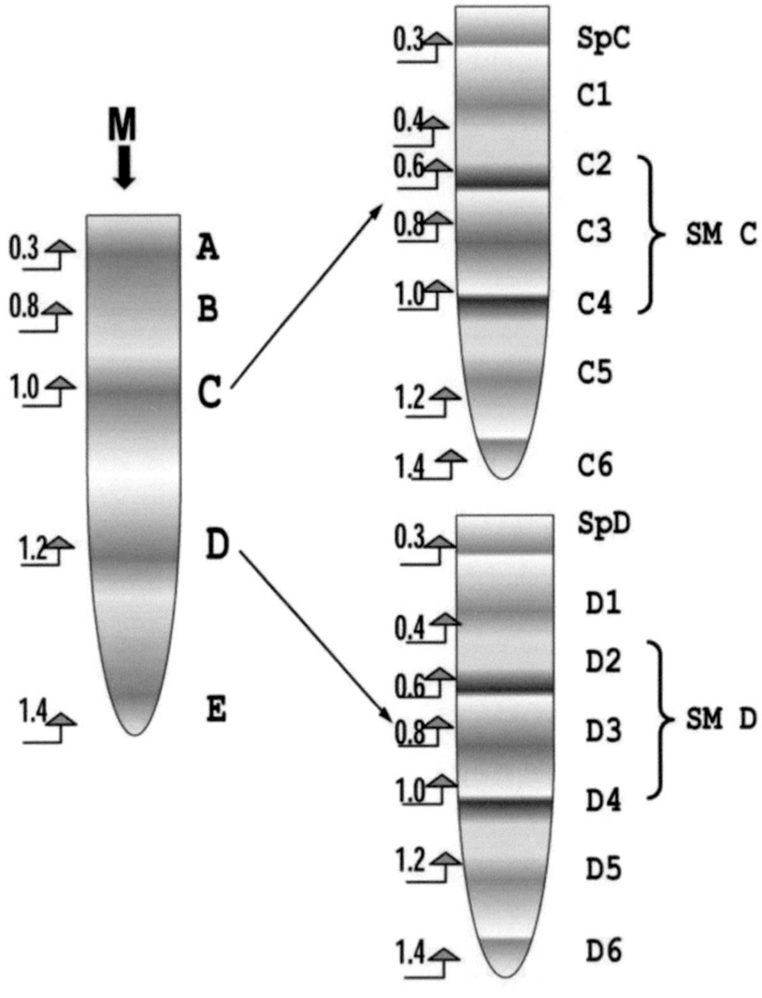

To the left of the tubes are marked the density of sucrose layers (in moles). Fractions obtained from crude mitochondrion fraction (by the method of De Robertis et al., 1962): myelin (A), neuronal and glial membrane and possibly small synaptosomes (B), light (C) and heavy (D) synaptosomes, cell mitochondria (E). Subsynaptic fractions obtained from light and heavy synaptosomes fractions (by the method of Whittaker et al., 1964): synaptoplasm (Sp), synaptic vesicles (1), synaptic membranes (2, 3, 4), non-disrupted synaptosomes (5), synaptic mitochondria (6).

Figure 1. Scheme of distribution of the fractions and subfractions of synaptosomes in discontinuous sucrose-density gradients.

2. Synaptosomes as an object of study in vitro and in vivo

Since these techniques were developed, new technologies in brain research have emerged. However, synaptosomes and their components remain a unique object of study. The reasons for this are as follows:

- the synapse is a unique structure specialized in the chemical transmission of nerve signals (chemical synapses are mainly in the mammalian brain).
- the synapse is always at the center of concepts about the adaptive properties of nervous tissue, such as learning and memory.
- the synapse is the most dynamic and labile structure of the nerve cell, and is an indicator of the reaction of the neuron to external stimuli.
- the synapse is an inherent structure of the neuron only.

It is now known that neurotransmitters and their key metabolic enzymes exist in some non-neuronal mammalian and human cells, including some cells of the neuroglia and vascular endothelium, epithelium and blood. In these cells, neurotransmitters perform specialized functions such as proliferation, differentiation, migration, organization of the cytoskeleton, cell-cell contact, secretion and transport of ions and water, blood-brain barrier maintenance and anti-inflammatory functions [14-17]. So, synaptomoses are the only object of molecular and biochemical studies that guarantees the investigation of neuronal function. Therefore, new technologies for the isolation of synaptosomes and their components continue to be developed, consistent with the purpose of science [18-20].

Using synaptosomes, one may study in vitro the molecular mechanisms of neurotransmitter secretion and the metabolism of neurotransmitter systems using the entire complexity of the molecular processes or using models of functional or pathological conditions in vitro and ex vivo.

Studies on synaptosomes in vivo are rarer but they are not less important. The brain is a very complicated organ in which a neuron exists in a permanent relationship with many other neurons. These interactions occur mainly through synapses. It is important not to forget about the signaling molecules that come into the brain through the blood, cerebrospinal fluid and intracellular matrix. The functional response of presynapses reflects the integrated response of the neuron to a stimulus. Therefore, it is important to know whether the patterns of synaptic functions are identical in vitro and in vivo.

In vivo models are used to investigate effects on the entire organism such as learning models and models of adapting and neuropathology. Then, the synaptosomes or subsynaptic components from the brain structures can be isolated. It is usually impossible to analyze the totality of the synaptic molecular and metabolic processes in these studies. The synaptic reaction is measured by the synaptic key indicators identified in studies in vitro. It is important that the biochemical methods allow the estimation of very fine metabolic and functional changes in synapses. The connection between nervous system function and synaptic processes has been investigated this way. It is possible to research the reaction of certain brain structures and even certain neuronal populations to external influences. Using neuromediators as markers, one can identify the participation of neuromediator systems in the mechanisms of various brain functions.

Furthermore, the in vivo study of synaptosomes has additional scope. Using biochemical parameters, not only metabolic changes can be evaluated, but also quantitative (synaptogenesis, reduction, degeneration) and morpho-structural (transformation) reorganizations in the synaptic pool. This is possible in comparative studies on the synaptic membrane and synaptoplasm subfractions. Subfractions of synaptic membranes and the synaptoplasm are the largest integral parts of the presynapse. Therefore, a correlation between the biochemical membrane (m) and cytosolic (c) biochemical parameters may reflect the reaction of the presynapse as a structural unit.

3. Natural markers of the neuronal systems

Neurotransmitters and some molecules of neurotransmitter metabolism are used as neuronal markers. These are natural indicators of functionally specialized brain systems, given to us by nature. Therefore, neuronal markers are widely used in biochemical studies, both in vitro and in vivo.

Neurotransmitter systems are named based on the main transmitter (glutamatergic, GABAergic, dopaminergic, etc.). Each mediator system consists of several neuronal populations. The neuronal populations in the brain are distributed topographically. Depending on the locus in the brain, neurons form specific neuronal connections using a specific combination of receptors. Moreover, these neurons can have specific metabolism dependent on their functional destination. Therefore, topography determines their metabolic and functional effects. Additionally, different neuronal populations often express comediators. These comediators influence the effects of mediators and metabolic pathways of the neuron in certain ways. It seems that future prospects in the study of brain function will be the investigation of the functional, metabolic and molecular features of distinct neuronal populations. It is necessary to understand the true mechanisms of the regulation, maintenance and recovery of brain functions. It should be noted that studies on synaptic fraction levels were carried out along these lines from the beginning [4, 18, 21-31].

In particular, regarding the cholinergic brain system, studies on this neurotransmitter system have been performed on synaptic fractions in vitro and in vivo. This review will present data from investigations into the molecular properties and metabolic and functional characteristics of cytosolic (c) and membrane-bound (m) choline acetyltransferase (ChAT) and of the use of cChAT and mChAT as cholinergic markers to establish brain function mechanisms. For the sake of completeness regarding modern notion, the characteristics of the molecular forms of ChAT will be presented using data from tissue cultures as well.

But first, a brief description of the cholinergic brain system.

4. Cholinergic brain system, cholinergic neuronal populations and their importance in health and disease

Cholinergic neurons use the classical neurotransmitter acetylcholine (ACh). ACh is a famous mediator. It was the first neurotransmitter discovered, by Otto Loewy in 1921-1926, and it proved the validity of the chemical nature of nervous communication [32]. ACh was quantified in P. Fatt's and B. Katz's experiments when the quantum nature of chemical neurotransmission was discovered [33]. S.O. Hebb and V.P. Whittaker used ACh and ChAT as indicators when they searched for and found subneuronal structures (synaptosomes) which accumulate mediators [2]. ACh was the first among the neuromediators found in the non-neuronal cells of mammals [34]. It would perhaps be helpful to add that ACh is also called "gentleman number one", for its non-neuronal function as well. It is clear that ACh is the most thoroughly examined neurotransmitter.

4.1. Metabolism of acetylcholine

ACh is an ester of acetic acid and choline with the chemical formula $CH_3COO(CH_2)_2N+(CH_3)_3$ and systematic name 2-acetoxy-N,N,N-trimethylethanaminium.The cycle of ACh synthesis, storage, release and degradation has been well-characterized at the cellular and molecular levels [26, 35, 36]. Briefly (Figure 2), ACh is synthesized in the cytoplasm of cholinergic neurons from the precursors choline and acetyl-coenzyme A by the enzyme choline acetyltransferase (ChAT), and is then taken up into synaptic vesicles for storage by the vesicular acetylcholine transporter (VAChT). Depolarization of the nerve terminal causes the fusion of synaptic vesicles with the presynaptic membrane at specialized release sites called active zones (named the junction complex in the subsynaptic fraction). Depositing and releasing ACh is a calcium-dependent process that involves the coordinated actions of many presynaptic proteins [26, 37]. When vesicles are linked up with the presynaptic membrane, ACh diffuses into the synaptic cleft where it can bind to subtypes of nicotinic and muscarinic receptors located on both post- and presynaptic membranes. ACh signaling is terminated by its diffusion away from the synaptic cleft and by its rapid hydrolysis into choline and acetate by acetylcholinesterase (AChE). The choline derived from ACh hydrolysis is recycled into the presynaptic terminal by the sodium-dependent high-affinity choline transporter (CHT) for resynthesis of ACh. After secretion of ACh, synaptic vesicles are recycled and are refilled with the neurotransmitter for another round of the depolarization-induced release. It should be noted that the details of the molecular mechanism of the regulation of these processes in both health and disease are lacking.

4.2. Topography and functions of cholinergic neuronal populations

Knowledge of the topography of mediator systems is basic for neurobiologists. The topography of the populations of cholinergic neurons and their projections has been studied in detail. ChAT has long been used as a marker of cholinergic structures in immunohistochemical studies. Initially, AChE was used as the cholinergic marker, but it was found that AChE coincides with ChAT only partially [38]. Later, colocalization of AChE was revealed in non-

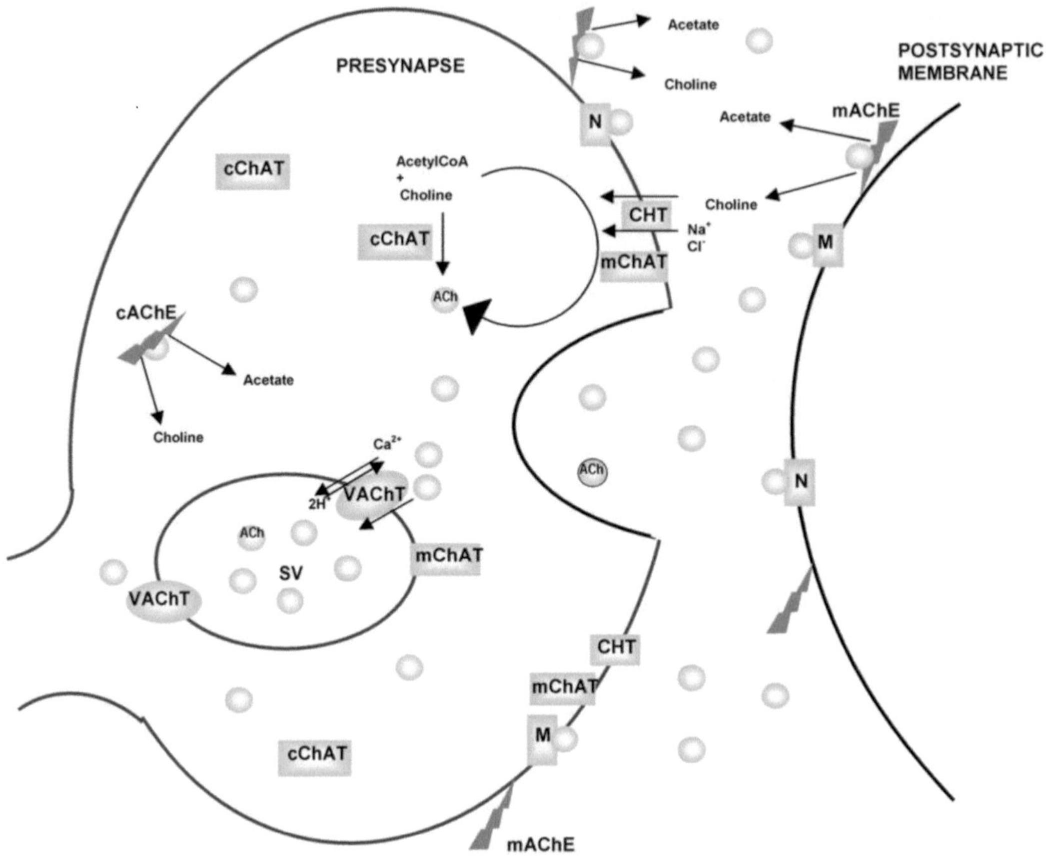

The idea of the scheme is taken from Black and Rylett [Black & Rylett, 2011]. Abbreviations: Presynapse, presynaptic part of nerve ending; SV, synaptic vesicle; ACh, acetylcholine; AcetylCo-A, acetylCoenzyme-A; cChAT and mChAT, cytoplasmic and membrane-bound choline acetyltransferase correspondingly; mAChE and cAChE, membrane-bound (extracellular isoform) and cytoplasmic acetylcholinesterase correspondingly; CHT, sodium-dependent, high-affinity choline transporter; M, muscarinic receptor; N, nicotinic receptor; VAChT, vesicular ACh transporter.
Some details of molecular mechanisms of the regulation of these processes are set out in sub-chapter 4.1.

Figure 2. Mechanisms involved in the synthesis, storage, release and degradation of ACh at the cholinergic synapse.

cholinergic neurons. For example, 36% of AChE-positive cells are GABA-immunoreactive [39]. VAChT, discovered after ChAT, is also used as a marker [40]. However, some discrepancies between VAChT and ChAT have been found [41].

Cholinergic neurons innervate almost all areas of the nervous system, both the central and peripheral systems. These areas can be innervated by either extrinsic projective neurons or by intrinsic interneurons. A very famous and major group of cholinergic projective neurons is found in the basal forebrain, which is comprised the nucleus basalis magnocellularis, also called the Meynert nucleus in primates and humans (a large bundle of cholinergic neurons encompassing the magnocellular preoptic nucleus, substantia innominata and globus pallidus), the medial septal nucleus and the vertical limb nucleus of the diagonal band of Broca.

The cortex, amygdaloid complex, hippocampus and olfactory bulb receive their cholinergic innervation principally from cholinergic projection neurons of the basal forebrain [40-49]. It is known that basal forebrain cholinergic projective neurons play a role in attention, learning, memory and consciousness. Another group of cholinergic projective neurons is found in the upper brainstem, which is comprised the pedunculopontine nucleus of the pontomesencephalic reticular formation and within the laterodorsal tegmental gray of the periventricular area. The thalamus and medulla receive their cholinergic innervation principally from cholinergic projection neurons of these brainstem nuclei. These neurons also present a minor component of the corticopetal cholinergic innervation of the frontal and visual cortical areas [43, 49-51]. The cholinergic projective neurons of the mesopontine region play a role in the primary treatment of some sensory information and memory (in the thalamus) and, hypothetically, in the central mechanisms regulating respiration and blood circulation (in the medulla). All immunohistochemical studies indicate the topographical arrangement of cholinergic projections. On the basis of connectivity patterns, M.M. Mesulam and coworkers proposed that the central cholinergic projective neurons to subdivide into six major sectors designated Ch1-Ch6 [43]. Moreover, the rostrocaudal and layerwise topographical arrangement of the cholinergic projections is indicated in the cerebral cortex [44-46, 48].

The most famous cholinergic interneurons are localized in the striatum, and they are involved in motor function and cognition [49]. As well, cholinergic interneurons have been detected in the cerebral cortex [46, 48, 52] and in the hippocampus [53-55]. Cortical and hippocampal interneurons perform associative functions and are presumably involved in learning and memory. Numerous electrophysiological studies have indicated this, but regarding cholinergic cortical and hippocampal neurons, such data are absent. In the human cerebral cortex, ChAT-immunoreactivity was found in some of the giant Betz and Meynert's pyramidal neurons [56].Cortical pyramidal neurons carry out motor functions. The medullar reticular formation has ChAT-positive neurons and their participation in the respiratory center is assumed [50].

Finally, ACh as a neurotransmitter is widely presented in the peripheral nerve system [40, 49, 57]. Acetylcholine is one of many neurotransmitters in the autonomic nervous system and is the only neurotransmitter used in the motor division of the somatic nervous system. The parasympathetic motoneurons of as the cranial nuclei of the caudal brainstem and postganglionic neurons and preganglionic sympathetic motoneurons of the spinal cord nuclei are ChAT- and VAChT-positive. Their efferents innervate all vegetative organs and glands, parasympathetic directly and sympathetic indirectly. ChAT- and VAChT-immunoreactivity has also been detected in the cell bodies of the spinal nerve motor neurons as well as in their axons and the endplates of the skeletal muscles.

It was found recently that the vagus (parasympathetic) nerve, involved in the control of heart rate, bronchomotor tone, hormone secretion and gastrointestinal motility, is also an immunomodulator. Its stimulation attenuates the production of proinflammatory cytokines and inhibits the inflammatory process via the $\alpha 7$ nicotinic acetylcholine receptor [58, 59]. It is possible that these studies are beginning to describe a new function of the cholinergic nerve system.

4.3. Comediators and other neuroactive components in some cholinergic neuronal populations

The functional effects of ACh are unique to each cholinergic population due to its targets and chemical composition. As a whole, ACh functions more often as a modulator in the central nervous system and as a mediator in the peripheral nervous system. Some populations of cholinergic neurons co-express vasoactive intestinal peptide (VIP) or/and nitric oxide (NO) or substance P. VIP has been found in cholinergic interneurons of the cortex [48, 60, 61] and in the parasympathetic efferents to the airways [62, 63]. Substance P is present in the majority of projections to the medial frontal cortex from ChAT-positive neurons in the midbrain [48]. ChAT-VIP-, NO synthase-ChAT- and NO synthase-ChAT-VIP-immunoreactive ganglionic cells have been detected in the sphenopalatine ganglia [64, 65].

All three substances as well as ACh are well-known vasodilators. Therefore, their co-localization with ACh is connected in the first place with blood flow regulation. The vasodilator action of ACh on the vessels of the vegetative organs was one of its first described effects [66]. With respect to cerebral vessels, it was detected in (1) direct contacts with small cortical vessels with vasodilator effects of the cholinergic projective neurons and interneurons, including ACh-VIP-containing interneurons [61, 67-69]; (2) ACh-, NO-ACh- and rarely ACh-VIP- containing fibers innervate the middle cerebral arteries composed of perivascular nerves of the sphenopalatine ganglia [64]; (3) ACh induces both direct vasodilation and atypical constriction in the internal cerebral arteries [64, 70, 71]; (4) brainstem ACh indirectly induces, via the stimulation of the dorsal facial area neurons of the medulla, a vasodilator effect in the common carotid and the internal cerebral arteries [72, 73].

The third vesicular glutamate transporter (VGLUT3) is present in a subset of cholinergic projective neurons in the basal forebrain and in cholinergic interneurons in the striatum [74]. It should be noted that both these cholinergic populations have similar large neurons. VGLUT3 is one of three transporter isoforms that fills synaptic vesicles with glutamate; however, VGLUT3 is also expressed in neurons and brain regions that were not previously thought to use glutamate as a neurotransmitter. It is possible that VGLUT3, because of its ionic balance, helps to load synaptic vesicles with ACh. In addition, the cholinergic projective neurons of the basal forebrain express the nerve growth factor (NGF) receptor [75, 76]. Basal forebrain neurons are trophically responsive to NGF. Neurotrophin is important for the development and maintenance of the basal forebrain cholinergic phenotype. In these neurons, NGF markedly increases ACh synthesis, content and release [77, 78].

4.4. Cholinergic functions and brain diseases

The brain cholinergic system is of permanent interest for neuroscientists because of its important role in cognitive, attention and motor functions. Dysfunction of cholinergic neurotransmission in the central nervous system is revealed in a number of neurological disorders. Dysfunction and degeneration of the cortical and hippocampal cholinergic projections from the basal forebrain nuclei is the basis of the pathogenesis of diseases such as Alzheimer's disease and Lewy body dementia, as well as diseases with other etiologies such as schizophrenia, Parkinson's disease and cerebral ischemia, in some cases aggravated by cognitive impairment [79-88]. The leading role of cholinergic afferent dysfunction in the development of ischemic pathology was suggested by data on the sensitivity of cortical and hippocampal cholinergic projections to ischemic exposure and a correlation between the development of cholinergic dysfunction, the delayed death of pyramidal neurons and cognitive impairments in rodents [89-91]. Dysfunction of cholinergic interneurons of the striatum is partly responsible for involuntary movements in Harrington's disease [80, 92]. Low expression of ChAT in the cholinergic neurons of the motor nuclei of the spinal cord is a specific early sign of amyotrophic lateral sclerosis [80, 92]. Multiple abnormalities in cholinergic function in the motor nuclei of the spinal cord a responsible for congenital myasthenic syndrome [93].

4.4.1. Synaptic soluble and membrane-bound choline acetyltransferase and their participation in cholinergic function in vitro and in vivo

Choline acetyltransferase (ChAT, E.C. 2.3.1.6) is a key enzyme in ACh synthesis and a marker of cholinergic neurons. It catalyzes the transfer of an acetyl group from acetyl-CoA to choline to form ACh. Studies in recent decades have revealed (1) the significant role of ChAT in the regulation of ACh synthesis and secretion and (2) that disturbances in the catalytic properties of ChAT may be the origin of some neuropathologies.

5. Forms of ChAT

It has been shown that ChAT has both a hydrophilic (cChAT) and hydrophobic state (stationary mChAT) in nerve endings. It has also been shown that ChAT is able to translocate from the cytosol to the synaptic membrane and to turn reversibly into the hydrophobic state associated with the synaptic membrane by ionic links (ionic-bound mChAT) [92, 94-96]. All this presupposes the existence of multiple forms or isoforms of the enzyme. Also, differences in the optimum pH, substrate specificity, sensitivity to the selective inhibitor 4-(1-naphthyl) pyridine (NVP) and some other molecular characteristics of the synaptoplasm and synaptic membrane fractions indicated this [97-99].

Research has revealed only one ChAT gene that encodes the multiple forms and isoforms of the enzyme [80, 83]. High homology has been detected between ChAT gene nucleotide sequences in the mouse, rat, pig and human brains with differences in the 5'-noncoding region. Polymorphisms of ChAT mRNAs are due to alternate splicing and various use of at least of five non-coding exons in the promoter region of the gene [100].

Five types of mRNA have been isolated from the rat brain ChAT (R1/2-, N1/2- transcripts and M-) [101] and six types from the human brain (R1/2-, N1/2-, S- and M-transcripts) [83]. All five ChAT transcripts generate ChAT with a molecular weight of 69 kDa (ChAT-69). This is the major form of ChAT in the CNS. In addition, the human M and S transcripts generate minor forms of ChAT with a molecular weight of 82-83 kDa (ChAT-82) and 74 kDa (ChAT-74) [80, 83, 93, 100, 102, 103]. Also, ChAT-69 and ChAT-82 are subdivided into a number of isoforms with differences in the isoelectric point [104].

The cytoplasm and plasma membranes of cholinergic neurons express only ChAT-69 [80, 83, 100]. In the human brain, ChAT is also found in the cell nucleus. Initially, ChAT-82 was selectively found in the nucleus in some brain structures [82, 95, 104, 105] and, later, ChAT-69 was also found [83]. In rat ganglia in the central nervous system at the level of the medulla oblongata, ChAT is expressed with a molecular mass of about 50 kDa and is called peripheral ChAT (pChAT). pChAT also exhibits alternative splicing of the mRNA [106].

The physiological significance of such a large number of isoforms of ChAT is not clear at present. Also, the relationship between of ChAT-69 isoforms in subsynaptic compartments is not known. Polymorphisms in ChAT transcripts suggest that ChAT isoforms or transcripts may vary in stability or translation efficiency or may be differentially expressed in response to trophic or pathological factors. Thus pChAT is not expressed in cholinergic neurons of the parasympathetic dorsal motor nucleus of the vagus nerve and nucleus ambiguus in the medulla of intact rats but pChAT- positive neurons were detected in these nuclei after axotomy against the background of almost disappearance of ChAT-69-positive neurons [107]. Furthermore, targeting of the enzyme to the cell nucleus suggests that ChAT may be able to perform other functions in addition to its essential role of synthesizing ACh in nerve terminals [102].

6. Features of ChAT phosphorylation

It is known that the genome does not provide the variety in the protein forms presented in a cell. In this regard, the post-genomic protein modifications are of special significance. Phosphorylation is one of the most studied pathways of the post-translational influence on the molecular properties of enzymes. Covalent modifications to serine, threonine and tyrosine residues in protein molecules can dynamically change their physicochemical nature, as well as regulate protein function and interactions with cellular components. This has been shown for the key enzyme in the synthesis of dopamine (tyrosine hydroxylase) and serotonin (tryptophan hydroxylase) and for glutamate decarboxylases GAD65 and GAD67, two synthetic enzymes of gamma-aminobutyric acid (GABA) [108].

For a long time, ChAT was not related to rate-limiting enzymes on the basis of kinetic calculations. It was believed that the ChAT synthesis rate dependents only on fluctuations in the levels of the substrate and the product of the synthesis, although ChAT is not saturated by choline and acetyl-CoA in their physiological concentrations [35]. However, in recent decades, other intracellular factors have been revealed to regulate the activity of the enzyme. These data suggest an important regulatory role of ChAT in the synthesis and secretion of ACh [36, 82, 103, 108, 109]. It is assumed that the cause of several diseases is spontaneous point mutations in the molecule of ChAT or of its regulatory proteins which lead to dysregulation of the enzyme or to changes in its ability to communicate with regulatory factors [93, 108].

As a rule, the different effects of phosphorylation on synaptic soluble (hydrophilic) cChAT and membrane-bound (hydrophobic) mChAT occur even with non-specific stimulation by the substrates ATP or phosphorus (Pi). Increased ATP markedly affects the specific activity of mChAT compared with cChAT [37]. At rest, cChAT but not mChAT is phosphorylated in incubation medium enriched with Pi. Under these incubation conditions, veratridine depolarization selectively activated and dephosphorylated mChAT but had no influence on either the degree of phosphorylation nor the activity of cChAT. Removal of Ca^{2+} from the incubation medium significantly inhibited the phosphorylation of cChAT and the specific activity of mChAT [110].

It has been shown that, in vivo, ChAT exists as a phosphoprotein [36, 111]. In vitro, phosphatase inhibitors activate cChAT and mChAT a little, even under non-phosphorylation conditions (ATP absent in the incubation medium) [37]. ChAT is a substrate for certain protein kinases. The amino acid sequence of the enzyme suggests the existence of multiple sites for phosphorylation by protein kinases such as protein kinase C (PKC), α-Ca^{2+}/calmodulin-dependent protein kinase II (CaM2), casein kinase II (CK2) and some others [108]. ChAT-69 is phosphorylated by the serine/threonine kinases CK2, PKC and CaM2 [92, 95, 105, 112].

It should be noted that PKC and CaM2 are the well-known and important regulators of neuronal functions. CaM2 is an obligatory component of the cholinergic vesicular mechanism [37], and PKC plays an important role in the regulation of ChAT molecular properties [36]. The authors also make the conjecture that oxidative stress can alter the phosphorylation-dependent regulation of ChAT expression and ACh synthesis in the aging brain and in the early stages of vascular and Alzheimer's disease and related disorders. Both of these protein kinases interact with serine/threonine residues which the protein kinases use for ChAT phosphorylation [92, 95, 108, 112]. In different studies, PKC activated cChAT and mChAT with variable efficacy [37, 95, 104]. It has been shown that different protein kinase isoforms have distinct patterns and ChAT phosphorylation by PKC isoforms has a hierarchical construct [92, 95, 108, 112]. Thus, phosphorylation of Ser-476 had no effect on the molecular properties of ChAT but allows the possibility of phosphorylating other serine residues, such as Ser-440 and/ or Ser-346/347 which are necessary to maintain the catalytic activity of ChAT under basal and stimulated conditions. Also, Ser-346/347 modulates ChAT phosphorylation at other amino acid residues, and Ser-440 initiates the translocation of soluble ChAT to the cellular membrane and the formation of ionic-bound ChAT.

CaM2 and its inhibitors selectively regulate mChAT activity without affecting the activity of cChAT [37]. These data were also confirmed indirectly by experiments with total ChAT (actually cChAT), in which CaM2 phosphorylated but did not activate the enzyme [104]. Further investigations showed that CaM2 activated total ChAT in terms of the combined phosphorylation of Thr-456 by CaM2 and of Ser-440 by PKC [112]. It is assumed that this PKC feature of the potentiation of CaM2 action in cholinergic projection neurons of the hippocampus and the cortex is dramatically implicated in the pathogenesis of Alzheimer's disease [112]. Likewise, PKC inactivation of Ser-440 phosphorylation is implicated in the pathogenesis of myasthenic syndrome in the motor nuclei of the spinal cord [94, 113].

7. Role of cChAT and mChAT in regulation of acetylcholine synthesis and secretion – In vitro studies

In neurons, the principal place of synthesis of ACh is in the nerve endings. ChAT has long been recognized as a cytoplasmic enzyme, even after its detection on synaptic membranes in the 1960s [1, 114]. Later, it was shown that ChAT exists as a structural membrane protein [95, 115-117]. The long-term study of the properties of synaptic soluble (c) and membrane-bound (m) ChAT in vitro has shown that the relationship between ChAT activity and the secretion of ACh depends on the compartmentalization of the enzyme.

7.1. Functional properties of synaptic cChAT

Soluble cChAT activity is the prevalent activity of synaptic ChAT. cChAT regulates the dynamic equilibrium between the synthesis and degradation of ACh in the resting state [35, 99, 118, 119]. Under physiological conditions, cChAT is activated during stimulation by depolarizing agents such as K^+ and/or veratridine [37, 120, 121]. Another regulator of the level of free cytosolic ACh is AChE, the enzyme that mediates ACh splitting. A close interaction takes place between cChAT and soluble cAChE [120]. Thus, in calcium-free medium conditions, the quantum release of ACh is blocked, the activity of cChAT is not changed and cAChE is activated and cleaves an abundance of ACh [120, 122].

From these experiments, it follows that non-quantum, Ca^{2+}-independent "leak" of acetylcholine and its decay products, choline and acetate, is in direct dependence on the ratio of the activity of these two cytosolic enzymes [120, 122, 123]. In these studies, (1) K^+ stimulation in calcium-free medium causes the release of cytosolic choline due to disruption of cytosolic ACh by cAChE and (2) veratridine stimulation can cause the release of both choline and cytosolic ACh. (3) In mAChE and cAChE inhibition conditions by a tertiary inhibitor such as paraoxon coming through the plasma membrane, the release of choline is blocked under veratridine stimulation in calcium-free medium and its extracellular level is decreased. Instead of choline, the release of cytosolic ACh is observed. (4) Under cChAT and mChAT inhibition conditions by the selective inhibitor NVP, cChAT is selectively activated and the release of newly synthesized ACh is increased directly from the cytosol under veratridine stimulation in physiological medium (in the presence of Ca^{2+}). (5) A similar output of ACh is observed under the same conditions in calcium-free medium.

The choline and ACh concentrations could increase by 40-60% in the extracellular medium in such a non-quantum manner. Choline is a selective agonist of α-7 subtype of ACh nicotinic receptors [65, 124]. Thus, the "leak" of cytosolic choline and/or ACh, as well as changes in their relationship in the extracellular environment may have independent signaling effects in intercellular interactions.

7.2. Functional properties of synaptic mChAT

The functional purpose of mChAT has long been unclear [80, 125]. Investigation of this problem was difficult in the absence of selective inhibitors of cChAT and mChAT. Their separation is possible only by subsynaptic fractionation in combination with methods that destroy the synaptosome. The contribution of mChAT to general ChAT activity is low, i.e. 4-15% [1, 94, 95, 97, 119]. Therefore, for a long time, it was assumed that the association of ChAT with neuronal membranes was an artifact as the result of synaptoplasm contamination [1, 35, 114].It has now been shown that mChAT exists (1) as stationary membrane protein [99, 115, 117] and (2) as ionic-bound mChAT, a reversible form of cytosolic ChAT [95, 126].

In vitro, mChAT like cChAT are activated in response to K^+ or veratridine stimulation in physiological medium [37, 110, 120, 121]. Compelling data have accumulated regarding the direct involvement of mChAT in the mechanisms of quantum secretion of acetylcholine. This is indicated by a number of ultrastructural and functional characteristics of the enzyme.

mChAT is localized to synaptic vesicles [127]. Its activity, unlike cChAT, depends on the specific factors of ACh transfer into the vesicles, VAChT and the proton gradient, and on CaM2 activity, which is the main kinase associated with synaptic vesicles [37]. Activation and inhibition of mChAT are fully coupled with the activation or, respectively, blockade of ACh quantum release [120].

The non-vesicular Ca^{2+}-dependent pathway of the quantum secretion of ACh has been revealed [128-131]. It was shown that this pathway provides fast secretion of ACh by a synaptic membrane structural protein [132] called mediatophore [128]. It was found that mediatophore is functional linked to ChAT [133]. This suggests that mChAT located on the synaptic membrane participates in the regulation of the quantum secretion of ACh, similar to vesicular mChAT. This agrees with the preferential sensitivity of mChAT to the functional state of CHT that is selectively localized to the neuronal membrane of cholinergic neurons [94, 134].

mChAT is selectively sensitive to the balance of ions. It is known that ions are important regulators of quantum neurotransmitter release and other transmembrane functions. Control of quantum ACh release is carried out by the interaction of the Ca^{2+} and H^+ balance (vesicular Ca^{2+}/H^+ antiporter), Zn^{2+} and K^+ (K^+ channels) [131, 135-138]. mChAT activity is selectively or preferably (1) inhibited in calcium-free medium [118, 120, 121], (2) is increased at a high concentration of Ca^{2+} and/or K^+ [37, 110, 121, 123, 139], (3) is dose-dependently inhibited by the intracellular concentration of Cl^- [118, 125] and increases in conditions of a high Cl^- concentration and chloride conductivity stimulation [125]. (5) Zn^{2+} regulates both pathways of the quantum secretion of ACh. High concentrations of Zn^{2+} block ACh release from vesicles and through mediatophore [135, 140]. Similarly, the direction of ChAT translocation depends on Zn^{2+} ions. Zn^{2+} blocks the "anchoring" of ChAT on the membrane [126]. The last argument indicates the involvement of ionic-bound mChAT in the quantum release of ACh.

So, the catalytic properties of cChAT and mChAT depend on phosphorylation and possibly on the type of splicing. Moreover, the specific activity of mChAT, unlike cChAT, also depends on the ionic environment and on other factors affecting the quantum secretion of ACh. The functional significance of mChAT is not nearly as clear as cChAT. The relationship between cChAT and mChAT and their dependence on external influences are poorly understood [138]. Nevertheless, it seems that the compartmentalization of the enzyme ensures the involvement of cChAT and mChAT in different functional-metabolic cycles, which may contribute to the fine regulation of the mediator actions of ACh.

8. cChAT and mChAT as markers of functional and structural reorganization in cholinergic nerve endings following external exposure — In vivo studies

The synaptosomal subfractions of the synaptic membranes and synaptoplasm of the cortex, hippocampus and some other rat brain structures are used for research in vivo cholinergic mechanisms of brain functions by biochemical methods (radiometric and spectrophotometric). Subsynaptic fractions gave according to the scheme shown in Figure 1. Respectively, mChAT and cChAT activity and the m-protein and c-protein content have been measured to estimate cholinergic function. In addition, in some experiments, mAChE and cAChE and Na^+/K^+-ATPase activity was measured. The Na^+/K^+-ATPase activity and content of synaptic proteins, as universal synaptic parameters, as well AChE activity were correlated with ChAT activity in those cases when the cholinergic reaction following exposure was dominant in the synaptosomal fraction. Generally, models of acute (3 hours) and chronic (11-14 days) brain ischemia (bilateral occlusion of the carotid arteries, the 2VO model) or acute hypobaric hypoxia with variable intensity (10% O_2, 60 min; 6.5% O_2, 15 min; 4.5% O_2, 1-3 minutes or 10-20 minutes) were used as the exposure methods.

8.1. Biochemical equivalents of activation and inhibition of cholinergic mediator function

In in vivo investigations, ChAT activity was found to be the most mobile parameter. So, ChAT has become the main landmark for analysis of the cholinergic reaction to exposure.

cChAT activation was observed under acute ischemia or hypoxia at all intensities [27, 29, 141]. mChAT or both mChAT and cChAT activation was revealed under acute and chronic ischemia and only in severe hypoxia (4.5% O_2) [27-29, 141]. When the activation of ChAT was observed (165-170%), extracellular mAChE (the predominant isoform of mAChE) was simultaneously activated [141]. cChAT activation positively correlated with the activation of Na^+/K^+-ATPase and negatively correlated with the decrease in the c-protein content [27]. All these reactions of the synaptic biochemical parameters and their combinations are regarded as the activation of cholinergic synaptic function, because they conform to the characteristics of synaptic activation.

Compared to cChAT, the selective activation of mChAT has been revealed (1) under equal experimental conditions (3 hours of ischemia) in rats less resistant to hypoxia [141], and (2) under hypoxic conditions with variable intensity only in severe hypoxia [27] and was not observed in the subcritical and moderate hypoxia (6.5% or 10% O_2) [27, 29]. A parallel study of the ultrastructure of the synapses in the cortex revealed the dependence of swelling synapses and synaptic mitochondria on the duration of severe hypoxia [27]. Taken together, these data suggest that the activation of mChAT in vivo occurs due to an imbalance of synaptic $Ca2^+$, while cChAT activation is apparently initiated in the natural physiological way, under neuronal influences [27].

The inhibitory reactions of ChAT under ischemic/hypoxic conditions were revealed as well. It was found that these conditions decrease cChAT or mChAT or both cChAT and mChAT activity [27-29, 141]. Also, a negative correlation has been found between cChAT activity and the c-protein content and a positive correlation has been found between mChAT activity and the m-protein content [27, 29, 141].

A parallel study of the ultrastructure of the synapses in the cortex revealed a significant decrease in the number of vesicles docked to the presynaptic active zone in the rat with a profound decrease in both cChAT and mChAT activity in acute hypoxia [27, 142].Taken together, these data suggest that such a decrease in ChAT activity in vivo may reflect the deep inhibition of cholinergic synaptic function as result of the superexcitation, the equivalent of the well-known "depression of neurons" in electrophysiology, i.e. reduced neuronal excitability due to the depletion of mediator substrates.

Selective inhibition of mChAT, as well as its activation, is likely a consequence of a disturbance in the ion balance. Based on the dominance of the hypoxic factors in these experiments, it is supposed that the decrease in mChAT activity is due to the accumulation of H^+ ions in the presynapses [27, 29]. It can be induced (1) by acidosis in the case of severe hypoxia and (2) by the weak increase in H^+ ion concentrations as the primary response to hypoxia in the case of moderate hypoxia (10% O_2). It has been shown that such primary H^+ ion accumulation is subthreshold for the initiation of cellular acidosis and can disrupt the function of the Ca^{2+}/H^+ antiporter [143].

Finally, cAChE activation has been detected under acute ischemia [141]. This is probably another means of regulating the abundance of free cytosolic ACh during the inhibition of ACh quantum transmission. The simultaneous increase in the c-protein content in the same synaptosomal fraction corroborates this supposition. It is well-known that numerous fibrillar synaptic proteins are soluble at rest and quickly form a structure under stimulation conditions.

So, the high reactivity as cChAT and mChAT and the peculiarities in the manifestation of ChAT (and AChE) activity according to the compartmentalization of the enzyme and to the experimental situation in vivo testify to the naturalness of functional properties cChAT and mChAT (and also c- and mAChE) revealed in vitro.

8.2. Biochemical equivalents of the quantitative changes in the cholinergic synaptic pool

The correlations in the activation or inhibition of cChAT and mChAT may reflect changes in a number of cholinergic synapses, namely synaptogenesis (the growth of new synapses) or their elimination, retraction or another means of reduction in the quantity of nerve endings. As was described above, the correlation between the biochemical synaptic membrane and cytosolic parameters may reflect the reaction of the presynapse as a structural unit. The most reliable criterion of the quantitative reorganization of cholinergic synapses is the positive correlation between ChAT activity and the c-protein content, since their functional changes have contrasting directionality.

A reduction in the number of presynapses was provoked by acute hypoxia of variable severity [27, 29]. It was shown by various methods, including non-invasive video technology, that a reduction in the number of synapses can occur within minutes or tens of minutes [144-148].

Sprouting as well as destruction with the swelling of neurons and their terminals, including cholinergic neurons, predominates in late brain ischemia or postischemic reoxygenation (over days and months) [149-152]. In biochemical studies, the activation of ChAT was observed in the majority of the synaptic subfractions of the cortex and hippocampus following chronic brain ischemia [28]. The correlated increase between mChAT activity and m-protein content could indicate synaptogenesis and hyperfunction of the cholinergic synapses, whereas the correlated increase between cChAT/mChAT activity and the c-protein content indicates synaptogenesis only.

8.3. Biochemical equivalents of the morpho- structural reorganization in the cholinergic synaptic pool

Under the influence of moderate hypoxia (10% of O_2, 60 min), an increase in the activity of cChAT and the c-protein content was observed in the “light” synaptosomes from the caudal structures of the brainstem [29]. This indicated an increase in quantity of the corresponding synapses; however, synaptogenesis was impossible in such a brief period. Additional analysis revealed a decrease in the activity of mChAT and the m-protein content in the "heavy" synaptosomal fraction of the same brain structures. This decrease in the “m” biochemical parameters in the "heavy" fraction negatively correlated with the increase in the corresponding “c” biochemical parameters in the "light" fraction.These data indicate the transformation of presynapses from one morphological type to another.

This phenomenon of the transformation of synapses was found in electron microscopic experiments during 90 minutes of severe hypoxia [144, 145]. It was shown that the change of a morphological type occurs due to the changes in the area, density and configuration of the network elements of the presynapses and in their configuration [153]. Almost all of these parameters can affect the density of the presynapses. Therefore, it is possible that some population of the cholinergic presynapses from the "heavy" synaptosomal fraction transformed into presynapses with the less density and was located in the “light" fraction of the sucrose density gradient. Apparently, this transformation resulted in a morphological type more resistant to hypoxia.

In such studies on synaptic subfractions in vivo, various cholinergic synaptic reactions have been revealed in response to hypoxic/ischemic exposures. The responsiveness of synaptic cChAT and mChAT allows the study of synaptic reactions depending on the exposure conditions, the functional specificity of different brain structures and neuronal populations. It was noticed that a reaction to the hypoxia had phase type of change in the course of intensification of hypoxic exposure [27]. As well a diversity of the plastic possibilities of the brain is detected. For example, under the same moderate hypobaric hypoxic conditions (10% O_2, 60 min) which initiated an increase in resistance to hypoxia, three alternative cholinergic adaptive pathways were obtained in the same brain structure (the caudal brainstem) in three different groups of rats. Transformation and activation of the presynapses was seen in one of the rat groups and the inhibition of cholinergic activity in different populations of presynapses (in the light or heavy synaptosomes) was seen in the other two groups [29]. The mechanisms behind this plastic diversity are unknown, although it is clear that it is associated with individual neuronal organization of brain functions.

8.4. Cholinergic organization of brain functions under normal conditions and patterns of adaptive reorganization under the influence of stress stimuli or pathological conditions

Synaptic ChAT activity can be used as an instrument to study the cholinergic mechanisms of brain functions in vivo. Biochemical (radiometric) methods to estimate synaptic ChAT activity are very sensitive and allow for assessing fine individual differences between experimental animals. In turn, this method allows for successful correlation analysis between ChAT activity and indicators of brain function and performance. Moreover, it is possible to study certain populations of cholinergic neurons using, for example, the synaptic fractions of the cortex and hippocampus.

As mentioned above, according to immunohistochemical data, both the cortex and the hippocampus have two basic sources of cholinergic innervation. The first major source is neuronal projections from the forebrain nuclei. The second minor source is interneurons (intrinsic neurons). The third source to the frontal and visual cortical areas from the meso-pontine region is weak and biochemical methods can detect it only when the frontal or visual area is assessed separately. In these brain structures, ChAT activity was estimated in the fractions of the light and heavy synaptosomes (isolated as in [4]), and it appeared that these fractions both in the cortex and in the hippocampus differ in terms of functional activity. From this, it follows that in both brain structures, the cholinergic presynapses from different sources are isolated in different synaptosomal fractions during preparation in the sucrose density gradient.

Next, it was revealed that the ratio of ChAT activity in the light and heavy synaptosomal fractions corresponded to the ratio of the immunoreactivity of the enzyme in the projections and interneurons [46, 48, 52, 53, 154].This and some other data promoted the conclusion that, in the cortex and hippocampus, the presynapses of cholinergic projections from the forebrain nuclei accumulate mainly in the light synaptosomal fractions, whereas the presynapses of cholinergic interneurons accumulate mainly in the heavy synaptosomal fractions [27, 27, 155].

This differential approach was used to study rat and cat brain cholinergic synaptic organization of cognitive functions such as learning, different forms of memory and inherited abilities in some experimental situations. mChAT and cChAT activities of the light and heavy synaptosomes of the hippocampus and/or cortex were used as markers of forebrain projections and interneurons, respectively. These studies revealed some patterns in the relationship between cognitive functional mechanisms that have not been sufficiently analyzed or defined by any other methods.

Thus, under normal brain conditions, it was shown that (Figure 3, a):

1. Both the cholinergic projective systems and interneurons of the rat cortex and hippocampus are actively involved in learning and memory processes in the Morris water maze

model [28]. The presynapses of cholinergic interneurons in the cat temporal associative cortical area do not participate in inherited abilities for the analysis of images [25] but all of other associative cortical areas (frontal and parietal) active participated in cognitive processes [153].

2. The cholinergic system participates not only in the mechanisms of learning and working memory, which has been repeatedly observed [151, 157-160], but also in the mechanisms of long-term memory [28]. The involvement of cholinergic projective systems in the mechanisms of long-term memory is usually denied [161-164] or has been discussed in only a few studies [165-167].

3. Each form of memory has an individual cholinergic synaptic composition [28]. This conclusion agrees with the results of investigations into cholinergic and monoaminergic systems obtained in the Morris water maze and some other behavioral models [165, 168-170].

4. Cholinergic projective neurons and interneurons of the rat cortex and hippocampus can have both positive and negative connections with cognitive functions [28]. Identical results were obtained in all cat cortical areas except the temporal zone. Cholinergic projections in the temporal area had only negative connections with inherited cognitive functions. The number of cholinergic presynapses may be more than doubled in this brain area of cats with weak cognitive abilities as compared with cats with strong abilities [25]. Negative connections with cognitive functions are not specific for only the cholinergic system. In morphological research on hippocampal mossy fibers (glutamatergic) in the rat and mouse brain, feedback was also found between the quantity of synapses which mossy fibers create and learning [171].

Taken together, these data demonstrate that the cholinergic mechanisms of learning and memory are more complex than is currently perceived.

Stress and pathological stimuli initiate a considerable reorganization of the normal cholinergic synaptic connections in cognitive functions. As an illustration, it was revealed during chronic 2VO conditions in the Morris water maze models that [28] (Figure 3, b):

1. The majority of normal cholinergic connections are lost and new connections arise.

2. Cholinergic link was considerably reduced in mechanisms of cognitive functions and proportion of negative connections increased.

3. In addition to reduction, the structural isolation of cholinergic links in cognitive functions and performance takes place; cortical cholinergic influences are completely removed from spatial contextual functions as are hippocampal influences from spatially cued functions.

In general, cholinergic synaptic influences disappear in some forms of cognition. It is clear that the consequences of different exposures on the cholinergic composition of cognitive functions are individual; however, the itemized consequences of 2VO are general for other stress stimuli such as acute severe hypoxia (4.5% O_2, Figure 3, c) [141, 156] and changes in season from warm to cold [25] (Figure 4).

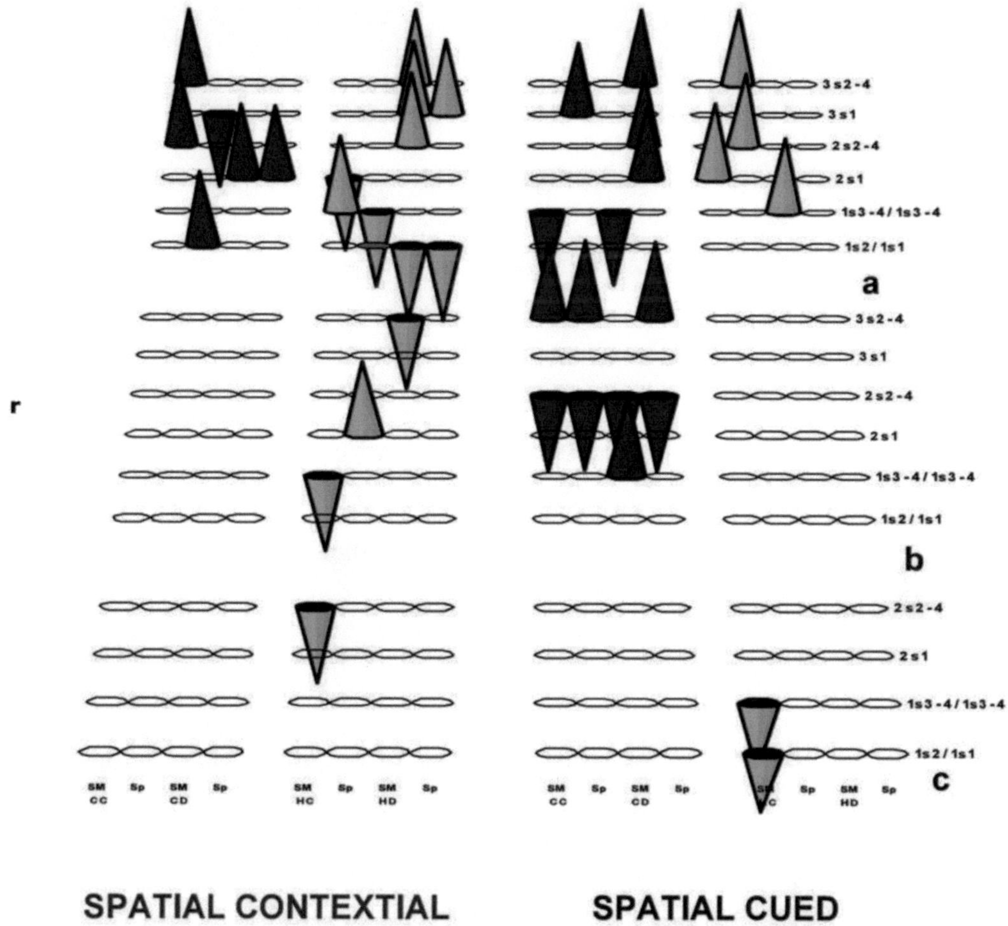

Abbreviations: 1s2(Contextual)/1s1 (Cued), the inherited abilities, the first non-casual attempt of making decision in the task (respectively, the second/ the first trial in the first session, "s " inclued in the abbreviations of the forms of cognition); 1s3-4 (Contextual)/1s2-4 (Cued), the working memory (averaged from the following trials in the first session); 2s2-4 and 3s2-4, the learning (average of trials in the second and the third sessions respectively); 2s1 and 3s1, the long-term memory (the first trials on the next days after the first and the second sessions of training respectively). SM and Sp, subfractions of the synaptic membranes and the synaptoplasm, respectively, of the cortical light (CL) and heavy synaptosomes (CH) and hippocampal light (HL) and heavy synaptosomes (HH).
Pyramids towards up indicate a positive correlation between behavioural performance and ChAT activity; inverted pyramidы indicate a negative correlation between behavioural performance and ChAT activity. In the rat groups n=4-7. Correlations between behavioural performance and ChAT activity are represented with only valid values and with the Bonferroni correction (p<0.02-0.001).

Figure 3. Values of *r*-criterion by the Pearson's test of behavioural performance and ChAT activity in rats in the Morris water maze in the spatial contextual and the spatial cued behavioural models under control (a, sham operated rats), ischaemic (b, 2VO operated rats) and one month after a single severe hypobaric hypoxia (c, sham operated rats) conditions.

It is logical to assume that the reduction in cholinergic links in cognitive mechanisms is a consequence of the degeneration of cholinergic fibers. However, the reverse was actually

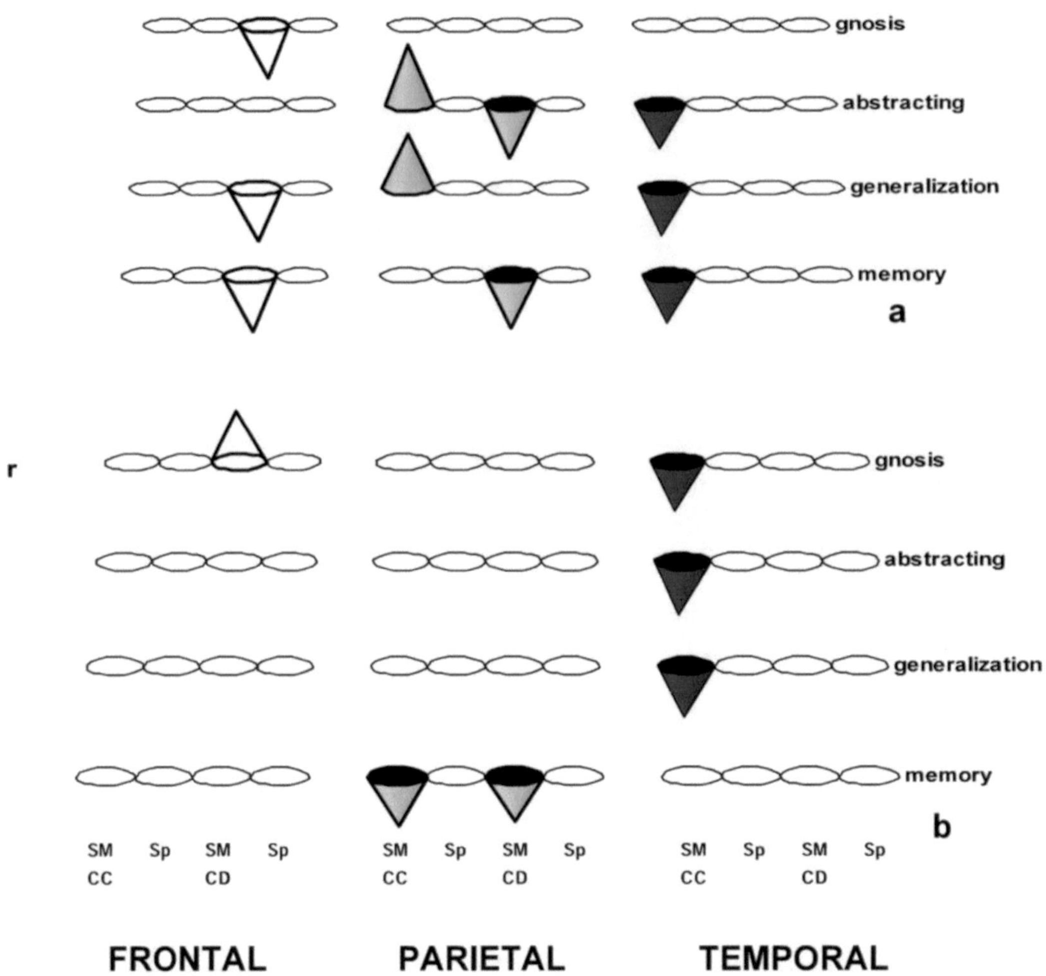

Abbreviations: SM, Sp, CL, CH, the same abbreviations of the subfractions as on Figure 3.
As on Figure 3, the pyramids towards up indicate a positive correlation between behavioural performance and ChAT activity; inverted pyramids indicate a negative correlation between behavioural performance and ChAT activity. In the cat groups n=6-8. Correlations behavioural performance and ChAT activity are represented with only valid values and with the Bonferroni correction (p<0.02-0.001).

Figure 4. Values of r-criterion by the Pearson's test of behavioural performance and ChAT activity in cats in the inherited abilities of generalisation, abstracting and gnosis of images tested on the basis of the food reflex (memory) in the summer (a) and winter (b).

observed. As was noted above, activation of ChAT was detected in the majority of the synaptic subfractions, and this may reflect cholinergic hyperfunction or synaptogenesis in the 2VO rat brain [28]. Moreover, ChAT activity showed a five- to ten-fold increase in the winter as compares with the summer in synaptic subfractions of both projection and interneurons in the temporal [25] as well in other cat cortical areas [156]. No quantitative distinctions in ChAT activity were found in the synaptic subfractions of the cortex and the hippocampus of rats in a month after a single acute hypoxic stress [156].

The new cholinergic connections with cognitive functions that arise after 2VO are not necessarily the consequence of degeneration or dysfunction in the presynapses of key cholinergic populations, i.e. these new connections could arise for other, indirect reasons. Therefore, it was assumed that noticeable weakening of cholinergic synaptic influences on cognitive processes is a consequence of adaptation. It seems that the cholinergic synaptic components of the highest brain structures, besides their participation in cognition, are necessary for the functions connected with survival under stress conditions.

At the same time, some cognitive functions were not affected by cholinergic reduction after 2VO [28]. All the more the inherited cognitive processes are preserved with annual seasonal cholinergic reorganization [25, 156]. From this, it was concluded that, during stress conditions, other mediator systems replace the cholinergic system in cognitive processes.

At least four questions follow from these data:

1. In what nervous functions are the cholinergic neuronal populations of the cortex and the hippocampus involved, both projective and intrinsic, for the maintenance of viability of an organism? Is it a function of regulation of the regional blood vessels or some other factor?

2. Why are cholinergic synaptic influences lost from cognitive mechanisms? Is it a negative dependence between vital and cognitive functions or low resistance of this neuronal population to stress conditions?

3. Is the structural isolation of cholinergic links in cognitive functions presumes a functional disbalance between the cortex and hippocampus? Is it a consequence of loss of cholinergic modulating influences?

4. What mediator systems mediate the execution of cognitive functions instead of the cholinergic system?

The answers to these questions are important for the restoration, maintenance and regulation of cognitive and vital brain functions under stress and pathological conditions.

9. Conclusion

The synapse is a unique and the most dynamic and labile structure specialized in the chemical transmission of nerve signals, an inherent structure of the neuron only.

Cholinergic system is essential constituent of the mammalian brain. Due to research using the synaptosomal and other synaptic fractions, knowledge behind the metabolism and secretory function of ACh and some new notion concerning the cholinergic mechanisms of cognitive functions under normal conditions and stress stimuli were gained. Today, however, accumulated data does not provide answers to the all questions as many more questions are asked. We have tried to outline some of the outstanding problems in the course of presenting the material.

The experimental cell physiology began to develop after the invention of the microscope by A. van Leeuwenhoek and his discoveries in the middle of the 17th century. Experimental synaptology began to develop after the invention of the electron microscope in the 1930s by M. Knoll and E. Ruska, ie three centuries later! Prior to this, researchers for the longest time, following two great neurohistologists, S. Ramón y Cajal and C. Golgi, in general could not reach a consensus, whether the brain is a cellular structure or syncytium? Only the electron microscope proved that a synapse exists.

Thus the science of the synapse is very young neuroscience.

Acknowledgements

We are grateful to all the mentors and colleagues, co-authors of our publications, especially to Prof. M.D. E.I. Mukhin, doctor of biology Z.I. Storozheva and Ph.D. M.Y. Monakov. Special thanks to Academician RAMS A.A. Kubatiev for supporting our research.

Author details

E.I. Zakharova and A.M. Dudchenko

*Address all correspondence to: zakharova-ei@yandex.ru

Institute of General Pathology and Pathophysiology, Russian Academy of Medical Sciences, Moscow, Russia

References

[1] Whittaker V P, Michaelson I A, Kirkland R J. The separation of synaptic vesicles from nerve-ending particles ('synaptosomes'). Biochemical Journal 1964; 90(2) 293-303.

[2] Hebb C O, Wh ittaker V P. Intracellular distributions of acetylcholine and choline acetylase. Journal of Physiology 1958; 142 (1) 187-196.

[3] Whittaker V P. The isolation and characterization of acetylcholine-containing particles from brain. Biochemical Journal 1959; 72, 694-706.

[4] De Robertis E, Pellegrino De Iraldi A, Rodrigues De Lores A G, Salganicoff L. Cholinergic and non-cholinergic nerve endings in rat brain. Journal of Nerochemistry 1962; 9, 23-35.

[5] Rodríguez de Lores A, Alberic M, De Robertis E. Ultrastructural and enzymic studies of cholinergic and non-cholinergic synaptic membranes isolated from brain cortex. Journal of Nerochemistry 1967; 14(2) 215-225.

[6] Cotman C W, Matthews D A. Synaptic plasma membranes from rat brain synaptosomes: isolation and partial characterization. Biochimica et Biophysica Acta 1971; 249(2) 380-394.

[7] De Robertis E. Ultrastructure and cytochemistry of the synaptic region. The macromolecular components involved in nerve transmission are being studied. Science 1967; 156(3777) 907-914.

[8] Davis G A, Bloom F E. Isolation of synaptic junctional complexes from rat brain. Brain Research 1973; 62(1) 35-53.

[9] Balázs R, Dahl D, Harwood J R. Subcellular distribution of enzymes of glutamate metabolism in rat brain. Journal of Nerochemistry 1966; 13(10) 897-905.

[10] Whittaker V P. The morphology of fractions of rat forebrain synaptosomes separated on continuous sucrose density gradients. Biochemical Journal 1968; 106(2) 412-417.

[11] Fonnum F. The distribution of glutamate decarboxylase and aspartate transaminase in subcellular fractions of rat and guinea-pig brain. Biochemical Journal 1968; 106(2) 401–412.

[12] Jones D G. Synapses and synaptosomes: Morphological aspects. London and New York: Chapman and Hall; 1975.

[13] Glebov RN, Kryzhanovskii G N. [Functional biochemistry of synapses]. Moscow: Meditsina; 1978. Russian.

[14] Wessler I, Kirkpatrick C J, Racké K. The cholinergic 'pitfall': acetylcholine, a universal cell molecule in biological systems, including humans. Clinical and Experimental Pharmacology and Physiology 1999; 26(3) 198-205.

[15] Wessler I, Bittinger F, Kamin W, Zepp F, Meyer E, Schad A, Kirkpatrick C J. Dysfunction of the non-neuronal cholinergic system in the airways and blood cells of patients with cystic fibrosis. Life Sciences 2007; 80(24-25) 2253-2258..

[16] Brust P, Friedrich A, Krizbai I A, Bergmann R, Roux F, Ganapathy V, Johannsen B. Functional expression of the serotonin transporter in immortalized rat brain microvessel endothelial cells. Journal of Nerochemistry 2000; 74(3) 1241-1248.

[17] Kirkpatrick C J, Bittinger F, Unger R E, Kriegsmann J, Kilbinger H, Wessler I. The non-neuronal cholinergic system in the endothelium: evidence and possible pathobiological significance. Japan Journal of Pharmacology 2001; 85(1) 24-28.

[18] Gorini A, D'Angelo A, Villa R F. Energy Metabolism of Synaptosomal Subpopulations from Different Neuronal Systems of Rat Hippocampus: Effect of L-Acetylcarnitine Administration In Vivo. Neurochemical Research 1999; 24(5) 617-624.

[19] Sokolow S, Henkins K M, Williams I A, Vinters H V, Schmid I, Cole G M, Gylys K H. Isolation of synaptic terminals from Alzheimer's disease cortex. Cytometry Part A 2012; 81(3) 248-254. doi: 10.1002/cyto.a.22009. http://www.ncbi.nlm.nih.gov/pubmed/?term=Sokolow+S%2C+Henkins+K+M%2C+Williams+I+A%2C+Vinters+H+V%2C+Schmid+I%2C+Cole+G+M%2C+Gylys+K+H (accessed 2011 Dec 28).

[20] Ammons D, Manrrique J, Rampersad J. An apparatus to control and automate the formation of continuous density gradients. Analytical Biochemistry 2012; 427(2) 124-126. doi: 10.1016/j.ab.2012.05.012. http://www.ncbi.nlm.nih.gov/pubmed/?term=Ammons+D%2C+Manrrique+J (accessed 2012 May 22).

[21] Laverty R, Michaelson I A, Sharman D F, Whittaker V P. The subcellular localization of dopamine and acetylcholine in the dog caudate nucleus. British Journal of Pharmacology and Chemotherapy 1963; 21, 482-490.

[22] Mangan J L, Whittaker V P. The distribution of free amino acids in subcellular fractions of guinea-pig brain. Biochemical Journal 1966; 98(1) 128-137.

[23] Sheridan M N, Whittaker V P, Israël M. The subcellular fractionation of the electric organ of Torpedo. Zeitschrift für Zellforschung und Mikroskopische Anatomie 1966; 74(3) 293-307.

[24] Robinson M B. Examination of glutamate transporter heterogeneity using synaptosomal preparations. Methods in Enzymology 1998; 296, 189-202.

[25] Mukhin E I, Zakharova E I, Kikteva E A. Comparison of the cholinergic system in neocortical field Ep in cats with strong and weak cognitive abilities. Neuroscience of Behavioral and Physiology 2002; 32(4) 379-387.

[26] Whittaker V P. Some Currently Neglected Aspects of Cholinergic Function. Journal of Molecular Neuroscience 2010; 40(1-2) 7–11.

[27] Zakharova E I, Dudchenko A M, Svinov M M, Fedorova M M, Germanova E L. Cholinergic Systems of the Rat Brain and Neuronal Reorganization under Conditions of Acute Hypoxia. Neurochemical Journal 2010; 4(4) 290–303.

[28] Zakharova E I, Storozheva Z I, Dudchenko A M, Kubatiev A A. Chronic Cerebral Ischaemia Forms New Cholinergic Mechanisms of Learning and Memory. International Jornal of Alzheimers Disease 2010; 2010: 954589. doi: 10.4061/2010/954589. http://www.ncbi.nlm.nih.gov/pmc/articles/PMC3010649/ (accessed 2010 December 20).

[29] Zakharova E I, Germanova E L, Kopaladze R A, Dudchenko A. M. Central Cholinergic Systems in the Mechanisms of Hypoxic Preconditioning: Diverse Pathways of Synaptic Reorganization in Vivo. Neurochemical Journal 2013; 7(1) 45–55.

[30] Villa R F, Ferrari F, Gorini A. Effect of in vivo L-acetylcarnitine administration on ATP-ases enzyme systems of synaptic plasma membranes from rat cerebral cortex. Neurochemical Research 2011; 36(8) 1372-1382. doi: 10.1007/s11064-011-0462-x. http://www.ncbi.nlm.nih.gov/pubmed/21479591 (accessed 2011 Apr 9).

[31] Villa R F, Ferrari F, Gorini A. ATP-ases of synaptic plasma membranes in striatum: Enzymatic systems for synapses functionality by in vivo administration of l-acetyl-carnitine in relation to Parkinson's Disease. Neuroscience 2013; 248C, 414-426.

[32] Dale H. Transmission of Nervous Effects by Acetylcholine. Harvey Lecture, May 20, 1937. Bulletin of the New York Academy of Medicine 1937; 13(7) 379–396.

[33] Fatt P, Katz B. Spontaneous subthreshold activity at motor nerve endings. Journal of Physiology 1952; 117(1) 109-128.

[34] Chang H C, Gaddum J H. Choline esters in tissue extracts. Journal of Physiology 1933; 79(3) 255-285.

[35] Tuček S. Regulation of Acetylcholine Synthesis in the Brain. Journal of Nerochemistry 1985; 44(1) 11-24.

[36] Black S A G, Rylett R J. Impact of Oxidative - Nitrosative Stress on Cholinergic Presynaptic Function, In: De La Monte S. (Ed.) Alzheimer's Disease Pathogenesis-Core Concepts, Shifting Paradigms and Therapeutic Targets. InTech; 2011. p345-368.

[37] Sha D, Jin H, Kopke R D, Wu J Y. Choline acetyltransferase: regulation and coupling with protein kinase and vesicular acetylcholine transporter on synaptic vesicles. Neurochemical Research 2004; 29(1) 199-207.

[38] Levey A I, Wainer B H, Rye D B, Mufson E J, Mesulam M M. Choline acetyltransferase-immunoreactive neurons intrinsic to rodent cortex and distinction from acetylcholinesterase-positive neurons. Neuroscience 1984; 13(2) 341-453.

[39] Hallanger A E, Wainer B H, Rye D B. Colocalization of gamma-aminobutyric acid and acetylcholinesterase in rodent cortical neurons. Neuroscience 1986; 19(3) 763-769.

[40] Arvidsson U, Riedl M, Elde R, Meister B. Vesicular acetylcholine transporter (VAChT) protein: a novel and unique marker for cholinergic neurons in the central and peripheral nervous systems. Journal of Comparative Neurology and Psychology 1997; 378(4) 454-467.

[41] Ichikawa T, Ajiki K, Matsuura J, Misawa H. Localization of two cholinergic markers, choline acetyltransferase and vesicular acetylcholine transporter in the central nervous system of the rat: in situ hybridization histochemistry and immunohistochemistry. Journal of Chemical Neuroanatomy 1997; 13(1) 23-39.

[42] McKinney M, Coyle J T, Hedreen J C. Topographic analysis of the innervation of the rat neocortex and hippocampus by the basal forebrain cholinergic system. Journal of Comparative Neurology and Psychology 1983; 217(1) 103-121.

[43] Mesulam M M, Mufson E J, Wainer B H, Levey A I. Central cholinergic pathways in the rat: an overview based on an alternative nomenclature (Ch1-Ch6). Neuroscience 1983; 10(4) 1185-1201.

[44] Saper C B. Organization of cerebral cortical afferent systems in the rat. II. Magnocellular basal nucleus. Journal of Comparative Neurology and Psychology 1984; 222(3); 313-342.

[45] Woolf N J, Eckenstein F, Butcher L L. Cholinergic systems in the rat brain: I. projections to the limbic telencephalon. Brain Research Bulletin 1984; 13(6) 751-784.

[46] Houser C R, Crawford G D, Salvaterra P M, Vaughn J E. Immunocytochemical localization of choline acetyltransferase in rat cerebral cortex: a study of cholinergic neurons and synapses. Journal of Comparative Neurology and Psychology 1985; 234(1) 17-34.

[47] Anderson K J, Gibbs R B, Salvaterra P M, Cotman C W. Ultrastructural characterization of identified cholinergic neurons transplanted to the hippocampal formation of the rat. Journal of Comparative Neurology and Psychology 1986; 249(2) 279-292.

[48] Eckenstein F P, Baughman R W, Quinn J. An anatomical study of cholinergic innervation in rat cerebral cortex. Neuroscience 1988; 25(2) 457-474.

[49] Butcher L L, Oh J D, Woolf N J, Edwards R H, Roghani A. Organization of central cholinergic neurons revealed by combined in situ hybridization histochemistry and choline-O-acetyltransferase immunocytochemistry. Neurochemistry International 1992; 21(3) 429-445.

[50] Jones B E. Immunohistochemical study of choline acetyltransferase-immunoreactive processes and cells innervating the pontomedullary reticular formation in the rat. Journal of Comparative Neurology and Psychology 1990; 295(3) 485-514.

[51] Higo S, Matsuyama T, Kawamura S. Direct projections from the pedunculopontine and laterodorsal tegmental nuclei to area 17 of the visual cortex in the cat. Neuroscience Research 1996; 26(2) 109–118.

[52] Parnavelas J G, Kelly W, Franke E, Eckenstein F P. Cholinergic neurons and fibers in rat visual cortex. Journal of Neurocytology 1986; 15(3) 329-336.

[53] Matthews D A, Salvaterra P M, Crawford G D, Houser C R, Vaughn J E. An immunocytochemical study of choline acetyltransferase-containing neurons and axon terminals in normal and partially deafferented hippocampal formation. Brain Research 1987; 402(1) 30-43.

[54] Kanaya-Ida S, Ben Ari Y. Transient increase in the number of cholinergic neurons in the developing rat dentate gyrus. Neuroscience Letters 1989; 101(1) 23-28.

[55] Frotscher M, Vida I, Bender R. Evidence for the existence of non-GABAergic, cholinergic interneurons in the rodent hippocampus. Neuroscience 2000; 96(1) 27-31.

[56] Motavkin PA, Okhotin V E, Sulimov G Iu. [Cholinergic pyramidal Betz's and Meynert's neurons in human cerebral cortex]. Zhornal Nevropatologii i Psikhiatrii im. S.S. Korsakova 1990; 90(10) 14-16. Russian.

[57] Houser C R, Crawford G D, Barber R P, Salvaterra P M, Vaughn J E. Organization and morphological characteristics of cholinergic neurons: an immunocytochemical study with a monoclonal antibody to choline acetyltransferase. Brain Research 1983; 266(1) 97-119.

[58] De Jonge W J, Ulloa L. The alpha7 nicotinic acetylcholine receptor as a pharmacological target for inflammation. British Journal of Pharmacology 2007; 151(7) 915-929. http://www.ncbi.nlm.nih.gov/pubmed/17502850 (accessed 2007 May 14)

[59] Gallowitsch-Puerta M, Pavlov V A. Neuro-immune interactions via the cholinergic anti-inflammatory pathway. Life Sciences 2007; 80(24-25) 2325-2329. http://www.ncbi.nlm.nih.gov/pubmed/17289087 (accessed 2007 Jan 13).

[60] Miao F J, Lee T J. Cholinergic and VIPergic innervation in cerebral arteries: a sequential double-labeling immunohistochemical study. Journal of Cerebral Blood Flow and Metabolism 1990; 10(1) 32-37.

[61] Chédotal A, Cozzari C, Faure M P, Hartman B K, Hamel E. Distinct choline acetyltransferase (ChAT) and vasoactive intestinal polypeptide (VIP) bipolar neurons project to local blood vessels in the rat cerebral cortex. Brain Research 1994; 646(2) 181-193.

[62] Fischer A, Canning B J, Kummer W. Correlation of vasoactive intestinal peptide and nitric oxide synthase with choline acetyltransferase in the airway innervation. Annals of the New York Academy of Sciences 1996; 805, 717-722.

[63] Kc P, Mayer C A, Haxhiu M A. Chemical profile of vagal preganglionic motor cells innervating the airways in ferrets: the absence of noncholinergic neurons. Journal of Applied Physiology 2004; 97(4) 1508-1517.

[64] Yu J G, Kimura T, Chang X F, Lee T J. Segregation of VIPergic-nitric oxidergic and cholinergic-nitric oxidergic innervation in porcine middle cerebral arteries. Brain Research 1998; 801(1-2) 78-87.

[65] Si M L, Lee T J. Alpha7-nicotinic acetylcholine receptors on cerebral perivascular sympathetic nerves mediate choline-induced nitrergic neurogenic vasodilation. Circulation Research 2002; 91(1) 62-69.

[66] Mikhelson M Ya, Zeimal E V. [Achetylcholine]. Leningrad: Nauka; 1970. Russian.

[67] Dauphin F, Lacombe P, Sercombe R, Hamel E, Seylaz J. Hypercapnia and stimulation of the substantia innominata increase rat frontal cortical blood flow by different cholinergic mechanisms. Brain Research 1991; 553(1) 75-83.

[68] Vaucher E, Hamel E. Cholinergic basal forebrain neurons project to cortical microvessels in the rat: electron microscopic study with anterogradely transported Phaseolus vulgaris leucoagglutinin and choline acetyltransferase immunocytochemistry. Journal of Neuroscience 1995; 15(11) 7427-7441.

[69] Lacombe P, Sercombe R, Vaucher E, Seylaz J. Reduced cortical vasodilatory response to stimulation of the nucleus basalis of Meynert in the aged rat and evidence for a control of the cerebral circulation. Annals of the New York Academy of Sciences 1997; 826, 410-415.

[70] Miao F J, Lee T J. VIP-ergic and cholinergic innervations in internal carotid arteries of the cat and rat. Journal of Cardiovascular Pharmacology 1991; 18(3) 369-378.

[71] Dauphin F, Ting V, Payette P, Dennis M, Hamel E. Vasocontractile muscarinic M1 receptors in cat cerebral arteries: pharmacological identification and detection of mRNA. European Journal of Pharmacology 1991; 207(4) 319-327.

[72] Nakai M, Tamaki K, Ogata J, Matsui Y, Maeda M. Parasympathetic cerebrovasodilator center of the facial nerve. Circulation Research 1993; 72(2) 470-475.

[73] Kuo J S, Leung Y M, Lin N N, Lee T J, Gong C L. Nicotine stimulation of the medulla increases blood flow of the common carotid artery in cats. Autonomic Neurosience 2010; 152(1-2) 49-54. doi: 10.1016/j.autneu.2009.08.019. http://www.ncbi.nlm.nih.gov/pubmed/19767248 (accessed 2009 Sep 19).

[74] Commons K G, Serock M R. Coincidence of Neurokinin 1 Receptor with the Vesicular Glutamate Transporter 3 (VGLUT3) in the Rat Forebrain. Neuroscience Letters 2009; 464(3) 188–192. doi: 10.1016/j.neulet.2009.08.042. http://www.ncbi.nlm.nih.gov/pubmed/?term=Commons+K+G%2C+Serock+M+R (accessed 2009 Aug 21).

[75] Batchelor P E, Armstrong D M, Blaker S N, Gage F H. Nerve growth factor receptor and choline acetyltransferase colocalization in neurons within the rat forebrain: response to fimbria-fornix transection. Journal of Comparative Neurology and Psychology 1989; 284(2) 187-204.

[76] Schnitzler A C, Lopez-Coviella I, Blusztajn J K. Differential modulation of nerve growth factor receptor (p75) and cholinergic gene expression in purified p75-expressing and non-expressing basal forebrain neurons by BMP9. Brain Research 2008; 1246, 19–28. doi: 10.1016/j.brainres.2008.09.085. http://www.ncbi.nlm.nih.gov/pubmed/18952073 (accessed 2008 Oct 14).

[77] Auld D S, Mennicken F, Day J C, Quirion R. Neurotrophins differentially enhance acetylcholine release, acetylcholine content and choline acetyltransferase activity in basal forebrain neurons. Journal of Nerochemistry 2001; 77(1) 253-262.

[78] Pongrac J L, Rylett R J. Differential effects of nerve growth factor on expression of choline acetyltransferase and sodium-coupled choline transport in basal forebrain cholinergic neurons in culture. Journal of Nerochemistry 1996; 66(2) 804-810.

[79] Zakharov V V, Khatiashvily I T, Iakhno N N. [Dementia with Lewy bodies]. Neurologicheskii Journal 1998; (6) 7-11. http://memorylab.ru/for_specialists/nejrozabolevania/demencia_s_telcam/ Russian.

[80] Oda Y. Choline acetyltransferase: the structure, distribution and pathologic changes in the central nervous system. Pathology International 1999; 49(11) 921-937.

[81] Mosimann U P, McKeith I G. Dementia with Lewy bodies – diagnosis and treatment. Swiss Medical Weekly 2003; 133(9-10) 131-142.

[82] Dobransky T, Rylett R J. Functional regulation of choline acetyltransferase by phosphorylation. Neurochemical Research 2003; 28(3-4) 537-542.

[83] Gill S K, Ishak M, Dobransky T, Haroutunian V, Davis K L, Rylett R J. 82-kDa choline acetyltransferase is in nuclei of cholinergic neurons in human CNS and altered in aging and Alzheimer disease. Nerobiology of Aging 2007; 28(7) 1028-1040.

[84] Wang J, Zhang H Y, Tang X C. Cholinergic deficiency involved in vascular dementia: possible mechanism and strategy of treatment. Acta Pharmacologica Sinica 2009; 30(7) 879-888.

[85] Nardone R, De Blasi P, Seidl M, Höller Y, Caleri F, Tezzon F, Ladurner G, Golaszewski S, Trinka E. Cognitive function and cholinergic transmission in patients with subcortical vascular dementia and microbleeds: a TMS study. Journal Of neuronal Pransmission 2011; 118(9) 1349-1358.

[86] Rochester L, Yarnall A J, Baker M R, David R V, Lord S, Galna B, Burn D J. Cholinergic dysfunction contributes to gait disturbance in early Parkinson's disease. Brain 2012; 135(9) 2779-2788.

[87] Shin J, Choi S, Lee J E, Lee H S, Sohn Y H, Lee P H. Subcortical white matter hyperintensities within the cholinergic pathways of Parkinson's disease patients according to cognitive status. Journal of neurology, neurosurgery and psychiatry 2012; 83(3) 315-321.

[88] Yarnall A, Rochester L, Burn D J. Mild cognitive impairment in Parkinson's disease. Age Ageing 2013; 42(5) 567-576.

[89] Onodera H, Sato G, Kogure K. Quantitative autoradiographic analysis of muscarinic and adenosine A1 binding sites after transient forefrain ischemia in the gerbil. Brain Research 1987; 415(2) 309-322.

[90] Ogawa N, Haba K, Asanuma M, Mizukava K, Mori A. Super-delayed changes of muscarinic acetylcholine receptors in the gerbil hippocampus following transient ischemia. In: Kito S. et al. (Eds) Advances in Experimental Medicine and Biology Volume 287: Neuroreceptor Mechanisms in Brain. New York: Plenum Press; 1991. p343-347.

[91] Ishimaru H, Takahashi A, Ikarashi Y, Maruiama Y. NGF delays rather then prevents the colinergic terminal and delayed neuronal death in the hippocampus after ischemia. Brain Research 1998; 789(2) 194-200.

[92] Dobransky T, Doherty-Kirby A, Kim A R, Brewer D, Lajoie G, Rylett R J. Protein kinase-C isoforms differentially phosphorylate human choline acetyltransferase regulating its catalytic activity. Journal of Biological Chemistry 2004; 279(50) 52059-52068.

[93] Ohno K, Tsujino A, Brengman J M, Harper C M, Bajzer Z, Udd B, Beyring R, Robb S, Kirkham F J, Engel A G. Choline acetyltransferase mutations cause myasthenic syndrome associated with episodic apnea in humans. Proceedings of the National Academy of Sciences of the United States of America-Physical Sciences 2001; 98, 2017–2022.

[94] Rylett R J. Synaptosomal "membrane-bound" choline acetyltransferase is most sensitive to inhibition by choline mustard. Journal of Nerochemistry 1989; 52(3) 869-875.

[95] Dobransky T, Davis W L, Rylett R J. Functional Characterization of Phosphorylation of 69-kDa Human Choline Acetyltransferase at Serine 440 by Protein Kinase C. Journal of Biological Chemistry 2001; 276(25) 22244-22250.

[96] Pahud G, Medilanski J, Eder-Colli L. Cytosolic Choline Acetyltransferase Binds Specifically to Cholinergic Plasma Membrane of Rat Brain Synaptosomes to Generate Membrane-Bound Enzyme. Neurochemical Research 2003, 28(3-4) 543–549.

[97] Fonnum F, Malthe-Sorenssen D. Membrane affinities and subcellular distribution of the different molecular forms of choline acetyltransferase from rat. Journal of Nerochemistry 1973; 20(5) 1351-1359.

[98] Smith C P, Carroll P T. A comparison of solubilized and membrane bound forms of choline-O-acetyltransferase (EC 2.3.1.6) in mouse brain nerve endings. Brain Research 1980; 185(2) 363-371.

[99] Benishin C G, Carroll P T. Multiple forms of choline-O-acetyltransferase in mouse and rat brain: solubilization and characterization. Journal of Nerochemistry 1983; 41(4) 1030-1039.

[100] Misawa H, Matsuura J, Oda Y, Takahashi R, Deguchi T. Human choline acetyltransferase mRNAs with different 5_-region produce a 69-kDa major translation product. Molecular Brain Research 1997; 44, 323–433.

[101] Kengaku M, Misawa H, Deguchi T. Multiple mRNA species of choline acetyltransferase from rat spinal cord. Molecular Brain Research 1993; 18(1-2) 71-76.

[102] Kim A R, Rylett R J, Shiton B H. Substrate binding and catalytic mechanism of human choline acetyltransferase. Biochemistry 2006; 45(49) 14621-14631.

[103] Matsuo A, Bellier J P, Nishimura M, Yasuhara O, Saito N, Kimura H. Nuclear choline acetyltransferase activates transcription of a high-affinity choline transporter. Journal of Biological Chemistry 2011; 286(7) 5836-5845.

[104] Dobransky T, Davis W L, Xiao G H, Rylett R J. Expression, purification and characterization of recombinant human choline acetyltransferase: phosphorylation of the enzyme regulates catalytic activity. Biochemical Journal 2000; 349(1) 141-145.

[105] Resendes M C, Dobransky T, Ferguson S S G, Rylett R J. Nuclear localization of the 82-kDa form of human choline acetyltransferase. Journal of Biological Chemistry 1999; 274, 19417–19421.

[106] Tooyama I, Kimura H. A protein encoded by an alternative splice variant of choline acetyltransferase mRNA is localized preferentially in peripheral nerve cells and fibers. Journal of Chemical Neuroanatomy 2000; 17(4) 217-226.

[107] Saito A, Sato T, Okano H, Toyoda K, Bamba H, Kimura S, Bellier J P, Matsuo A, Kimura H, Hisa Y, Tooyama I. Axotomy alters alternative splicing of choline acetyltransferase in the rat dorsal motor nucleus of the vagus nerve. Journal of Comparative Neurology and Psychology 2009; 513(2) 237-248.

[108] Dobransky T, Rylett R J. Protein kinase C isoforms differentially phosphorylate human choline acetyltransferase regulating its catalytic activity. Journal of Nerochemistry 2005; 95(2) 305-313.

[109] Dobransky T, Rylett R J. A model for dynamic regulation of choline acetyltransferase by phosphorylation. Journal of Nerochemistry 2005; 95, 305–313.

[110] Schmidt B M, Rylett R J. Phosphorylation of rat brain choline acetyltransferase and its relationship to enzyme activity. Journal of Nerochemistry 1993; 61(5) 1774-1781.

[111] Bruce G, Hersh L B. The phosphorylation of choline acetyltransferase. Neurochemical Research 1989; 14(7) 613-620.

[112] Dobransky T, Brewer D, Lajoie G, Rylett R J. Phosphorylation of 69-kD choline acetyltransferase at threonine-456 in response to short-term exposure to amyloid-b peptide 1-42. Journal of Biological Chemistry 2003; 278(8) 5883–5893.

[113] Rylett R J, Goddard S, Lambro A. Regulation of expression of cholinergic neuronal phenotypic markers in neuroblastoma LA-N-2.. Journal of Nerochemistry 1993; 61, 1388–1397.

[114] Fonnum F. The 'compartmentation' of choline acetyltransferase within the synaptosome. Biochemical Journal 1967; 103(1) 262-270.

[115] Eder-Colli L, Briand P A, Dunant Y. Membrane-bound choline acetyltransferase of the torpedo has characteristics of an integral membrane protein and can be solubilized by proteolysis. Brain Research 1992; 573(2) 284-292.

[116] Pahud G, Salem N, Van de Goor J, Medilanski J, Pellegrinelli N, Eder-Colli L. Study of subcellular localization of membrane-bound choline acetyltransferase in Drosophila central nervous system and its association with membranes. European Journal of Neuroscience 1998; 10(5) 1644-1653.

[117] Pahud G, Pahud G, Eder-Colli L. Cytosolic Choline Acetyltransferase Binds Specifically to Cholinergic Plasma Membrane of Rat Brain Synaptosomes to Generate Membrane-Bound Enzyme. Neurochemical Research 2003; 28(3-4) 543–549.

[118] Schmidt B M, Rylett R J. Basal synthesis of acetylcholine in hippocampal synaptosomes is not dependent upon membrane-bound choline acetyltransferase activity. Neuroscience 1993; 54(3) 649–656.

[119] Salem N, Medilanski J, Pellegrinelli N, Eder-Colli L. Hydrophilic and amphiphilic forms of Drosophila choline acetyltransferase are encoded by a single mRNA. European Journal of Neuroscience 1994; 6(5) 737-745.

[120] Carroll P T, Badamchian M, Craig P, Lyness W H. Veratridine-induced breakdown of cytosolic acetylcholine in rat hippocampal minces: an intraterminal form of acetylcholinesterase or choline O-acetyltransferase? Brain Research 1986; 383(1-2) 83-99.

[121] Carroll P T. Veratridine-induced activation of choline-O-acetyltransferase activity in rat hippocampal tissue: relationship to the veratridine-induced release of acetylcholine. Brain Research 1986; 414(2) 401-404.

[122] Carroll P T, Benishin C G. Depolarization of mouse forebrain minces with veratridine and high K+: failure to stimulate the Ca2+ independent, spontaneous release of acetylcholine from the cytoplasm due to hydrolysis of the acetylcholine stored there. Brain Research 1984; 291(2) 261-272.

[123] Carroll P T. Evidence to suggest that extracellular acetate is accumulated by rat hippocampal cholinergic nerve terminals for acetylcholine formation and release. Brain Research 1997; 753(1) 47-55.

[124] Alkondon M, Pereira E F, Cortes W S, Maelicke A, Albuquerque E X. Choline is a selective agonist of alpha7 nicotinic acetylcholine receptors in the rat brain neurons. European Journal of Neuroscience 1997; 9, 2734-2742.

[125] Rylett R J, Schmidt B M. Regulation of the synthesis of acetylcholine. Progress in Braim Research 1993; 98, 161-166.

[126] Smith L K, Carroll PT. Membrane-bound choline-O-acetyltransferase in rat hippocampal tissue is anchored by glycosyl-phosphatidylinositol. Brain Research 1993; 605(1) 155-163.

[127] Carroll P T. Membrane-bound choline-O-acetyltransferase in rat hippocampal tissue is associated with synaptic vesicles. Brain Research 1994; 633(1-2) 112-118.

[128] Birman S, Israël M, Lesbats B, Morel N. Solubilization and partial purification of a presynaptic membrane protein ensuring calcium-dependent acetylcholine release from proteoliposomes. Journal of Nerochemistry 1986; 47(2) 433-444.

[129] Israël M, Lesbats B, Morel N, Manaranche R, Le Gal la Salle G. Is the acetylcholine releasing protein mediatophore present in rat brain? FEBS Letters 1988; 233(2) 421-426.

[130] Falk-Vairant J, Corrèges P, Eder-Colli L, Salem N, Roulet E, Bloc A, Meunier F, Lesbats B, Loctin F, Synguelakis M, Israel M, Dunant Y. Quantal acetylcholine release induced by mediatophore transfection. Proceedings of the National Academy of Sciences of the United States of America-Physical Sciences 1996; 93(11) 5203-5207.

[131] Dunant Y, Cordeiro J M, Gonçalves P P. Exocytosis, mediatophore, and vesicular Ca2+/H+ antiport in rapid neurotransmission. Annals of the New York Academy of Sciences 2009; 1152, 100-112.

[132] Dunant, Y.; Israël M. Neurotransmitter release at rapid synapses. (2000). Biochimie, Vol. 82, No. 4, pp. 289-302.

[133] Bloc A, Bugnard E, Dunant Y, Falk-Vairant J, Israël M, Loctin F, Roulet E. Acetylcholine synthesis and quantal release reconstituted by transfection of mediatophore and choline acetyltranferase cDNAs. European Journal of Neuroscience 1999; 11(5) 1523-1534.

[134] Black S A, Rylett R J. Choline transporter CHT regulation and function in cholinergic neurons. Central Nervous System Agents in Medicinal Chemistry 2012; 12(2) 114-121.

[135] Dunant Y, Loctin F, Vallée J P, Parducz A, Lesbats B, Israël M. Activation and desensitisation of acetylcholine release by zinc at Torpedo nerve terminals. Pflügers Archiv 1996; 432(5) 853-858.

[136] Bancila V, Nikonenko I, Dunant Y, Bloc A. Zinc inhibits glutamate release via activation of pre-synaptic K channels and reduces ischaemic damage in rat hippocampus. Journal of Nerochemistry 2004; 90(5) 1243-1250.

[137] Medvedeva Y V, Lin B, Shuttleworth C W, Weiss J,H. Intracellular Zn2+ accumulation contributes to synaptic failure, mitochondrial depolarization, and cell death in an acute slice oxygen-glucose deprivation model of ischemia. Journal of Neuroscience 2009; 29(4) 1105-1114.

[138] Cordeiro J M, Gonçalves P P, Dunant Y. Synaptic vesicles control the time course of neurotransmitter secretion via a Ca^{2+}/H+ antiport. Journal of Physiology 2011; 589(1) 149-167.

[139] Carroll P T. Evidence to suggest that cytosolic acetylcholine in rat hippocampal nerve terminals is not directly transferred into synaptic vesicles for release. Brain Research 1996; 725(1) 3-10.

[140] Parducz A, Corrèges P, Sors P, Dunant Y. Zinc blocks acetylcholine release but not vesicle fusion at the Torpedo nerve-electroplate junction. European Journal of Neuroscience 1997; 9(4) 732-738.

[141] Zakharova E I. Storojeva Z I, Germanova E L, Monakov M Y, Proshin A T, Dudchenko A M, Lukyanova L D. Characteristics of cholinergic and cognitive functions in rats with individual resistance to the cerebral ischemia. In: Lukyanova L., Takeda N. and Singal P.K. (Eds.) Adaptation Biology and Medicine Volume 5: Health Potentials. New Delhi: Narosa Publishing House Pvt. Ltd.; 2008. p122-141,

[142] Svinov M M, Zakharova E I, Kositsyn N S. Ultrastructure of synapses in cerebral cortex layer i in rats with low and high resistance to hypoxia. Biulleten eksperimentalnoi biologii i meditsini 2001; 131(5) 499-501.

[143] Samoilov M O. [Reaction of brain neurons to hypoxia]. Leningrad: Nauka; 1985. Russian.

[144] Semchenko V V, Stepanov S S. [Effect of hypoxia on the structure of the presynaptic grid of the interneuronal contacts of the rat neocortex]. Tsitologia 1985; 27(11) 1235-1239. Russian.

[145] Semchenko V V, Stepanov S S. [Electron microscopic cytochemical and morphometric study of the cerebral cortex synapses in postmortem autolysis]. Biulleten eksperimentalnoi biologii i meditsini 1986; 102(7) 100-102. Russian.

[146] Gallo G. RhoA-kinase coordinates F-actin organization and myosin II activity during semaphorin-3A-induced axon retraction. Journal of Cell Science 2006; 119(16) 3413-3423.

[147] Keck T, Scheuss V, Jacobsen R I, Wierenga C J, Eysel U T, Bonhoeffer T, Hübener M. Loss of sensory input causes rapid structural changes of inhibitory neurons in adult mouse visual cortex. Neuron 2011; 71(5) 869-882.

[148] Woods G F, Oh W C, Boudewyn L C, Mikula S K, Zito K. Loss of PSD-95 enrichment is not a prerequisite for spine retraction. Journal of Neuroscience 2011; 31(34) 12129-12138.

[149] Semchenko V V, Bogolepov N N, Stepanov S S, Maksimishin S V, Khizhnyak A S. Synaptic plasticity of the neocortex of white rats with diffuse-focal brain injuries. Neuroscience of Behavioral and Physiology 2006; 36(6) 613-618.

[150] Bueters T, Von Euler M, Bendel O, Von Euler G. Degeneration of newly formed CA1 neurons following global ischemia in the rat. Experimental Neurology 2008; 209(1) 114-124.

[151] Mufson E J, Counts S E, Perez S E, Ginsberg S D. Cholinergic system during the progression of Alzheimer's disease: therapeutic implications. Expert Reviews of Neurotherapeutics 2008; 8(11) 1703–1718.

[152]] Sun M K, Hongpaisan J, Nelson T J, Alkon D L. Poststroke neuronal rescue and synaptogenesis mediated in vivo by protein kinase C in adult brains. Proceedings of the National Academy of Sciences of the United States of America-Physical Sciences 2008; 105(36) 13620-13625.

http://dx.doi.org/10.5772/58307

[153] Semchenko V V, Stepanov S S. [The system of subsynaptic units as an universal system-organizing and regulating factor of brain synapses]. Biulleten eksperimentalnoi biologii i meditsini 1997; 124(7) 4-12. Russian.

[154] Rossor M N, Svendsen C, Hunt S P, Mountjoy C Q, Roth M, Iversen L L. The substantia innominata in Alzheimer's disease: an histochemical and biochemical study of cholinergic marker enzymes. Neuroscience Letters 1982; 28(2) 217-222.

[155] Zakharova E I, Dudchenko A M, Svinov M M. Ivanov D S. Ignatiev I V. [The comparative characteristics of the cholinergic systems in the brains of the low and high resistant to the oxygen deficit rats]. Neurokhimia 2001; 18(2) 119-131. Russian.

[156] Zakharova E I, Storozheva Z I, Mukhin E I, Dudchenko A M. [Regulation of cognitive functions: cholinergic mechanisms and their variability]. In: Falikman M.V. & Pechenkova E.V. (Eds.) Cognitive Science in Moscow: new researches. Moscow: Buki-Vedi; 2011. p120-124. Russian.

[157]] Ni J W, Matsumoto K, Li H B, Murakami Y, Watanabe H. Neuronal damage and decrease of central acetylcholine level following permanent occlusion of bilateral common carotid arteries in rat. Brain Research 1995; 673(2) 290-296.

[158] Watanabe H, Ni J W, Sakai Y, Matsumoto K, Murukami Y, Tohda M. Permanent occlusion of bilateral internal carotid arteries produces cognitive deficits in two learning behavior tasks. Nihon Shinkei Seishin Yakurigaku Zasshi 1996; 16(1) 19-24.

[159] Rogers D C, Hunter A J. Photothrombotic lesions of the rat cortex impair acquisition of the water maze. Pharmacology, Biochemistry and Behavior 1997; 56(4) 747-754.

[160] Higashi H, Meno J R, Marwaha A S, Winn H R. Hippocampal injury and neurobehavioral deficits following hyperglycemic cerebral ischemia: effect of theophylline and ZM 241385. Journal of Neurosurgery 2002; 96(1) 117-126.

[161] Casamenti F, Bracco L, Bartolini L, Pepeu G. Effects of ganglioside treatment in rats with a lesion of the cholinergic forebrain nuclei. Brain Research 1985; 338(1) 45-52.

[162] Wenk G, Sweenay J, Hughey D, Carson J, Olton D. Cholinergic function and memory: extensive inhibition of choline acetyltransferase fails to impair radial maze performance in rats. Pharmacology, Biochemistry and Behavior 1986; 25(3) 521-526.

[163] Wisman L A, Sahin G, Maingay M, Leanz G, Kirik D. Functional convergence of dopaminergic and cholinergic input is critical for hippocampus-dependent working memory. Journal of Neuroscience 2008; 28(31) 7797-7807.

[164] Lee B, Shim I, Lee H, Hahm D H. Effect of Bupleurum falcatum on the stress-induced impairment of spatial working memory in rats. Biological and Pharmaceutical Bulletin 2009; 32(8) 1392-1398.

[165] Barros D M, Pereira P, Medina J, Izquierdo I. Modulation of working memory and of long- but not short-term memory by cholinergic mechanisms in the basolateral amygdala. Behavioural Pharmacology 2002; 13(2) 163-167.

[166] Vuckovich J A, Semel M E, Baxter M G. Extensive lesions of cholinergic basal forebrain neurons do not impair spatial working memory. Learning & Memory (2004); 11(1) 87-94.

[167] Lee B, Choi E J, Lee E J, Han S M, Hahm D H, Lee H J, Shim I. The Neuroprotective Effect of Methanol Extract of Gagamjungjihwan and Fructus Euodiae on Ischemia-Induced Neuronal and Cognitive Impairment in the Rat. Evidence-Based Complementary and Alternative Medicine 2011; 2011:685254. doi: 10.1093/ecam/nep028. http://www.ncbi.nlm.nih.gov/pmc/articles/PMC3137009/ (accessed 2011 March 10).

[168] Izquierdo I, Izquierdo L A, Barros D M, Mello e Souza T, De Souza M M, Quevedo J, Rodrigues C, Sant'Anna M K, Madruga M, Medina J H. Differential involvement of cortical receptor mechanisms in working, short-term and long-term memory. Behavioural Pharmacology 1998; 9(5-6) 421-427.

[169] Izquierdo I, Medina J H, Izquierdo L A, Barros D M, De Souza M M.; Mello e Souza T. Short- and long-term memory are differentially regulated by monoaminergic systems in the rat brain. Neurobiology of Learning and Memory 1998; 69(3) 219-224.

[170] Brown R W, Beale K S, Jay Frye G D. Mecamylamine blocks enhancement of reference memory but not working memory produced by post-training injection of nicotine in rats tested on the radial arm maze. Behavioural Brain Research 2002; 134(1-2) 259-265.

[171] Schweigler H, Lipp H P. Hereditary covariations of neuronal circuity and behavior: Correlation between the proportions of hippocampal synaptic fields in the region inferior and two-way avoidance in mice and rats. Behavioural Brain Research 1983; 7(1) 1-38.

Chapter 6

Neurochemical Communication: The Case of Endocannabinoids

Thomas Heinbockel

Additional information is available at the end of the chapter

http://dx.doi.org/10.5772/58410

1. Introduction

The brain is equipped with a magnificent diversity of molecules that allow neurons to communicate with each other. Some of these molecules have been known to function as neurotransmitters for several decades such as GABA and glutamate while for others their involvement in brain signaling has been demonstrated more recently. Cannabinoids fall into the latter group. Even though the effects of cannabinoids as active ingredients in marijuana on human psyche and behavior have been experienced by humans for centuries or possibly millennia, their existence and production in the brain was described only some thirty years ago. Even more recently, their functional role in neural circuits of the brain has been discerned. This review focuses on these endogenously produced signaling molecules, endogenous cannabinoids or endocannabinoids (eCBs). Their functional role in the nervous system and interaction with other neurotransmitter systems will be described. One hallmark feature of endocannabinoid signaling is their ability to act as retrograde messengers in neural circuits. Two examples, one from the hippocampus and one from the main olfactory bulb, illustrate in detail this intercellular communication pathway.

Several features underscore the importance to understand the endocannabinoid system. Increasing evidence demonstrates the relevance of endocannabinoids in normal behaviors, including pain reception [1] and feeding [2, 3]. The therapeutic potential of cannabinoids has received increasing attention over the past few years [4]. endocannabinoids play a role in neuroprotection against acute excitotoxicity [5] and functional recovery after brain injury [6]. Endocannabinoids regulate human airway function and provide a means to treat respiratory pathologies [1]. Cannabinoids are in widespread use recreationally as psychoactive drugs and interact with other drugs of abuse. This fact emphasizes even more the need to understand the endocannabinoid system and the neurobiological substrate of their mood-altering capacity [7,

8]. Furthermore, the endocannabinoid system is crucially involved in processes of learning and memory, e.g., in the extinction of aversive memories [9].

2. The endocannabinoid system

Endocannabinoids are small lipids that regulate various aspects of brain function such as learning and memory including synaptic transmission and different forms of short-and long-term plasticity [10]. They also influence growth and development such as synapse formation and neurogenesis. Other biological functions modulated by endocannabinoids include eating and anxiety. Principally, two endocannabinoids, N-arachidonoylethanol-amide (anandamide, AEA) and 2-arachidonoylglycerol (2-AG) are the natural agonists/ligands of the most widely expressed cannabinoid receptor in the brain, CB1R [11] (Figure 1).

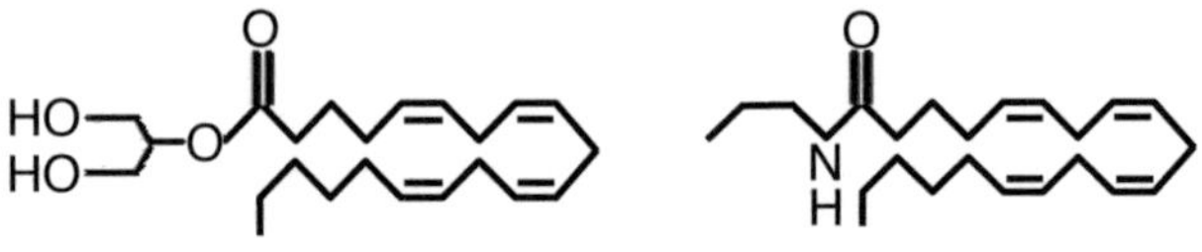

Figure 1. Two endocannabinoids, 2-arachidonoylglycerol (2-AG) and N-arachidonoylethanol-amide (anandamide, AEA), are the natural agonists/ligands of cannabinoid receptors, CB1Rs, in the brain.

Endocannabinoids, as fatty-acid derived endogenous ligands, together with their G-protein coupled cannabinoid receptors form the endocannabinoid system. This system also includes associated biochemical machinery with endocannabinoid precursors, synthetic and degradative enzymes for these lipidic neurotransmitters, and transporters [12-15]. Two different cannabinoid receptors have been cloned, CB1 and CB2 receptors. They share 44% amino acid sequence homology [16, 17]. The expression pattern of the two cannabinoid receptors in various body parts is distinctly different. In the brain, CB1R is the most abundant G-protein coupled receptor [18]. CB2R is primarily expressed in immune cells and peripheral tissues [17]. Some level of CB2R expression has also been detected in the brainstem, cortex and cerebellar neurons and microglia [19, 20].

Cannabinoid receptors are found at high levels in the brain [21, 22], specifically at presynaptic nerve terminals [23, 24]. They can be activated by cannabis-derived drugs. Δ9-Tetrahydrocannabinol, THC, is the bioactive ingredient of the drugs marijuana and hashish [25] and can artificially activate cannabinoid receptors as exogenous cannabinoids. Cannabinoid receptors exist in all normal brains [18, 21, 22] where they subserve many essential brain functions when activated by their natural ligands. Cannabinoid receptors in the nervous system are predominantly $G_{i/o}$-protein-coupled type 1 cannabinoid receptors (CB1 receptors, CB1Rs). Their ligands, endocannabinoids are synthesized from membrane lipids [26]. Endocannabinoids can diffuse through membranes and are thus able to activate receptors in the same manner as exogenously applied cannabinoids such as cannabis. Anandamide and 2-AG were discovered in the early 1990s [27-29, reviewed in 30] while their functional role in neuronal communication remained obscure for years. Since their discovery, the role of endocannabinoids as retrograde messengers that suppress both excitatory and inhibitory transmission has been well-established. Endocannabinoids mediate retrograde signals in the hippocampus [31-35], cerebellum [36-38], neocortex [39, 40], amygdala [41, 42], and olfactory bulb [43]. Termination of endocannabinoidsignalling is accomplished by reuptake into both neurons and glia. Subsequently, anandamide and 2-AG are hydrolyzed intracellularly by fatty acid amide hydrolase (FAAH) and monoacylglycerol lipase (MAGL), respectively [44].

3. Unusual and novel neurotransmitters

Endocannabinoids are different from conventional neurotransmitters because they are lipids that are not stored but rather are rapidly synthesized on demand at the site of need from components of the cell membrane. Upon cellular activation, they are released from places all over the cell. They are arachidonic acid-containing messengers generated by phospholipase action [45]. Stimuli that trigger release of endocannabinoids include rise of intracellular calcium levels inside the neuron or activation of certain G-protein-coupled receptors such as metabotropic glutamate receptors (mGluR5). Subsequent to their non-synaptic, non-vesicular release, endocannabinoids bind to cannabinoid receptors on nearby neurons such as presynaptic interneurons where they regulate presynaptic neurotransmitter release, e.g., through closure of specific ion channels.

Endocannabinoids are members of a loose family of unusual and novel neurotransmitters. Similar to endocannabinoids, other novel neurotransmitters such as nitric oxide (NO), carbon monoxide (CO), and hydrogen sulfide (H2S) do not adhere to the classic definition of neurotransmitters and challenge the notion of what constitutes a neurotransmitter [46, 47]. These synaptic molecules have changed markedly the definition of a neurotransmitter. They satisfy key neurotransmitter criteria but differ radically from classical transmitters. For example, endocannabinoids, nitric oxide and carbon monoxide are neither stored in synaptic vesicles nor released by exocytosis. Nitric oxide does not act via traditional receptors on postsynaptic membranes.

Like endocannabinoids, nitric oxide can serve as an intercellular messenger in the brain [48]. It acts as a retrograde factor at synapses and presynaptically regulates both glutamatergic and GABAergic synapses to alter release-probability in synaptic plasticity. Nitric oxide influences the synaptic machinery involved in transmitter release and, in a coordinated fashion, also the vesicular recycling mechanisms. Nitric oxide has a role in the coordination of local pre-and post-synaptic function during plasticity at individual synapses. It is involved in experience-dependent plasticity in the cerebral cortex. Likewise, cannabinoids mediate a variety of forms of short-and long-term synaptic plasticity that have been reviewed in detail elsewhere [49-51].

4. Depolarization-induced suppression of inhibition

The relevance of the endocannabinoid system for neural signaling and brain function in general has been explored only recently [13]. Endocannabinoids mediate a new type of neuronal communication, called DSI, **D**epolarization-induced **S**uppression of **I**nhibition (Fig. 2) (reviewed in [10, 12, 30]. A short rise in intracellular calcium concentration in a principal neuron, e.g., a pyramidal cell of the hippocampus, results in a transient decline of incoming inhibitory signals in the form of GABA arriving from other neurons. This observation led to the hypothesis that during DSI, some unknown messenger must travel from the postsynaptic cell to the presynaptic GABA-releasing one and somehow turns off neurotransmitter release. Conventional chemical synaptic signaling between two neurons involves activation of a presynaptic neuron resulting in transmitter release and subsequent activation of the postsynaptic neuron, e.g., a GABAergic inhibitory interneuron makes synaptic contacts with a glutamatergic pyramidal cell in the hippocampus. When the interneuron is activated it releases the inhibitory neurotransmitter GABA and inhibits the pyramidal cell. In contrast, during DSI, when a pyramidal cell is activated, e.g., through direct current injection, the inhibitory input onto that pyramidal cell is reduced. As a major breakthrough in our understanding of endocannabinoid signaling, endocannabinoids were found to act as retrograde signaling molecules that mediate communication between postsynaptic pyramidal cells and presynaptic inhibitory interneurons and evoke the reduction in GABA release. Since endocannabinoids are lipids, they do not diffuse over great distances in the watery extracellular environment of the brain. Rather, DSI acts as a short-lived local effect that enables individual neurons to disconnect briefly from their neighbors and encode information [12].

The announcement of this breakthrough has been given the Latin term 'Dies mirabilis' (wonderful day) by Alger [10]. In March of 2001 four independent labs described in three different journals their studies culminating in the conclusion that endocannabinoids function mainly as retrograde messengers. Elphick and Egertova [52] analyzed prior pharmacological and anatomical studies of the actions of cannabinoid receptor agonists and combined this with their knowledge of the localization of cannabinoid receptors and degradative enzymes for anandamide, fatty acid amide hydrolase (FAAH) to reason that endocannabinoids act as retrograde messengers. Pivotal work by Wilson and Nicoll [34] and Ohno-Shosaku et al. [32] established that DSI was mimicked by activating cannabinoid receptors whereas blockade of cannabinoid receptors prevented DSI. A corresponding phenomenon, DSE, **D**epolarization-induced **S**upression of **E**xcitation, mediated by retrograde action of endocannabinoids, was identified by Kreitzer and Regehr [36] at cerebellar excitatory synapses. DSI and DSE are based on a presynaptic effect as shown by an increase in calcium in the postsynaptic cells and corresponding changes in paired pulse ratio of neurotransmitter release.

G-protein coupled receptors (GPCRs) are involved in mediating the transduction of extracellular stimuli, such as neurotransmitters, into intracellular signaling cascades. Activation of specific G-protein coupled receptors triggers the release of endocananbinoids for many minutes, e.g., dopamine [53], metabotropic glutamate [33, 37, 54] or muscarinic M1/M3 acetylcholine receptors [55, 56]. Even though endocannabinoids are typically released in a

http://dx.doi.org/10.5772/58410

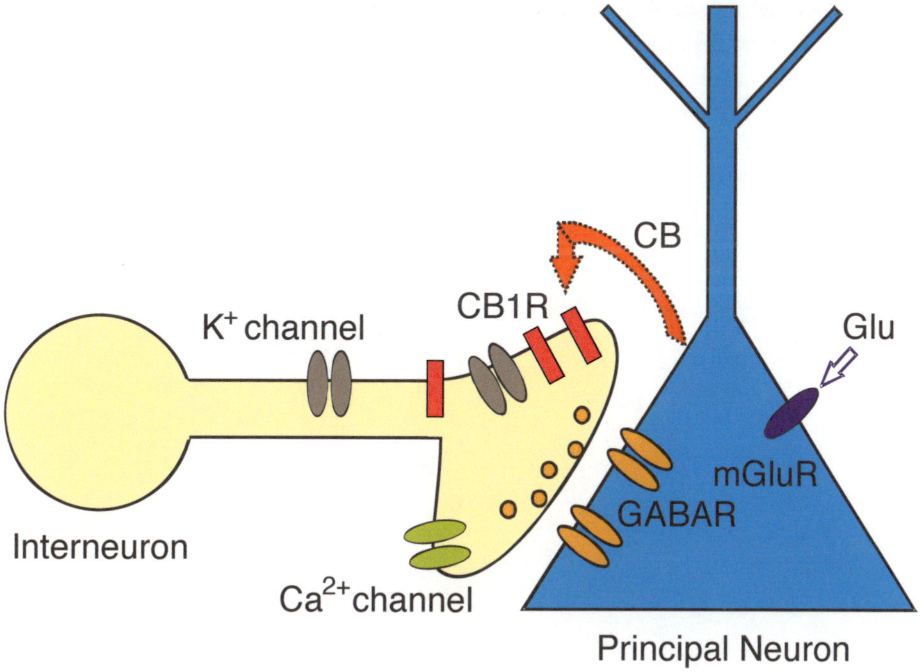

Figure 2. **D**epolarization-induced **S**uppression of **I**nhibition (DSI) is a model for retrograde signaling in the brain and allows assaying real time release of endocannabinoids from principal neurons as a brief cessation of GABA ouput. Activation of metabotropic glutamate receptors (mGluRs) on principal neurons or depolarization of postsynaptic principal cells evokes synthesis and release of cannabinoids (CBs). Cannabinoids bind to presynaptic cannabinoid receptors (CB1R) on GABAergic interneurons and transiently reduce GABA release from synaptic terminals. As a consequence, $GABA_A$ receptor-mediated synaptic currents and GABAergic inhibition are temporarily suppressed in postsynaptic principal neurons.

calcium-dependent manner [57, 58], in the mGluR-and mAChR-dependent pathways, no clear rise in intracellular calcium $[Ca^{2+}]_i$ [37, 55] is necessary. The release of endocananbinoids can be initiated even in the presence of high intracellular concentrations of calcium chelators, although endocannabinoids may nevertheless be sensitive to the ambient intracellular calcium concentration [59]. Studies by the Alger lab and others indicate that G-protein coupled receptor activation of postsynaptic cells leads to enhancement of DSI, e.g., glutamate acting on group I metabotropic glutamate receptors (mGluRs) directly generates endocannabinoids and enhances DSI ([37, 33]. It is now established that activation of many G-protein coupled receptors is linked to the use of endocannabinoids to deliver or fine-tune their messages to target cells [11].

The discovery of DSI has been a major advance in our understanding of the endocannabinoid system for brain function [60]. DSI is a type of short-term synaptic plasticity originally observed in the cerebellum and hippocampus [12, 14]. Endocannabinoids are retrograde signaling molecules that are released from depolarized principal neurons and travel to presynaptic inhibitory interneurons to reduce GABA release. DSI is a novel, regulatory process that manifests itself as a transient suppression of synaptic $GABA_A$ responses mediated by retrograde signaling of endocannabinoids from principal neurons (Fig. 3). Through the retrograde signaling process neurons alter the strength of synapses made onto them and thereby control their own synaptic excitability in an activity-dependent manner, which is functionally important in information processing by neuronal networks [14]. In the cerebellum, a retrograde signaling process that is similar to DSI reduces synaptic excitation by suppressing presynaptic glutamate release and is called DSE [61], see above.

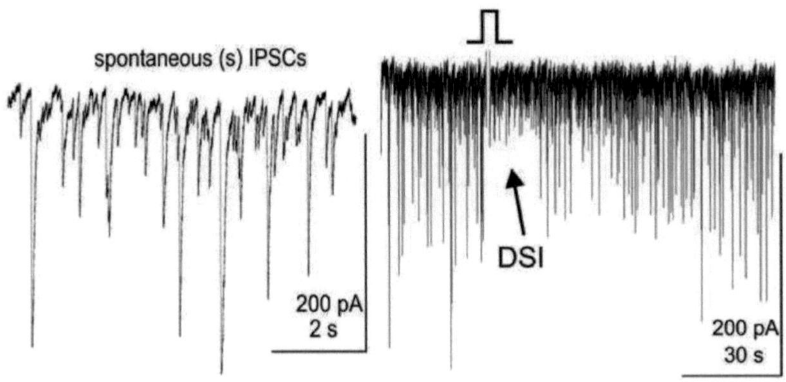

Figure 3. Right panel: Hippocampal pyramidal cells show spontaneous inhibitory postsynaptic currents (IPSCs). Left panel: In response to a 1-s voltage pulse the pyramidal cell reveals DSI, a transient reduction in IPSC activity as a result of endocannabinoids acting on CB1R on presynaptic GABAergic interneurons.

5. Hippocampal depolarization-induced suppression of inhibition

Endocannabinoids are lipids and, unlike classic neurotransmitters, are not stored but rather rapidly synthesized from components of the cell membrane. They are synthesized in, and released from, postsynaptic somatodendritic domains that are readily accessible to whole-cell patch electrodes. The effects of these lipid signals are detected electrophysiologically as CB1R-dependent alterations in conventional synaptic transmission, which, therefore, provide a sensitive means of bioassay in gendocannabinoid levels and actions. Endocannabinoid release can be triggered through Ca^{2+}-dependent or relatively Ca^{2+}-independent pathways, with different down-stream effects. As discussed above, endocannabinoids are released non-synaptically, non-vesicular from places all over cells when levels of calcium rise inside the neuron or when certain G-protein-coupled receptors are activated. After cellular release, endocannabinoids travel to cannabinoid receptors on nearby neurons and evoke a reversible, short-term depression of synaptic transmission, DSI. In activated hippocampal pyramidal cells, DSI leads to a transient reductionof GABA release from presynaptic terminals of inhibitory interneurons. Direct insights into the actions of endocannabinoids have been based primarily on pharmacological experiments. The hydrophobicity of endocannabinoids severely limits their penetration into brain tissue, and endocannabinoids are rapidly degraded by abundant endogenous lipases. These intrinsic properties of endocannabinoids make it difficult to directly study physiological effects of endocannabinoids. The development of a highly water-soluble caged anandamide that is inert to lipases circumvents these problems [62]. When perfused into hippocampal slice preparations, the caged anandamide serves as a latent endocannabinoid pool, and focal photolysis rapidly liberates highly hydrophobic anandamide *in situ* to activate CB1R. Photolysis is an alternative experimental approach to chemically stimulate synapses, cells, or circuits by directly applying neurotransmitter or neuromodulators. Often pharmacological approaches yield little control of the stimulation in terms of timing, space and specificity. However, photo-uncaging of caged neurotransmitters has made the pharmacological approach more sophisticated. Photo-uncaging uses localized, patterned light and yields higher spatial and temporal resolution. One application of photostimulation, the flash photolysis technique, can be used to determine signaling kinetics of the endocannabinoid system [60, 62]. The endocannabinoid system can be used as a tool for bioassaying the temporal dynamics or kinetics of lipid signaling. Combining whole-cell voltage patch-clamp recording, intracellular calcium measurements, and photorelease of caged glutamate and a novel, caged cannabinoid, anandamide (AEA) allows determining endocannabinoid signaling kinetics. Flash photolysis of caged compounds (photolysis using so-called molecular optical probes or photoprobes) is an important tool in this endeavor. Caged compounds are inert, biologically inactive (e.g., a caged cannabinoid or caged glutamate) until a flash of laser light breaks open the molecular cage, releases the caged molecule and generates a biologically active effector molecule in situ [63]. Chemically, the caged compound is a modified signal molecule. The modification of the molecule prevents its bioactivity until light absorption results in a photochemical change of the signal molecule such that its bioactivity is restored.

The lipid signaling pathway comprises several temporal components that can be determined to quantify the time that it takes from the DSI-inducing stimulus to the onset of DSI. These components contribute to the latency to onset of DSI (start of DSI-inducing stimulus to initial suppression of IPSCs). Among them is the rise of calcium to initiate endocannabinoid synthesis (t-Ca). The rise in intracellular calcium leads to endocannabinoid synthesis and release, followed by travel of these molecules to cannabinoid receptors on presynaptic interneurons, t-EC. The next step is the activation of CB1R and downstream effects, t-CB1R (t-DSI = t-Ca + t-EC + t-CB1R). Experiments carried out using the above-mentioned technological advances allowed determining the time for synthesis and release of eCB from the postsynaptic neuron, which was estimated to be around 150 ms at room temperature, comparable with the timescale of metabotropic signaling and at least an order of magnitude faster than previously thought. A major portion of the DSI onset time, t-DSI, reflects activation of presynaptic CB1Rs and downstream consequences. The data suggest that, far from simply serving long-term neuromodulatory functions, endocannabinoid signaling is sufficiently fast to exert moment-to-moment control of synaptic transmission. The DSI onset latency after a voltage step, t-DSI, is 350 to 400 ms. t-CB1R, the direct activation of CB1R by photoreleasing anandamide which results in suppression of sIPSCs, takes ~180ms (Fig. 4). A transient rise in intracellular calcium sufficient to obtain minimal DSI, t-Ca, is evoked by a 50-ms voltage step and takes ~60 ms. The time needed for endocannabinoid synthesis and release to occur, t-EC, is about 150 ms.

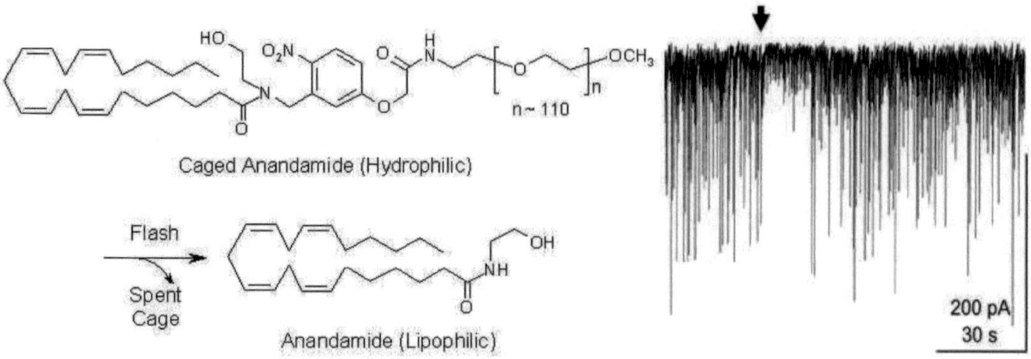

Figure 4. Left panel: Photolysis of caged anandamide yields bioactive anandamide. Right panel: Photorelease of anandamide suppresses sIPSCs after a delay of ~180 ms. Modified from [62] with permission of the Society for Neuroscience.

Voltage-activated DSI works through a rise in intracellular calcium concentration. However, release of endocannabinoids can be triggered even in the presence of high intracellular concentrations of calcium chelators, although they may nevertheless be sensitive to ambient intracellular calcium [59]. To test if these two pathways function on the same time scale, the dynamic components of the mGluR-induced endocannabionoid response on sIPSC frequency in pyramidal cells are compared (Fig. 5) [62]. The mean onset latency, duration and magnitude of the IPSC suppression evoked by uncaged glutamate are similar to that caused by uncaged AEA (Figs. 4, 5). No reduction in sIPSCs occurred for 221 ms (determined by extrapolation of the exponential fit to the control sIPSC level). The time-to-onset of IPSC suppression evoked by the mGluR-induced endocannabinoid process (time to mGluR-dependent suppression of inhibition, $t_{mGluRSI}$) is described by: t-mGluR-SI = 221 ms = t-eCB(mGluR) + t-CB1R, where t-eCB(mGluR) is the time for activation of the mGluR-dependent endocannabinoid synthesis and release, and t-CB1R is ~180 ms (see above). This leaves t-eCB(mGluR) to be < 50 ms, which is even faster than endocannabinoid synthesis and released evoked by a voltage step.

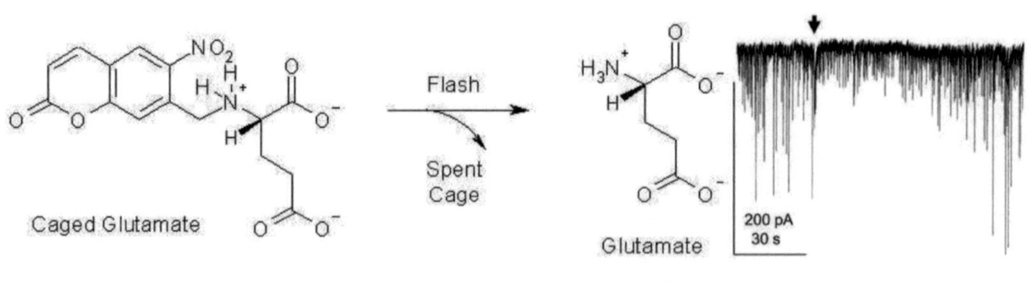

Figure 5. Dynamics of mGluR-dependent endocannabinoid suppression of sIPSCs in cultured hippocampal slices. Left panel: Photorelease of glutamate. Right panel: Recording from a pyramidal cell illustrates the transient reduction in spontaneous (s) IPSC frequency of CA1 pyramidal cells after flash photorelease of caged glutamate (photolysis induced suppression of inhibition, PSI). Arrow indicates laser flash. From [62] with permission of the Society for Neuroscience.

Anandamide can be released from its caged form by a UV-laser flash and rapidly activates presynaptic CB1Rs to suppress the release of GABA [62]. A specific CB1R antagonist, AM 251, blocks the suppression of spontaneous IPSCs. This establishes that uncagedanandamide can be used as a CB1R agonist to study activation of CB1R in the brain. Similarly, uncaged glutamate acts at mGluRs on hippocampal pyramidal cells to evoke cannabinoid release and subsequent suppression of presynaptic GABA release [62]. The data provide the first detailed attempt to determine the minimal time required for activation of an intercellular neuronal lipid messenger system. This signaling system requires a major portion of DSI onset time, t-DSI, for activation of presynaptic CB1R and downstream consequences. Endocannabinoids, and by extension similar lipid messengers, can be mobilized and evoke responses as quickly as conventional metabotropic, G-protein receptor-coupled neurotransmitters. The speed with which neuromodulators such as endocannabinoids act places critical constraints on the physiological roles they can play. Endocannabinoids and other lipids function in brain signaling not simply in homeostatic processes or slowly-activating forms of regulation, but rather lipids can affect neuronal excitability in moment-to-moment information processing.

6. Depolarization-induced suppression of inhibition in glomerular circuits of the olfactory bulb

The olfactory bulb is the first relay station in the CNS for processing of sensory information that comes from olfactory receptor cells in the nasal epithelium. Cannabinoid receptors are expressed at high levels in the olfactory bulb, specifically in the input region, the glomerular layer [21, 64-66]. Neurons in the glomerular layer are immunoreactive for enzymes that synthesize endocannabinoids [67-69]. Our understanding of the physiological role of endocannabinoids and cannabinoid receptors for neural signaling in the olfactory system is just emerging. Recent electrophysiological evidence has established that the endocannabinoid system plays a functional role in regulating neuronal activity and signaling in olfactory bulb glomeruli [43].

Neurons in the glomerular fall into three subpopulations: periglomerular (PG), external tufted (eTC), and short-axon (SA) cells. Periglomerular cells are neurochemically and functionally heterogeneous [70-72]. Periglomerular cells are GABAergic, short-axon cells express both GABA and dopamine, and external tufted cells are glutamatergic [72, 73]. Periglomerular cells receive input from the olfactory nerve or dendrodendritic glutamatergic input from external tufted or mitral cells, e.g., as spontaneous bursts of EPSCs [70, 73-74]. Periglomerular cells presynaptically inhibit olfactory receptor neurons through GABAergic transmission [76, 77]. External tufted cells receive spontaneous bursts of inhibitory postsynaptic currents (sIPSCs) from periglomerular cells at inhibitory GABAergic synapses as well as spontaneous glutamatergic EPSCs [74; 78]. In the glomerular layer, external tufted cells can be a potential source of endocannabinoids.

Cannabinoid receptors directly regulate membrane properties of periglomerular cells as shown by the effects of CB1R antagonist AM251 and agonist WIN in the presence of ionotropic glutamate and $GABA_A$ receptor blockers (synaptic blockers: CNQX, APV, gabazine) [43]. This indicates that the actions of cannabinoids on periglomerular cells are mediated through CB1R expressed by periglomerular cells. AM251 directly activates periglomerular cells and enhances their GABA release. Periglomerular cells are synaptically connected to external tufted cells. Therefore, any CB1R-mediated regulation of activity of periglomerular cells could affect GABA release and synaptic transmission to external tufted cells. CB1R is also expressed in external tufted cells and may participate in modulating external tufted cell activity.

In external tufted cells, neither AM251 nor WIN influences firing frequency or membrane potential [43]. However, in the presence of synaptic blockers cannabinoid drugs have a modest effect on external tufted cells. In this condition, AM251 slightly increases the firing rate of external tufted cells without membrane depolarization. In synaptic blockers, WIN slightly decreases firing of external tufted cells without a clear change in membrane potential. The effects of AM251 and WIN in the presence of synaptic blockers, i.e., during pharmacological isolation of external tufted cells, indicate that CB1R mediates a direct effect on external tufted cells. The direct excitatory effect of a CB1R antagonist on external tufted cells is opposed by increased GABAergic synaptic input from periglomerular cells onto external tufted cells, i.e., the enhanced GABA release from periglomerular cells triggered by a CB1R antagonist may dominate and mask the CB1R antagonist-evoked direct excitation of external tufted cells.

The CB1R effects on periglomerular and external tufted cell prompt the questions if DSI is present in the glomerular layer of the olfactory bulb. In external tufted cells, DSI can be induced with a 5-sec depolarizing voltage step from a holding potential of -60 mV to 0 mV (Fig. 5). In external tufted cells DSI is visible as a decrease in the amplitude and frequency of sIPSCs. The response to a single depolarizing step is a suppression of sIPSC area by ~40 % of control which then gradually recoveres. External tufted cells exhibit a distinct intrinsic bursting pattern [74]. In order to mimic spontaneous rhythmic bursting of an external tufted cell a train of depolarizing steps can be applied to the cell. This experimental paradigm allows determining a possible functional role of DSI in glomeruli. A train of depolarizing steps results in a transient 60% reduction in sIPSC area (20 steps, 0.75 Hz) (Fig. 4B, F). DSI can be completely eliminated in the presence of AM251, indicating that DSI is mediated by CB1R (Fig. 5C, F). The bursting frequency of external tufted cells ranges from 0.5 to 6.5 Hz with a mean frequency of 2.7 bursts/sec [74]. Depolarizing voltage pulses at 2 Hz (20 steps, pulse duration: 250 ms) evoke DSI as a reduction of sIPSCs in external tufted cells, similar to the results obtained with voltage steps at 0.75 Hz to 0 mV. In external tufted cells, single depolarizing voltage steps as well as a train of voltage steps evoke suppression of inhibition (DSI). This suggests that spontaneous rhythmic bursting of these cells triggers the release of endocannabinoids which function as retrograde messengers to reduce GABA release from periglomerular cells which in turn, regulates the activity of periglomerular cell synaptic targets such as external tufted cells.

Endocannabinoids regulate neuronal activity and signaling in olfactory bulb glomeruli. They function in the form of DSI through CB1R-mediated retrograde signaling among glomerular neurons. Endocannabinoids are released from external tufted cells and act as retrograde messengers to control the excitability of presynaptic neurons, i.e., periglomerular cells, and to regulate their transmitter release. Endocannabinoids are synthesized and

http://dx.doi.org/10.5772/58410

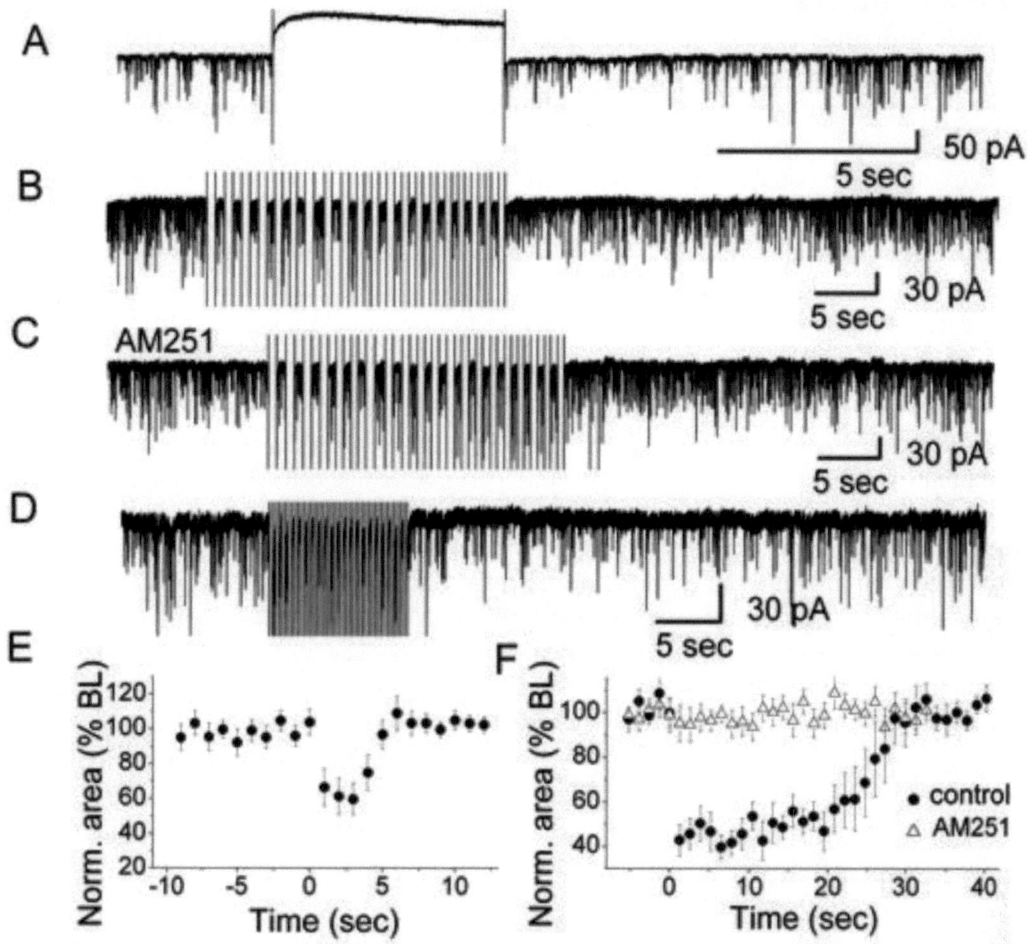

Figure 6. **D**epolarization-induced **S**uppression of **I**nhibition (DSI) in olfactory glomeruli. **A** A depolarizing voltage step evoked DSI in a representative external tufted cell. High Cl^--based pipette solution was used for recording sIPSCs. Depolarization was achieved by stepping from-60 mV holding potential to 0 mV for 5 sec. **B** In the presence of CNQX and 5-AP, a train of 20 voltage steps to 0 mV (0.75 Hz; step duration: 667 ms) transiently reduced sIPSCs in an external tufted cell. Holding potential was-60 mV. **C.** In the presence of AM251, no sIPSC suppression was observed. **D** A train of 20 voltage steps to-30 mV (2 Hz; step duration: 250 ms) transiently reduced sIPSCs in an external tufted cell (in CNQX and 5-AP). **E** Normalized sIPSCs area illustrating the magnitude and time course of DSI elicited by a 5-sec depolarizing pulse (n=7). The averaged values between 0 – 5 sec after the end of the voltage step were significantly different from the baseline (ANOVA and Bonferroni post-hoc analysis, $p< 0.05$). **F** Normalized sIPSC area illustrating the magnitude and time course of DSI elicited by a train of depolarizations to 0 mV (n=12) in control and in the presence of AM251 (n=10). In control conditions, the averaged values between zero to 2 5 seconds after the end of the train of voltage steps were significantly different from the baseline (ANOVA and Bonferroni post-hoc analysis, $p< 0.05$). From [43] with permission of the Society for Neuroscience.

released from neuronal cell bodies as a result of cellular excitation [11]. One potential source of endocannabinoids in the olfactory bulb is neurons that synapse onto presynaptic cells, i.e., periglomerular cells, and receive feedback synaptic inputs. This profile fits external tufted cells and they could be a potential endocannabinoid source in the olfactory bulb which is supported by the fact that DSI is found in external tufted cells. DSI in external tufted cells is subject to the level of cellular activation, i.e., voltage step duration and step number. DSI cannot be evoked with step durations of 1 sec or less while a step duration closer to 5 seconds evokes transient DSI. A train of depolarizing voltage steps (>3) generates particularly prominent DSI and strengthens the inhibition of sIPSCs. This suggests that excitation of external tufted cells in the form of rhythmic bursting triggers the release of endocannabinoids and regulates glomerular activity. Bursting is intrinsic to external tufted cells and mediated by several cell intrinsic conductances [79]. Bursting of neurons may modulate endocannabinoid release not only in the olfactory bulb but also in other brain systems and constitute a general phenomenon of endocannabinoidsignaling.

Olfactory sensory neurons form direct synaptic contacts with external tufted cells. Sensory or synaptic input to external tufted cells can trigger the release of endocannabinoids which have an inhibitory effect on CB1Rs in presynaptic periglomerular cells. Endocannabinoids thus reduce inhibitory input to external tufted cells and enhance external tufted cell sensitivity to weak sensory inputs by depolarizing the membrane potential closer to spike threshold. This CB1R-mediated inhibition of periglomerular cells reduces their GABA release and, in turn, modifies the firing pattern of external tufted cells and, potentially, also reduces inhibition of mitral cells and presynaptic olfactory nerve terminals. The functional relevance of this signaling pathway lies in a potential increase of the overall sensitivity of the glomerulus to sensory inputs resulting from activation of CB1R on periglomerular cells.

7. Endocannabinoid-evoked physiological responses and crosstalk with other neurotransmitters

Endocannabinoids can evoke physiological responses that are not mediated by presynaptic CB1Rs but rather by postsynaptic CB1Rs [14], e.g., via regulation of K^+ conductances present on the extrasynaptic dendritic surface of neurons or modulation of postsynaptic NMDA receptors or even non-CB1R, e.g., [80]. Several conventional CB1R ligands have been reported to have CB1R unspecific effects or activate non-CB1 receptors [14]. Electrophysiological evidence suggests that the CB1R agonist WIN55,212-2 produces non-CB1R mediated effects on the excitability of principal neurons in the basolateral amygdala [81], thus providing evidence for a non-CB1R site of action of WIN55,212-2 [82, 83]. Cannabinoid drugs can activate other 'non-CB' receptors, such as GPR55, peroxisome proliferator-activated receptors (PPARs), and vanilloid type TRP channels [84, 85].

The accepted view of endocannabinoid action is based on hippocampal studies demonstrating that endocannabinoids reduce synaptic inhibition of the principal cell (DSI), see above. Endocannabinoids were found to possess other properties, namely, to mediate self-modulation of neocortical pyramidal neurons [86] or long-lasting self-inhibition in neocortical GABA-containing interneurons [87]. This self-inhibition is mediated by autocrine release of endocannabinoids and does not depend on glutamatergic and/or GABAergic neurotransmis-

http://dx.doi.org/10.5772/58410

sion but rather on activity-dependent long-lasting hyperpolarization due to the activation of a K^+-conductance. Endocannabinoids released by these interneurons target the same cells and mediate a lasting hyperpolarization that is blocked by a CB1R antagonist. Self-inhibited cells can become hyperpolarized below spike threshold and are effectively removed from the neural circuit in which they reside.

The endocannabinoid system reciprocally modulates other neurotransmitter systems [88]. Examples include interactive cross-talk with the endogenous opioid system [89, 90]. Incidentally, like the endogenous opiate system, the endocannabinoid system was first discovered because it can be activated by a plant-derived compound – in the case of the endocannabinoids, this is Δ9-tetrahydrocannabinol, the bioactive ingredient of the drugs marijuana and hashish [25]. Other studies detected an interaction of the endocannabinoid system at the molecular and functional levels with other neurotransmitters such as the dopaminergic and adenosinergic systems [91-93]. Recent evidence has suggested cross-modulation between the endocannabinoid and hypocretinergic system [88]. This idea is based on the overlap observed in the neuroanatomical distribution of both systems as well as their putative functions. Functionally, both endocannabinoids and hypocretins can contribute to the regulation of appetite, reward and analgesia. Furthermore, biochemical and functional studies have demonstrated heterodimers between CB1 cannabinoid receptor and hypocretin receptor-1. Activation of hypocretin receptor-1 stimulates the synthesis of 2-arachidonoyl glycerol which through retrograde endocannabinoid signaling results in inhibition of neighboring cells. This interaction would allow endocannabinoids to contribute to hypocretin effects and provide potential therapeutic applications to currently existing drugs targeting these systems [88]. However, these two neuromodulatory systems exert antagonistic effects in the regulation of the sleep/wake cycle and anxiety-like responses which contributes even more to the excitement of performing research targeting the endocannabinoid system.

Acknowledgements

This work was supported in part by U.S.-PHS grants GM08016 and MD007597. I would like to gratefully acknowledge current and former collaborators Drs. Bradley E. Alger, Joseph P. Y. Kao, and Ze-Jun Wang.

Author details

Thomas Heinbockel*

Address all correspondence to: theinbockel@howard.edu

Department of Anatomy, Howard University College of Medicine, Washington, DC, USA

References

[1] Calignano A, Katona I, Desarnaud F, Giuffrida A, La Rana G, Mackie K, Freund TF, Piomelli D. Bidirectional control of airway responsiveness by endogenous cannabinoids. Nature 2000; 408:96-101.

[2] Cota D, Marsicano G, Lutz B, Vicennati V, Stalla GK, Pasquali R, Pagotto. Endogenous cannabinoid system as a modulator of food intake. Internat J Obesity 2003; 27:289-301.

[3] Soria-Gómez E, Bellocchio L, Reguero L, Lepousez G, Martin C, Bendahmane M, Ruehle S, Remmers F, Desprez T, Matias I, Wiesner T, Cannich A, Nissant A, Wadleigh A, Pape HC, Chiarlone AP, Quarta C, Verrier D, Vincent P, Massa F, Lutz B, Guzmán M, Gurden H, Ferreira G, Lledo PM, Grandes P, Marsicano G. The endocannabinoid system controls food intake via olfactory processes. Nat Neurosci 2014; 17:407-415.

[4] Iversen L, Chapman V. Cannabinoids: a real prospect for pain relief. Curr Opin Pharmacol 2002; 2:50-55.

[5] Marsicano G, Goodenough S, Monory K, Hermann H, Eder M, Cannich A, Azad SC, Cascio MG, Gutierrez SO, van der Stelt M, Lopez-Rodriguez ML, Casanova E, Schutz G, Zieglgansberger W, Di Marzo V, Behl C, Lutz B. CB1 cannabinoid receptors and on-demand defense against excitotoxicity. Science 2003; 302:84-88.

[6] Panikashvili D, Simeonidou C, Ben-Shabat S, Hanus L, Breuer A, Mechoulam R, Shohami E. An endogenous cannabinoid (2-AG) is neuroprotective after brain injury. Nature 2001; 413:527-531.

[7] Katona I, Rancz EA, Acsady L, Ledent C, Mackie K, Hajos N, Freund TF. Distribution of CB1 cannabinoid receptors in the amygdala and their role in the control of GABAergic transmission. J Neurosci 2001; 21:9506-9518.

[8] Valjent E, Mitchell JM, Besson MJ, Caboche J, Maldonado R. Behavioural and biochemical evidence for interactions between Delta9-tetrahydrocannabinol and nicotine. Br J Pharmacol 2002; 135:564-578.

[9] Marsicano G, Wotjak CT, Azad SC, Bisogno T, Rammes G, Cascio MG, Hermann H, Tang J, Hofmann C, Zieglgansberger W, Di Marzo V, Lutz B. The endogenous cannabinoid system controls extinction of aversive memories. Nature 2002; 418:530-534.

[10] Alger BE. Endocannabinoids at the synapse a decade after the dies mirabilis (29 March 2001): what we still do not know. J Physiol 2012; 590.10:2203–2212.

[11] Kano M, Ohno-Shosaku T, Hashimotodani Y, Uchigashima M, Watanabe M. Endocannabinoid-mediated control of synaptic transmission. Physiol Rev 2009; 89:309–380.

[12] Alger BE. Retrograde signaling in the regulation of synaptic transmission: focus on endocannabinoids. Prog Neurobiol 2002; 68:247-286.

[13] Alger BE, Kim J. Supply and demand for endocannabinoids. Trends Neurosci 2011; 34:304-315.

[14] Freund TF, Katona I, Piomelli D. Role of endogenous cannabinoids in synaptic signaling. Physiol Rev 2003; 83:1017-1066.

[15] Howlett AC, Breivogel CS, Childers SR, Deadwyler SA, Hampson RE, Porrino LJ. Cannabinoid physiology and pharmacology: 30 years of progress. Neuropharmacol 2004; 47:345-358.

[16] Matsuda LA, Lolait SJ, Brownstein MJ, Young AC, Bonner TI. Structure of a cannabinoid receptor and functional expression of the cloned cDNA. Nature 1990; 346, 561-564.

[17] Munro S, Thomas KL, Abu-Shaar M. Molecular characterization of a peripheral receptor for cannabinoids. Nature 1993; 365, 61–65.

[18] Herkenham M, Lynn AB, Little MD, Johnson MR, Melvin LS, de Costa BR, Rice KC. Cannabinoid receptor localization in brain. ProcNatlAcadSci USA 1990; 87:1932–1936.

[19] Van Sickle, M.D., Duncan, M., Kingsley, P.J., Mouihate, A., Urbani, P., Mackie, K., et al. Identification and functional characterization of brainstem cannabinoid CB2 receptors. Science 2005; 310:329-332.

[20] Núñez, E., Benito, C., Pazos, M.R., Barbachano, A., Fajardo, O., González, S., et al. Cannabinoid CB2 receptors are expressed by perivascular microglial cells in the human brain: an immunohistochemical study. Synapse 2004; 53:208-213.

[21] Herkenham M, Lynn AB, Johnson MR, Melvin LS, de Costa BR, Rice KC. Characterization and localization of cannabinoid receptors in rat brain: a quantitative in vitro autoradiographic study. J Neurosci 1991; 11:563-583.

[22] Matsuda LA, Bonner TI, Lolait SJ. Localization of cannabinoid receptor mRNA in rat brain. J Comp Neurol 1993; 327:535-550.

[23] Katona I, Sperlagh B, Sik A, Kafalvi A, Vizi ES, Mackie K, Freund TF. Presynaptically located CB1 cannabinoid receptors regulate GABA release from axon terminals of specific hippocampal interneurons. J Neurosci 1999; 19:4544-4558.

[24] Tsou K, Mackie K, Sanudo-Pena MC, Walker JM. Cannabinoid CB1 receptors are localized primarily on cholecystokinin-containing GABAergic interneurons in the rat hippocampal formation. Neurosci 1999; 93:969-975.

[25] Ameri A. The effects of cannabinoids on the brain. Prog Neurobiol 1999; 58:315-348.

[26] Di Marzo V, Melck D, Bisogno T & De Petrocellis L. Endocannabinoids: endogenous cannabinoid receptor ligands with neuromodulatory action. Trends Neurosci 1998; 21:521–528.

[27] Devane WA, Hanus L, Breuer A, Pertwee RG, Stevenson LA, Griffin G, et al. Isolation and structure of a brain constituent that binds to the cannabinoid receptor. Science 1992; 258:1946–1949.

[28] Mechoulam R, Ben-Shabat S, Hanus L, Ligumsky M, Kaminski NE, Schatz AR, Gopher A, Almog S, Martin BR, Compton DR, Pertwee RG, Griffin G, Bayewitch M, Barg J, Vogel Z. Identification of an endogenous 2-monoglyceride, present in canine gut, that binds to cannabinoid receptors. Biochem Pharmacol 1995; 50, 83–90.

[29] Sugiura T, Kondo S, Sukagawa A, Nakane S, Shinoda A, Itoh K, Yamashita A, Waku K. 2-Arachidonoylgylcerol – a possible endogenous cannabinoid receptor-ligand in brain. Biochem Biophys Res Commun 1995; 215:89–97.

[30] Nicoll R, Alger BE. The brain's own marijuana. Sci Amer 2004; 291:68-75

[31] Maejima T, Ohno-Shosaku T, Kano M. Endogenous cannabinoid as a retrograde messenger from depolarized postsynaptic neurons to presynaptic terminals. Neurosci Res 2001; 40:205-210.

[32] Ohno-Shosaku T, Maejima T, Kano M. Endogenous cannabinoids mediate retrograde signals from depolarized postsynaptic neurons to presynaptic terminals. Neuron 2001; 29:729-738.

[33] Varma N, Carlson GC, Ledent C, Alger BE. Metabotropic glutamate receptors drive the endocannabinoid system in hippocampus. J Neurosci 2001; 21:(RC188) 1-5.

[34] Wilson RI, Nicoll RA. Endogenous cannabinoids mediate retrograde signalling at hippocampal synapses. Nature 2001; 410:588-592.

[35] Wilson RI, Kunos G, Nicoll RA. Presynaptic specificity of endocannabinoid signaling in the hippocampus. Neuron 2001; 31:1-20.

[36] Kreitzer AC, Regehr WG. Cerebellar depolarization-induced suppression of inhibition is mediated by endogenous cannabinoids. J Neurosci 2001; 21:RC174.

[37] Maejima T, Hashimoto K, Yoshida T, Aiba A, Kano M. Presynaptic inhibition caused by retrograde signal from metabotropic glutamate to cannabinoid receptors. Neuron 2001; 31:463-475.

[38] Yoshida T, Hashimoto K, Zimmer A, Maejima T, Araishi K, Kano M. The cannabinoid CB1 receptor mediates retrograde signals for depolarization-induced suppression of inhibition in cerebellar Purkinje cells. J Neurosci 2002; 22:1690-1697.

[39] Trettel J, Levine ES. Endocannabinoids mediate rapid retrograde signaling at interneuron pyramidal neuron synapses of the neocortex. J Neurophys 2003; 89:2334-2338.

[40] Trettel J, Fortin DA, Levine ES. Endocannabinoidsignalling selectively targets perisomatic inhibitory inputs to pyramidal neurones in juvenile mouse neocortex. J Physiol (London) 2004; 556:95-107.

[41] Zhu PY, Lovinger DM. Retrograde endocannabinoid signaling in a postsynaptic neuron/synaptic bouton preparation from basolateral amygdala. J Neurosci 2005; 25:6199-6207.

[42] Kodirov SA, Jasiewicz J, Amirmahani P, Psyrakis D, Bonni K, Wehrmeister M, Lutz B. Endogenous cannabinoids trigger the depolarization-induced suppression of excitation in the lateral amygdala. Learning & Memory 2009; 17:43-49.

[43] Wang Z-J, Sun L, Heinbockel T. Cannabinoid receptor-mediated regulation of neuronal activity and signaling in glomeruli of the main olfactory bulb. J Neurosci 2012; 32:8475-8479

[44] Muccioli GG. Endocannabinoid biosynthesis and inactivation, from simple to complex. Drug Discov Today 2010; 15:474-483

[45] Di Marzo V. The endocannabinoid system: its general strategy of action, tools for its pharmacological manipulation and potential therapeutic exploitation. Pharmacol Res 2009; 60:77-84.

[46] Barañano DE, Ferris CD, Snyder SH. Atypical neural messengers. Trends Neurosci 2001; 24:99-106.

[47] Boehning D, Snyder SH. Novel neural modulators. Annu Rev Neurosci 2003; 26:105-31.

[48] Hardingham N, Dachtler J, Fox K. The role of nitric oxide in pre-synaptic plasticity and homeostasis. Front Cell Neurosci 2013; 31, 7:190.

[49] Cachope R. Functional diversity on synaptic plasticity mediated by endocannabinoids. Philos Trans R Soc Lond B BiolSci 2012; 367:3242-3253

[50] Castillo PE, Younts TJ, Chávez AE, Hashimotodani Y. Endocannabinoidsignaling and synaptic function. Neuron 2012; 76:70-81

[51] Katona I, Freund TF. Multiple functions of endocannabinoid signaling in the brain. Annu Rev Neurosci. 2012; 35:529-558.

[52] Elphick MR, Egertova M. The neurobiology and evolution of cannabinoid signalling. Philos Trans R SocLond B BiolSci 2001; 356:381–408.

[53] Giuffrida A, Parsons LH, Kerr TM, Rodriguez de Fonseca F, Navarro M, Piomelli D. Dopamine activation of endogenous cannabinoid signaling in dorsal striatum. Nat Neurosci 1999; 2:358-363.

[54] Ohno-Shosaku T, Shosaku J, Tsubokawa H, Kano M. Cooperative eCB production by neuronal depolarization and group I metabotropic glutamate receptor activation. Eur J Neurosci 2002; 15:953-961

[55] Kim J, Isokawa M, Ledent C, Alger BE. Activation of muscarinic acetylcholine receptors enhances the release of endogenous cannabinoids in the hippocampus. J Neurosci 2002; 22:10182-10191.

[56] Ohno-Shosaku T, Matsui M, Fukudome Y, Shosaku J, Tsubokawa H, Taketo MM, Manabe T, Kano M. Postsynaptic M1 and M3 receptors are responsible for the muscarinic enhancement of retrograde endocannabinoidsignalling in the hippocampus. Eur J Neurosci 2003; 18:109-116.

[57] Di Marzo V, Fontana A, Cadas H, Schinelli S, Cimino G, Schwartz JC, Piomelli D. Formation and inactivation of endogenous cannabinoid anandamide in central neurons. Nature 1994; 372:686-691.

[58] Stella N, Schweitzer P, Piomelli D. A second endogenous cannabinoid that modulates long-term potentiation. Nature 1997; 388:773-778.

[59] Hashimotodani Y, Ohno-Shosaku T, Tsubokawa H, Ogata H, Emoto K, Maejima T, Araishi K, Shin HS, Kano M. Phospholipase C_{β} serves as a coincidence detector through its Ca^{2+}dependency for triggering retrograde endocannabinoid signal. Neuron 2005; 45:257-268.

[60] Heinbockel T. Electrophysiological recording and imaging of neuronal signals in brain slices. In: Neuroscience. Heinbockel T (ed.), Rijeka, Croatia: Intech, 2012,ch 2, pp. 19-48.

[61] Kreitzer AC, Regehr WG. Retrograde inhibition of presynaptic calcium influx by endogenous cannabinoids at excitatory synapses onto Purkinje cells. Neuron 2001; 29:717-727.

[62] Heinbockel T, Brager DH, Reich C, Zhao J, Muralidharan S, Alger BE, Kao JPY. Endocannabinoid signaling dynamics probed with optical tools. J Neurosci 2005; 25: 9449-9459.

[63] Kao JPY. Controlling neurophysiology with light and caged molecules. In: Optical control of neural excitability. Keshishian H (ed), Washington, DC: Society for Neuroscience; 2008, pp. 1-12.

[64] Pettit DA, Harrison MP, Olson JM, Spencer RF, Cabral GA. Immunohistochemical localization of the neural cannabinoid receptor in rat brain. J Neurosci Res 1998; 51:391-402.

[65] Tsou K, Brown S, Sanudo-Pena MC, Mackie K, Walker JM. Immunohistochemical distribution of cannabinoid CB1 receptors in the rat central nervous system. Neurosci 1998; 83:393-411.

[66] Moldrich G, Wenger T. Localization of the CB1 cannabinoid receptor in the rat brain. An immunohistochemical study. Peptides 2000; 21:1735-1742.

[67] Allen Institute for Brain Science. Allen Mouse Brain Atlas [Online]. Seattle, WA. http://mouse.brain-map.org.; 2009

[68] Okamoto Y, Wang J, Morishita J, Ueda N. Biosynthetic pathways of the endocannabinoid anandamide. Chem Biodivers 2007; 4:1842-1857.

[69] Piomelli D. The molecular logic of endocannabinoid signaling. Nat Rev Neurosci 2003; 4:873-884.

[70] Ennis M, Hayar A, Hamilton KA. Neurochemistry of the main olfactory system. In: Handbook of Neurochemistry and Molecular Neurobiology (ed. Lajtha A), Sensory Neurochemistry, ed. Johnson DA. Springer: Heidelberg.; 2007, pp. 137-204.

[71] Shao Z, Puche AC, Kiyokage E, Szabo G, Shipley MT. Two GABAergic intraglomerular circuits differentially regulate tonic and phasic presynaptic inhibition of olfactory nerve terminals. J Neurophysiol 2009; 101:1988-2001.

[72] Kiyokage E, Pan YZ, Shao Z, Kobayashi K, Szabo G, Yanagawa Y, Obata K, Okano H, Toida K, Puche AC, Shipley MT. Molecular identity of periglomerular and short axon cells. J Neurosci 2010; 30:1185-1196.

[73] Hayar A, Karnup S, Ennis M, Shipley MT. External tufted cells: a major excitatory element that coordinates glomerular activity. J Neurosci 2004; 24:6676-6685.

[74] Hayar A, Karnup S, Shipley MT, Ennis M. Olfactory bulb glomeruli: external tufted cells intrinsically burst at theta frequency and are entrained by patterned olfactory input. J Neurosci 2004; 24:1190-1199.

[75] Hayar A, Shipley MT, Ennis M. Olfactory bulb external tufted cells are synchronized by multiple intraglomerular mechanisms. J Neurosci 2005; 25:8197-8208.

[76] Aroniadou-Anderjaska V, Zhou F-M, Priest CA, Ennis M, Shipley MT. GABA-B receptor-mediated presynaptic inhibition of sensory input to the olfactory bulb. J Neurophysiol 2000; 84:1194-1203.

[77] Murphy GJ, Darcy DP, Isaacson JS. Intraglomerular inhibition: Signaling mechanisms of an olfactory microcircuit. Nat Neurosci 2005; 8: 354-364.

[78] Hayar A, Ennis M. Endogenous GABA and glutamate finely tune the bursting of olfactory bulb external tufted cells. J Neurophysiol 2007; 98:1052-1056.

[79] Liu S, Shipley MT. Multiple conductances cooperatively regulate spontaneous bursting in mouse olfactory bulb external tufted cells. J Neurosci 2008; 28:1625-1639.

[80] Lozovaya N,Yatsenko N, Beketov A, Tsintsadze T, Burnashev N. Glycine receptors in CNS neurons as a target for nonretrograde action of cannabinoids. J Neurosci 2005; 25:7499-7506.

[81] Pistis M, Perra S, Pillolla G, Melis M, Gessa GL, Muntoni AL. Cannabinoids modulate neuronal firing in the rat basolateral amygdala: evidence for CB1-and non-CB1-mediated actions. Neuropharmacol 2004; 46:115-25.

[82] Breivogel CS, Griffin G, Di Marzo V, Martin BR. Evidence for a new G protein-coupled cannabinoid receptor in mouse brain. Mol Pharmacol 2001; 60:155-63.

[83] Hajos N, Ledent C, Freund TF. Novel cannabinoid-sensitive receptor mediates inhibition of glutamatergic synaptic transmission in the hippocampus. Neurosci 2001; 106:1-4.

[84] Kukkonen JP. A ménage à trois made in heaven: G-protein-coupled receptors, lipids and TRP channels. Cell Calcium 2011; 50:9-26.

[85] Pertwee RG, Howlett AC, Abood ME, Alexander SP, Di Marzo V, Elphick MR, et al. International Union of Basic and Clinical Pharmacology. LXXIX. Cannabinoid receptors and their ligands: beyond CB1 and CB2. Pharmacol Rev 2010; 62, 588-631.

[86] Marinelli S, Pacioni S, Cannich A, Marsicano G, Bacci A. Self-modulation of neocortical pyramidal neurons by endocannabinoids. Nat Neurosci 2009; 12, 1488–1490.

[87] Bacci A, Huguenard JR, Prince DA. Long-lasting self-inhibition of neocortical interneurons mediated by endocannabinoids. Nature 2004; 431:312-316.

[88] Flores A, Maldonado R, Berrendero F. Cannabinoid-hypocretin cross-talk in the central nervous system: what we know so far. Front Neurosci 2014; 7:256.

[89] Parolaro D, Rubino T, Viganò D, Massi P, Guidali C, Realini N. Cellular mechanisms underlying the interaction between cannabinoid and opioid system. Curr Drug Targets 2010; 11:393-405.

[90] Robledo P, Berrendero F, Ozaita A, Maldonado R. Advances in the field of cannabinoid-opioid cross-talk. Addict Biol 2008; 13:213-224.

[91] Carriba P, Ortiz O, Patkar K, Justinova Z, Stroik J, Themann A, et al. Striatal adenosine A2A and cannabinoid CB1 receptors form functional heteromeric complexes that mediate the motor effects of cannabinoids. Neuropsychopharmacol 2007; 32:2249-2259.

[92] Ferré S, Lluís C, Justinova Z, Quiroz C, Orru M, Navarro G, et al. Adenosine-cannabinoid receptor interactions. Implications for striatal function. Br J Pharmacol 2009; 160:443-453.

[93] Fernández-Ruiz J, Hernández M, Ramos JA. Cannabinoid-dopamine interaction in the pathophysiology and treatment of CNS disorders. CNS Neurosci Ther 2010; 16:e72-91.

Chapter 7

High Temporal Resolution Brain Microdialysis as a Tool to Investigate the Dynamics of Interactions Between Olfactory Cortex and Amygdala in Odor Fear Conditioning

Chloé Hegoburu, Luc Denoroy,
Anne-Marie Mouly and Sandrine Parrot

Additional information is available at the end of the chapter

http://dx.doi.org/10.5772/57490

1. Introduction

Fear conditioning is one of the most widely used paradigms for studying the neurobiology of emotional learning. In this paradigm, an emotionally neutral stimulus (the conditioned stimulus or CS) is paired with an aversive unconditioned stimulus (US), generally a mild foot shock. After a few trials, re-exposure to the CS alone elicits a fear response, proceeding through the necessary connecting structures, and ending with the autonomic and motoric effector outputs. This fear response is part of an anticipatory response to danger [1], initiating a range of defensive reactions that counter threats to survival [2]. The most universal response is a postural immobility, called freezing [3, 4]. Moreover, the threatening stimulus also triggers the activation of the hypothalamic subnuclei to induce an increase in blood pressure, ultrasonic vocalizations emission, or the release of stress hormones.

The vast majority of studies devoted to investigate the neural basis of fear conditioning have used auditory cues as conditioned stimuli and the neural pathways involved in auditory fear conditioning have been well characterized [5-8]. The information carried by the auditory CS can take one of two pathways: either directly from the thalamus to quickly reach the amygdala or the CS can travel from the auditory thalamus to the auditory cortex before reaching the amygdala. These thalamic and cortical areas send projections to the lateral nucleus of the amygdala, which is a site of CS-US convergence. The lateral nucleus, in turn, projects to the central amygdala, which controls the expression of fear responses by way of projections to brainstem areas. The major conclusion of these studies is that the amygdala plays a critical role in linking external stimuli to defense responses through synaptic plasticity. However, although the amygdala seems to be essential to the formation and storage of fear memories, it might not store all aspects of the aversive event. Indeed, plasticity also occurs in cortical areas during fear conditioning, which could support declarative memories of the learning episode mainly through interactions with the medial temporal lobe memory system [9-13]. Thus, the amygdala may store some aspects of fear memory and facilitate the storage of other, more sensory-related, aspects of fear memory in cortical areas [14]. Yet few studies have investigated this question [15].

Intriguingly, whereas olfaction plays a dominant role in rat behavior from birth throughout adulthood, very few studies have used odor cues as CS in fear conditioning paradigms. Yet, odors have a rather unique status for eliciting emotional memories.[16]. This particularity might be linked to the uniqueness of the anatomy of the olfactory system. Indeed, in contrast to the other sensory pathways, olfactory information has a direct access to the amygdala and olfactory (piriform) cortex with no obligatory thalamic relay [17-19]. The literature suggests that, similarly to what is observed in auditory fear conditioning, the amygdala is a key brain structure involved in the acquisition, consolidation and expression of odor fear conditioning [20-26]. Recently, some studies also suggest that the posterior piriform cortex (PPC) may play a critical role in this associative learning [23, 26, 27]. Therefore, the olfactory system constitutes a particularly relevant model for studying the relative contribution of sensory cortices and amygdalar nuclei to odor fear learning.

For several years now, the glutamatergic transmission in the amygdala is known to play a critical role in the acquisition of fear conditioning [28, 29]. Indeed, pharmacological studies show that NMDA and AMPA subclasses of glutamate receptors are crucial for synaptic plasticity and long-term potentiation to occur in the amygdala, sustaining the formation of the CS-US association [25, 30-35]. In addition, the GABAergic transmission seems to be also involved in the acquisition of fear learning. Intra-amygdala infusion of the $GABA_A$ receptor agonist muscimol before training impairs learning [36, 37]. Therefore, glutamate and GABA neurotransmission are thought to play a critical role in the acquisition and expression of fear memories (for review, see [38]).

Beside these neuropharmacological studies, a few neurochemical studies have directly measured glutamate or GABA levels in the amygdala during auditory fear conditioning, using a 10-min sampling rate [39, 40]. However, this sampling rate is too long as compared to the rapid neurobiological events underlying fear conditioning. An approach allowing rapid, sub-minute sampling is required to better characterize the dynamics of neurotransmitter changes evoked by the stimuli involved in fear conditioning experiments [41]. Until now, the precise time course of the differential involvement of the amygdala and sensory cortices in fear conditioning has received little investigation. The aim of this chapter is to show that intra-cerebral in vivo microdialysis with high temporal resolution is an interesting tool to investigate the time course of activation of amygdala and sensory cortices in this learning.

2. Monitoring neurotransmitters using microdialysis

2.1. Principle of the technique and analytical considerations

Microdialysis has become a conventional technique for sampling low molecular weight molecules present in the extracellular medium of many organs from animals or humans [42]. In the brain, it has been used *in vivo* or *ex vivo* to monitor amino acids neurotransmitters as excitatory or inhibitory amino acids as glutamate and GABA, monoamines as dopamine, noradrenaline, serotonin and/or neuropeptides for instance. The microdialysis relies on a semi-permeable membrane that allows free diffusion of solutes between the extracellular space and an artificial fluid. A microdialysis probe consists of two concentric tubes with the distal part (1–5 mm) covered by a dialysis hollow fibre whose cut-off ranges between 6,000 and 100,000 Da. Such a probe is inserted into a living brain tissue and is perfused by an isotonic physiological fluid. Molecules diffuse down their concentration gradient across the dialysis membrane in a bidirectional way ("dialysis" for collecting endogenous molecules or "reverse dialysis" for applying exogenous compounds) (Figure 1). In the case of collection, the relative recovery across the probe membrane, defined as the ratio between the extracellular concentration and the concentration of a compound in the dialysate collected at the outlet of the probe, depends on several factors: it increases with the surface of the membrane, it decreases with higher flow rate of the perfusion fluid, and it varies with the chemical and physical characteristics of the membrane [43]. The choice of the dialysis membrane can be crucial for compounds present at trace concentration or when the limit of detection of the analytical method is relatively moderate. For instance, a short length (i.e. 1-2 mm) of the membrane chosen to sample a very small brain area in rats, such as the periaqueductal grey matter, the locus coeruleus, the amygdala and hypothalamic nuclei leads to a low recovery of sampling, making difficult the monitoring of low concentrated compounds as monoamines or neuropeptides. Depending on the methodological parameters, recovery values usually reported in literature are between 5 and 25 % for amino acids or monoamines and can reach < 1 % for neuropeptides. Another point to take into account is the choice of the geometry of the probe tubings when considering the sampling rate, especially when designing in vivo microdialysis on awake animals. These latter peculiar points will be explained and detailed in the next section part of the manuscript.

As the microdialysis probe is continuously perfused at a constant flow rate, continuous sampling of neurotransmitters is possible with no loss. Indeed, neurotransmitters present in the microdialysate can be directly analyzed without clean-up procedures as high molecular weight proteins cannot cross the dialysis membrane thanks to the cut-off of the membrane used. However, manipulation of microdialysis samples requires precaution in case of amino acids: use of sterile tubes, filtered aCSF and wear of gloves avoiding contamination due to the ubiquitous presence of free amino acids on labware and skin. Eventually, samples may be usually analyzed by a separative method like high performance liquid chromatography (HPLC) or capillary electrophoresis (CE) [44, 45]. Microdialysates can be analyzed on-line, i.e., at the outlet of the probe, through an analytical interface, or off-line i.e., after sample collection in micro-tubes, in combination with a separative method [44, 46, 47]. Thus, the determination

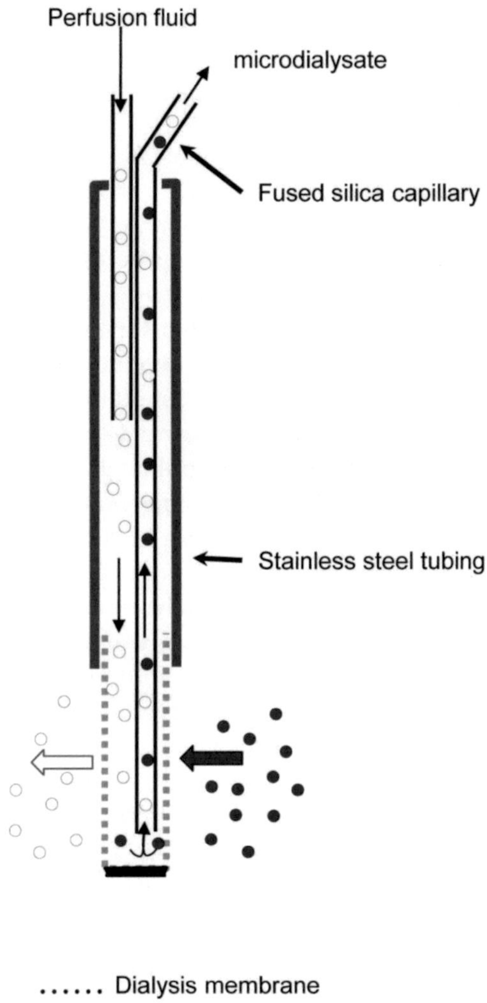

Figure 1. Schematic representation of a microdialysis probe. The probe is continuously perfused by an isotonic physiological fluid. Endogenous compounds (filled circles) diffuse through the dialysis membrane (filled arrow) and are sampled in the microdialysate collected at the outlet of the probe. Drugs (open circles) can be added to the perfusion medium and can diffuse out of the probe into the extracellular medium (open arrow) providing a means of local administration. From [109], with permission from John Wiley and Sons.

of concentrations in each sample reflects the average concentration over the defined sampling duration. Data are classically expressed as % of the average of the first samples collected, corresponding to baseline. As a consequence, microdialysis (except in very peculiar methodological contexts not explained in this chapter) is considered as a semi-quantitative method as it permits to monitor precisely relative variations of neurotransmitters.

Analysis of microdialysates has commonly used HPLC with electrochemical [48, 49] or fluorometric detection [50, 51], and also enzymatic methods [52]. However, these analytical techniques exhibit poor mass sensitivity and require large volume samples to determine neurotransmitter contents. As a consequence, despite constant improvements in HPLC [50, 51, 53], the required sample volume may still be too large, leading to lengthy dialysis sampling times and poor temporal resolution. Consequently, most microdialysis experiments were severely limited by the temporal resolution of microdialysis (5–30 min) compared to rapid changes occurring in the extracellular concentrations of neurotransmitters. In contrast, microdialysis coupled to CE, a more recent technique, allows the monitoring of rapid changes in the extracellular concentration of neurotransmitters by analysing nanovolume dialysates with low limits of detection. At present, it appears to be suitable for microdialysis with high sampling rate. Often coupled to laser-induced fluorescence (LIF) detection or mass spectrometry (MS), capillary electrophoresis has become one of the most powerful analytical tools for the routine determination of neurotransmitters because it offers the advantage of rapidity, high resolution and sensitivity, while requiring very small sample sizes [44, 54, 55]. In brain microdialysates, glutamate and GABA [56-64] were often analysed using CE with LIF detection. However, as amino acid neurotransmitters are not fluorescent at wavelengths of most commercially available lasers, derivatization prior to the separation is needed. Fluorescent reagents, as naphthalene-2,3-dicarboxaldehyde (NDA), orthophtaldehyde (OPA) or fluorescein isothiocyanate, reacting with the primary amine function of neurotransmitters, allow their detection following laser excitation at 442, 325, or 488 nm, respectively [63-65]. Several groups, including our own, have developed methodologies for the CE–LIF analysis of brain microdialysates after a derivatization of samples with fluorogenic agents, even on sub-microliter dialysates obtained with high temporal resolution microdialysis (5s – 1 min, [44] for minireview).

2.2. Set-up for high temporal microdialysis on behaving animal

According to the neurophysiological question asked, the experimental set-up for microdialysis experiments has to be carefully designed: the choice of microdialysis probe according to the targeted brain area, the choice of the analytical method to quantify dialysate neurotransmitters and the coupling of the experimental set-ups or approaches are all crucial to succeed in neurochemical studies. The aim of the study described here [66] was to monitor amino acid neurotransmitters as glutamate and GABA in brain areas involved in emotional learning and memory using odor fear conditioning. Indeed, while a few studies have investigated the time course of events separately in the auditory cortex and the amygdala during auditory fear conditioning [11, 12], no study up to date has been conducted to investigate simultaneously the changes in amygdala and sensory cortical areas in the same animal during fear conditioning.

Our group previously reported lasting changes in electrophysiological field potential signals in both posterior piriform cortex (PPC) and amygdala (basolateral nucleus, BLA) after a session of odor fear conditioning [23]. As a consequence, we conducted an experiment using a dual-microdialysis probe implantation, in order to compare the time courses of changes in GABA and glutamate concentrations, monitored simultaneously in BLA and PPC during odor fear conditioning. Very few groups have developed dual (or triple) implantation of microdialysis probes on the same animal [67, 68]. Indeed in most studies using brain microdialysis, dialysates collection is usually performed in one brain structure at a time, sometimes on different days. Literature on microdialysis experiments in BLA is rather abundant, mainly for monoamines.

There are only a few papers in the literature reporting microdialysis studies in the piriform cortex in an epileptic model [69] or during a feeding/diet procedure [70]. Two other studies were devoted to glutamate monitoring at 20 or 30-min sampling rate in anesthetized [71] or awake rats [72]. In order to target the centre of each brain structure and avoid excluding rats with inaccurate implantation on one hand, and in order to optimize the amount of collected glutamate and GABA in the microdialysates for analytical quantification on the other hand, 1.5-mm microdialysis probes were used for both BLA and PPC. However, due to the size of the probes and the vicinity of amygdala and olfactory cortex, we implanted one probe per hemisphere, BLA probe on one side, PPC probe contralaterally (Figure 2). As the acquisition session of odor fear conditioning was short-lasting (30 min), we monitored glutamate and GABA at high sampling rate using CE-LIFD as analytical technique. When performing high sampling rate, it is crucial to optimize the geometry of the probe tubings.

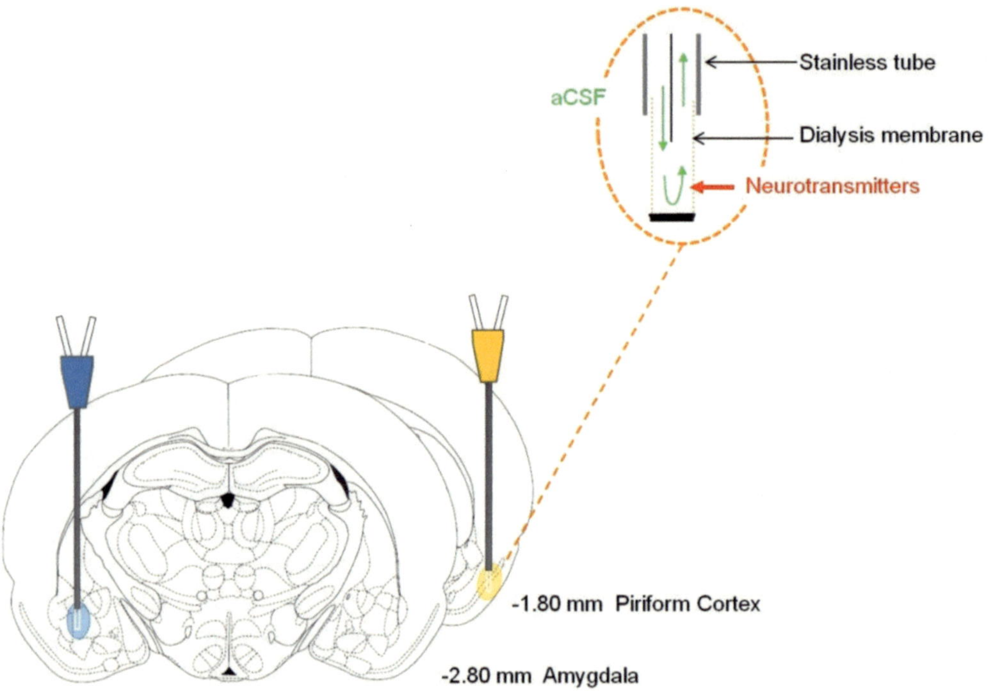

Figure 2. Brain sections from Paxinos & Watson's atlas with a schematic probe implanted in the left basolateral amygdala and the other implanted in the right posterior piriform cortex of the same freely-moving rat for simultaneous glutamate and GABA monitoring.

Indeed, a high sampling rate requires appropriate probe tubings since solutes could undergo more longitudinal diffusion in the outlet probe tubing if the interval of time between dialysis and collection, also called 'dead time, is superior to the sampling time [56]. As a consequence, to avoid mixing of analytes between successive samples, the dead volume of these tubings has to be minimized. This is particularly relevant when microdialysis experiments are carried out on awake animals because the setting requires long inlet and outlet probe tubings in order to let the animals move freely. In our odor fear conditioning, the set-up includes specific

http://dx.doi.org/10.5772/57490

characteristics: an experimental chamber with a grid for electrical stimulation which is a mild footshock (Unconditioned Stimulus, US) and with an ventilation system bringing and removing the odor (Conditioned Stimulus, CS); besides, this experimental chamber has to be placed in a soundproof box in which we can position cameras to record the behavior of the animal. Material for microdialysis (perfusion pump) and collection have to be placed outside the box for not disturbing the animal in learning. In our set-up, the height of the box reaches almost one meter (Figure 3). The dead volume can be greatly minimized by using capillary tubings with sub-50 μm inner diameters, as previously demonstrated by our group [56]. By using a 40-μm inner diameter, we have optimized the microdialysis set-up for odor conditioning by adapting methods that our group previously used for an accurate monitoring of 30-s pharmacologically-induced increases [73] or 20-s behaviourally-induced variations [56] in extracellular levels of amino acids neurotransmitters. We showed that the experimental determination of the dead time is necessary in order to adapt each set-up to the sampling rate required (Figure 4). The final length of the outlet tubing is 120 cm with a dead time of 1 min 30 at 2μL/min as sampling rate and the final sampling resolution is 1 min. The time scale in the figures corresponds to the real time of collection of the fractions. Administration of odor was timed to take into account the outlet dead time of the dialysate system.

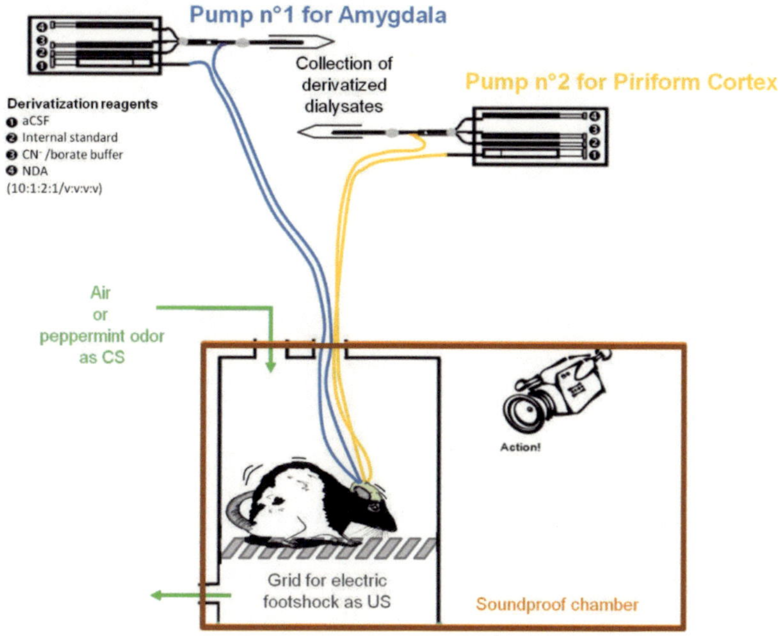

Figure 3. Experimental set-up for both microdialysis sampling and dialysates derivatization during the acquisition of odor fear conditioning. The dual probe-implanted animal is placed in an experimental chamber for odor (conditional stimulus) and shock (unconditional stimulus) deliveries, required in the learning procedure. This chamber is soundproof in order to prevent external noise to interfere with the animal's behaviour. Microdialysis and derivatization are performed simultaneously using one pump per brain area and four syringes delivering artificial cerebrospinal fluid (aCSF) in the inlet of the probe or reagents (NDA as derivatization agent in presence of cyanide ions at pH 8.7 and internal standard for better quantification by capillary electrophoresis with laser-induced fluorescence detection) to tag the neurotransmitters at the outlet of the probe.

Another analytical constraint is to tag the sample in order to detect the amino acids collected during the dialysis experiment. As glutamate and GABA are not fluorescent, we employed a validated home-made on-line system able to deliver the derivatization reagents directly in the collection tube [56], allowing to derivatize the dialysate while dialyzing, without sample loss, noticeable dilution or contamination and without increasing the dead volume of the probe. Thus, the collection tube is not only the micro-reactor of derivatization, but also the injection tube for capillary electrophoresis analysis (Figure 3).

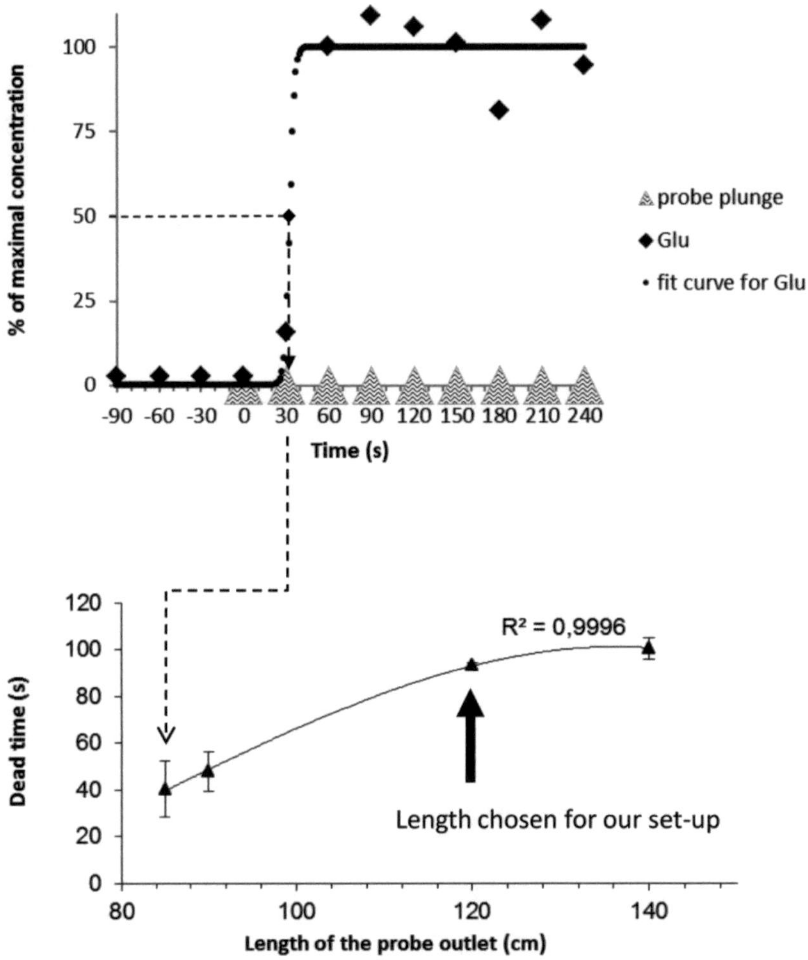

Figure 4. Example of determination of the dead time of an 85-cm outlet home-made probe perfused at 2µL/min by plunging the probe into a known concentration of glutamate at t=0s. The dead time is determined as the time when 50% of the maximal response is reached using a sigmoid curve fitting the 30-s glutamate monitoring (up). By varying the length of the outlet tubing of customized probes (n=3), the dead time of probes can be interpolated and the final length of outlet tubing (here, 120 cm for a dead time of 1 min 30 s) can be chosen according to the height of our experimental set-up and the 1-min sampling rate (bottom). As a consequence, administration of odor was timed to take into account the outlet dead volume of the dialysate system.

Figure 5 presents an example of typical electropheregramm obtained from 1 minute sampling rate of brain microdialysate in freely-moving rat during the acquisition of fear conditioning. Note that the concentrations for GABA and glutamate are similar in PPC or in BLA.

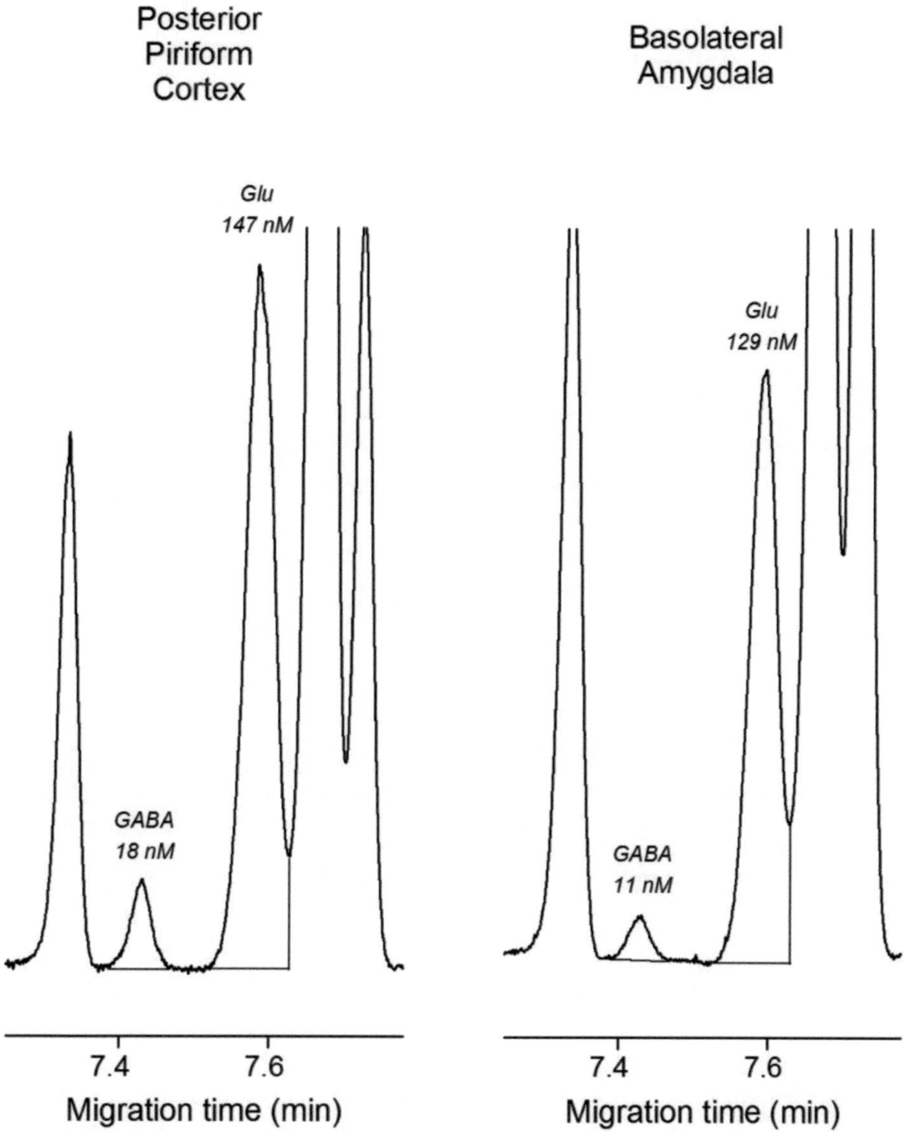

Figure 5. Typical electropherograms from microdialysates obtained in posterior piriform cortex and basolateral amygdala on the same freely-moving Long-Evans rat. Samples were collected every minute at 2μL/min and derivatized online as described in Figure 3 of this chapter. Adapted from [110].

3. Neurochemistry of odor fear conditioning

3.1. Interactions between amygdala and piriform cortex in odor fear conditioning

The odor fear conditioning paradigm consisted of six 20-s odor/ 2-s shock associations presented with an interval of 4 minutes between each pairing. In the amygdala, the first odor-shock association is accompanied by a significant but transient +40%-increase of glutamate release. During the next trials, the concentrations returned to the baseline levels or slightly below. In contrast, in piriform cortex, each odor-shock association is followed by a transient +25%-increase in glutamate release. The comparison of the pattern of release observed in the two structures has also shown that the increase in the amygdala during the first association occurred 1-2 min before the first response in the piriform cortex (Figure 6).

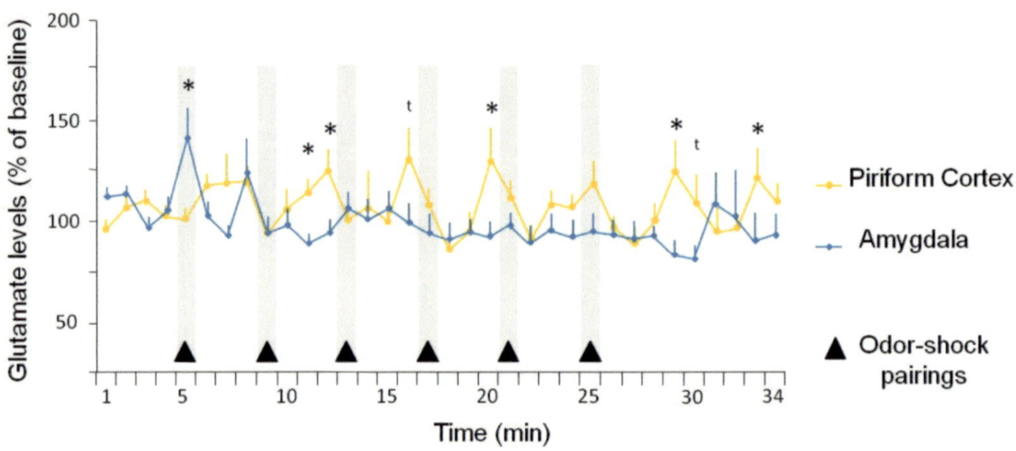

Figure 6. Comparison of glutamate concentration fluctuations in the amygdala and the piriform cortex during odor fear acquisition session. Glutamate concentrations were measured throughout the session and expressed as a percentage of baseline calculated as the mean of concentration for the four points preceding the first pairing. Black arrowheads above the x-axis symbolize trial occurrence. Light gray vertical bars indicate the timing of the 4-min intertrial intervals. (*) Significant difference between the two structures ($p < 0.05$); (#) tendency toward significant difference ($p < 0.09$). Adapted from [66].

The profile of GABA variations during odor fear conditioning was similar in duration and amplitude to that obtained for glutamate presented in Figure 6, i.e. with an enhancement of GABA levels in the amygdala during the first pairing and increases of GABA concentrations in piriform cortex 1-2 min after each pairing. As glutamate and GABA fluctuations were not overall significantly different throughout the experiment, it can be suggested that GABA increases could be induced by glutamate increases, as shown by [74, 75] in the prefrontal cortex.

The high temporal resolution microdialysis allowed us to highlight a differential dynamics of neurotransmitters release in the piriform cortex and amygdala during odor fear acquisition. Taken together, these results suggest that there is a temporal sequence of neurochemical events in the amygdala and piriform cortex, a very precise dynamics of neurotransmitters during the early stages of the acquisition session, which could be involved in the initiation of plastic changes supporting the formation of the memory.

3.2. Functional significance of neurochemical data

Glutamate collected from the BLA and PPC may have originated from both extrinsic and intrinsic sources. Indeed, the BLA receives afferences from primary olfactory cortex [76-78] and from other associative areas [19, 79], providing an extrinsic source of glutamate. Similarly, PPC receives a strong glutamatergic input from the olfactory bulb as well as inputs from the BLA, prefrontal cortex, and hippocampus [80-82]. In addition, both the BLA and PPC contain glutamatergic pyramidal cells that send axon collaterals to neighboring cells, thus providing an intrinsic source of glutamate [79, 83, 84]. Concerning GABA origin, in both BLA and PPC, GABA is released by local inhibitory interneurons [79, 85].

While *in vivo* microdialysis is a useful method for monitoring the neurotransmitters present in the brain extracellular fluid [86], many studies have questioned to what extent dialysate glutamate concentration reflects the amount of glutamate released by the presynaptic neuron. Indeed, due to the ubiquitous localization of its metabolism enzymes and transporters in all brain cells and its paramount role in protein synthesis and general metabolism, numerous works attempted to determine the origin of extracellular glutamate. If the proportion of extracellular glutamate taken up by astrocytes is about 80–90% of the whole glutamate pool [87], the part of the neuronal glutamate, i.e. released for the only neurotransmission purpose, is still matter of debate, because glutamate may come from many sources of effluxes as neuronal "classical" release [88], exchange via cysteine/glutamate transporters [89-92], inversion of transporters [93] and glial release via exocytosis or non-exocytosis [94-96]. Former methodological strategies used for monoamine neurotransmitters to impair the vesicular neuronal release by lowering or removing calcium in aCSF or by blocking nerve impulse Na^+-dependent channels with tetrodotoxine (TTX) gave contradictory answers: some studies reported decreases in basal level of glutamate in dialysate, which is in favour of the neuronal origin of basal extracellular glutamate. In contrast, other studies described no change or even increases under such experimental conditions [97]. Consequently, it was suggested that most part of neurotransmitter glutamate released into synaptic cleft in basal conditions may be taken up into surrounding glia and diffuses poorly to the dialysis probe. The same question can be asked for extracellular GABA because its metabolism is tightly linked to glutamate. As for glutamate, unsuccessful conclusions were also reported regarding the origin of dialysate GABA in basal conditions [97]. However, increasing the microdialysis sampling rate had been proposed in order to observe the rapid variations in glutamate extracellular level which are expected to occur in neurophysiological events [73, 98]. Recent studies using high sampling rate microdialysis showed that NMDA application [99] or electrical stimulation of the prefrontal cortex [100] increases dialysate glutamate concentrations in brain regions receiving projections from this area and that the increase is suppressed or partly altered by TTX [99, 100]. These studies strongly suggest that the transient increase in dialysate glutamate detected under these conditions really represents evoked neurotransmitter glutamate release [101].

Extracellular (or dialysate) concentrations of glutamate and GABA may not always provide a reliable index of their synaptic exocytotic release. Indeed, a strict compartment between intra-synaptic and extra-synaptic was evidenced with poor spill-over from synaptic compartment to extra-synaptic part [102, 103], mainly due to a strong glial uptake. So that, the changes in extracellular concentrations of glutamate and GABA under specific pharmacological and behavioural stimuli should not be only interpreted as a consequence of the activation of specific neurochemical circuits, but as an expression of the activity of the neuron-astrocyte unit in specific circuits of the brain. Several authors proposed that dialysate changes in glutamate and GABA could be used as an index of volume transmission mediated actions of these two neurotransmitters. This hypothesis is based firstly on the assumption that the activity of neurons is functionally linked to the activity of astrocytes, which can release glutamate and GABA to the extracellular space [94, 104]; secondly, on the existence of extrasynaptic glutamate and GABA receptors with functional properties different from those of receptors located in the synapse [105, 106]; and thirdly, on the experimental evidence reporting specific electro-physiological and neurochemical effects of glutamate and GABA when their levels are increased in the extracellular space [107]. Thus, glutamate and GABA, once released into the extracellular compartment, can diffuse and have long-lasting effects modulating glutamatergic and/or GABAergic neuron-astrocytic networks and interact with neurons containing other neurotransmitters and located in the same areas of the brain. In conclusion, monitoring of glutamate and GABA concentrations in the extracellular space using microdialysis may provide an indirect index of amino acids synaptic neurotransmission while giving direct indications of amino acids volume neurotransmission [101].

A few studies have specifically measured extracellular glutamate or GABA in brain structures involved in fear conditioning, investigating the neurotransmitters changes in amygdala during auditory fear learning. More precisely, these microdialysis studies have described a long-lasting decrease in GABA during expression of conditioned fear [39] and a small increase in glutamate during auditory fear conditioning [40]. However, these studies suffer from poor (10–20 min) temporal resolution associated with traditional microdialysis. Only one study has used high temporal resolution microdialysis to measured glutamate and GABA into the amygdala during the acquisition of auditory fear conditioning [108] and suggests that the co-variations of glutamate and GABA may be explained as a glutamate-induced increase in GABA. This study also showed an increase in neurotransmitters levels in the amygdala only for the first association after which the concentration returned to baseline levels. This last result is in agreement with our microdialysis data for the amygdala in odor fear conditioning. Unfortunately, microdialysis was not performed in the auditory cortex, thus precluding any comparison with our own data on the piriform cortex. Nevertheless, there are some electro-physiological data which show that the amygdala is activated before the auditory cortex in auditory fear learning [9, 11]. These data are in accordance with our findings and confirm the differential activation of the amygdala and sensory cortices within the acquisition session of fear conditioning.

http://dx.doi.org/10.5772/57490

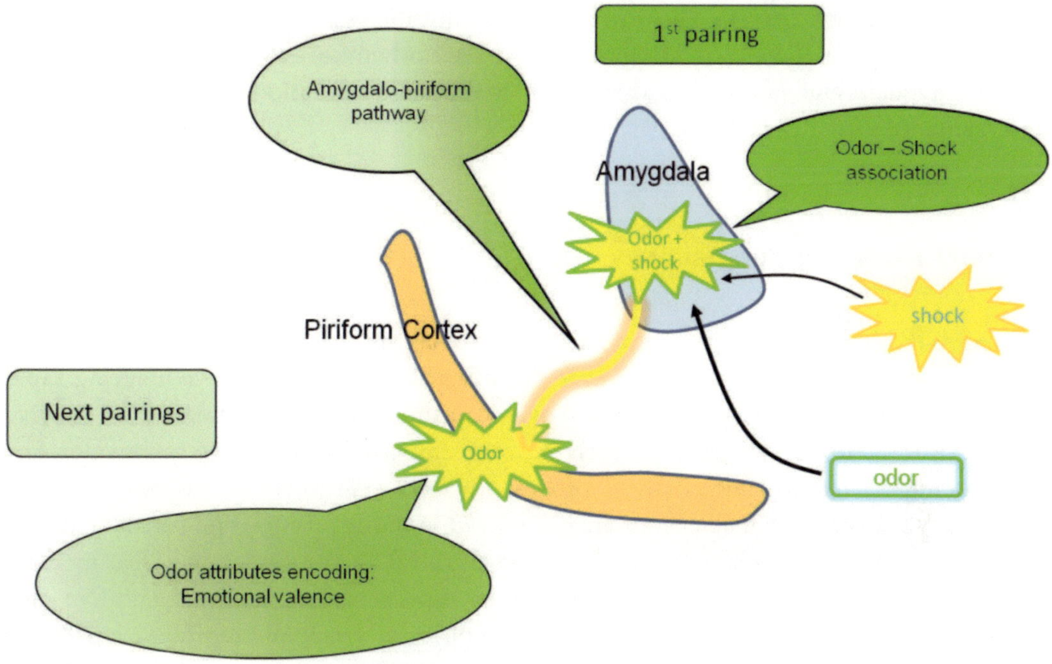

Figure 7. Functional hypotheses on the interactions between the amygdala and the piriform cortex during the acquisition of odor fear learning. An early transient response in the amygdala may allow fast signaling following the first CS-US pairing. Projections from the amygdala to the piriform cortex may provide a pathway through which the amygdala can modulate cortical processing of olfactory information and initiate the storage of the various attributes of the learned odor. The piriform cortex might store certain aspects of the conditioning experience, including the learned hedonic value of the CS odor.

Our microdialysis data led us to formulate the following working hypothesis (Figure 7). During the first pairing, the amygdala glutamatergic transmission would allow the formation of the memory of the CS-US association as it is the case for auditory fear conditioning. The new idea brought by our data is that this could be initiated by a single trial, since no further increase in glutamate was detected in the amygdala for the next pairings. In parallel, the amygdala would trigger the first glutamate increase detected in the olfactory cortex. This would be achieved through the involvement of a direct projection pathway between the amygdala and the piriform cortex [82]. After that, the piriform cortex would progressively build the memory of the different attributes of the learned odor across the next trials.

What are the strengths of our data? This work was aimed at studying the neurochemical interaction between the amygdala and the piriform cortex in odor fear conditioning. We described a differential activation dynamics between the amygdala and the olfactory cortex within the acquisition session. This dynamic reveals an early and transient involvement of the amygdala, restricted to the first odor-shock association followed by the activation of the olfactory cortex during the next associations, which persists until the end of the acquisition session. Until now, most studies questioning the role of the amygdala and sensory areas in fear conditioning have used local lesions or inactivation before or after the acquisition session. Our technical approach is one of the very few allowing online monitoring of neurochemical events occurring in parallel in the amygdala and olfactory cortex, using a temporal resolution compatible with the observation of very transient changes.

4. Conclusion and perspectives

The recent development of high sampling rate microdialysis coupled with high-performance separative microtechniques able to handle sub-microliter sample allows monitoring rapid changes in extracellular levels of amino acid neurotransmitters. Such a platform allows in vivo investigating neurotransmission in freely-moving animals learning fear as in odor fear conditioning. Using two microdialysis probes, we were able to study the neurochemical interactions between two major brain areas involved in the acquisition and consolidation of odor fear conditioning: the amygdala which role is crucial for the formation of fear memory and the piriform cortex which could encode other aspects of the aversive event. Our data suggest that projections from the amygdala to the piriform cortex might provide a pathway via which the amygdala could modulate the cortical processing of olfactory information and initiate the progressive storage of the different attributes of the learned odor in long-term memory.

Author details

Chloé Hegoburu[1,2,4], Luc Denoroy[3,4], Anne-Marie Mouly[2,4] and Sandrine Parrot[4,5]

*Address all correspondence to: sandrine.parrot@univ-lyon1.fr

1 Present address: Center for Psychiatric Neuroscience, Prilly, University of Lausanne, Lausanne, Switzerland

2 CNRS, UMR 5292, Lyon Neuroscience Research Center, Olfaction: From Coding to Memory Team, Lyon, France

3 University Lyon, Lyon Neuroscience Research Center, BioRaN team, Lyon, France

4 University Lyon , Lyon, France

5 INSERM, U1028, Lyon Neuroscience Research Center, NeuroDialyTics, Lyon, France

References

[1] Bevins RA, Ayres JJB. One-trial context fear conditioning as a function of the interstimulus interval. Animal Learning & Behavior. 1995;23 (4):400-10.

[2] Davis M, Shi C. The amygdala. Current biology : CB. 2000;10(4):R131.

[3] Blanchard RJ, Blanchard DC. Crouching as an index of fear. J Comp Physiol Psychol. 1969;67(3):370-5.

[4] Blanchard DC, Blanchard RJ. Innate and conditioned reactions to threat in rats with amygdaloid lesions. J Comp Physiol Psychol. 1972;81(2):281-90. Epub 1972/11/01.

[5] LeDoux JE. Emotion circuits in the brain. Annu Rev Neurosci. 2000;23:155-84. Epub 2000/06/09.

[6] Maren S. Neurobiology of Pavlovian fear conditioning. Annu Rev Neurosci. 2001;24:897-931. Epub 2001/08/25.

[7] Maren S, Quirk GJ. Neuronal signalling of fear memory. Nat Rev Neurosci. 2004;5(11):844-52. Epub 2004/10/22.

[8] Myers KM, Davis M. Mechanisms of fear extinction. Molecular psychiatry. 2007;12(2):120-50. Epub 2006/12/13.

[9] Edeline JM, Pham P, Weinberger NM. Rapid development of learning-induced receptive field plasticity in the auditory cortex. Behav Neurosci. 1993;107(4):539-51. Epub 1993/08/01.

[10] McClelland JL, McNaughton BL, O'Reilly RC. Why there are complementary learning systems in the hippocampus and neocortex: insights from the successes and failures of connectionist models of learning and memory. Psychol Rev. 1995;102(3): 419-57. Epub 1995/07/01.

[11] Quirk GJ, Armony JL, LeDoux JE. Fear conditioning enhances different temporal components of tone-evoked spike trains in auditory cortex and lateral amygdala. Neuron. 1997;19(3):613-24. Epub 1997/10/23.

[12] Armony JL, Quirk GJ, LeDoux JE. Differential effects of amygdala lesions on early and late plastic components of auditory cortex spike trains during fear conditioning. J Neurosci. 1998;18(7):2592-601. Epub 1998/04/16.

[13] Weinberger NM. Specific long-term memory traces in primary auditory cortex. Nat Rev Neurosci. 2004;5(4):279-90. Epub 2004/03/23.

[14] Maren S. Building and burying fear memories in the brain. Neuroscientist. 2005;11(1):89-99. Epub 2005/01/06.

[15] Sacco T, Sacchetti B. Role of secondary sensory cortices in emotional memory storage and retrieval in rats. Science. 2010;329(5992):649-56. Epub 2010/08/07.

[16] Chu S, Downes JJ. Odour-evoked autobiographical memories: psychological investigations of proustian phenomena. Chem Senses. 2000;25(1):111-6. Epub 2000/02/11.

[17] Price JL. An autoradiographic study of complementary laminar patterns of termination of afferent fibers to the olfactory cortex. J Comp Neurol. 1973;150(1):87-108. Epub 1973/07/01.

[18] Savander V, LeDoux JE, Pitkanen A. Topographic projections from the periamygdaloid cortex to select subregions of the lateral nucleus of the amygdala in the rat. Neurosci Lett. 1996;211(3):167-70. Epub 1996/06/28.

[19] McDonald AJ. Cortical pathways to the mammalian amygdala. Prog Neurobiol. 1998;55(3):257-332. Epub 1998/06/27.

[20] Cousens G, Otto T. Both pre- and posttraining excitotoxic lesions of the basolateral amygdala abolish the expression of olfactory and contextual fear conditioning. Behav Neurosci. 1998;112(5):1092-103.

[21] Rosenkranz JA, Grace AA. Dopamine-mediated modulation of odour-evoked amygdala potentials during pavlovian conditioning. Nature. 2002;417(6886):282-7.

[22] Kilpatrick L, Cahill L. Modulation of memory consolidation for olfactory learning by reversible inactivation of the basolateral amygdala. Behav Neurosci. 2003;117(1): 184-8.

[23] Sevelinges Y, Gervais R, Messaoudi B, Granjon L, Mouly AM. Olfactory fear conditioning induces field potential potentiation in rat olfactory cortex and amygdala. Learn Mem. 2004;11(6):761-9. Epub 2004/11/13.

[24] Sevelinges Y, Moriceau S, Holman P, Miner C, Muzny K, Gervais R, et al. Enduring effects of infant memories: infant odor-shock conditioning attenuates amygdala activity and adult fear conditioning. Biol Psychiatry. 2007;62(10):1070-9. Epub 2007/09/11.

[25] Walker DL, Paschall GY, Davis M. Glutamate receptor antagonist infusions into the basolateral and medial amygdala reveal differential contributions to olfactory vs. context fear conditioning and expression. Learn Mem. 2005;12(2):120-9.

[26] Jones SV, Stanek-Rattiner L, Davis M, Ressler KJ. Differential regional expression of brain-derived neurotrophic factor following olfactory fear learning. Learn Mem. 2007;14(12):816-20.

[27] Sevelinges Y, Sullivan RM, Messaoudi B, Mouly AM. Neonatal odor-shock conditioning alters the neural network involved in odor fear learning at adulthood. Learn Mem. 2008;15(9):649-56. Epub 2008/09/06.

[28] Fanselow MS, Kim JJ. Acquisition of contextual Pavlovian fear conditioning is blocked by application of an NMDA receptor antagonist D,L-2-amino-5-phosphono-

valeric acid to the basolateral amygdala. Behav Neurosci. 1994;108(1):210-2. Epub 1994/02/01.

[29] Maren S, Aharonov G, Fanselow MS. Retrograde abolition of conditional fear after excitotoxic lesions in the basolateral amygdala of rats: absence of a temporal gradient. Behav Neurosci. 1996;110(4):718-26.

[30] Miserendino MJ, Sananes CB, Melia KR, Davis M. Blocking of acquisition but not expression of conditioned fear-potentiated startle by NMDA antagonists in the amygdala. Nature. 1990;345(6277):716-8. Epub 1990/06/21.

[31] Campeau S, Miserendino MJ, Davis M. Intra-amygdala infusion of the N-methyl-D-aspartate receptor antagonist AP5 blocks acquisition but not expression of fear-potentiated startle to an auditory conditioned stimulus. Behav Neurosci. 1992;106(3): 569-74. Epub 1992/06/01.

[32] Gewirtz JC, Davis M. Second-order fear conditioning prevented by blocking NMDA receptors in amygdala. Nature. 1997;388(6641):471-4. Epub 1997/07/31.

[33] Kim JJ, Lee HJ, Han JS, Packard MG. Amygdala is critical for stress-induced modulation of hippocampal long-term potentiation and learning. J Neurosci. 2001;21(14): 5222-8.

[34] Walker DL, Davis M. The role of amygdala glutamate receptors in fear learning, fear-potentiated startle, and extinction. Pharmacol Biochem Behav. 2002;71(3):379-92. Epub 2002/02/07.

[35] Goosens KA, Maren S. NMDA receptors are essential for the acquisition, but not expression, of conditional fear and associative spike firing in the lateral amygdala. Eur J Neurosci. 2004;20(2):537-48. Epub 2004/07/06.

[36] Muller J, Corodimas KP, Fridel Z, LeDoux JE. Functional inactivation of the lateral and basal nuclei of the amygdala by muscimol infusion prevents fear conditioning to an explicit conditioned stimulus and to contextual stimuli. Behav Neurosci. 1997;111(4):683-91. Epub 1997/08/01.

[37] Wilensky AE, Schafe GE, LeDoux JE. Functional inactivation of the amygdala before but not after auditory fear conditioning prevents memory formation. J Neurosci. 1999;19(24):RC48. Epub 1999/12/14.

[38] Ehrlich I, Humeau Y, Grenier F, Ciocchi S, Herry C, Luthi A. Amygdala inhibitory circuits and the control of fear memory. Neuron. 2009;62(6):757-71. Epub 2009/06/27.

[39] Stork O, Ji FY, Obata K. Reduction of extracellular GABA in the mouse amygdala during and following confrontation with a conditioned fear stimulus. Neurosci Lett. 2002;327(2):138-42. Epub 2002/07/06.

[40] Yokoyama M, Suzuki E, Sato T, Maruta S, Watanabe S, Miyaoka H. Amygdalic levels of dopamine and serotonin rise upon exposure to conditioned fear stress without elevation of glutamate. Neurosci Lett. 2005;379(1):37-41.

[41] Young AM. Increased extracellular dopamine in nucleus accumbens in response to unconditioned and conditioned aversive stimuli: studies using 1 min microdialysis in rats. J Neurosci Methods. 2004;138(1-2):57-63. Epub 2004/08/25.

[42] Ungerstedt U. Microdialysis--principles and applications for studies in animals and man. J Intern Med. 1991;230(4):365-73. Epub 1991/10/01.

[43] Benveniste H, Huttemeier PC. Microdialysis--theory and application. Prog Neurobiol. 1990;35(3):195-215. Epub 1990/01/01.

[44] Parrot S, Bert L, Mouly-Badina L, Sauvinet V, Colussi-Mas J, Lambas-Senas L, et al. Microdialysis monitoring of catecholamines and excitatory amino acids in the rat and mouse brain: recent developments based on capillary electrophoresis with laser-induced fluorescence detection--a mini-review. Cell Mol Neurobiol. 2003;23(4-5): 793-804. Epub 2003/09/30.

[45] Zapata A, Chefer VI, Parrot S, Denoroy L. Detection and quantification of neurotransmitters in dialysates. Current protocols in neuroscience / editorial board, Jacqueline N Crawley [et al]. 2013;Chapter 7:Unit7 4. Epub 2013/04/06.

[46] Westerink BH. Brain microdialysis and its application for the study of animal behaviour. Behav Brain Res. 1995;70(2):103-24. Epub 1995/10/01.

[47] Watson CJ, Venton BJ, Kennedy RT. In vivo measurements of neurotransmitters by microdialysis sampling. Anal Chem. 2006;78(5):1391-9. Epub 2006/03/31.

[48] Abercrombie ED, Finlay JM. Monitoring extracellular norepinephrine in brain using in vivo microdialysis and HPLC-EC. In: Robinson TE, Justice JBJ, editors. Microdialysis in Neurosciences. Amsterdam: Elsevier; 1991. p. 253–74.

[49] Smolders I, Sarre S, Michotte Y, Ebinger G. The analysis of excitatory, inhibitory and other amino acids in rat brain microdialysates using microbore liquid chromatography. J Neurosci Methods. 1995;57(1):47-53. Epub 1995/03/01.

[50] Kehr J. Determination of gamma-aminobutyric acid in microdialysis samples by microbore column liquid chromatography and fluorescence detection. J Chromatogr B Biomed Sci Appl. 1998;708(1-2):49-54. Epub 1998/07/08.

[51] Kehr J. Determination of glutamate and aspartate in microdialysis samples by reversed-phase column liquid chromatography with fluorescence and electrochemical detection. J Chromatogr B Biomed Sci Appl. 1998;708(1-2):27-38. Epub 1998/07/08.

[52] Obrenovitch TP, Zilkha E. Microdialysis coupled to online enzymatic assays. Methods. 2001;23(1):63-71. Epub 2001/02/13.

[53] McKenzie JA, Watson CJ, Rostand RD, German I, Witowski SR, Kennedy RT. Automated capillary liquid chromatography for simultaneous determination of neuroactive amines and amino acids. J Chromatogr A. 2002;962(1-2):105-15. Epub 2002/08/30.

[54] Lunte SM, Lunte CE. Microdialysis sampling for pharmacological studies: HPLC and CE analysis. Adv Chromatogr. 1996;36:383-432. Epub 1996/01/01.

[55] Kennedy RT, Watson CJ, Haskins WE, Powell DH, Strecker RE. In vivo neurochemical monitoring by microdialysis and capillary separations. Curr Opin Chem Biol. 2002;6(5):659-65. Epub 2002/11/05.

[56] Parrot S, Sauvinet V, Riban V, Depaulis A, Renaud B, Denoroy L. High temporal resolution for in vivo monitoring of neurotransmitters in awake epileptic rats using brain microdialysis and capillary electrophoresis with laser-induced fluorescence detection. J Neurosci Methods. 2004;140(1-2):29-38. Epub 2004/12/14.

[57] Touret M, Parrot S, Denoroy L, Belin MF, Didier-Bazes M. Glutamatergic alterations in the cortex of genetic absence epilepsy rats. BMC Neurosci. 2007;8:69. Epub 2007/08/30.

[58] Bergquist J, Vona MJ, Stiller CO, O'Connor WT, Falkenberg T, Ekman R. Capillary electrophoresis with laser-induced fluorescence detection: a sensitive method for monitoring extracellular concentrations of amino acids in the periaqueductal grey matter. J Neurosci Methods. 1996;65(1):33-42. Epub 1996/03/01.

[59] Dawson LA, Stow JM, Palmer AM. Improved method for the measurement of glutamate and aspartate using capillary electrophoresis with laser induced fluorescence detection and its application to brain microdialysis. J Chromatogr B Biomed Sci Appl. 1997;694(2):455-60. Epub 1997/07/04.

[60] Lada MW, Vickroy TW, Kennedy RT. High temporal resolution monitoring of glutamate and aspartate in vivo using microdialysis on-line with capillary electrophoresis with laser-induced fluorescence detection. Anal Chem. 1997;69(22):4560-5. Epub 1998/01/07.

[61] Li YM, Qu Y, Vandenbussche E, Arckens L, Vandesande F. Analysis of extracellular gamma-aminobutyric acid, glutamate and aspartate in cat visual cortex by in vivo microdialysis and capillary electrophoresis-laser induced fluorescence detection. J Neurosci Methods. 2001;105(2):211-5. Epub 2001/03/29.

[62] Robert F, Bert L, Parrot S, Denoroy L, Stoppini L, Renaud B. Coupling on-line brain microdialysis, precolumn derivatization and capillary electrophoresis for routine minute sampling of O-phosphoethanolamine and excitatory amino acids. J Chromatogr A. 1998;817(1-2):195-203. Epub 1998/10/09.

[63] Tucci S, Rada P, Sepulveda MJ, Hernandez L. Glutamate measured by 6-s resolution brain microdialysis: capillary electrophoretic and laser-induced fluorescence detec-

tion application. J Chromatogr B Biomed Sci Appl. 1997;694(2):343-9. Epub 1997/07/04.

[64] Zhou SY, Zuo H, Stobaugh JF, Lunte CE, Lunte SM. Continuous in vivo monitoring of amino acid neurotransmitters by microdialysis sampling with on-line derivatization and capillary electrophoresis separation. Anal Chem. 1995;67(3):594-9. Epub 1995/02/01.

[65] Hernandez L, Joshi N, Murzi E, Verdeguer P, Mifsud JC, Guzman N. Colinear laser-induced fluorescence detector for capillary electrophoresis. Analysis of glutamic acid in brain dialysates. J Chromatogr A. 1993;652(2):399-405. Epub 1993/10/22.

[66] Hegoburu C, Sevelinges Y, Thevenet M, Gervais R, Parrot S, Mouly AM. Differential dynamics of amino acid release in the amygdala and olfactory cortex during odor fear acquisition as revealed with simultaneous high temporal resolution microdialysis. Learn Mem. 2009;16(11):687-97. Epub 2009/10/30.

[67] Del Arco A, Segovia G, Prieto L, Mora F. Endogenous glutamate-taurine interaction in striatum and nucleus accumbens of the freely moving rat: studies during the normal process of aging. Mechanisms of ageing and development. 2001;122(4):401-14. Epub 2001/03/10.

[68] Hernandez LF, Segovia G, Mora F. Chronic treatment with a dopamine uptake blocker changes dopamine and acetylcholine but not glutamate and GABA concentrations in prefrontal cortex, striatum and nucleus accumbens of the awake rat. Neurochemistry international. 2008;52(3):457-69. Epub 2007/09/21.

[69] Layton ME, Pazdernik TL. Reactive oxidant species in piriform cortex extracellular fluid during seizures induced by systemic kainic acid in rats. Journal of molecular neuroscience : MN. 1999;13(1-2):63-8. Epub 2000/02/26.

[70] Wang CX, Erecius LF, Beverly JL, 3rd, Gietzen DW. Essential amino acids affect interstitial dopamine metabolites in the anterior piriform cortex of rats. The Journal of nutrition. 1999;129(9):1742-5. Epub 1999/08/25.

[71] Tanaka K, Graham SH, Simon RP. The role of excitatory neurotransmitters in seizure-induced neuronal injury in rats. Brain research. 1996;737(1-2):59-63. Epub 1996/10/21.

[72] Wade JV, Samson FE, Nelson SR, Pazdernik TL. Changes in extracellular amino acids during soman- and kainic acid-induced seizures. Journal of neurochemistry. 1987;49(2):645-50. Epub 1987/08/01.

[73] Bert L, Parrot S, Robert F, Desvignes C, Denoroy L, Suaud-Chagny MF, et al. In vivo temporal sequence of rat striatal glutamate, aspartate and dopamine efflux during apomorphine, nomifensine, NMDA and PDC in situ administration. Neuropharmacology. 2002;43(5):825-35. Epub 2002/10/18.

[74] Del Arco A, Mora F. Effects of endogenous glutamate on extracellular concentrations of GABA, dopamine, and dopamine metabolites in the prefrontal cortex of the freely

moving rat: involvement of NMDA and AMPA/KA receptors. Neurochem Res. 1999;24(8):1027-35.

[75] Del Arco A, Mora F. Endogenous dopamine potentiates the effects of glutamate on extracellular GABA in the prefrontal cortex of the freely moving rat. Brain Res Bull. 2000;53(3):339-45. Epub 2000/12/13.

[76] Haberly LB, Price JL. Association and commissural fiber systems of the olfactory cortex of the rat. II. Systems originating in the olfactory peduncle. J Comp Neurol. 1978;181(4):781-807. Epub 1978/10/15.

[77] Ottersen OP. Connections of the amygdala of the rat. IV: Corticoamygdaloid and intraamygdaloid connections as studied with axonal transport of horseradish peroxidase. J Comp Neurol. 1982;205(1):30-48. Epub 1982/02/10.

[78] Luskin MB, Price JL. The laminar distribution of intracortical fibers originating in the olfactory cortex of the rat. J Comp Neurol. 1983;216(3):292-302. Epub 1983/05/20.

[79] Sah P, Faber ES, Lopez De Armentia M, Power J. The amygdaloid complex: anatomy and physiology. Physiol Rev. 2003;83(3):803-34.

[80] Haberly LB, Price JL. The axonal projection patterns of the mitral and tufted cells of the olfactory bulb in the rat. Brain research. 1977;129(1):152-7. Epub 1977/06/24.

[81] Datiche F, Cattarelli M. Reciprocal and topographic connections between the piriform and prefrontal cortices in the rat: a tracing study using the B subunit of the cholera toxin. Brain Res Bull. 1996;41(6):391-8. Epub 1996/01/01.

[82] Majak K, Ronkko S, Kemppainen S, Pitkanen A. Projections from the amygdaloid complex to the piriform cortex: A PHA-L study in the rat. J Comp Neurol. 2004;476(4):414-28.

[83] Luskin MB, Price JL. The topographic organization of associational fibers of the olfactory system in the rat, including centrifugal fibers to the olfactory bulb. J Comp Neurol. 1983;216(3):264-91. Epub 1983/05/20.

[84] Datiche F, Litaudon P, Cattarelli M. Intrinsic association fiber system of the piriform cortex: a quantitative study based on a cholera toxin B subunit tracing in the rat. J Comp Neurol. 1996;376(2):265-77. Epub 1996/12/09.

[85] Suzuki N, Bekkers JM. Inhibitory interneurons in the piriform cortex. Clin Exp Pharmacol Physiol. 2007;34(10):1064-9. Epub 2007/08/24.

[86] Benveniste H. Brain microdialysis. Journal of neurochemistry. 1989;52(6):1667-79. Epub 1989/06/01.

[87] Kanamori K, Ross BD, Kondrat RW. Glial uptake of neurotransmitter glutamate from the extracellular fluid studied in vivo by microdialysis and (13)C NMR. Journal of neurochemistry. 2002;83(3):682-95. Epub 2002/10/23.

[88] Fonnum F. Glutamate: a neurotransmitter in mammalian brain. Journal of neurochemistry. 1984;42(1):1-11. Epub 1984/01/01.

[89] Melendez RI, Vuthiganon J, Kalivas PW. Regulation of extracellular glutamate in the prefrontal cortex: focus on the cystine glutamate exchanger and group I metabotropic glutamate receptors. J Pharmacol Exp Ther. 2005;314(1):139-47. Epub 2005/03/17.

[90] Xi ZX, Shen H, Baker DA, Kalivas PW. Inhibition of non-vesicular glutamate release by group III metabotropic glutamate receptors in the nucleus accumbens. Journal of neurochemistry. 2003;87(5):1204-12. Epub 2003/11/19.

[91] Baker DA, Xi ZX, Shen H, Swanson CJ, Kalivas PW. The origin and neuronal function of in vivo nonsynaptic glutamate. J Neurosci. 2002;22(20):9134-41. Epub 2002/10/22.

[92] Xi ZX, Ramamoorthy S, Baker DA, Shen H, Samuvel DJ, Kalivas PW. Modulation of group II metabotropic glutamate receptor signaling by chronic cocaine. J Pharmacol Exp Ther. 2002;303(2):608-15. Epub 2002/10/22.

[93] Nicholls D, Attwell D. The release and uptake of excitatory amino acids. Trends Pharmacol Sci. 1990;11(11):462-8. Epub 1990/11/01.

[94] Araque A, Li N, Doyle RT, Haydon PG. SNARE protein-dependent glutamate release from astrocytes. J Neurosci. 2000;20(2):666-73. Epub 2000/01/13.

[95] Bezzi P, Gundersen V, Galbete JL, Seifert G, Steinhauser C, Pilati E, et al. Astrocytes contain a vesicular compartment that is competent for regulated exocytosis of glutamate. Nat Neurosci. 2004;7(6):613-20. Epub 2004/05/25.

[96] Malarkey EB, Parpura V. Mechanisms of glutamate release from astrocytes. Neurochemistry international. 2008;52(1-2):142-54. Epub 2007/08/03.

[97] Timmerman W, Westerink BH. Brain microdialysis of GABA and glutamate: what does it signify? Synapse. 1997;27(3):242-61. Epub 1997/11/05.

[98] Drew KL, Pehek EA, Rasley BT, Ma YL, Green TK. Sampling glutamate and GABA with microdialysis: suggestions on how to get the dialysis membrane closer to the synapse. J Neurosci Methods. 2004;140(1-2):127-31. Epub 2004/12/14.

[99] Parrot S, Bert L, Renaud B, Denoroy L. Glutamate and aspartate do not exhibit the same changes in their extracellular concentrations in the rat striatum after N-methyl-D-aspartate local administration. J Neurosci Res. 2003;71(3):445-54. Epub 2003/01/15.

[100] Lada MW, Vickroy TW, Kennedy RT. Evidence for neuronal origin and metabotropic receptor-mediated regulation of extracellular glutamate and aspartate in rat striatum in vivo following electrical stimulation of the prefrontal cortex. Journal of neurochemistry. 1998;70(2):617-25. Epub 1998/02/07.

[101] Parrot S, Renaud B, Zimmer L, Denoroy L. Monitoring Neurotransmitter Amino Acids by Microdialysis: Pharmacodynamic Applications. In: Tsai T-H, editor. Appli-

cations of Microdialysis in Pharmaceutical Science: John Wiley & Sons, Inc.; 2011. p. 151-206.

[102] Obrenovitch TP, Urenjak J, Zilkha E, Jay TM. Excitotoxicity in neurological disorders--the glutamate paradox. Int J Dev Neurosci. 2000;18(2-3):281-7. Epub 2000/03/15.

[103] Rusakov DA, Kullmann DM. Extrasynaptic glutamate diffusion in the hippocampus: ultrastructural constraints, uptake, and receptor activation. J Neurosci. 1998;18(9): 3158-70. Epub 1998/05/09.

[104] Schousboe A, Waagepetersen HS. Glial modulation of GABAergic and glutamat ergic neurotransmission. Curr Top Med Chem. 2006;6(10):929-34. Epub 2006/06/22.

[105] Sierra-Paredes G, Sierra-Marcuno G. Extrasynaptic GABA and glutamate receptors in epilepsy. CNS Neurol Disord Drug Targets. 2007;6(4):288-300. Epub 2007/08/19.

[106] Galvan A, Kuwajima M, Smith Y. Glutamate and GABA receptors and transporters in the basal ganglia: what does their subsynaptic localization reveal about their function? Neuroscience. 2006;143(2):351-75. Epub 2006/10/25.

[107] Del Arco A, Segovia G, Fuxe K, Mora F. Changes in dialysate concentrations of glutamate and GABA in the brain: an index of volume transmission mediated actions? Journal of neurochemistry. 2003;85(1):23-33. Epub 2003/03/19.

[108] Venton BJ, Robinson TE, Kennedy RT, Maren S. Dynamic amino acid increases in the basolateral amygdala during acquisition and expression of conditioned fear. Eur J Neurosci. 2006;23(12):3391-8. Epub 2006/07/06.

[109] Denoroy L, Bert L, Parrot S, Robert F, Renaud B. Assessment of pharmacodynamic and pharmacokinetic characteristics of drugs using microdialysis sampling and capillary electrophoresis. Electrophoresis. 1998;19(16-17):2841-7. Epub 1998/12/31.

[110] Denoroy L, Renaud B, Parrot S. Capillary Electrophoresis Analysis in Neuroscience. In: He Z, editor. Capillary Electrophoresis: Fundamentals, Techniques and Applications: NOVA Science Publishers; 2012. p. 211-51.

Section 3

Growth, Development and Differentiation

Chapter 8

Participation of Neurochemical Signaling in Adult Neurogenesis and Differentiation

E.V. Pushchina, A.A. Varaksin and D.K. Obukhov

Additional information is available at the end of the chapter

http://dx.doi.org/10.5772/58306

1. Introduction

The revealed peculiarities of structural and neurochemical organization and description of basic histogenetic processes (proliferation, migration and neuronal cell differentiation) during the brain forming in fish, which have signs of fetal organization, widen the existing knowledge about histogenesis of these structures in postembryonic development. It seems conceivable, that during postembryonic development in teleost fishes some neurotransmitters and gaseous mediators (NO and H_2S) act as factors, which initiate and regulate the cellular and the tissues processes of genetic program during the brain development. We suppose the presence of epigenetic control of adult neurogenesis in salmon brain via highly coordinated nonsynaptic cell–cell signaling. This communication engages the neurotransmitters GABA and dopamine whose extracellular concentrations depend on neuroblasts number and high affinity uptake systems in neural stem cells. Neuroblasts release GABA providing a negative feedback control of stem cell proliferation and instructing them on the size of the neuroblast pool. We suggest that in salmon brain exist strong control mechanisms of neuroblast production. The data provided by our study add to our general understanding, that peculiarities of distribution of classical neuromediators (GABA, catecholamines) and gasotransmitters (NO and H_2S) are directly connected with ability of the fishes brain to grow during the animal entire life. We suggest, that some classical neuromediators (GABA, catecholamines) and gasotransmitters (NO and H_2S) not only regulate functional activity of neurons and modulate synaptic transmission in mature neural networks, but also are regarded as inductors of the fishes brain development (morphogenetic factors) in postembryonic ontogenesis. We propose that dopamine and GABA act as homeostatic signals to regulate neuroblast production. This confirmation is proved by finding of the phenotypically immature elements, expressing the above mentioned molecules in proliferating brain areas, in the three-year-old salmon brain, and of elements, which owe morphology of radial glia. The presence of enzymes, synthesizing gasotransmitters in the brain areas, which are expressing proliferative cell nuclear antigen PCNA, have proved their participation in regulation of postembryonic neurogenesis.

In the fishes, which preserve fetal state during long time (salmon and carp), such markers as NO and H_2S in periventricular proliferative areas may present in different ratios. This is consistent with the hypothesis that in functionally similar complexes in animals the different signal transduction systems may be involved. In contrast to widespread neurogenetic model *Danio rerio,* the development of the salmon and sturgeon nervous system occurs during long time. As it follows from our data, the development of different CNS structures in the *Oncorhynchus masou* brain is characterized by evident heterochrony, so the cells of caudal brain regions gain features of phenotypical specialization earlier than in the forebrain structures. We suggest that the brain of these animals during a long time preserves the signs of fetal organization and low differentiated cells presence confirms this hypothesis.

Last years, certain attention of neuroscientists of different profile was turned to participation in the work of the brain «gaseous intermediaries»: nitric oxide (NO) and hydrogen sulphide (H_2S). Their presence is found in the brains of representatives of different groups of vertebrates: from the Agnatha to human. The few data points to a high degree of variability in the distribution of NO-ergic neurons in the fish brain [1-3], and information about the involvement of nitric oxide and hydrogen sulphide in the functional activity of nervous system of fish is unordered and contradictory. This draws attention to the fact that the relative number of NO-synthesizing neurons and glial cells in the sensory, motor and integrative centers of the brain fish significantly exceeds that of terrestrial vertebrates, in particular, mammals [1, 4, 5]. This implies a wide and varied participation of NO in the metabolism of neurons and glial cells in the central nervous system of fish compared with mammals. However, information about the relationship of the NO-producing neurons of the brain of fish with the systems of classical neurotransmitters such as acetylcholine, catecholamines and GABA, are practically absent. Virtually nothing is known about the distribution of H_2S-producing systems in the CNS of bony fishes. These investigations are of particular importance in connection with the emerging data on morphogenetic the role of classical and gas intermediary in the formation of the central nervous system of vertebrates [6].

The brain of fish has a unique vertebrates feature - it grows with the organism during all life. In connection with this fish is a model object for the study of embryonic and postembryonic development of the CNS, to influence these processes of various factors. It is shown that in the brain of adult vertebrate a system of cambial elements remains, the activity of which allows to replenish the population of neurons and glial cells in the course of a long period after birth [7]. Currently the mechanisms of pre-and postnatal morphogenesis of the brain in the fish, which for a long time secures the larval state, virtually have not been studied [8-10].

Especially it concerns the role of the so-called «radial glial cells» in the processes of morphogenesis of the brain, the availability and distribution of proliferative areas in the brain of adult fish. The results of the research on *Danio rerio* showed that the newly formed cells moving from periventricular areas deep inside the brain, where they differentiate into neurons [11]. It was found that the centers of proliferation are localized along the rostro-caudal axis of the brain [7].

The interest to the study of these processes in fish is caused by the fact that the «radial glia» may be connected with the processes of migration and differentiation of neurons and glial cells in the prenatal period, large quantities present in the brain of a fish and in the adult state (unlike other vertebrates). However, in spite of the available literature information, participation of the radial glia (RG) is in the process of neurogenesis adult animals and little studied. One of the reasons for the lack of such information is a small number of examined in the terms of species and groups of fish, the absence of reliable markers of the RG in lower vertebrates.

Sturgeon and salmon fish, which have become the main objects of our research, represent the most ancient group of vertebrates, which are the most primitive branches ray-finned fish [12-13]. The information about the development of the brain sturgeon and salmon, the relations of embryonic and a definitive parts in the structure of the pre-and postnatal neurogenesis, organization and formation of the neuromediating and modulating brain systems in the literature are extremely limited. This concerns especially the sturgeon fishes, the evolution of which was carried on the pedomorphosis way, which is characterized by the slowing of organs or of their systems and the preservation of the adult embryonic status of relevant features.

The purpose of this chapter is to explore the organization, projection features and relationships of signal-transduction systems, producing a classic neurotransmitters (catecholamines, acetylcholine, gamma-aminobutyric acid-GABA) and gazotransmitters (nitric oxide and hydrogen sulphide), in the brain of fish and evaluate their participation in the processes of the post-embryonic morphogenesis the CNS.

2. Methods

Molecular-biological approaches associated with identifying of histochemical and immunohistochemical activity of mediators or enzymes of their synthesis were used for characteristics of neurotransmitter systems structures of the brain and spinal cord fish. Specific antibodies are also used by us in identifying of proliferative cell nuclear antigen (PCNA), transcription factor Pax6 and calcium binding protein parvalbumin. To investigate the relationship of brain applied marking nerve fibers using carbocyanin dye DiI. To track ascending mediatorically specific projections of catecholaminergic cells was used the immunofluorescence method of marking tyrosine hydroxylase in combination with the marking of the DiI.The **histochemical reaction on NADPH-diaphorase** (NADPH-d, NF 1.6.99.1). Experimental procedures were conducted in accordance with European Community guidelines on animal care and experimentation. The animals were deeply anesthetized with 0.03% tricain methanesulfonate (MS-222, Sandoz) and perfused transcardially with 50 ml of 0,63% saline followed by 200 ml of a fixative containing 4% paraformaldehyde in 0.1 M phosphate buffer (PB), pH 7.4. The brains were then removed from the skull, postfixed in the same fixative for 5 hours, washed in PB at 4°C overnight and then placed in a 30% sucrose solution for cryoprotection.

Fifty-micron-thick transverse sections were cut on a cryostat and collected in cold PB and, after several washes in PB, processed for NADPH-diaphorase histochemistry. Free-floating sections were incubated in a medium made up of 1mM β-NADPH, 0.8 mM nitro blue tetrazolium, and

0.06% Triton X-100 in 0.1 M phosphate buffer (pH 7.6), at 37°C for 2 hours [14]. All chemicals were purchased from Sigma. After incubation, the sections were rinsed in PB, mounted on gelatin-coated glass slides, and air-dried overnight. The following day they were dehydrated cleared in xylene, and coverslipped with Entellan (Merck, Darmstadt, Germany).

In order to determine the specificity of the histochemical reaction, the following controls were carried out: incubation without the substrate β-NADPH, and incubation without the chromogen nitro blue tetrazolium in order to rule out possible nonspecific formation of reaction product. In all cases, no residual reaction was observed.

For **histochemical staining of cholinergic neurons** in the brain of fish we used marking of choline acetyltransferase (ChAT; NF 2.3.1.6.). Method was performed on fishes whose brains were fixed at 4°C for 2 h in 1% solution of paraformaldehyde based on cacodylate buffer (0.1 M) with sucrose (0.32 M; pH 5.0). The material was washed out in cacodylate buffer (pH 5.2) with sucrose for 18 h with sevenfold change of this solution. Frontal and sagittal 50-μm-thick slices were prepared with a freezing microtome. To exclude nonspecific transferase activity, 20 mM diisopropyl fluorophosphate (DFP), 10 % sucrose, and 25 mM cacodylate buffer were added to the incubation medium (pH 6.0) cooled to 4°C ; this medium was placed on an ice bath (0-4°C) for 1 h. After preincubation, the slices were placed in the incubation medium (pH 6.0) with the following final concentrations (mM): cacodylate buffer, 25; DFP, 1.0; choline chloride, 4.0; lead nitrate, 1.0; acetyl-CoA, 0.3, and 5% sucrose. The sliced were thermostated at 37°C for 2 h, washed out in distilled water, and treated in 5% solution of ammonium sulfide. Then, the slices were post-fixed for 5 min in 5% solution of formaldehyde based on cacodylate buffer (0.1 M; pH 5.2) with sucrose (0.32 M), dehydrated, and embedded in balsam. To estimate the specificity of reactions to ChAT, we carried out a few control experiments. In the first control series, we excluded DFP from the incubation medium. In the second control series, cetyl-CoA or choline chloride were absent in the incubation medium. In the third control series, we added chloracetylcholine-perchlorate (10 mM) to the DFP-containing pre-incubation medium; the incubation period was increased to 1.5-2 h. In all control experiments, a positive reaction was absent.

Immunohistochemical methods. Fishes were kept in aquaria with aerated seawater at 15-17°C. Before experiments, fishes were anesthetized in the cuvette with 0.1% solution of tricaine methanesulfonate (MS-222; Sigma, USA) in seawater for 10-15 min. The brains of fishes were fixed for 2 h at 4°C in 4% solution of paraformaldehyde dissolved in phosphate buffer (0.1 M, pH 7.2). For morphological analysis, the obtained material was embedded in paraffin according to a standard technique and stained by Nissl. In the course of immunohistochemical studies, we identified the elements containing GABA, tyrosine hydroxylase (TH), parvalbumin (PA), neuronal nitric oxide synthase (nNOS), proliferative cells nuclear antigen (PCNA), transcription factor Pax6 and cystathionine β-synthase (CBS). For this purpose, we used indirect avidin-biotin-peroxidase (ABC technique) or streptavidin-biotin staining. The material was washed out for 24 h in 30% sucrose solution. Transverse 50-μm-thick slices of the fish brain were prepared using a freezing microtome. Free-floating slices were incubated at 4°C for 48 h in the presence of monoclonal mouse antibodies against GABA (ICN Biomedicals, USA; dilution 1:4000) and tyrosine hydroxylase, TH (Vector Laboratories, USA; dilution

1:5000), PCNA (Dako, Denmark; 1:4000), monoclonal antibodies against human transcription factor Pax6 (Chemicon, USA; 1:3000), monoclonal antibodies frog against PA (ICN, Biomedicals, USA; 1:4000), rabbit polyclonal antibodies against nNOS (ICN, Biomedicals, USA; 1:5000), monoclonal antibodies mouse against CBS (Abcam ab54883, England 1:5000). Then, the slices were incubated with secondary biotin-conjugated horse antibodies against mouse immunoglobulins (Vector Laboratories, USA) for 2 h at room temperature and washed out three times in 0.1 M phosphate buffer. To reveal localization of NO-ergic neurons and fibers, we used a technique of indirect streptavidinbiotin immunohistochemical labeling of NOS. The slices were incubated with primary polyclonal rabbit antibodies against nNOS (ICN Biomedicals, USA; dilution 1:5000) at 4°C for 24 h. After three washings out in phosphate buffer, the slices were incubated with secondary biotin-conjugated goat antibodies against rabbit immunoglobulins (Biomedicals, Germany) at room temperature for 2 h. The material was washed out three times in phosphate buffer. Then, the slices were incubated in the presence of the streptavidin-peroxidase complex (Biomedicals, Germany) at room temperature for 2 h and again washed out three times in phosphate buffer. Immunohistochemical reactions were visualized using a standard avidinbiotin system (ABC; Vectastain Elite ABC Kit; Vector Laboratories, USA). To identify the reaction products, the slices were incubated in a substrate for detection of peroxidase (VIP Substrate Kit; Vector Laboratories, USA); the process of staining was controlled under a microscope. Then, the slices were washed out in three changes of phosphate buffer, mounted on slides, dehydrated using a standard technique, and embedded in balsam. To estimate the specificity of the immunohistochemical reaction, we used a technique of negative control. The masu brain slices were incubated in a medium containing 1% nonimmune horse serum (instead of primary antibodies) for 48 h, and then all procedures were performed as was described above. In all control experiments, the immunopositivity in the studied cells was absent.

To study projections of the preglomerular complex and glomerular nucleus, we used the carbocyanine dye 1,1'-dioctadecyl-3,3,3',3'-tetramethylindocarbocyanine perchlorate, DiI (Aldrich, Sigma, USA). The brains of fishes were fixed for 24 h in 4% solution of paraformaldehyde; then, crystals of the above dye were introduced in the region of the anterior and medial preglomerular and mammillary bodies. The obtained preparations were incubated in 4% solution of paraformaldehyde with the addition of 0.01% ethylenediamine tetraacetic acid (EDTA) at room temperature. Frontal, sagittal, and horizontal slices (50 μm thick) were prepared using a vibratome (VIBRATOME 3000; Sectioning system, Germany) and embedded in glycerine. To visualize the marker, we used an optical system, AXIOPLAN-2, Imaging (Gerinang, Germany). Preparations with DiI-marked structures were photographed using a optical system AXIOPLAN-2, Imaging (Gerinang).

Immunofluorescent labeling of tyrosine hydroxylase (TH) combined with retrograde labeling of neurons with the carbocyanine stain DiI was used to study the brains of Amur bitterlings *Rhodeus sericeus*. Specimens were fixed in 4% paraformaldehyde for one day, after which crystals of stain were placed in the ventral part of the telencephalon. Specimens were incubated in 4% paraformaldehyde supplemented with 0.01% ethylenediaminetetraacetate (EDTA) at room temperature for one day. Frontal, sagittal, and horizontal vibratome sections of thickness

50 μm were cut and incubated with primary mouse monoclonal antibodies against TH (Vector Laboratories, Burlingame, USA) diluted 1:1000 at 4°C for two days. Sections were then incubated with secondary fluorescent antibodies conjugated with Alexa 546 (Invitrogen Molecular Probes, USA) diluted 1:300 overnight. TH localization was studied using a Leica DM 4500 fluorescent microscope (Germany). Labeled TH and the carbocyanine label were visualized using a Leica TSC SPE confocal laser system (Germany).

Immunoperoxidase labeling of fragmented DNA chains, (TUNEL-labeling). To reveal apoptotic cells, we used a technique for immunoperoxidase labeling of fragmented DNA chains. After 2-h-long fixation in 4% solution of paraformaldehyde based on 0.1 M phosphate buffer (pH 7.2), dissected parts of the brain were washed out for 24 h in 0.1. M phosphate buffer. Then, these samples were put in 30% solution of sucrose based on phosphate buffer (0.1 M) for cryoprotection and kept in this solution up to full immersion. Frontal and horizontal slices (20 μm thick) were prepared using a freezing microtome. To identify TUNEL-positive structures, we used a immuno-peroxidase identification system, ApopTag Peroxidase In Situ Apoptosis Detection Kit (Chemicon International Inc., USA). For blocking endogenous peroxidase, the slices were incubated in 1% solution of hydrogen peroxide for 3 min and then washed out two times for 5 min in phosphate buffer. The slices were covered with a smoothing buffer (75 μl) and kept for 10 sec at room temperature. Then, the slices were slightly dried, subjected to the action of TdT enzyme (55 μl/5 cm^2), incubated in a humid chamber for 1 h at 37°C, and immersed in a stop buffer for 10 min. The slices were washed out in phosphate buffer at room temperature (three times for 1 min with changing of the solution), again dried, covered with antidioxygenin conjugate (65 μl/5 cm^2), and incubated in a humid chamber for 30 min. To detect the reaction products, cerebral slices were incubated in the substrate for identification of peroxidase (VIP Substrate Kit; Vector Labs, USA) with control of the development of color under a microscope, washed out in three changes of phosphate buffer, and mounted on glass slides. The cell nuclei were subjected to final staining with methyl green according to the technique of Brasher [15]. The preparations obtained were dewatered using a conventional technique and embedded in balsam. Morphometric processing was performed using an inverted-stage microscope, Axiovert 200M, equipped with a module, ApoTome, and digital cameras, Axio Cam MRM and Axio Cam HRC (Carl Zeiss, Germany).

The measurements were performed at ×400 magnification in five randomly chosen fields of vision for each studied region. The proliferation index (PI) and apoptosis index (AI) were calculated per 1 mm^2 of the section using the following formulas:

PI = (n of the PCNA-positive nuclei × 100%) ÷ total n of the nuclei and

AI = (n of TUNEL-positive fragments × 100%) ÷ total n of nuclei

Parametric comparison (Student's t-test) was used for estimation of the intergroup differences. The data obtained were processed using Statistica and Excel software. Numerical data are presented below as Means ± s.e.m.

http://dx.doi.org/10.5772/58306

3. Participation of classic neurotransmitters in the postembryonic neurogenesis in the fish brain

Studies suggest that in the salmon's brain at different stages of postembryonic development two forms of intercellular communications exist. The first form occurs in the early stages of postembryonic development and represents cells cooperation, carried out paracrinic in the period when cells have not developed processes and synaptic structure yet. However, such little differentiated cells are already able to express the specific synthetic machinery for some neurotransmitters and their synthesizing enzymes, gaseous intermediates, transcription factors and other substances (Fig. 1A-D). We suppose that most of the synthesized signals in this period are involved in the regulation of neuronal targets, differentiation and expression of their specific phenotype, acting as a morphogenetic factors. This is consistent with the Ugryumov concept [6] regarding the development of the mammalian brain in the embryonic period of ontogenesis. Already in the early stages of post embryonic morphogenesis of masou salmon, simultaneously two systems of neurochemical signaling exist, the dopaminergic and GABA-ergic systems, providing paracrinic and perhaps autocrinic influence on target cells until the formation of synaptic contacts and the beginning of neurotransmission with specific interneuronal connections. Study on the eal *Anguilla anguialla* showed that the maximum concentration of dopamine D_1 receptors is found in periventricular zones [16] which represent a matrix areas of the brain, where neurogenesis continues throughout the life of the animal. Consequently, the cells located in proliferating areas are targeted for the regulatory impact of dopamine. These cells are localized on the territory of the largest vascular plexus (forebrain and caudal medullar), and synthesize in these regions some substances, like a dopamine and GABA, which then may be excreted in the portal system blood flow and further into the general circulation system, providing regulatory endocrine effects on the peripheral organs [17]. Thus, there is considerable justification to suggest that in the hypophysotrophic areas of the diencephalon and medulla oblongata of the brain of juvenile salmons *O. masou*, dopamine and GABA in undifferentiated cells of periventricular and subventricular areas are inducers of development (morphogenetic factors).

Along with the specified form of intercellular signaling in salmon brain, in ontogenesis there is the development of specific system of forebrain activation and development of the system of remote intercellular signaling. The source of these directed connections are the nuclei of preglomerular complex [18]. Development of projective systems of salmon take place simultaneously with the formation of the structure of preglomerular complex [19]. In the brain of non mammalian vertebrates the volume of sensory projection zones increases during all their life and is provided due to the proliferation of neural stem cells located in the areas of special neurogenetic niches [10]. It is connected with the necessity of adaptation of the CNS of such animals to increase the size of the body and increased inflow of primary sensory information. We believe that a dopamine, GABA-and NO-ergic systems in the brain of salmon participate in regulation of some basis histogenetic processes, such as a cell migration and differentiation of neuro- and gliospecific lines, because the nuclei of preglomerular complexes contain morphologically and neurochemically heterogeneous cell populations (table. 1) represented

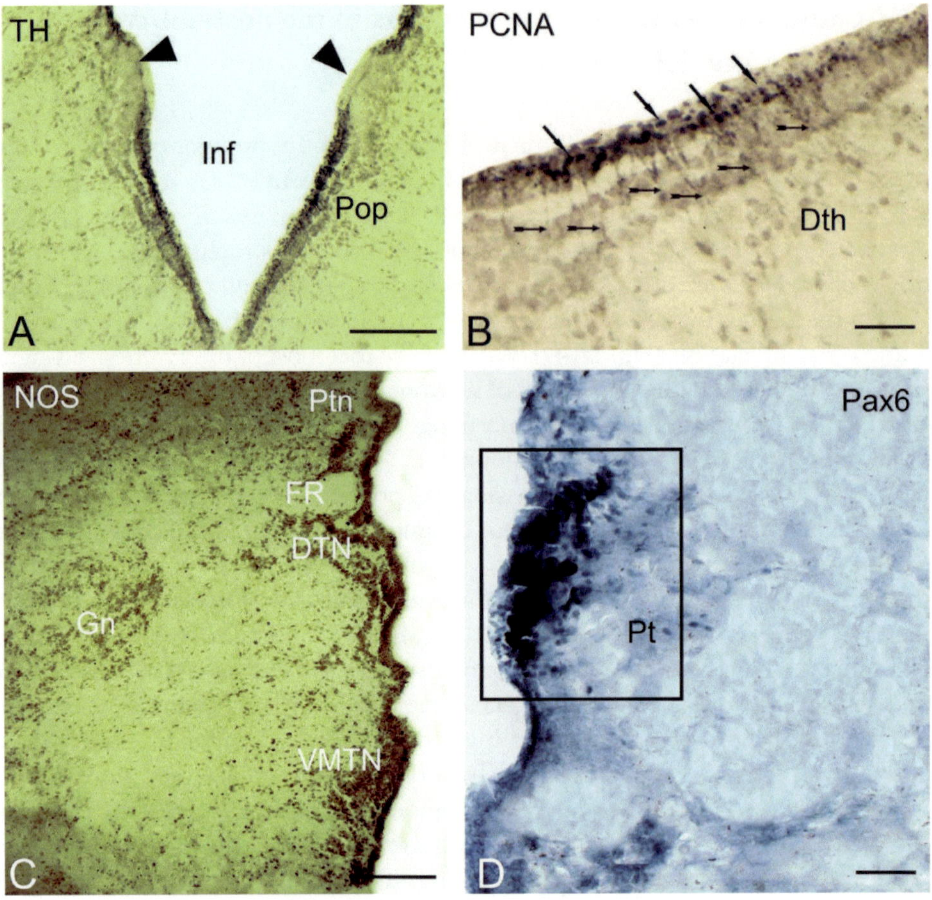

Figure 1. A - immunolocalisation of tyrosine hydroxilase (TH) in parvocellular preoptic nucleus (Pop), B - proliferative nuclear antigen (PCNA) in dorsal thalamus (DTh), C - neuronal nitric oxide synthase (NOS) in pretectal (Ptn), dorsal (DTN), ventro-medial (VMTN) thalamic nuclei, D - transcriptional factor Pax6 in periventricular diencephalon of 6-month-old *Oncorhynchus masou*. Immunonegative border of dorsal neuromers on A, delineated by a triangle, the cluster of immunopositive cells on D, delineated by rectangle. Inf – infundibulum, FR – fasciculus retroflexus, Pt – pretectum. Scale: A, C – 100 μm, B, D – 50 μm.

by the different stages of ontogenesis of major cell types. Cells formed in the proliferative (PCNA-containing) diencephalic areas migrate to the region of preglomerular complex, where their subsequent differentiation and growth take place. These processes are regulated by dopamine and GABA, that indicates the presence of D_1 and D_2 dopamine receptors [16, 20] and $GABA_B$ benzodiazepine receptors [21] in these nucleus of fish. A critical step prevalence of paracrinic relations in the salmons brain can be considered the period before the formation of the blood brain barrier (BBB), which in salmon brain is formed during the first year of life (according to [22]). In the next period of ontogenesis, the formation of the specific connections and the development of cellular processes of neurons and synaptogenesis take place. Today much data exist about the participation of radial glia in the processes of postembryonal neurogenesis by asymmetric mitoses in which one daughter cell remains in the periventricular area and has a rounded shape, while the other has a long process, which may later be eliminated through somal translocation [23]. It was shown that during embryogenesis of human, the predecessors of dopaminergic neurons in the basal part of the midbrain have the morphology of radial glia [24]. Immunolabeling of radial glia cells in salmon's brain in different ages (Fig. 2 (A-D), as well as evidence that the TH-and GABA-ip cells were located on the territory of PCNA-ip proliferative zones and together with PCNA marked the neuromeric structure of diencephalon and medullar part of the brain, certainly shows that dopamine and GABA-ergic signaling participates in the processes of postembryonic neurogenesis of the salmon's brain, as inductors of development. Our data are consistent with the labeling of some rhombomeres in the brain in an embryo of sharks *Scyliorhinus canicula* [25].

Nuclei	**Neuronal nitric oxide synthase (nNOS)**		**Choline acetyltransferase (ChAT)**		**GABA**		**Tyrosine hydroxylase (TH)**		**Parvalbumine (PA)**	
	Size of cells (μm)	Total number (%)	Size of cells (μm)	Total number (%)	Size of cells (μm)	Total number (%)	Size of cells (μm)	Total number (%)	Size of cells (μm)	Total number (%)
Glomerular	8-7 II 10-8 II 12-10 III	30±4	20-12 I 18-12 I 14-6 IV	18±2	9-6 II 7-7 II 12-6 IV 14-7 IV	50±6	9-7 II 10-6 II 15-6 III 17-8 IV	12±2	6-6 II 11-7 II 12-9 III 13-6 IV	48±4
Anterior Preglomer.	10-8 I 12-7 III 14-8 III 15-6 IV	24±3	12-9 III 13-8 III	9±1	20-13 I 12-12 III	47±5	8-6 II 10-7 II 12-9 III 14-6 III 12-6 IV	14±2	10-8 II 11-7 II 13-10 III	45±5
Medial Preglomer.	10-8 II 12-9 III 13-8 III	21±3	12-9 III 13-10 III 14-11 III	12±1	8-7 II 10-7 II 12-9 III	32±4	9-9 II 10-7 II 12-9 III 14-7 IV	8±1	9-7 II 10-8 II 13-10 III	30±3

Footnotes. Roman numerals (in brackets) indicate the cell type. Mean values of the large and small diameters of neurons (M ± m, μm) are separated by slashes.

Table 1. Morphometric characteristics and relative numbers of neurons belonging to different neurochemical types in the nuclei of the Preglomerular complex and also in the Glomerular nucleus of the *Oncorhynchus masou* brain.

Differentiation of cells in various parts of the salmon's brain presents a heterochronical process. In caudal part of brain some reticulospinal cells, cells of nucleus raphi, nuclei of V, VII, IX and X pairs of cranial nerves, much earlier acquire the features of phenotypic specialization than in the structures of forebrain. Measurements of fractal dimension and some morphometric parameters (total length of branches, number of terminal branches, number of branching points, and cell area) were used for the quantification of morphological patterns of two spinal neuron groups in young *Oncorhynchus masou* at two ontogenetic stages [26]. During the 1st and 2nd years of life, the neurons of brainstem and spinal cord have enough developed dendrites and axons, which, however, have growth cones, indicating the continued postembryonic period of growth and development of these structures and their further differentiation. During the second year of life, the values of morphometric parameters and fractal dimension of neurons increased in both groups. Basic morphometric values correlated with fractal dimensions and conformed to morphological changes in the dendritic tree of the investigated neurons in ontogenesis. During the third year of life, in the nuclei of the brain and spinal cord large-differentiated cells expressing TH, GABA and parvalbumine in the motoneurons of ventral spinal column, nuclei of craniocerebral nerves, reticulospinal cells and some diencephalic nuclei were revealed [27].

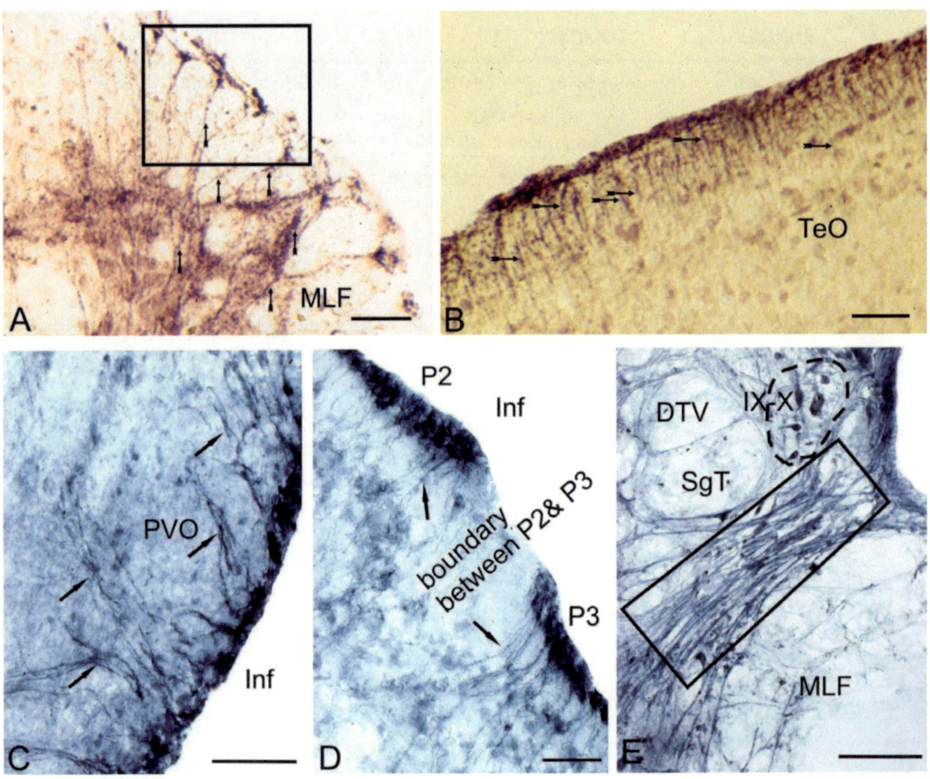

Figure 2. Immunohistochemistry of tyrosine hydroxylase in a spinal cord (A) and tectum (B) of a one-year old *O. masou*, in the periventricular diencephalic (C, D) and the medullar (D) departments of a 3-year-old fish. The arrows show the radial fiber; and: rectangle delineated areas of radial fibers, forming the «end feet»; D: on the border between dorsal neuromeres the immunolabeling of TH is absent; E: rectangle delineated by interfascicular area containing the radial fiber. Scale: A, B, D-50 μm; D-100 μm.

Along with systems synthesis of classical neurotransmitters, immunolocalisation of transcription factor Pax6 was investigated, the marking of which adequately reflects neuromeric structure of the salmon's brain in different ages (Fig 3 A, B). The early juveniles (3 and 6 months old) are the Pax6-ip cells do not have any processes and formed a small clusters corresponding to forebrain prosomeres (P1-P3), and in the medulla, such accumulations marked the rostral (R1-R2) rhombomeres (Fig. 3B). On the boundary of neuromeres labeling of PCNA and Pax6 were absent (Fig.3 A, D). In three-year old salmons the marking Pax6 was found in the cells and radial fibers, located in the periventricular and subventricular areas of diencephalon that corresponds to the data of labeling of Pax6 radial glia in the areas of postnatal neurogenesis of mammals [10]. On borders of the forebrain neuromeres the immunolabeling Pax6 in 3-years old individuals was absent. Expression of Pax6 was also found in glomerular nucleus and nuclei preglomerular complex that suggests about morphogenetic processes on the territory of the largest sensory center during postembryonal period. Immunolocalisation of Pax6 in specific cell clusters of glomerular nucleus, appropriated to some neuroanatomical zones, in which the differentiation of neurons, conducting various types of sensory signalization was revealed (Fig 3C. D). Studies suggest that factor Pax6 participates in the regionalization of the structure of the brain in postembryonal period, and its expression in different ages of salmon brain shows that the processes of neurodetermination and migration of cells, formed in proliferative areas of the brain in these age periods are regulated by means of this transcriptional factor. In the literature there are discrepancies regarding the organization and topography of dopamine, GABA-and NO-ergic complexes in the brain of different teleost fishes. Significant differences in the organization of the mediator systems in different fish species become more explainable, given the above mentioned scheme. We believe that neurotransmitter systems in the brain fish should be considered not only from the standard point of view of their definitive neuroanatomical structure, but must also take into account data on heterogeneous molecular phenotype of dopaminergic, GABA and, apparently, NO-ergic systems. Thus, for the establishment of homology, along with the systematic position, it is advisable to take into account the age, stage of development, physiological status and sex of the animal. In adult masou salmon and chum salmon the cells of Dc area of the telencephalon reach a high level of specialization and corresponding to the Ramon-Molener classification can be attributed to allodendric type.

Such cells have been found only in the most mature individuals (of 4-5 years old) going to spawn. One of the forms of specialization of these cells is that they have a network of basal spiny dendrites. This corresponds to the estimated specialization of such cells as associative spiny interneurons participated in communications with other parts of the dorsal area in telencephalon. Widespread TH and GABA in the telencephalon of adult chum salmon indicates that species to this period of development, along with paracrinic (volume) neurotransmission, there is a distant form of neurotransmission, which is becoming the predominant further ontogenetic development and ageing of the animal. We suggest that the acquisition of spiny apparatus by the neurons in the dorsal (Vd) and internal (Vi) areas ventral zone can be considered as one of the stages of ontogenetic development of neurons in the brain, indicating the age-related changes in the organization of the salmon's dopaminergic system. Formation of the system of neurochemical communication in the CNS of masou salmon in postembryonal period consists of two main stages. At the first stage the undifferentiated cells are located in matrix areas of the brain and expressed of specific syntheses (catecholamenes, GABA, NO,

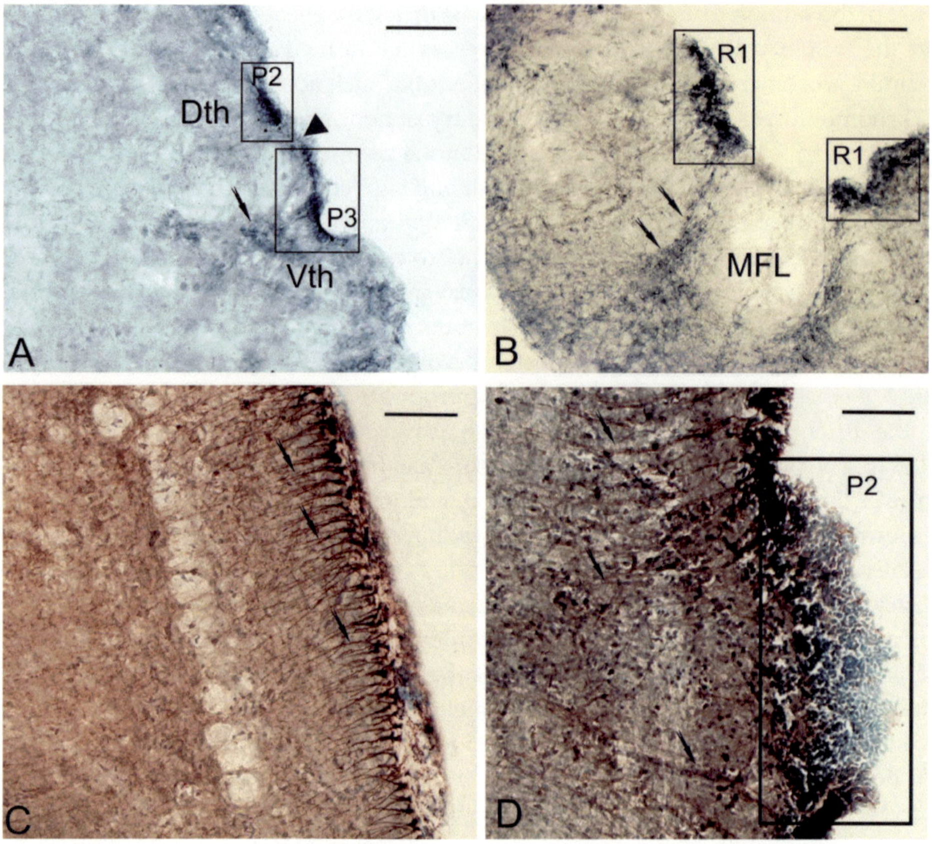

Figure 3. Expression of transcription factor Pax6 in the brain of 3-month-old salmon *O. masou* (A and B) and 3-year-old trout (C and D) (immunoperoxidase staining, light microscopy). Accumulations of immunopositive cells in the diencephalon (A) and medulla (B). Part of the brain (in rectangles) labels its neuromeric structure, the sites without immunolabeling constitute the borders of forebrain P2 and P3 prosomers (black edges of arrows), arrows with a cut show accumulations of migrating cells. Radial glia in the optical tectum (C) and around dorsal neuromer (P2) in the diencephalon (D). Scale: A-100 μm, B-200 μm, C and D – 50 μm.

some transcription factors). These substances are acting in paracrinic interaction and involved in regulating basis histogenetic processes: cell proliferation, cell migration, differentiation of target cells and expression of a specific phenotype. Under the influence of these factors on the second step is the formation of specific relations, development of processes of neurons and sinaptogenesis.

As a model to test an alternative hypothesis, we studied the CNS of amur bitterling *Rhodeus sericeus* (Cyprinidae), coming to sexual maturity in the first year of life. The literature of the late twentieth century actively discussed some issues relating to the organization and topography catecholaminergic system of vertebrate's brain detectable by methods formaldehyde-induced fluorescence (FIF) and IHC labeling of tyrosine hydroxylase. In this period, a hypothesis was formulated about the existence of dopamine deposited system in the brain of fish [28]. Data about neuromeric organization and molecular markers that define dopaminergic phenotype of neurons in *Danio rerio*, had recently published [29]. In the bitterling brain 3 main types of cells were verified. The first type consists of small round cells in the periventricular nucleus of the diencephalon and second one are formed by large pear-shaped or fusiform cells [30]. The cerebrospinalliquor-contacting cells (CSL) are the most common third type of catecholaminergic cells. According to the Meek classification [28], large cells and CSL-contacting cells at Amur bitterling can be attributed to the elements of dopamine deposited system. In the hypothalamus of bitterling were discovered a few CSL-contacting cells with a low level of activity TH, but cells were marked by gliocsalic acid. Some fish have similar features morphology of CSL-contacting cells (in particular, the presence of apical dendrite, turned into the lumen of the cerebral ventricle), and these cells are a FIF-positive, but do not contain enzymes synthesis of catecholamines (TH-negative). It was the reason for the assumption that such cells are not synthesizes catecholamines by themselves, but receives CE from external sources, in particular, liquor or from large dopaminergic neurons [31]. Data labeling catecholaminergic systems on other groups of vertebrates show that dopamine and norepinephrine dissolved in the cerebrospinal fluid are of greater importance for non mammalian vertebrates; but in mammals, the CSL-contacting cells at all have not been identified [32]. These confirm the observations obtained by us on the masou salmon.

Lack of Cyprinidae fish glomerular nucleus largely hinders establishing of homology between ascending sensory projections in the telencephalon with those of other fishes [33]. To identify sources of CA-ergic innervation of the ventral part of the telencephalon of bitterling investigated the projection of this area of the brain. Tracing part of dopaminergic fibers in the ventral telencephalon bitterling showed that along with intratelencephalic cell groups exists the extratelencephalic sources of innervation of the dorsal and ventral nuclei [30]. Sources of dopaminergic projections in the ventral part of the telencephalon are two populations of cells in posterior tuberculum of bitterling, namely large cells and small rounded cells. Such cells are projected on the dorsal and ventral areas of ventral telencephalic part respectively and are considered by us as the morpho-functional equivalents of meso-striatal and meso-limbic systems of mammals. Identification dopaminergic fibers in the dorsal region of telencephalon of *D. rerio* [31] suggests that teleostea have also equivalents of meso-pallial system.

The peculiarities of localization of medullary neurons, morphology of the dendrites, and trajectories of the axon projections in the medulla of the Amur bitterling allow us to differentiate three groups of TH-positive neurons, namely interfascicular cells, units related to the *lobus vagus*, and cells localized within the *area postrema* (Fig. 4 A-D). The 3-year-old masou salmon in all the above mentioned areas of the brain stem were also identified large TH-ip cells with clear features of phenotypic differentiation. However, along with differentiated TH-positive elements of masou salmon we revealed previously not described alternative TH-positive elements, namely small undifferentiated cells, located on the territory of proliferative periventricular and subventricular zones [27]; numerous radial fibers, having different localizations in medullar part of CNS (Fig. 2E). We believe that the presence of such elements with clear features of fetal organization, as well as radial fibers in the brain 3-year-old masou salmon connected with the processes of postembryonic (adult) morphogenesis of the brain. The differentiated TH-ip neurons in salmon brain are functionally active to this period of

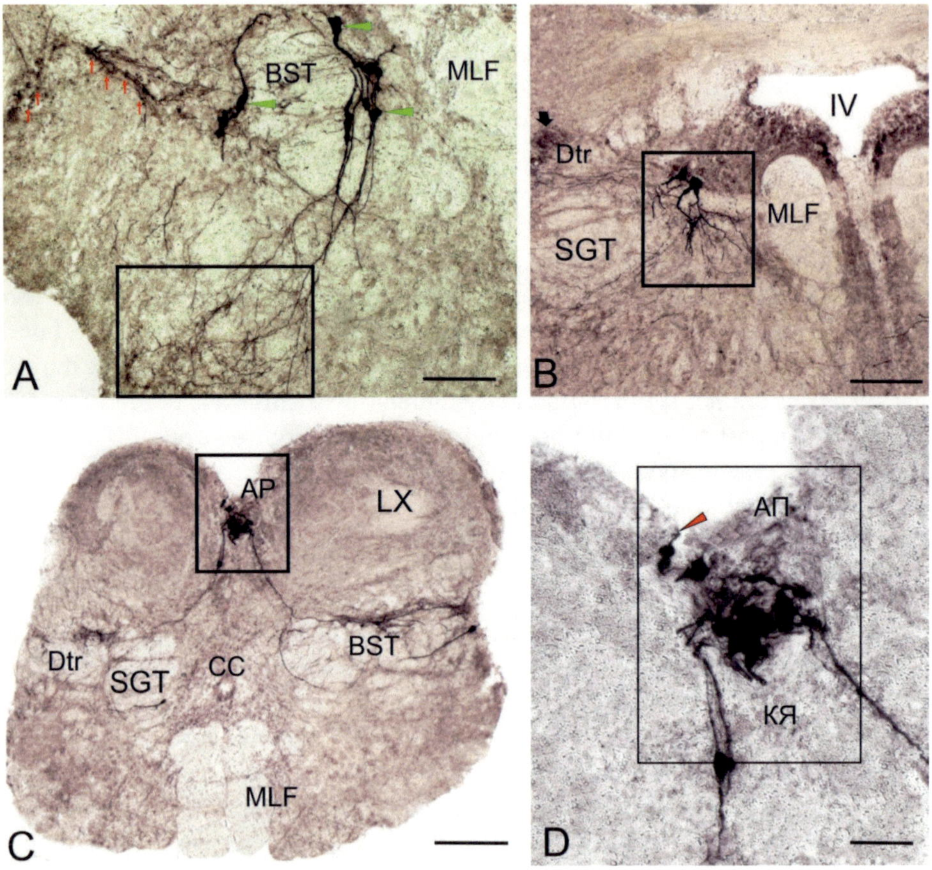

Figure 4. Tyrosine hydroxylase in the neurons of the medulla oblongata Amur bitterling *Rhodeus sericeus*. A and B-neurons of interfascicular group, C, D-neurons of area postrema. Scale: A-C-100 μm; D-50 μm.

ontogenesis elements of CA-ergic system. Study of the CA-ergic system in the medullary part of bitterling found pronounced features of specialization associated with the organization of medullary CA-ergic complexes. Analysis of these characteristics showed that of bitterling CA-ergic cells in neuronal networks of the medulla can fulfill the functions of local interneurons, projection long axon neurons, neurosecretory units, or sensory units. The morphology of interfascicular TH-positive cells in the Amur bitterling brain allows one to regard their functional specialization as local interneurons, since they form intensely branched dendritic networks (Fig. 4A, B). All three groups of medullary TH-ip neurons of bitterling project their terminals to the longitudinal catecholaminergic tract. Therefore, it is appropriate to hypothesize that all these cells are relatively long-axon neurons projecting to the rostral part of reticular formation, isthmus, and secondary gustatory nucleus which are relay centres, between the primary sensory nuclei of medulla oblongata and sensory centers of the ventral thalamus. The TH-positive cells of the vagus region and *area postrema* (supposedly dopaminergic) have access to the fourth ventricle; likely, these neurons are chemosensory units responsible for the relations between the cerebrospinal fluid and neuronal medullary systems (Fig. 4C, D). On the other hand, these two neuronal groups in the Amur bitterling differ from others in an extremely high level of TH activity; it cannot be ruled out that they can serve as a source of dopamine coming to the cerebrospinal fluid. The morphology of these neurons allows one to hypothesize that each of the three groups of medullary CA-ergic neurons in the Amur bitterling is involved in realization of at least two functions of the above-listed ones, while the cells associated with the lobus vagus can combine all three functions. In the masou salmon brain phenotypically mature types of TH-ip cells localized in similar areas of the medulla oblongata, can have a similar functional specialization (Fig. 2E). However, part of the identified by us TH-ip elements is located in the proliferative (PCNA-marked) areas of medulla oblongata [27] at the earlier stages of ontogenesis mark neuromeric structure of medulla oblongata. At later stages localization TH found in the fibres of radial glia in interfascicular region, on the territory of fossa romboidea, as well as in populations of small cells in periventricular and subventricular areas (Fig. 2E).

In the Amur bitterling the density of the distribution of such phenotypically not mature cell forms in the periventricular area of the brain is significantly lower than the masou salmon. We believe that the features allocation in medullar part of masou salmon and Amur bitterling confirm the assumption about the participation of dopamine as a morphogenic factor regulating brain development of fish in postembryonal period.

4. Participation gaseous intermediators in the modulation of classical neurotransmitters in fishes brain

Study of the modulating influence gaseous intermediators to the classical system of neurotransmitters in the brain of fish previously had not been carried out. In our studies showed that the total nitroxidergic products in the nuclei of the brain stem in different fish species significantly exceeded the measure set for other groups of vertebrates and, particularly mammals. So, it is normal for different fish species NO-producing neurons were verified somato- and viscerosensor and visceromotor nuclei of medulla oblongata (V, VII, IX, X nuclei of craniocerebral nerves, Fig. 5), efferent octavo-lateral neurons, the nuclei of the isthmus, secondary gustatory nuclei, the nuclei of oculomotor complex (III, IV and VI nuclei of cranial nerves). Most of these nuclei in fish brain are cholinergic centers of brain stem involved in the innervation of brachiomotor muscles and some sensory inputs from the somatosensory, gustatory extra- and intraoral system, mechanosensory, octavolateral receptors. In fish due to low level of cephalization brain the most of the sensory inputs from the somatosensory (nucleus V), octavolateral, gustatory extraoral (nucleus VII), intraoral (nucleus IX) are concentrated on the territory of medullary part; therefore this sector is perceived by a large volume of incoming sensory information (see the diagram on Fig. 5). Despite significant interspecific morpho-adaptative differences, in Perciformes and Cyprinoid fish were identified similarities in the organization of medullar and spinal NO-producing centres. Participating NO in modulation of sensor systems in forebrain of mammals it was proved today [34]. We assume that in the medulla fish NO performs modulation of primary sensory centers, located in the nuclei of craniocerebral nerves. In the masou salmon brain all of the above mentioned nuclei, located in the stem and isthmus region are cholinergic and express nNOS (see the diagram on Fig. 5). Primary sensory nuclei (V, VII, VIII, IX and X), and secondary relay nuclei (secondary gustatory nucleus, the nucleus of the isthmus) in tha masou salmon brain, processing hetero-modal sensory the information in the nuclei of preglomerular complex modulated by NO (Fig. 5). We assume that in the masou salmon brain NO is modulator of sensory and motor cholinergic centers.

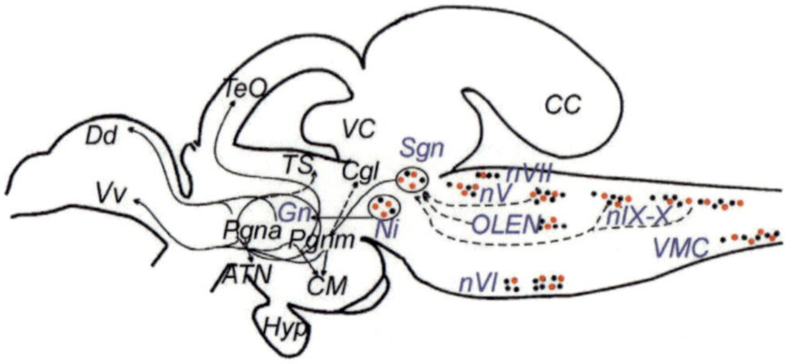

Figure 5. Schematic diagram of sensory signals ascending from the nuclei V, VII, IX, X and octavo-lateral nerves of medulla oblongata to the telencephalon. In the left part are demonstrated the efferent ascending and descending projection, anterior, medial preglomerular nuclei and mammilar body O. masou labeling by the DiI [19]. NO-ergic nuclei of brainstem are shown by black, cholinergic-red circles. The other explanation see text.

The most important sensory center, conducting nociceptive information in fish's brain is a nucleus raphi. We found that in different species of teleost fish the most of the neurons of the nucleus raphi superior and nucleus raphi inferior are expressed NADPH-d. This confirms the data installed on mammalian and human brain, that NO is a mediator of nociception [35]. The presence of nNOS-producing neurons and high level of activity NADPH-d in the nuclei of raphi, dorsal spinal cord fibers and sensory part of the nucleus of trigeminal nerve indicates participation of nitric oxide in the modulation signals of nociceptive and somatosensor centers of the medulla oblongata in fishes brain. Study of the localization of nNOS in some periventricular hypophysotropic nuclei in diencephalon of adult specimens of Amur bitterling showed that TH-ip and NO-producing system in periventricular and subventricular nuclei in general have similar localization and area of colocalisation these transmitters is periventricular nucleus of posterior tuberculum, where nNOS and TH were localized in small cells, forming ascending projections on the ventral telencephalon. In these cells NO can modulate synaptic plasticity of dopaminergic neurons and regulate the excretion of dopamine.

Study of physiological activity of hydrogen sulfide in the nervous system of mammals began recently [36], and identifying its role in the central nervous system of fish previously had not been carried out. The results of researches conducted on fish suggest that hydrogen sulfide acts as an intermediary, regulating a number of enzymatic reactions cells. Distribution of the enzyme synthesis of H_2S in the CNS of fish is expressed species-specific features, perhaps reflecting their adaptation character and functional status of the animal. Cystathionine β-synthase in the brain of masu salmon *Oncorhynchus masou* and carp *Cyprinus carpio* was found

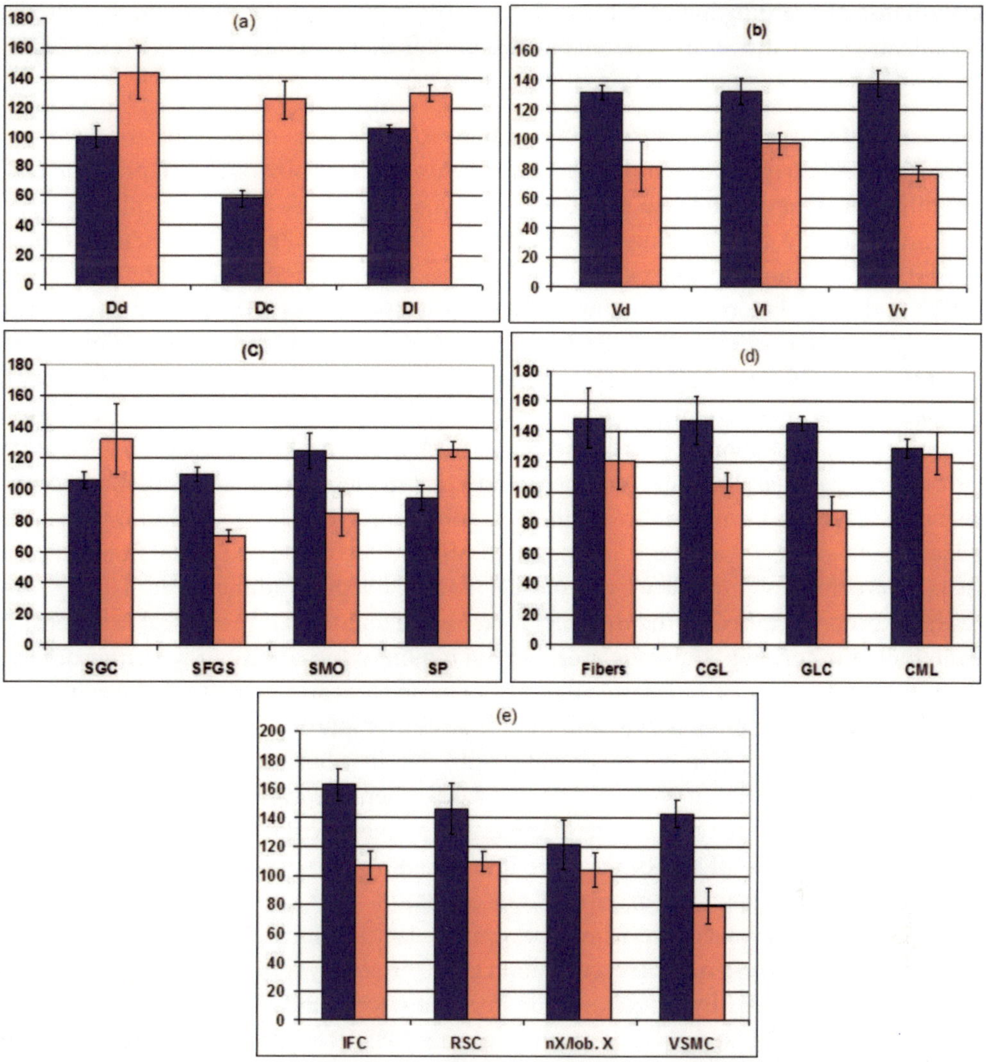

Figure 6. Densitometric analysis of the CBS activity in different brain areas of masu salmon Oncorhynchus masou and carp Cyprinus carpio. Abscissa axis, brain areas; Ordinate axis, optical density (OD). Data are shown as M ± m. (a) CBS activity in neurons of dorsal telencephalon; (b) CBS activity in neurons of ventral telencephalon; (c) CBS activity in the optic tectum; (d) CBS activity in the cerebellum; (e) CBS activity in the spinal cord and medulla oblongata. Designations: Vv, Vd, Vl, ventral, dorsal, and lateral cell nuclei of the ventral telencephalon; Dd, Dc, Dl, dorsal, central, and lateral cell nuclei of dorsal telencephalon. blue columns-masu salmon; pink columns-carp.

in neurons of the ventral spinal column and medulla oblongata, fibers and cells of the cerebellum, optic tectum, and telencephalon. In all brain areas, the intensity of CBS labeling in neurons varied between moderate and high. We found interspecies differences in the immunolocalizatoin and optical density of CBS in different brain structures of masu salmon and carp. In carp, the medulla oblongata and spinal cord contained intensely marked vessels that were absent in masu salmon. In the brain of carp, H_2S presumably functions as a predominant vasoregulator. H_2S-producing systems in the brain of bony fishes have specific characteristics of organization and strong species-related differences that correlate with the specificities of neuromediators, for example, NO-producing, systems.

Comparative studies of localization CBS and densitometric data in various structures of the masu salmon and carp showed interspecific differences, having obviously adaptive value (Fig. 10). In different areas of the masu salmon brain revealed varicose or smooth microcytosculpture of afferents and their endings, which may indicate to synaptic or paracrinic (volume) methods of H2S release in different areas of the fishes brain.Currently shows the involvement of GABA in the regulation of the endocrine activity of hormones preoptico-pituitary complex at the early juveniles *Salmo trutta fario* [37]. On larval and early juvenile of this salmon species showed the participation of GABA-ergic innervation in the regulation of synthesis of peptide hormones of the pituitary, namely metencephalin and galanin [37]. In our research on different age groups of masu salmon, it was found that GABA-ip neurons are present in various parts of the brain: in the medulla oblongata, periventricular nuclei of diencephalon, mesencephalic tegmentum, the brain stem, the cerebellum and spinal cord (Fig. 11). In addition to the neural localization of GABA, it was identified small undifferentiated cells and radial fibers, localized in areas where the proliferative activity of cells persists in adults animals (Fig. 11A, D). These zones have been identified in the diencephalon on the territory of preoptical area, posterior tuberal, thalamic and hypothalamic areas; in the region of the central gray matter of mesencephalic tegmentum; in the interfascicular area of brain stem and in the periventricular zones in nuclei IX-X pairs of cranial nerves and the spinal cord. Patterns of distribution GABA-ergic elements in the masu salmon brain is similar with the distribution of TH-ip structures. This similarity manifests itself in the presence of both phenotypically mature cell forms and undifferentiated elements with periventricular and subventricular localization and marking of neuromeric structure of the brain. This immunomorphology of GABA-ergic structures, discovered in the different age groups of masu salmon, may indicate that, like dopamine, GABA should be also considered as morphogenetic factor affecting of postembryonic brain development.GABA-ergic neurotransmission characterized by a high variability of synaptic responses. In mammals, hydrogen sulfide regulates the condition of GABA-receptor of different subtypes, localized pre-and postsinapticaly [38]. In adult masu salmon in different areas of the brain and spinal cord, containing large projection cells, namely the dorsal tegmental nuclei, medial reticular formation, reticulospinal cells, neurons in the ventral spinal column were installed joint localization of GABA, PA and CBS (Fig. 7). These large-cells structures in the fish brain participate in the organization of fast motor responses [39]. In medullary regions of the medial RF and VSC of the masu salmon, the level of colocalization of CBS, GABA, and PA is rather high. It is believed that the presence of PA promotes the formation of buffer calcium systems that provide generation of repeated action potentials in neurons with high-frequency discharges (Fig. 7). The high level of colocalization of PA, cytochrome oxidase, and 2-deoxyglucose also indicates that the PA content is typical of neuronal systems characterized by a high level of oxidative metabolism [40]. It was demonstrated that the concentration of intracellular calcium in neurons and glial cells upon the action of H_2S reversibly increases (due to the release of calcium from intracellular stores and its entry into the cell through the plasma membrane) [41, 42]. Such adenylate cyclase-dependent

http://dx.doi.org/10.5772/58306

mechanisms of activation can also be realized in the magnocellular CBS-and PA-ip populations of myelencephalic cells of the masu salmon brain identified in our experiments. As was found, inhibition of H_2S synthesis results in a significant decrease in the level of intracellular calcium. This confirms the conclusion on the appreciable effect of H_2S-dependent pathways on the time characteristics of processes related to calcium homeostasis in the neurons [41].

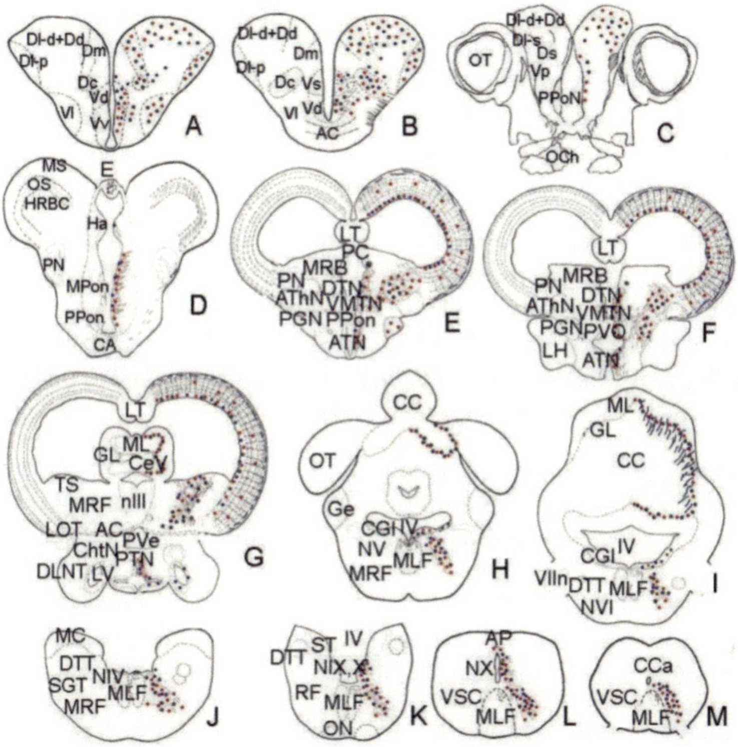

Figure 7. Schematic diagrams of distribution of cystathionine-β-synthase (CBS)-, GABA-, and parvalbumin (PA)-immunopositive loci in frontal CNS slices of the masu salmon, Oncorhynchus masou (A-M). Zones of immunopositivity with respect to CBS, GABA, and PA are indicated by blue circles, red diamonds, and black asterisks, respectively. AC) Ansular commissure, AP) area postrema, Vv, Vd, Vl, and Vs) ventral, dorsal, lateral, and supracommissure zones of the ventral region, respectively, SGT) secondary gustatory tract, VMTN) ventromedial thalamic nucleus, VSC) ventral spinal column, Ha) habenula, GE) granular eminence, Gl) granular layer, Dd, Dl, Dm, and Dc) dorsal, lateral, medial, and central zones of the dorsal region, respectively, DLNT) dorsolateral nucleus of the tegmentum, DTN) dorsal thalamic nucleus, PVe) posterior ventricle, PC) posterior commissure, PTN) posterior tuberal nucleus, rV) root of the trigeminal (V cranial) nerve, MPoN) magnocellular preoptic nucleus; LH) lateral hypothalamus, LVe) lateral ventricle, LOT) lateral optic tract, CC) corpus cerebelli, MeRF) mesencephalic reticular formation, CeV) cerebellar valve, CeCh) cerebellar chiasm, PPoN) parvicellular preoptic nucleus, MLF) medial longitudinal fascicle, MRF) medial reticular formation, CeMl) cerebellar molecular layer, DTT) descending tract of the trigeminal nerve, OLen) octavolateral efferent neurons, MRB) Meynert's retroflex bundle, OT) optic tectum, OCh) optic chiasm, ON) olivary nucleus, SlT) semilunar torus, PVO) paraventricular organ, PGN) preglomerular nucleus, AC) anterior commissure, LT) longitudinal torus, ATN), anterior thalamic nucleus, ATbN) anterior tuberal nucleus, PN) pretectal nucleus, RF) reticular formation, ST) solitary tract, CHtN) central hypothalamic nuclei, CC) central canal, CGl) central gray layer, NIII) oculomotor nucleus, NIV) nucleus of the trochlear nerve, NIX-X), nuclei of the glossopharyngeal and vagus nerves, respectively, NV) nucleus of the trigeminal nerve, NVII) nucleus of the facial nerve, IIIn) oculomotor nerve, IV) fourth ventricle, and VIIn) facial nerve.

Significant heterogeneity of CBS-ip, GABA-ip,and PA-containing subpopulations of neurons in all regions of the masu brain is indicative of the fact that such units belong to different neurochemical and electrophysiological systems. The density of CBS-, PA-, and GABA-ip cells in the masu salmon is maximum and constant in the magnocellular caudal cerebral regions, namely in the regions of localization of the reticulo-spinal neurons, "high-frequency" Mauthner cells, and ventral spinal cord (VSC) neurons. Cells of these types in fishes are involved in the organization and control of rapid motor reactions [43]. H_2S-dependent regulation of calcium release with participation of PA can influence the parameters of impulse activity due to shortening of the refractory period in the corresponding neurons after generation of action potentials and, therefore, can provide the animal with certain behavioral evolutionary preference. Thus, in the population of large inhibitory neurons containing enhanced concentration of intracellular Ca^{2+}, the excretion of GABA in our opinion can be arranged with the help of hydrogen sulphide.

Study of the relationship between NO and H_2S-producing systems in the masu salmon brain revealed that they were separate, non-overlapping system of intra-and intercellular signaling. The study of the distribution of NADPH-d positive, nNOS-and CBS-ip elements in different areas of the masu salmon brain, and some features immunolabeling of cells and fibers indicate that NO and H_2S-producing systems are independent neural complexes that perform specialized functions in the work of local neural networks.

In the dorsal region of the telencephalon in masu salmon NO is predominant gasotransmitter, the effects of which release by paracrinical way. In the ventral region of the telencephalon prevails system of hydrogen sulfide synthesis. In the ventral region of the telencephalon high activity CBS was revealed. Perhaps this system has synaptic localization, significant morphological heterogeneity of cells in the dorsal nucleus (Vd) and varicose cytosculpture of the afferents. Apparently, in the telencephalon of masu salmon way to release the gasotransmitters affect the nature of their neuromodulatory effects.

In the periventricular area of diencephalon and optic tectum masu salmon were populated by both CBS and nNOS and NADPH-d-producing cells. The presence of NO and H_2S-producing elements in these areas indicates possible participation of hydrogen sulfide and nitric oxide in morphogenesis these compartments of a brain. In masu salmon brain has been identified CBS-ip fibers of varicose type that penetrate the layer of Purkinje cells. The presence of such fibers and CBS-ip endings in interganglionic plexus of corpus cerebelli, possibly reflecting the sinaptical method of release of H_2S in this area of the masu salmon brain. The presence of NO-ergic cells and fibers was shown in the cerebellum on different species of fish by histochemical marking of NADPH-d [4, 44, 45]. Detection of nNOS in eurydendroid cells of masu salmon cerebellum confirms received our earlier data on histological labelling of NADPH-d in the neurons of this type of fish [46]. According to Ikenaga with co-authors [47], most of the eurydendroid cells in fish are aspartat-ergic and receive GABA-ergic impulses from the Purkinje cells. According to our data, the population of eurydendroid cells of masu salmon in cerebellum contains GABA-ergic and PA-ergic cells. Identified in the of masu salmon cerebellum thin nNOS-ip fibers, in our opinion, are the axons of eurydendroid neurons. Thus, nitric oxide, and being located in the projection eurydendroid cells, can acts as a modulator of aspartat-ergic signals in structure of efferent fibres to various parts of the masu salmon brain. Localization of nNOS, NADPH-d and CBS in interfascicular cells of masu salmon, by the classification [48], identified for the first time. We believe that interfascicular CBS-and nNOS-ip neurons of masu salmon are separate subpopulations of cells of the reticular formation, which modulating GABA-and cholinergic system in the medulla oblongata, respectively.

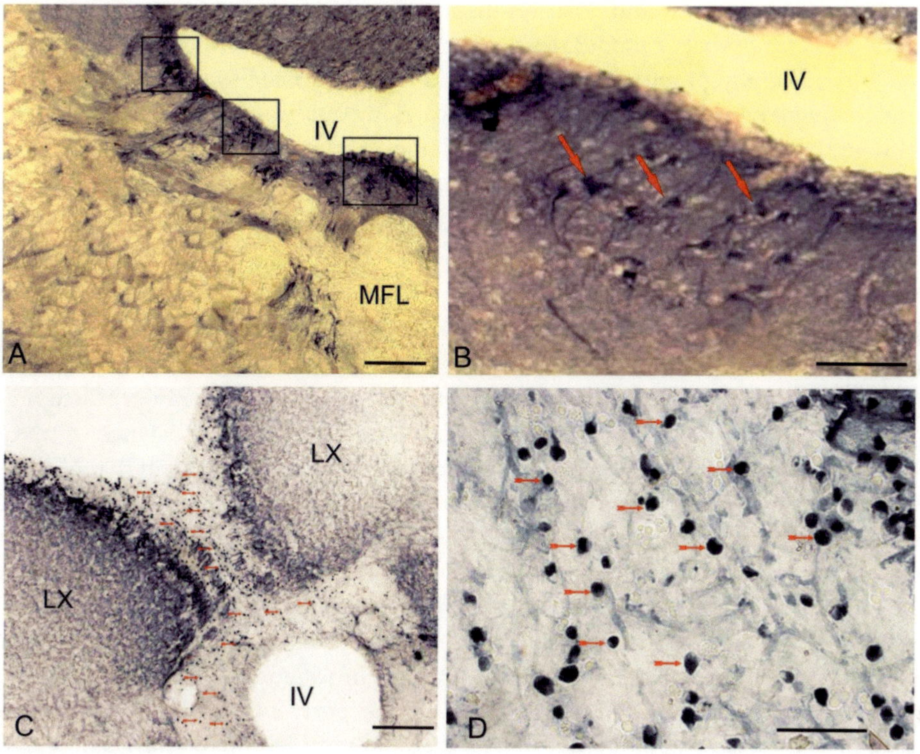

Figure 8. A – clusters of NADPH-d-producing cells (delineated by rectangles) in periventricular area of medulla oblongata of Oncorhynchus masou; on B in a large magnification. C - cystathionine β-synthase (CBS) producing cells (red arrows) in periventricular area of Cyprinus carpio brain, on D in a large magnification. LX – lobus of vagal nerve, IV – forth ventricle, MLF – medial longitudinal fascicle. Scale: A, C – 200 μm, B, D – 50 μm.

Secondary gustatory nucleus is seen as a visceral integrative centre in medulla oblongata in fishes brain [46]. In Carp in this nucleus was found the CBS immunolocalization, and in the masu salmon the secondary gustatory nucleus is CBS-immunonegative, but contains NADPH-d and nNOS. We believe that with the participation of H_2S and NO-producing systems in the brain fish is carried out sensory modulation functions related to the evaluation of food in space and coordination of mechanosensor, visual and gustatory features. In Carp brain the main neurotransmitter of the gustatory system is hydrogen sulfide, and in the masu salmon brain is nitric oxide, which confirms the assumption about the use of fish of various signal transductor systems to transfer the neurochemical information in functionally similar complexes.

We have revealed the existence of NO and H_2S-producing neurons in brainstem and isthmus regions of masu salmon brain. nNOS-ip and NADPH-d positive neurons were discovered in the composition of somato- and viscerosensoric (V, VII, IX-X) and visceromotoric (III, IV and VI) of craniocerebral nerves, octavo-lateral efferent complex, medial reticular formation. CBS in the medulla of masu salmon was detected in neurons of the nucleus X nerve, reticulospinal cells and ventro-lateral reticular formation. Distribution of NO and H_2S-producing neurons in the nuclei of medulla oblongata of masu salmon indicates that NO is the predominant neuromodulator of somato-and viscerosensoric and visceromotoric systems of medulla oblongata, and H_2S probably modulates viscerosensoric systems associated with the nucleus X nerve, and descending motor systems. NO and H_2S-producing systems in the fishes brain: 1) are independent neural complexes which are carrying out specialized functions in the work of local neural networks; 2) represent separate, non-overlapping systems of intra-and inter-cellular signaling, modulating the activity of choline-, GABA-and catecholaminergic systems, respectively; 3) regulate the processes of adult neurogenesis in the matrix areas of the brain.

5. Gaseous mediators as a regulators of adult neurogenesis

Unlike mammals, the fish brain has a high neuronal plasticity and can produce new cells throughout life [49]. The results of our investigations indicate the existence of nNOS and NADPH-d in neurons and glial cells in the masu salmon brain. It is shown that NO plays the role of signaling agent, regulating the processes directed growth of axons and dendrites and migration of differentiating neurons [50]. It is established that in the subventricular zone of mammalian forebrain is surrounded by NO-producing neurons [51, 52]. Cells expressing nNOS were identified among progenitor cells of dentate girus in the hippocampus of Guinea pig [53]. These areas of the brain are considered zones adult neurogenesis in which the proliferation of the cells is maintained throughout the life of animals and human. The results of our investigation (Fig. 8A, B) suggest that in the periventricular area of the medulla oblongata in masu salmon containing PCNA-ip proliferating cells in different age periods, NO can act as a regulator of adult neurogenesis, which confirms the data obtained on mammals.

In the periventricular area of the medulla oblongata, ventral and lateral areas of the cerebellum of carp are considered matrix areas of the brain of this species [54], identified highly CBS-immunogenic cells, without any processes (Fig. 8C, D). The sizes of cells, their location in the brain and correlations with H_2S-producing neurons indicate the presence of H_2S-producing of glia in the matrix zone of carp brain. In similar areas of the masu salmon brain such cells were not found. As currently participation of gaseous mediators in the regulation of post-embryonal neurogenesis of mammals was shown [55], we believe that in carp brain H_2S can act as such an agent, as the presence of CBS in proliferative areas of brain we consider as one of the proofs of this. One of the mechanisms regulating the in fish producing the large number of cells, educated including postembryonal period is apoptosis [7]. Study of a 60-day old sturgeon fry showed the presence of intensively proliferating zones containing PCNA-ip cells in forebrain. The active proliferation of cells in this period of the sturgeon's development is complemented by the formation of secondary neurogenetic zones.

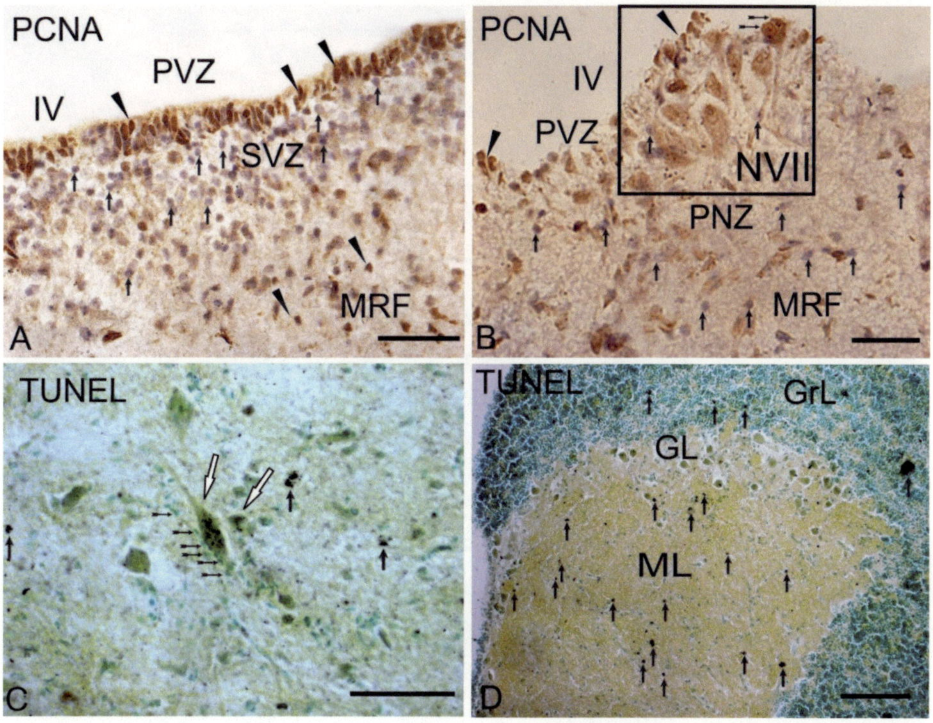

Figure 9. Proliferative activity (A and B) and apoptosis (C and D) in the brain of a three-year sturgeon *A. schrenckii*. PCNA-ip cells are shown triangular arrow, TUNEL labeled elements – are shown black arrows. Scale: A, B-100 μm; C-50 μm; D-200 μm.

The 3-year olds sturgeons' zone proliferation and apoptosis in various parts of the intact CNS saved (Fig. 9A, B). The highest proliferative activity was detected in periventricular zone of medulla oblongata, that allows considering this area as a major area of adult neurogenesis (Fig. 14A, 15B). In the medial reticular formation, dorsal nuclei of the thalamus, the inner fibrous layer of tectum opticum and lateral hypothalamus were discovered maximum number of apoptotic elements. This circumstance allows us to suppose that these regions in the sturgeon brain correspond with the areas of postmitotic neuroblasts localization. In the sensory centers (tectum opticum and nuclei V, VII and X nerves were revealed variable ratio processes of proliferation and apoptosis (Fig. 10A), which indicates different rates of growth and differentiation of visual and chemosensory centers of the sturgeon brain. In contrast to mammals in which central divisions of sensory systems are completely formed and correspond strictly to the number of sensory receptors at the moment of birth and/or immediately after this event, sensory projections in the fish brain continue their growth and development during the entire life. Such a peculiarity of the fishes is related to the fact that the CNS organization must adapt to a significant permanent increase in the size of the body and, correspondingly, to a rise in the volume of incoming sensory information. Our studies of projections of the somato- and viscerosensory nuclei of the myelencephalon and tectum opticum of the sturgeon confirmed in general the hypothesis that adult neurogenesis and apoptosis exert significant effects on the

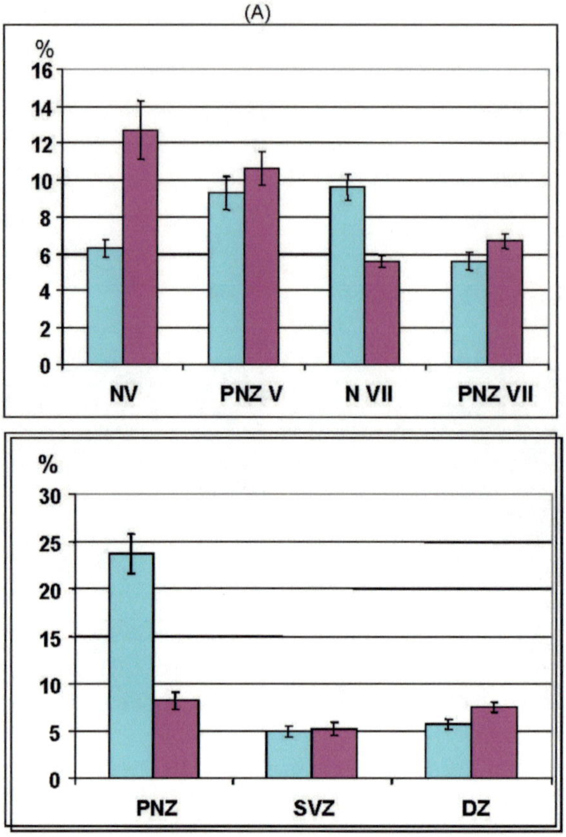

(B)

Figure 10. Intensity of the processes of proliferation and apoptosis in different parts of the myelencephalon of the Amur sturgeon Acipenser schrenckii. Data are shown as M ± m. A) In the nuclei of trigeminal and facial nerves (NV and NVII, respectively) and perinuclear zones adjacent to these nuclei (PNZ V and PNZ VII, respectively). B) In the lobe of the vagus nerve. PVZ, SVZ, and DZ-periventricular, subventricular, and deep zones, respectively. Ordinate axis-proliferation index, PI (blue columns) and apoptosis index, AI (pink columns), %.

peculiarities of postnatal development of the sensory systems. Our findings agree with the published data on intensification of differential growth in primary sensory regions in the lobe of the nucl. vagus of the carp, as well as in the Danio retina and tectum, compared with other cerebral regions [56].

Up to now, it remains unknown whether all types of neurons develop and are integrated into the corresponding networks of the growing brain of fishes. It seems probable that some initial level of organization of neuronal networks in fishes is already preformed at the moment of their hatching, and only some types of neurons continue their formation and integration into existing networks during the later period of life. It is believed that the weak ability for substitution or development of new neurons in the mammalian brain is related to the limited ability of such cells in animals of this class to be integrated into mature neuronal networks [58]. It is hypothesized that neurons formed de novo in adult animals are distinguished by a higher plasticity compared with that of preexisting cells [59, 60]. This viewpoint agrees well with our findings on the sturgeon and allows us to suppose that postembryonic (adult) neurogenesis correlates with coordinated growth of the sensory systems and sensory structures of the brain. Therefore, this phenomenon can open possibilities for the processing of new ontogenetic experience. Incorporation of new cells into the neuronal networks existing earlier in the sensory regions is directly related, first of all, to an increase in the size of the brain in the course of growth of the fish. However, it should be taken into account that fishes, immediately after hatching, possess relatively well preformed sensory and motor systems making possible rather rapid training for complex behavioral habits, e.g., active catching of food and avoidance of predators. This indicates that some parts of the CNS of fishes, which are responsible for information processing and realization of functional needs of the organism necessary within a certain life period, begin to function before hatching. The later postembryonic growth can be considered a process of delayed development related to the maintenance of the functions necessary in future, e.g., for the formation of zoosocial communication or sexual behavior. Therefore, our conclusion that some parts of the sturgeon brain remain, in fact, in the neotenic state over a rather long postembryonic period seems to be quite logical. This hypothesis explains the high indices of proliferative activity in some brain regions in cartilaginous ganoid fishes.

The particular relevance of the results obtained acquire the communications regulatory functions of nitric oxide and hydrogen sulfide, regarded as regulators of adult neurogenesis in the fish brain. We have highlighted nNOS-ip fiber varicose type in subventricular area of the spinal cord, as well as the presence of PCNA-and nNOS-ip cells in the composition of the periventricular area of diencephalon and medulla oblongata in sturgeon and salmon indicates the presence of NO-producing elements in zones containing proliferating cells. On the other hand, detection of NO-ergic activity in TUNEL positive areas of the brain sturgeon indicates the involvement of nitric oxide in the regulation of apoptosis. Thus, it is possible that in the brain sturgeon NO is as proapoptogenic and regulatory proliferation factor exercising to maintain a balance between the two processes. Cytotoxic and neuroprotective effects NO can be viewed as interrelated elements of a single action: if the excess output of NO potentiates the mechanisms of apoptosis in the zones of localization of postmitotic neuroblasts, the factors reducing NO production can be considered as compensatory. In the basis of post embryonic morphogenesis of sturgeon's A. schrenckii brain, and particular, development of sensor systems are founded on certain ratio of the processes of proliferation and apoptosis, having NO-dependent mechanism of regulation.

6. Conclusion

Thus, we believe that the peculiarities of the distribution of the investigated systems synthesis of classic neurotransmitters (GABA, catecholamines), as well as gaseous mediators (NO and H_2S) is directly linked to the ability of the brain fish grow throughout life. We interpret the obtained results in this context. This led us to the conclusion that some of the classic neurotransmitters (dopamine, GABA), as well as gaseous intermediaries (NO and H_2S) are not only regulators of the functional activity of neurons and modulators of synaptic transmission in mature neural networks, but also are considered as inductors of development (morphogenetic factors) in the brain during postembryonic fish ontogenesis. Proof of this is a detection of the phenotypic immature elements in the masou salmon brain adult age, expressing the above mentioned molecules in proliferative areas of the brain, as well as elements that have the morphology of the radial glia. Presence of markers of gaseous intermediaries in the areas of expressing proliferative nuclear antigen (PCNA), proves the involvement of gaseous intermediaries in the regulation of post-embryonal neurogenesis. The fish with the prolonged cycle of development (salmon, and carp) such markers (NO and H_2S) in periventricular proliferative areas of the brain may differ, which is consistent with the notion that in functionally similar complexes in animals can be used different signal transduction systems. Development of the nervous system salmon and sturgeon, in contrast to the widespread neurogenetic model D. rerio occurs over a long period of time. According to our data, the different structures of the CNS of masou salmon characterized by severe heterochrony, i.e. the cells of caudal parts of the brain in much earlier than neurons of forebrain departments, acquire the features of phenotypic specialization. We are convinced that the brains of these animals for a long time keeps features of fetal organization, and the presence of first and second years of life low differentiated phenotypically immature cell forms, confirms this hypothesis. The data presented in this study open a new trend in investigation of cellular mechanisms of shaping in structural organization in the postembryonic fishes brain and in examination of morpho-functional manifestations concerning histogenetic processes in different periods of postembrionic ontogenesis. The new priority data received are connected with development of nervous tissue in the pacific salmon brain and with dynamic of the brain shaping and distribution of classical neurotransmitters and gaseous mediators in a context of incessant postembryonic neurogenesis.

Acknowledgements

This work was supported by the Grant of Far Eastern Branch of Russian Academy of Sciences № 12-III-A-06-095.

Author details

E.V. Pushchina[1*], A.A. Varaksin[1] and D.K. Obukhov[2]

*Address all correspondence to: puschina@mail.ru

1 A. V. Zhirmunski Institute of Marine Biology, Far East Division, Russian Academy of Sciences, St. Petersburg, Russia

2 St. Petersburg State University, St. Petersburg, Russia

References

[1] Villani L., Guarnieri T. Localization of NADPH-diaphorase in the Goldfish Brain. Brain Res. 1995; 679(2) 261-266.

[2] Anken R.H., Rahmann H. An Atlas of the Distribution of NADPH-diaphorase in the Brain of the Highly Derived Swordtail Fish Xiphophorus Helleri (Atherinoformes: Teleostei). J Hirnforsch. 1996; 37(3) 421-49.

[3] Villani L. Development of NADPH-diaphorase activity in the Central Nervous System of the Cichlid Fish Tilapia Mariae. Brain Behav. Evol. 1999; 54(3) 147-58

[4] Arévalo R., Alonso J.R., García-Ojeda E., Briñón J.G., Crespo C., Aijón J. NADPH-diaphorase in the Central Nervous System of the Tench (Tinca tinca L., 1758). J. Comp. Neurol. 1995; 352(3) 398-420.

[5] Bordieri L., Persichini T., Venturini G., Cioni C. Expression of Nitric Oxide Synthase in the Preoptic-Hypothalamo-Hypophyseal System of the Teleost Oreochromis Niloticus. Brain Behav. Evol. 2003; 62(1) 43-55.

[6] Ugrumov M.V. Developing Brain as an Endocrine Organ: a Paradoxical Reality. Neurochem. Res. 2010; 35(6) 837-850.

[7] Zupanc G.K. Towards Brain Repair: Insights From Teleost Fish. Semin Cell Dev Biol. 2009; 20 (6) 683-690.

[8] Zupanc G.K. Neurogenesis, Cell Death and Regeneration in the Adult Gymnotiform Brain. J. Exp. Biol. 1999; 202 (Pt 10) 1435-1446.

[9] Grandel H., Kaslin J., Ganz J., Wenzel I., Brand M. Neural Stem Cells and Neurogenesis in the Adult Zebrafish Brain: Origin, Proliferation Dynamics, Migration and Cell Fate. Dev. Biol. 2006; 295(1) 263-277.

[10] Kaslin J., Ganz J., Brand M. Proliferation, Neurogenesis and Regeneration in the Non-mammalian Vertebrate Brain. Phil. Trans. R. Soc. B. 2008; 363(1489) 101-122.

[11] Zupanc G.K. Neurogenesis and neuronal regeneration in the adult fish brain. J. Comp. Physiol. A Neuroethol. Sens. Neural Behav. Physiol. 2006; 192(6) 649-670.

[12] Dorofeeva E.A. Modern Controversial Issues in Systematics of Salmon. Modern problems of systematics of fishes. Ed. by A.V. Balushkin, O.S. Voskoboynikova. SPb., 1998.

[13] Artyukhin E.N. Sturgeons (Ecology, Geographic Distribution and Phylogeny). SPb.: Izd-vo SPbGU. 2008.

[14] Hope B.T., Vincent S.R. Histochemical characterization of neuronal NADPH-diaphorase. J. Histochem. Cytochem. 1989; 37(5) 653-661.

[15] Merkulov G.A. Course Pathologohistological Technology. HP: Medicine. 1969. 423 C.

[16] Kapsimali M., Vidal B., Gonzalez A., Dufour S., Vernier P. Distribution of the mRNA Encoding the Four Dopamine D(1), Receptor Subtypes in the Brain of the European Eel (Anguilla Anguilla): Comparative Approach to the Function of D(1), Receptors in Vertebrates. J. Comp. Neurol. 2000; 419(3) 320-343.

[17] Trudeau V.L. Neuroendocrine Regulation of Gonadotropin II Release and Gonadal Growth in the Goldfish, Carassius auratus. Rev. Reprod. 1997; 2(1) 55-68.

[18] Northcutt R.G. Forebrain Evolution in Bony Fishes. Br. Res. Bull. 2008; 75 (2-4) 191-205.

[19] Puschina E.V. Neurochemical Organization and Connections of the Cerebral Preglomerular Complex of the Masu Salmon. Neurophysiology. 2012; 43(6) 437-451.

[20] Vernier P., Wullimann M.F. Evolution of the Posterior Tuberculum and Preglomerular Nuclear Complex. Encyclopedia of Neurosciences. Part 5. Eds. M.D. Binder, N. Hirokawa, U. Windhorst. Berlin: Springer-Verlag. 2009.

[21] Mueller T., Guo S. The Distribution of GAD67-mRNA in the Adult Zebrafish (teleost) Forebrain Reveals a Prosomeric Pattern and Suggests Previously Unidentified Homologies to Tetrapods. J. Comp. Neurol. 2009; 516(6) 553-568.

[22] Horsberg T.E. Avermectin use in Aquaculture. Curr. Pharm. Biotechnol. 2012; 13(6) 1095-1102.

[23] Noctor S.C., Martínez-Cerdeño V., Ivic L., Kriegstein A.R. Cortical Neurons Arise in Symmetric and Asymmetric Division Zones and Migrate through Specific Phases. Nat. Neurosci. 2004; 7(2) 136-44.

[24] Hebsgaard J.B., Nelander J., Sabelström H., Jönsson M.E., Stott S., Parmar M. Dopamine Neuron Precursors within the Deveoping Human Mesencephalon Show Radial Glial Characteristics. Glia. 2009; 57(15) 1648-1658.

[25] Rodríguez Díaz M.A., Candal E., Santos-Durán G.N., Adrio F., Rodríguez-Moldes I. Comparative analysis of Met-enkephalin, galanin and GABA immunoreactivity in the developing trout preoptic-hypophyseal system. Gen. Comp. Endocrinol. 2011. 173(1) 148-158.

[26] Isaeva V.V., Puschina E.V., Karetin Yu.A. Changes of the Morphometric Indices and Fractal Dimension of the Spinal Cord Neurons During Ontogenesis of the Cherry Salmon Oncorhynchus Masou. Rus. Journal of Marine Biology. 2006; 32(2) 106-114

[27] Pushchina E.V., Obukhov D.K. Varaksin A.A. Features of Adult Neurogenesis and Neurochemical Signaling in the Cherry Salmon Oncorhynchus masou Brain. Neural Regen. Res. 2013; 8(1) 13-23.

[28] Meek J. Catecholamines in the Brains of Osteichtyes (Bony Fishes). Phylogeny and Development of Catecholamine Systems in the CNS of Vertebrates. Cambridge: Cambrifge Univ. Press. 1994.

[29] Yamamoto K., Vernier P. The Evolution of Dopamine Systems in Chordates. Front. Neuroanat. 2011; 5 1-21. doi: 10.3389/fnana.2011.00021

[30] Pushchina E.V. Tyrosine Hydroxylase in Telencephalon and Diencephalon of Rhodeus sericeus (Cyprinidae). Tsitologiia. 2009; 51(1) 63-77.

[31] Rink E., Wullimann M.F. The Teleostean (Zebrafish) Dopaminergic System Ascending to the Subpallium (Striatum) is Located in the Basal Diencephalon (Posterior Tuberculum). Brain Res. 2001; 889(1-2) 316-330.

[32] Smeets W.J., González A. Catecholamine Systems in the Brain of Vertebrates: New Perspectives through a Comparative Approach. Brain Res. Brain Res. Rev. 2000; 33 (2-3) 308-379.

[33] Wullimann M.F. The Central Nervous System. The Physiology of Fishes. Boca Raton. New-York: CRS Press. 1998.

[34] Kiss J. P. Role of Nitric Oxide in the Regulation of Monoaminergic Neurotransmition. Brain Res. Bull. 2000; 52(6) 459-466.

[35] Boldyrev A.A., Yeshchenko N.D., Ilukha V.A. Neurochemistry. M: Drofa. 2010.

[36] Kimura H. Hydrogen Sulfide Induces Cyclic AMP and Modulates the NMDA Receptor. Biochem. Biophys. Res. Commun. 2000; 267(1) 129-133.

[37] Diaz J., Ridray S., Mignon V., Griffon N., Schwartz J.C., Sokoloff P. Selective Expression of Dopamine D3 Receptor mRNA in Proliferative Zones During Embryonic Development of the Rat Brain. J. Neurosci. 1997; 17(11) 4282-4292.

[38] Han Y., Qin J., Chang X., Yang Z., Bu D., Du J. Modulating Effect of Hydrogen Sulfide on Gamma-aminobutyric Acid B Receptor in Recurrent Febrile Seizures in Rats. Neurosci. Res. 2005; 53 (2) 216-219.

[39] Grillner S. Motor Control Systems of Fish. Encyclopediya of Fish Fisiology from Genom to Environment. Ed.-in-Chi. Farrel A.P. Elsevier: Academic Press: 2011; 56-65.

[40] Braun K., Scheich H., Schachner M. et al. Distribution of Parvalbumin, Cytochrome Oxidase Activity and 14C-2-deoxyglucose Up-take in the Brain of the Zebra Finch. I. Auditory and Vocal Motor Systems. Cell Tissue Res. 1985; 240(2) 101-115.

[41] Dedman J.R., Kaetzel M.A. Calcium as an Intracellular Second Messenger: Mediation by Calcium Binding Proteins. Cell Physiology Source Book. Academic Press: London. 1995.

[42] Lee S.W., Hu Y.S., Hu L.F., Lu Q., Dawe G.S., Moore P.K., Wong P.T., Bian J.S. Hydrogen Sulphide Regulates Calcium Homeostasis in Microglial Cells. Glia. 2006; 54(2) 116-124.

[43] Korn H., Faber D.S., Triller A. Convergence of Morphological, Physiological, and Immunocytochemical Techniques for the Study of Single Mauthner Cells. Handbook of

Chemical Neuroanatomy. Eds. A. Björklund, T. Hökfelt, F.G. Wouterlood, A. N. van der Pol. Amsterdam: Elsevier. 1990.

[44] Brüning G., Katzbach R., Mayer B. Histochemical and Immunocytochemical Localization of Nitric Oxide Synthase in the Central Nervous System of the Goldfish, Carassius auratus. J. Comp. Neurol. 1995; 358(3) 353-382.

[45] Giraldez-Perez R.M., Gaytan S.P., Ruano D., Torres B., Pasaro R. Distribution of NADPH-diaphorase and Nitric Oxide Synthase Reactivity in the Central Nervous System of the Goldfish (Carassius Auratus). J Chem Neuroanat. 2008; 35(1) 12-32.

[46] Pushchina E.V., Varaksin A.A. Argyrophilic and Nitric Oxidergic Bipolar Neurons in Cerebellum of the Opisthocentrus Pholidapus dybowskii. J. Evol. Biochem. Physiol. 2001; 37(5) 569-575.

[47] Ikenaga T., Yoshida M., Uematsu K. Cerebellar Efferent Neurons in Teleost Fish. Cerebellum. 2006; 5(4) 268-274.

[48] Ma P.K. Catecholaminergic Systems in the Zebrafish. III. Organization and Projection Pattern of Medullary Dopaminergic and Noradrenergic Neurons. J. Comp. Neurol. 1997; 381(4) 411-427.

[49] Wulliman M.F., Puelles L. Postembryonic Neural Proliferation in the Zebrafish Forebrain and its Relationship to Prosomeric Domains. Anat. Embryol. (Berl). 1999; 199(4) 329-348.

[50] Platel J.C., Stamboulian S., Nguyen I., Bordey A. Neurotransmitter Signaling in Postnatal Neurogenesis: the First Leg. Brain Res. Rev. 2010; 63(1-2) 60-71.

[51] Moreno-López B., Noval J.A., González-Bonet L.G., Estrada C. Morphological Bases for a Role of Nitric Oxide in Adult Neurogenesis. Brain Res. 2000; 869(1-2) 244-250.

[52] Romero-Grimaldi C., Moreno-López B., Estrada C. Age-dependent Effect of Nitric Oxide on Subventricular Zone and Olfactory Bulb Neural Precursor Proliferation. J. Comp. Neurol. 2008; 506(2) 339-346.

[53] Islam A.T., Kuraoka A., Kawabuchi M. Morphological Basis of Nitric Oxide Production and its Correlation with the Polysialylated Precursor Cells in the Dentate Gyrus of the Adult Guinea Pig Hippocampus. Anat. Sci. Int. 2003; 78(2) 98-103.

[54] Extröm P., Johnsson C.M., Ohlin L.M. Ventricular Proliferation Zones in the Brain of an Adult Teleost Fish and Their Relation to Neuromeres and Migration (Secondary Matrix) Zones. J. Comp. Neurol. 2001; 436(1) 92-110.

[55] Zhou L., Zhu D.Y. Neuronal Nitric Oxide Synthase: Structure, Subcellular Localization, Regulation, and Clinical Implications. Nitric Oxide. 2009; 20(4) 223-230.

[56] Brandstätter R., Kotrschal K. Brain Growth Patterns in Four European Cyprinid Fish Species (Cyprinidae, Teleostei): Roach (Rutilus Rutilus), Bream (Abramis brama),

Common Carp (Cyprinus Carpio) and Sabre Carp (Pelecus Cultratus). Brain Behav. Evol. 1990; 35(1) 195-211.

[57] Marcus R.C., Delaney C.L., Easter S.S. Neurogenesis in the Visual System of Embryonic and Adult Zebrafish (Danio Rerio) off. Vis. Neurosci. 1999; 16(3) 417-424.

[58] Rakic P. Elusive Radial Glial Cells: Historical and Evolutionary Perspective. Glia. 2003; 43(1) 19-32.

[59] Song H., Kempermann G., Overstreet Wadiche L., Zhao C., Schinder A.F., Bischofberger J. New Neurons in the Adult Mammalian Brain: Synaptogenesis and Functional Integration. J. Neurosci. 2005; 25(45) 10366-10368.

[60] Lledo P.M., Alonso M., Grubb M.S. Adult Neurogenesis and Functional Plasticity in Neuronal Circuits. Nat. Rev. Neurosci. 2006; 7(3) 179-193.

Chapter 9

Physiological Role of Amyloid Beta in Neural Cells: The Cellular Trophic Activity

M. del C. Cárdenas-Aguayo, M. del C. Silva-Lucero,
M. Cortes-Ortiz, B. Jiménez-Ramos,
L. Gómez-Virgilio, G. Ramírez-Rodríguez,
E. Vera-Arroyo, R. Fiorentino-Pérez, U. García,
J. Luna-Muñoz and M.A. Meraz-Ríos

Additional information is available at the end of the chapter

http://dx.doi.org/10.5772/57398

1. Introduction

Amyloid is a term for the build-up of protein deposits or plaques in the body. Thus amyloid are extracellular insoluble fibrous protein aggregates. One characteristic is that these fibrils acquire β-sheet structure. Therefore the structure of the proteins that form deposits is altered and often exhibits inappropriate folding. The misfolded proteins, interact with each other and with other proteins, forming aggregates and the accumulation of these amyloid fibrils in particular organs is call amyloidosis, which is characteristic of several pathologies, including neurodegenerative diseases, such as Alzheimer's Disease (AD), transmissible spongiform encephalopathies, type II diabetes, familial amyloidoses and other variants of systemic amyloidoses [1].

2. APP processing

There are two pathways (Figure 1) for processing amyloid precursor protein (APP): An amyloidogenic pathway and a non-amyloidogenic, constitutive secretory pathway. Different APP fragments are generated after secretase cleavage.

In the non-amyloidogenic pathway, part of the extracellular domain of APP is cleaved by the α-secretases, that belong to the disintegrin and metalloproteinase (ADAM, including ADAM9,

ADM10 and ADAM17, also known as TACE), releasing a soluble extracellular fragment know as sAPP-α, that has neurotrophic and neuroprotective functions [2, 3]. Then γ-secretase [4, 5] that is present at the plasma membrane, can generate an intracellular APP fragment that is known as APP intracellular C-terminal domain (AICD) [6]. In the amyloidogenic pathway, APP is cleaved by β-secretase (BACE1) [7, 8] at its extracellular domain, giving rise to two fragments; sAPP-β (N-terminal fragment) and CT99 or CT89. Then CT99 could be cleaved by the γ-secretase complex (including Nicastrin, Anterior Pharynx defective 1, Presenilin enhancer 2, Presenilin 1 and or Presenilin 2) within the plasma membrane. These two cleavages (β-secretase and γ-secretase cleavages) generate Amyloid beta (Aβ) and more AICD fragment. The length of the AICD fragment could vary due to heterogeneous γ-secretase cleavage, and subsequent ε-secretase and ζ-secretase activity. AICD has physiological and pathological actions, particularly in signaling from the membrane to the nucleus through epigenetic modulation of gene expression [9]. Moreover inside the cell, AICD fragment can undergo more processing by caspases giving rise to a fragment called CT31, which is a potent inducer of apoptosis [10].

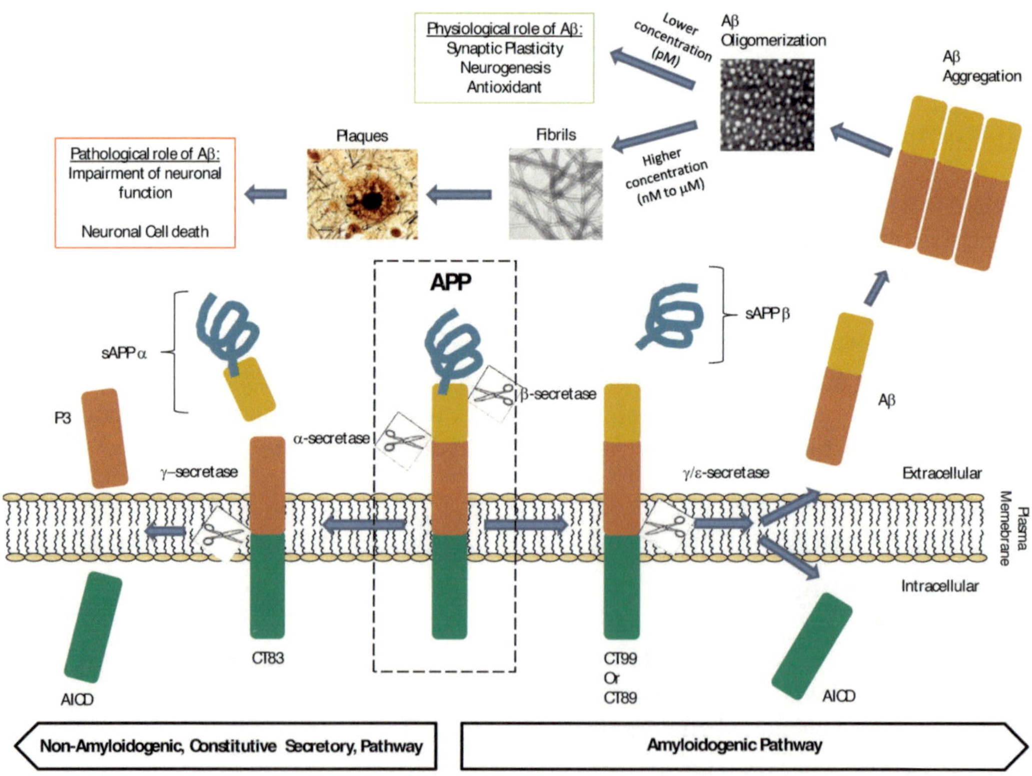

Figure 1. APP processing.

3. Amyloid Beta

Amyloid Beta (Aβ) is a peptide generated by the amyloidogenic pathway of APP processing [11]. As we mentioned before, initially APP, a transmembrane protein, is cleaved by α- or β-secretases (Figure 1), generating large, soluble, secreted fragments (sAPPα and sAPPβ) and membrane associated carboxy-terminal fragments (CTFs). Aβ peptides could vary in size, from 38 to 43 aminoacids, being the predominant isoforms the Aβ 1-40, 90%, and the more fibrilogenic Aβ 1-42, 10% and they are generated after β-secretase (also known as BACE1, β-site APP cleaving enzyme) cleavage, followed by γ-secretase cleavage [12]. Aβ peptide has the ability of auto-aggregate, so it could exist as monomers, dimers or oligomers; which in turn can generate fibrils, that have β-sheet structure, and could deposit to form extracellular plaques (neuritic plaques) [13].

As we mentioned above, the amyloidosis is a condition in which normally soluble proteins become insoluble and are deposited in the extracellular space of various tissues. The extracellular deposits of Aβ are characteristic of several neurological conditions including: Alzheimer's Disease [14], Down's syndrome [15], brain traumatic injuries [16], and ageing [17]. Particularly Aβ is the predominant protein in the plaques, which are one of the principal histological hallmarks of Alzheimer's disease brains. Alzheimer's disease is the most common cause of dementia among older people, and is characterized by a progressive cognitive decline and loss of memory and the inability to perform common tasks.

4. Physiologycal role of Aβ

Although Aβ peptides are produced at high amounts in pathological conditions, they are also present in low levels in normal brains, particularly during synaptic activity. For many years it has not been clear the role of APP and Aβ in non-pathological conditions, and it was thought that Aβ was an incidental product of the catabolism of APP without a physiological role (Figure 2). APP is an integral membrane protein with high affinity to copper, ubiquitously expressed and it has been reported that APP is involved in neurodevelopment and is required for neuronal growth [18]. APP also participates in synaptogenesis [19] and cell adhesion. Moreover, anti-APP antibodies block memory formation [20].

At high concentrations (nanomolar to micromolar) Aβ causes neurotoxicity and cell death [21]. However, it has been proposed that low concentrations (picomolar) of Aβ could act as trophic signal [22] and as modulator of synaptic activity, with implications in memory and learning. In addition, picomolar levels of Aβ had been determined in interstitial fluid of normal brain by microdialysis [23]. According to Cirrito and colleagues, the Aβ peptide levels in the brain are dynamically and directly influenced by synaptic activity. Furthermore, low amounts of Aβ, could work as antioxidants, due to its ability to capture redox metals, such as Cu, Fe and Zn, and thus, preventing their participation in redox cycling with other ligands [24]; hence Aβ has the ability to function as a chelator and antioxidant molecule.

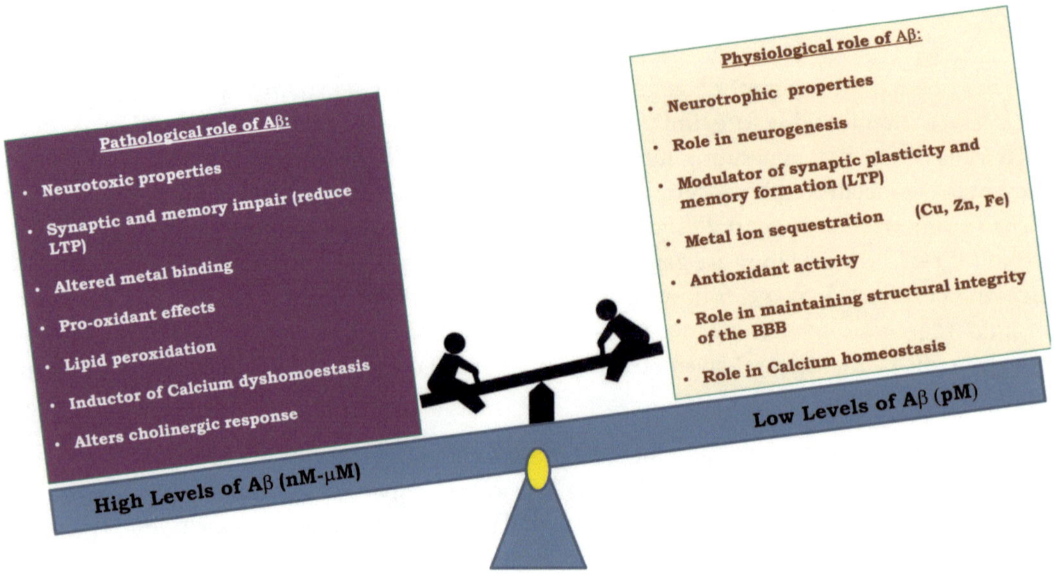

Figure 2. Balance between physiological and pathological effects of Aβ. Like a seesaw in a park, the levels of Aβ change due to environmental factors or genetic background. In normal healthy conditions, Aβ is at lower concentration (pM), and exerts its physiological functions, but in disease conditions the levels of Aβ are elevated (nM to μM) and it switches it functions to pathological effects.

Aβ has been extensively studied due to its association with neuritic plaques in AD brains [25]. However, in non-pathological conditions the existence of Aβ has also been reported. Considering it, many attempts have been addressed to find the physiological function of Aβ in the brain, particularly its role in synaptic plasticity and neuronal survival. The physiological levels of Aβ are essential for synaptic plasticity in normal individuals [26]. Taking into account the positive- or negative- effects of Aβ, it is proposed that the peptide exhibits dual effects: neurotrophic or neurotoxic. These effects may be attributed to different aspects such as its relative concentration, the cellular environment and is also related to the age of the individuals. The low physiological concentrations of Aβ could play a key role for regulating synaptic plasticity and improve cognitive functions, whereas the accumulation of high concentrations of Aβ, coupled with the effects of age, causes dysregulation and loss of synaptic function, as shown in the AD [27].

The functional properties of the Aβ have not been completely elucidated; however numerous studies have suggested that the peptide possesses neurotrophic properties [22, 28]. Recently it was suggested that soluble Aβ plays important roles in the facilitation of neuronal growth, cellular survival, in the modulation of synaptic function and defense against oxidative stress. Also, the physiological concentrations of Aβ favor the learning and memory processes [29]. In addition, it has been suggested that monomers of Aβ40, which is the most abundant species found in the brain, could function as antioxidant natural molecule by preventing the neuronal death caused by metal-induced oxidative damage.

Also, it is known that low picomolar concentrations of a preparation containing both monomers and oligomers of $A\beta_{42}$ cause a marked increase of hippocampal long-term potentiation (LTP), whereas high nanomolar concentrations lead to the well-established reduction of potentiation. The picomolar levels of $A\beta_{42}$ also produce a pronounced enhancement of both reference and contextual fear memory.

Thus, these findings here described strongly support a duality for Aβ effects in which low concentrations play a novel positive role on neurotransmission and memory, whereas high concentrations produce the well-known detrimental effect culminating in dementia [30].

5. APP and Aβ as modulators of synaptic activity

APP levels increase during synaptogenesis suggesting its role in neuronal communication [9]. There are evidences that suggest that APP interacts with the calcium sensor of synaptic vesicles possibly regulating synaptic vesicle exocytosis, and calcium homeostasis [31, 32]. The role of APP in learning and memory has been evidenced by studies showing that regulation of its levels of expression can modulate synaptic spine density, an effect that is mediated by its soluble α-cleaved fragment sAPPα [33, 34]. APP is also essential for the synapses and required for spatial learning and long-term potentiation (LTP, which correlate with memory formation) [35]. Moreover, APP participates in axonal outgrowth and restoration of neuronal functions [36, 37].

Although it is thought that Aβ impairs synaptic plasticity, it mostly depends on its concentration. High levels of Aβ have been found to markedly reduce long-term potentiation (LTP) [38], as we mentioned before, this is the type of synaptic plasticity that correlates with learning and memory, therefore, causing memory loss [25, 39, 40]. However, Aβ peptides are not only present in elevated amounts; they are also present in low levels throughout life, suggesting a possible physiological role of Aβ in normal healthy individuals [41, 42]. Recently it has been suggested that Aβ levels are likely to be regulated by synaptic activity in an endocytosis dependent manner depressing synaptic function [43, 44]. The group of Ottavio Arancio demonstrated first that low picomolar amounts of exogenous applied $A\beta_{42}$ enhance synaptic plasticity and memory [30], and second, that endogenously produced Aβ is critical for normal synaptic plasticity and memory [41]. For these latest experiments, this group used wild type mice, in which endogenous Aβ function was blocked by utilization of rodent-specific monoclonal antibody (JRF/rAb2) and by blocking the production of Aβ with the use of siRNA against APP. They concluded that endogenous Aβ is required for synaptic plasticity and memory, and that this effect is mediated via α7-nAChRs [41].

Cirrito and colleagues found that synaptic activity rapidly and dynamically regulates ISF (Interstitial fluid) Aβ levels *in vitro* in an acute brain slice model. Accordingly, the relationship between synaptic activity and extracellular Aβ levels appears to be related to synaptic vesicle release: Thus extracellular Aβ levels are increased when synaptic vesicles undergo exocytosis, even in the absence of neuronal activity. This data suggest that the rapid effects of synaptic activity on Aβ are mediated at the presynaptic side of the synaptic cleft [44].

6. Antioxidant role of Aβ

Aβ belongs to a group of proteins (metalloproteins) that capture redox metal ions (even under mildly acidotic conditions), thus preventing them from participating in redox cycling with other ligands [45, 46]. It has the ability to bind Cu, Fe and Zn [47].

Although the product of Aβ's oxidant activity is the hydrogen peroxide (H_2O_2), that is likely to mediate toxicity as the levels of oxidant rise with the increased accumulation of Aβ in the AD brain, the excessive removal of Aβ is not beneficial, since the absence of Aβ may prevent adequate chelation of metal ions and appropriate removal of O_2^- leading to an enhanced rather than a reduced neuronal oxidative stress, and this has to be taken in account when designing therapeutic strategies that use drugs that lower Aβ levels. Oxidative stress promotes Aβ generation, and in these conditions, the formation of amyloid plaques could be a compensatory response to remove reactive oxygen species [24].

One of the pathological early events that occur in the brains of AD affected individuals is the oxidative damage [48]. And also both Amyloid deposits (Plaques) and neurofribillar tangles accumulate oxidative modifications over time.

Aβ has two major sites that are important for its redox activity. The first site involves the binding of redox active Cu or Fe to human AB_{40} and AB_{42} via histidine residues that directly produce H_2O_2 by a mechanism that involves the reduction of these metal ions [49-51]. The second site is a Methionine at position 35 in the lipophilic C-terminal region [49]. The interaction of metal ions by Aβ is crucial for the redox activity and neurotoxicity of the peptide.

Several studies had evidenced the antioxidant properties of Aβ. Kontush and colleagues [52], showed Aβ prevents lipoprotein oxidation in CSF and Zou and colleagues [53], showed that monomeric $Aβ_{40}$ inhibits the reduction of Fe(III) induced by vitamin C and the generation of O_2^-. Moreover, the increased production of Aβ in mutant PS1 fibroblasts is accompanied by a decrease in the production of ROS (reactive oxygen species), particularly .OH formation [54]. Furthermore, the increased production of Aβ induced by the over-expression of wild type PS1 in brains of transgenic mice resulted in increased brain resistance to metal-induced oxidation [55]. Conversely, primary hippocampal neurons from PS1M146V mutant knock-in mice, exhibit increased superoxide production when treated with Aβ [56]. In addition to its cellular protective role, physiological concentrations of $Aβ_{40}$ and $Aβ_{42}$ have been shown to protect lipoproteins from oxidation in cerebrospinal fluid and plasma [52]. Taken together the results discussed in this section, we can conclude that Aβ can function as an antioxidant in normal neurons and many other cells, such as astrocytes, neuroblastoma cells, hepatoma cells, fibroblasts and platelets [24]. Besides, its intracellular functions, Aβ could have a metal ion binding/antioxidant role extracellularly in diffuse amyloid deposits, CSF and plasma. In this context, the release of Aβ in response to injury or disease appears to be purposive, by providing neuroprotection against oxidative stress, after which Aβ is cleared. If the clearance is insufficient (e.g. decreased neprolysin, insulin degrading enzyme or the presence of Apo e4 allele) to compensate the excessive production of Aβ, the progressive accumulation of Aβ:Cu in response to oxidative stress or in response to mutations of APP/PS1 that induce amyloidogenesis, may lead to the generation of H_2O_2 that exceeds the capacity of the antioxidant defense systems, further exacerbating amyloid deposition and ROS production. Thus the Aβ may not be directly toxic but the indirect generation of H_2O_2 [50] could be responsible for the oxidative damage and the neuronal dysfunction [24].

7. Aβ and neurogenesis

Current experiments in our laboratory have suggested that low concentrations of Aβ oligomers showed neurogenic effects on adult hippocampal neural stem/precursor cells (NSPCs). Currently, we are evaluating the effects of these peptides on the neuronal development *in vitro* and *in vivo* to better understand its role for the generation of new neurons under physiological conditions, based on previous work that points the trophic effect of Aβ peptides on NSPCs [57].

NSPCs are undifferentiated cells that originated from the neuroepithelium and are able to generate all cell types of the CNS (Central Nervous System): neurons and glial (hippocampus) in which neurogenesis occur during the adulthood [58]. NSPCs are of particular therapeutic interest, due to its pluripotentiality and plasticity. The idea of using NSPCs in cell therapy opens the possibility to replace damaged neuronal cells during neurodegeneration. Alternatively, the resident NSPCs in the brain could be activated and induce to differentiate through the use of growth factors, which are key regulators of the survival, proliferation and differentiation of these pluripotent cells. Trophic factors promote neuronal survival mainly through the PI3K/Akt proteins. The phospho-Akt phosphorylates and inhibits glycogen synthase kinase 3β (GSK-3β), which is one of the kinases that phosphorylates tau protein. There is evidence that suggests that this PI3K/Akt/GSK-3β signaling pathway is directly impacted by Aβ and it is altered in AD [59]. Trophic factors such as Neurotrophins (for example NGF, BDNF), IGF-1, GDNF, and hormones (insulin), are critical for neuronal survival and plasticity. Accumulations of Aβ can alter growth factor signaling and induce changes in trophic factors and its receptor (TrkA, TrkB, p75NTR, IGF-1R, Insulin receptor) expression and distribution which are characteristic of neurodegeneration [60].

a. Neurogenesis in the adult brain

Neurogenesis is a process that maintains dynamic proliferation, migration and maturation of new neurons in the adult brain and contrary to what was thought about the static nature of the brain, it has been demonstrated that the encephalon is able to generate new neurons that can be integrated into existing neural circuits. This process is finely modulated and responds to intrinsic and extrinsic factors [61-66] (Figure 3).

The formation of new neurons occurs constitutively in two well-characterized brain regions: the subventricular zone-olfactory bulb system (SVZ/OB) and the dentate gyrus (DG) of the hippocampus [65, 67-70]. However, reactive neurogenesis has also been reported in other brain regions after damage caused by harmful agents.

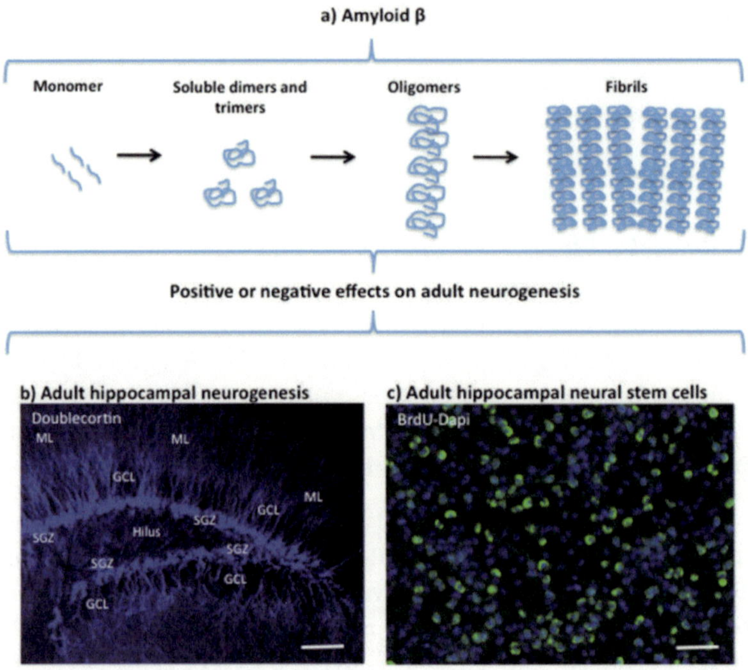

Figure 3. Role of amyloid-β in adult neurogenesis. a) Schematic cartoon indicating the different forms of Aβ (monomer, soluble dimmers and trimers, oligomers and fibrils). b) Representative picture of coronal section showing the hippocampus and stained for doublecortin (blue), a key marker for adult hippocampal neurogenesis. Doublecortin-cells line the subgranular zone (SGZ) and immature neurons migrate to the granular cell layer (GCL) to project dendrites to the molecular layer (ML). The picture also shows the hilus. Scale bar = 60 μm. c) Representative picture of proliferative adult hippocampal neural stem cells. Proliferative cells are identified by the BrdU-incorporation (green). The nuclei were stained with Dapi (blue). Scale bar = 50 μm.

Interestingly, constitutive adult neurogenic brain areas contain resident neural stem/progenitor cells (NSPCs), which have great potential for self-renewal and show multipotency [68, 71]. In the SVZ/OB system the resident stem cells located at the SVZ divide to form neuroblasts, a cellular population that migrates through the rostral migratory path to reach the OB, a place in which the immature cells become fully mature neurons [68]. A similar process occurs in the SGZ of the dentate gyrus in the hippocampus, a place in which the neural stem cells divide to form neuroblasts which will migrate a short distance into the granule cell layer to finally differentiate into hippocampal granular cells [63, 71] (Figure 3).

The fact that the stem cells of the SVZ and DG exist, makes possible their isolation to perform studies in a well-controlled cellular platform, thus many possibilities have opened to address relevant questions about the possible mechanism by which Aβ acts in a positive- or negative-manner on the neurogenic process.

b. Physiological role of Aβ in neurogenesis

Recent studies have shown that Aβ may be vital for neuronal development, plasticity, and survival due to its integral membrane interactions. Also, neuronal viability appears to be dependent on the Aβ, a peptide that possess neurogenic properties [22]. Thus, several studies have addressed the effects of Aβ on the different events of the neurogenic process using NSPCs [57, 72, 73].

Despite the controversy about the effects of the Aβ, it is known that $A\beta_{42}$ increased the differentiation of embryonic NSPCs, an effect that was not the result of changes at the level of cell proliferation. Interestingly, this effect was only seen with soluble oligomeric forms of the $A\beta_{42}$ peptide but not with the monomeric form of $A\beta_{42}$ or with $A\beta_{40}$ or $A\beta_{25-35}$ [57]. In a similar way, but in developing neurons, Aβ induced survival and protected mature neurons against excitotoxic cell death [74]. The Aβ peptide exerts a neurotrophic role when low concentrations of the peptide are added to undifferentiated hippocampal neurons [75]. In addition, the $A\beta_{40}$ and $A\beta_{42}$ isoforms stimulate proliferation of primary neural progenitor cells isolated from rat E18 cerebral cortices [73]. Concomitant to the increase in cell proliferation, $A\beta_{40}$ induces the neuronal differentiation, whereas Aβ drives glial differentiation of neural progenitor cells into neurons [73].

In adult NSPCs derived from the SVZ, Chaejeong and collaborators [72], conducted a study with $A\beta_{42}$ peptide. In this study the three aggregated forms: monomeric, oligomeric and fibrillar, were used to evaluate their effects on the cellular proliferation and differentiation. According to the degree of aggregation or concentration of the peptides, it was found that micromolar concentrations (1 μmol/L) of the oligomeric form of $A\beta_{42}$ remarkably increase adult SVZ NSPCs. The peptide also enhances neuronal differentiation and the ability of these cells to migrate. In a similar way, recently it was reported that Aβ increases NSPCs activity in senes cence- accelerated SAMP8 mice. In the same report, but using in vitro cultures of SVZ-NSPCs, it was confirmed that Aβ promotes cell proliferation partially through a cell autonomous mechanism, in which soluble $A\beta_{42}$ exerts autocrine and paracrine effects on NSPCs.

Furthermore, the mechanisms that explain the beneficial effects of $A\beta_{42}$ have been elucidated and involved the participation of key proteins for the PI3K-Akt pathway [76]. Also, $A\beta_{42}$ acts through the p75 neurotrophin receptor to stimulate neurogenesis in the SVZ in adult mice [77]. However, it remains to be determined whether the p75 receptor is involved in neurotrophic or in the neuroprotective effects of $A\beta_{42}$. Oligomeric forms of Aβ also increase neuronal differentiation of NSPCs, acting through tyrosin kinases and MEK, but not through PI3K [57]. Although, some mechanisms have been explored, the way by which Aβ peptide targets a signal to neurogenesis remains an open question.

In addition, the physiological significance of the early increase in cell proliferation caused by Aβ is still a matter of investigation in hippocampal NSPCs models because it has been proposed that this effect causes the cessation of the new neuron formation [78]. However, it is important to consider that during aging there are also changes in the brain- and systemic- milieu, thus the decrease in the levels of neurotrophins and growth factors may also impact the neurogenic process as was previously reported [79]. Interestingly, studies performed in animal models of AD have shown that the exposure to an environmental enrichment paradigm that is capable to increase the levels of neurotrophins and growth factors, promotes the decrease in the levels of Aβ peptides and favors the neurogenic process in the hippocampus [80]. Altogether, these evidences suggest that physiological concentrations of Aβ may be relevant for promoting or maybe to maintain adult neurogenesis. However, the direct impact of Aβ in the adult hippocampus and in hippocampal NSPCs needs to be investigated to get a full picture of Aβ roles in and during neuronal development (Figure 3).

8. Role of Aβ in maintaining the structural integrity of the blood brain barrier (BBB)

Interestingly, another Aβ trophic effect is due to its sealant properties that according to Atwood and colleagues, allows it to maintain the structural integrity of the blood brain barrier (BBB), and parenchymal structures during physiological and stress conditions [81]. In search for a therapeutic approach, the removal of Aβ (by vaccination) has been proposed, but accumulated evidence shows that low levels of Aβ had a role in maintaining the cellular homeostasis, thus complete removal of Aβ would have negative side effects. For example, Aβ could act as a sealant to maintain the integrity of the BBB, so its removal could cause leakage of serum components into the brain, resulting in an immune or autoimmune response characterized by inflammation and as a consequence it could cause also mini-strokes. In fact some clinical trials of Aβ immunization had to be halted, due to the development of encephalitis and meningitis in some patients under investigation [82].

9. Effects of high cholesterol diet on APP processing

Cholesterol is the main sterol in animal tissues, and has very important functions, as being a major component of eukaryotic membranes, and function as a biosynthetic precursor of important bioactive molecules such as steroid hormones and bile acids [83]. And also it has been shown that cholesterol can directly modulate the processing of APP [84, 85]. The main sources of cholesterol are the dietary intake and endogenous hepatic biosynthesis. Cholesterol levels and the cellular distribution of cholesterol have a major influence on amyloidogenesis [86]. The amyloidogenic processing of APP occurs in the lipid rafts (small membrane-adjacent heterogeneous domains, enriched in steroids and sphingolipids, with a role in multiple cellular processes). The β- and γ- secretases that (as mentioned before, Figure 1) participate in the amyloidogenic pathway, are located at the surface of these cholesterol-enriched regions. Accordingly, it has been reported that, increased cholesterol levels enhance β and γ- secretase activity therefore, promoting APP metabolism by the amyloidogenic pathway. Conversely a decrease in intracellular cholesterol, leads to structural rupture of the lipid rafts, favoring α-secretase non-amyloidogenic APP cleavage, leading to a significant decrease in Aβ levels [83].

Cholesterol also plays an important role in atheroesclerosis as a major component of atheroma plaques. Hypercholesterolemia is associated with the formation of atheroma plaques that progressively could cause ischemic brain damage. Brain ischemia induce an increase in APP expression, and damages the BBB [83], and as a result the clearance of cerebral Aβ is affected (Figure 4).

http://dx.doi.org/10.5772/57398

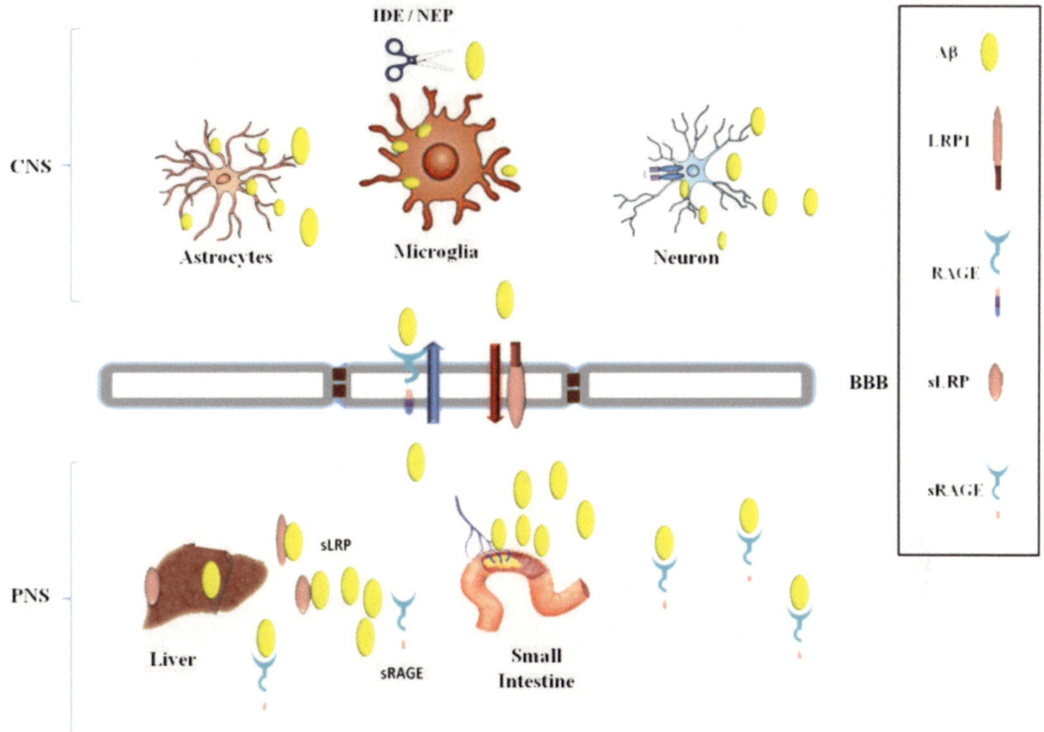

Figure 4. Clearance of Aβ peptides.A) Aβ produced by APP processing in neurons and astrocytes in the central nervous system (CNS), can be cleared by microglia phagocytosis, and further degraded by the enzymatic action of the insulin degrading enzyme (IDE) or by nephrilysin (NEP). Moreover, Aβ could be also removed by efflux through the low density lipoprotein receptor (LRP) at the blood brain barrier (BBB). **B)** Aβ peptides in the peripheral circulation could be generated at amyloidogenic organs, mainly the small intestine and the liver. In these cases, the clearing mechanisms, could involve the soluble forms of sLRP1 and the receptor of the advanced glycation end products (sRAGE). The full length form of this receptor (RAGE), is located at the BBB, and allows the influx of Aβ to the cerebral parenchyma.

The deregulation of cholesterol homeostasis and metabolism, is frequently observed in AD patients [87]. Thus it is important to consider the inappropriate diet (e.g. a diet rich in cholesterol) as a risk factor.

A set of experiments of our laboratory are focused on the evaluation of the effect of a high cholesterol diet on APP processing and generation of Aβ, based on the fact that statins (that lower cholesterol), diminish the risk of AD [83, 88]. Moreover, several reports support the possibility of a link between abnormal cholesterol metabolism and AD [86, 89-92]. According to Thirumangalakudi and colleagues, there are three principal evidences between cholesterol levels and Alzheimer disease: First, most of the genes associated with AD (that have polymorphism associated with the neurodegeneration), participate in the metabolism of cholesterol, such as ApoE, cyp46 and ABCA1. The second evidence comes from the clinical studies, which had shown that patients with high cholesterol, are more susceptible to AD [86, 93], and the third evidence comes from animal models transgenic and non-transgenic (rabbits, mice and rats), in which a high cholesterol diet have shown an enhance in brain Aβ [94-96].

Taken together, all the evidences mentioned above, it is necessary to evaluate the relationship between a high cholesterol diet and the levels of systemic and brain Aβ. We are focusing our study in the principal amyloidogenic organs (like the intestine, the liver and the brain) in rats that undertake a cholesterol enriched diet for different time periods, and evaluating if the mechanisms of clearance of Aβ are compromised and the possibility that systemic Aβ could affect or induce brain Aβ deposits possible through alterations in the permeability of the BBB. If this study shows a correlation between high cholesterol diet and elevated Aβ levels in the brain it will be tempting to speculate clinical implications directed to propose a balance diet with low cholesterol as a preventive approach for AD, as well as the use of drugs that lower cholesterol levels concomitant with the possibility of lowering Aβ levels, preferentially at early stages of the disease.

10. $A\beta_{42}$ oligomers modulate intracellular Ca2+ transients evoked by cholinergic receptors

Finally our lab is also interested in the study of the effects of Aβ oligomers on cholinergic receptors: nicotinic and muscarinic; and the role of these oligomeric forms of Aβ in intracellular calcium homeostasis. It is well known that oligomers can bind extracellular receptors [97] and indirectly activate signaling pathways. Some of these pathways could be linked to the release of intracellular calcium and the induction of cell death in cases in which the oligomeric peptide is at high concentration [98]. We are focussed on studying the consequences of Aβ interaction with the cholinergic receptors, on the levels of intracellular calcium and its impact in cell viability and synaptic transmission, based on previous reports of the role of Aβ in potentiating nicotinic receptor function and promoting oxidative stress and cellular toxicity [99].

Cholinergic pathways serve important functions in learning and memory processes. Nicotinic and muscarinic receptors are widely expressed in the brain and implicated in the pathophysiology of AD, that is the most common form of dementia, characterized by loss of neurons and synapses in the cerebral cortex and subcortical regions. The correlation of clinical dementia ratings with the reductions in a number of cortical cholinergic markers such as choline acetyltransferase, muscarinic and nicotinic acetylcholine receptor binding as well as levels of acetylcholine, suggested an association of cholinergic hypofunction with cognitive deficit, which led to the formulation of the cholinergic hypothesis of memory dysfunction in senescence and in AD [100]. As we mentioned before, Aβ is the major protein component of neuritic plaques found in AD. Evidence suggests that the physical aggregation state of Aβ directly influences neurotoxicity and specific cellular biochemical events. In addition, it has been shown that Aβ oligimers are able to modulate the release of several neurotransmitters (dopamine, γ-aminobutyric acid, aspartate, glutamate) elicited by the stimulation of cholinergic muscarinic and nicotinic receptor (mAChR, nAChR) in different brain areas. Recently it was shown the activation of both $\alpha7$ and $\alpha4\beta2$ (nAChRs) as well as by the activation of mAChR modulate the Glycine release from hippocampal synaptosomes [101].

Sustained disruptions in Ca2+ signaling have significant implications for the health and functionality of neurons and form the basis of the Ca2+ hypothesis of AD [102]. Under resting conditions, cytosolic Ca2+ is maintained at low nanomolar concentrations by an array of pumps, buffers, and transport mechanisms. Ca2+ entry into the cytosol is rigorously regulated and originates from one of two major sources: the extracellular fluid via entry across the plasma membrane (through receptor-, voltage-, and store-operated channels and Ca2+ exchangers) and intracellular stores such as the endoplasmic reticulum (ER) and mitochondria [103, 104]. Interactions between Aβ and intracellular Ca2+ are particularly relevant to AD pathogenesis, as Ca2+ perturbations are a causal factor in excitotoxicity, synaptic degeneration, and cell death, whereas reduced Ca2+ release is neuroprotective [105].

In our laboratory we investigate the effects of $A\beta_{42}$ oligomers on the transient rises in [Ca2+]i evoked by cholinergic receptors in the human neuroblastoma cell line SH-SY5Y. Our results indicate that mAChR type M3 increased 56% the transient rise in [Ca2+]i evoked by carbachol in the presence of $A\beta_{42}$ oligomers, whereas the nicotine response only increased in 21%.

The experimental procedures for these set of experiments were as follows:

Briefly, preparation of oligomers was performed as reported previously by Demuro and colleagues [98]

To be able to observe the Aβ oligomers, we used atomic force microscopy. Concentrated oligomers of $A\beta_{42}$ (1 μl ~ 250 ng) were added to 9 μl double-distilled water and placed on a freshly cleaved cover slip and air-dried taken for observation by atomic force microscopy. The samples were imaged in AC-mode using a JSPM-5200 instrument (JEOL scanning probe microscope) equipped with NSC15 n-type silicon probe Al coated (μMasch), in the tapping mode. The probe has nominal spring constant of 20 to 80 N/m and driving frequencies of 265 to 410 kHz. To determine oligomer sizes we used the WinSPM system computer program provided by the manufacturer (JEOL) and Gwyddion free software for 3D analysis.

Cell culture and immunocytochemistry assays were carried out as reported before [106]. The cell line used for these experiments was the human neuroblastoma SH-SY5Y. These cells were immunostained with anti-mAChR M1 or anti-mAChR M3 (Santa Cruz Biotechnology Inc.).

For the recording experiments, the cells were seeded on recording chambers pre-coated with Poly-L-Lys. [Ca2+]i determinations in single SH-SY5Y cells were performed as reported before [107] using the Ca^{2+} indicator Fura-2AM (Molecular Probes). Aβ1-42 oligomers were applied by pipetting a fixed aliquot (50 μl) of a diluted stock solution into the recording chamber (200 μl volume). Acetylcholine, nicotine and carbachol were freshly prepared in saline solution at the indicated final concentrations. All the experiments were done at room temperature.

In the following section, we will describe our results of the experiments in which we evaluate the effects of $A\beta_{42}$ oligomers on the modulation of intracellular Ca2+ transients evoked by cholinergic receptors.

Atomic force microscopy (AFM) is used to investigate the three-dimensional structure of aggregated Aβ and characterize aggregate/fibril size, structure, and distribution. Figure 5 shows the 3D analysis of $A\beta_{42}$ oligomers morphology using AFM. The packing densities correspond to the differential thickness of globular aggregates along a zeta axis (fiber height above the x-y imaging surface).

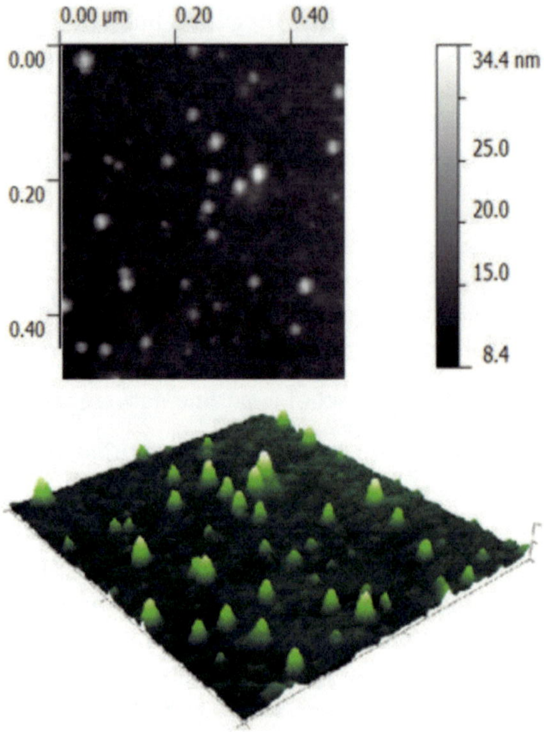

Figure 5. Aβ_{42} oligomers morphology, tapping mode AFM image that shows the characteristic globular texture (scan area 540 x 540 nm).

The human neuroblastoma SH-SY5Y cells express muscarinic cholinergic receptors (mAChRs) of predominantly the M_3 subtype, which are robustly coupled to phosphoinositide (PPI) hydrolysis and Ca^{2+} homeostasis [108]. Figure 6 shows immunoreactivity for M3 and M1 receptors in SH-SY5Y cells in culture. In addition, SH-SY5Y cells express two types of nicotinic cholinergic receptors (nAChRs), ganglionic AChRs, which are normally postsynaptic and are composed of α3, α5, β2, and β4 subunits, and neuronal αBgt-binding AChRs, which are probably normally extrasynaptic composed of α7 subunits [109].

[Ca2+]i determinations in single SH-SY5Y cells:

The application of a short pulse of ACh (100 µM) to SH-SY5Y cells produced a rise in [Ca2+]i that peaked in approximately 1 s and declined toward basal levels of [Ca2+]i at the end of ACh pulse (Figure 7). When a second pulse of ACh was applied 120 s after the first pulse, the [Ca2+]i response was lightly reduced, but it was after 3 min period in resting conditions when the response recovered the whole amplitude (signaled with the arrow). Repetitive applications with 1 min interval produce progressive desensitization in the ACh response.

http://dx.doi.org/10.5772/57398

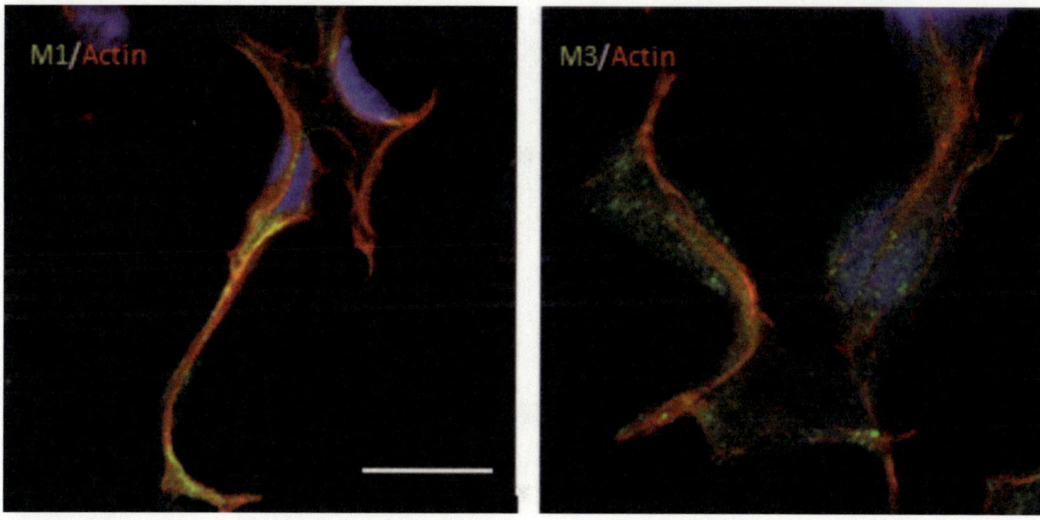

Figure 6. Confocal micoscopic localization of M3 (green staining, left panel) and M1 (green staining, right panel) immunoreactivity in SH-SY5Y neuroblastoma cells. M3 reactivity is enriched appearing finely granular and punctuate. Nuclear DNA was counterstained with Hoechst 33342 (blue staining) and the red signal corresponds to Actin inmunoreactvity. Scale bar 20 µm.

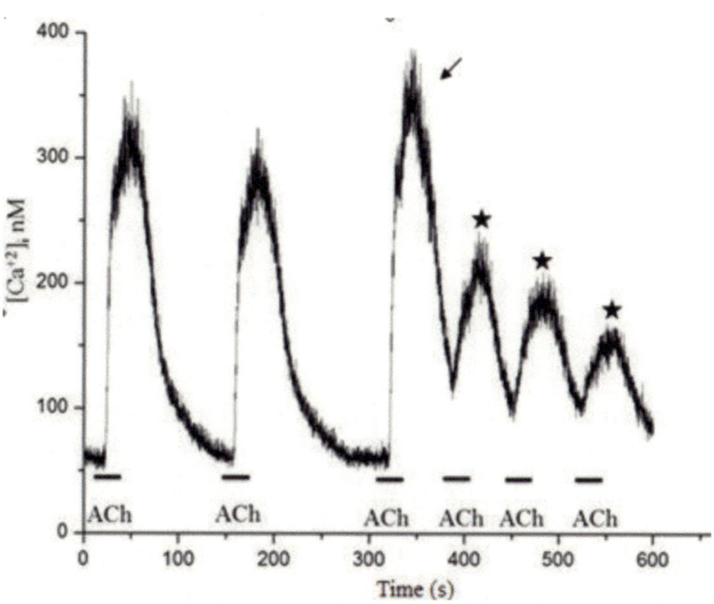

Figure 7. Transient rises in [Ca2+]i evoked by repetitive ACh pulses in SH-SY5Y cells. ACh pulses were applied during the continuous perfusion of normal saline solution (see text).

The rate of rise of the [Ca2+]i should reflect the number of activated nicotine and muscarinic receptors, however, in the most of the explored cells, the application of nicotine pulses (100 µM) was unable to produce any elevation of the [Ca2+]i, whereas in some cells the nicotinic response was approximately 20 times smaller than those evoked by carbachol (100 μM) suggesting that the cholinergic response is mediates mainly by muscarinic receptors (Figure 8).

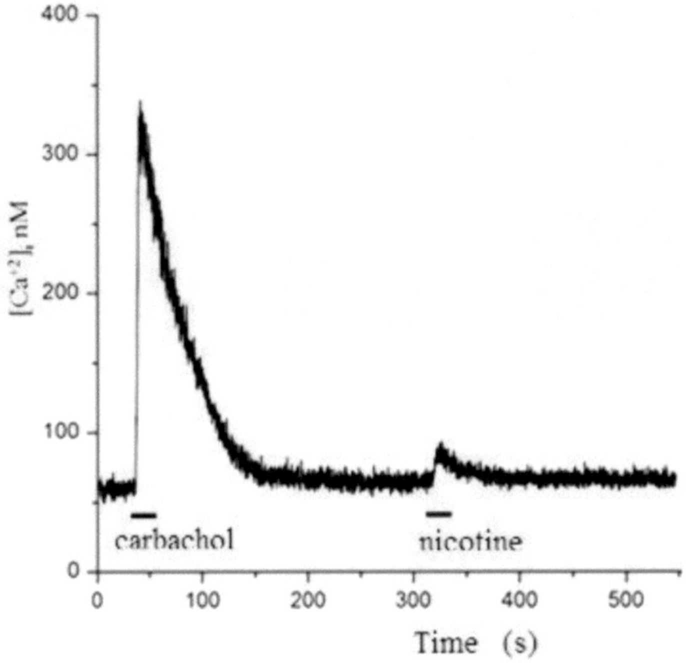

Figure 8. Transient rises in [Ca2+]i evoked by carbachol and nicotine pulses in the same SH-SY5Y cell. As in previous figure agonist pulses were applied during the continuous perfusion of normal saline solution (see text).

The incubation of SH-SY5Y cells with $A\beta_{42}$ oligomers (2.5 μg/ml) during 10 min increased 56% the transient rise in [Ca2+]i evoked by carbachol (see Figure 9), whereas the nicotine response only increased in 21%.

Taken together our results, we conclude that $A\beta_{42}$ oligomers are capable of inducing an increase in intracellular calcium levels in a dose dependent way, concomitant with an increase in intracellular Ca2+ transients evoked by cholinergic receptors. Thus the cholinergic response is potentiated by $A\beta_{42}$ oligomers. Based on previous reports (see below), our findings suggest that the increase in the transient rises of the [Ca2+]i after the incubation with the $A\beta_{42}$ oligomers evoked by carbachol, could be generated by a sustained increase of the IP3 levels, that induces a more efficient activation of IP3 receptors from the internal stores. Since ACh binding to mAChRs initiates the heterotrimeric G protein cycle, with the exchange of GTP for GDP on α-subunits and the subsequent dissociation of $\beta\gamma$ subunits, the activated, GTP-bound form of the α-subunit stimulates (or inhibits) its effector, then undergoes inactivation by intrinsic GTPase activity, which converts GTP to GDP by hydrolytic cleavage of the γ phosphate bond. Cholinergic agonist stimulation of M1, M3, and M5 receptors activates G proteins of the

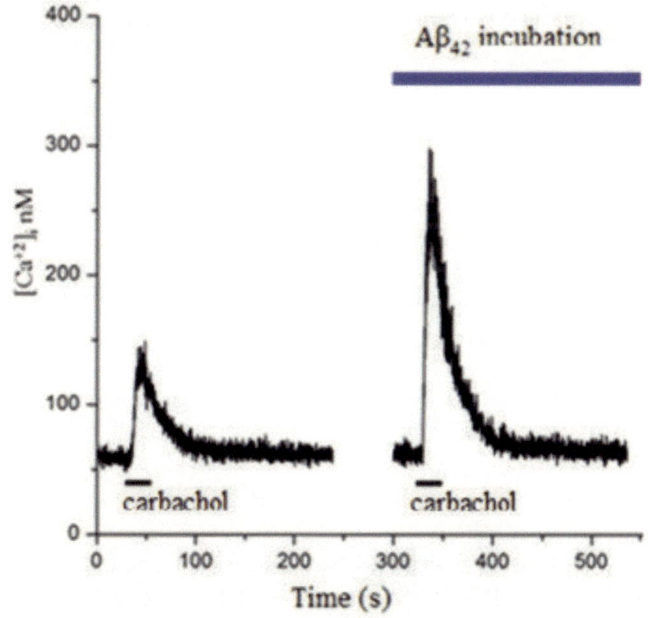

Figure 9. $A\beta_{42}$ oligomers potentiate the transient rises in [Ca2+]i evoked by carbachol in SH-SY5Y cell.

pertussis toxin-insensitive Gq/11 family. Gq/11 subunits stimulate phospholipase C, which catalyzes the hydrolysis of phosphatidylinositol-4,5-bisphosphate, resulting in the liberation of diacylglycerol and inositol triphosphate (IP3). Diacylglycerol activates protein kinase C (PKC), and IP3 induces the release of Ca2+ from endoplasmic reticulum [110]. Hence $A\beta_{42}$ induce a marked increase in the activation PKC and Ca2+/clamodulin-dependent kinase II (CaMKII) in cortical neurons, and the activation of mAChRs (M1 type) significantly inhibited the Aβ activation of PKC and CaMKII [111].

11. Conclusion

For years the Amyloid hypothesis was widely accepted as a cause of the neurodegeneration observed in AD. This hypothesis considers Aβ as a toxic factor that impairs neuronal function and leads to cell death. But recently our understanding of the physiological roles of Aβ is challenging this hypothesis.

The physiological roles of Aβ need to be taken in account in the development of therapies that intend to reduce its levels for diseases like Alzheimer's. Since excessively depleting Aβ could have negative effects, limiting its trophic functions could contribute, rather than delay the process of neurodegeneration. Furthermore, understanding the physiological functions of

APP and Aβ could help to elucidate its role during health vs disease. As we mentioned here, Aβ itself, might help to enhance synaptic plasticity and memory at appropriate concentration levels (Figure 2).

Author details

M. del C. Cárdenas-Aguayo[1], M. del C. Silva-Lucero[1], M. Cortes-Ortiz[1], B. Jiménez-Ramos[1], L. Gómez-Virgilio[1], G. Ramírez-Rodríguez[2], E. Vera-Arroyo[3], R. Fiorentino-Pérez[3], U. García[3], J. Luna-Muñoz[4] and M.A. Meraz-Ríos[1]

1 Department of Molecular Biomedicine, Centro de Investigación y de Estudios Avanzados del IPN, (CINVESTAV-IPN), México City, México

2 Laboratory of Neurogenesis, Instituto Nacional de Psiquiatría, México City, México

3 Department of Physiology, Biophysics and Neuroscience, Centro de Investigación y de Estudios Avanzados del IPN, (CINVESTAV-IPN), México City, México

4 National Brain Banking. Laboratorio Nacional de Servicios experimentales (LaNSE), Centro de Investigación y de Estudios Avanzados del IPN, (CINVESTAV-IPN), México City, México

References

[1] Ramirez-Alvarado, M., J.S. Merkel, and L. Regan, *A systematic exploration of the influence of the protein stability on amyloid fibril formation in vitro.* Proc Natl Acad Sci U S A, 2000. 97(16): p. 8979-84.

[2] Edwards, D.R., M.M. Handsley, and C.J. Pennington, *The ADAM metalloproteinases.* Mol Aspects Med, 2008. 29(5): p. 258-89.

[3] Pietri, M., et al., *PDK1 decreases TACE-mediated alpha-secretase activity and promotes disease progression in prion and Alzheimer's diseases.* Nat Med, 2013.

[4] Shoji, M., et al., *Production of the Alzheimer amyloid beta protein by normal proteolytic processing.* Science, 1992. 258(5079): p. 126-9.

[5] Golde, T.E., et al., *gamma-Secretase inhibitors and modulators.* Biochim Biophys Acta, 2013.

[6] Chang, K.A. and Y.H. Suh, *Possible roles of amyloid intracellular domain of amyloid precursor protein.* BMB Rep, 2010. 43(10): p. 656-63.

[7] Zhang, H., et al., *Proteolytic processing of Alzheimer's beta-amyloid precursor protein.* J Neurochem, 2011. 120 Suppl 1: p. 9-21.

[8] O'Brien, R.J. and P.C. Wong, *Amyloid precursor protein processing and Alzheimer's disease.* Annu Rev Neurosci, 2011. 34: p. 185-204.

[9] Nalivaeva, N.N. and A.J. Turner, *The amyloid precursor protein: a biochemical enigma in brain development, function and disease.* FEBS Lett, 2013. 587(13): p. 2046-54.

[10] Lu, D.C., et al., *A second cytotoxic proteolytic peptide derived from amyloid beta-protein precursor.* Nat Med, 2000. 6(4): p. 397-404.

[11] De Strooper, B., R. Vassar, and T. Golde, *The secretases: enzymes with therapeutic potential in Alzheimer disease.* Nat Rev Neurol, 2010. 6(2): p. 99-107.

[12] Kametani, F., *Epsilon-secretase: reduction of amyloid precursor protein epsilon-site cleavage in Alzheimer's disease.* Curr Alzheimer Res, 2008. 5(2): p. 165-71.

[13] Klein, W.L., *Abeta toxicity in Alzheimer's disease: globular oligomers (ADDLs) as new vaccine and drug targets.* Neurochem Int, 2002. 41(5): p. 345-52.

[14] Selkoe, D.J., *Toward a comprehensive theory for Alzheimer's disease. Hypothesis: Alzheimer's disease is caused by the cerebral accumulation and cytotoxicity of amyloid beta-protein.* Ann N Y Acad Sci, 2000. 924: p. 17-25.

[15] Glenner, G.G. and C.W. Wong, *Alzheimer's disease and Down's syndrome: sharing of a unique cerebrovascular amyloid fibril protein.* Biochem Biophys Res Commun, 1984. 122(3): p. 1131-5.

[16] Roberts, G.W., et al., *beta A4 amyloid protein deposition in brain after head trauma.* Lancet, 1991. 338(8780): p. 1422-3.

[17] Tomlinson, B.E., G. Blessed, and M. Roth, *Observations on the brains of non-demented old people.* J Neurol Sci, 1968. 7(2): p. 331-56.

[18] Luo, Y., et al., *Physiological levels of beta-amyloid peptide promote PC12 cell proliferation.* Neurosci Lett, 1996. 217(2-3): p. 125-8.

[19] Moya, K.L., et al., *The amyloid precursor protein is developmentally regulated and correlated with synaptogenesis.* Dev Biol, 1994. 161(2): p. 597-603.

[20] Mileusnic, R., et al., *APP is required during an early phase of memory formation.* Eur J Neurosci, 2000. 12(12): p. 4487-95.

[21] Jellinger, K.A., *Challenges in neuronal apoptosis.* Curr Alzheimer Res, 2006. 3(4): p. 377-91.

[22] Plant, L.D., et al., *The production of amyloid beta peptide is a critical requirement for the viability of central neurons.* J Neurosci, 2003. 23(13): p. 5531-5.

[23] Cirrito, J.R., et al., *In vivo assessment of brain interstitial fluid with microdialysis reveals plaque-associated changes in amyloid-beta metabolism and half-life.* J Neurosci, 2003. 23(26): p. 8844-53.

[24] Atwood, C.S., et al., *Amyloid-beta: a chameleon walking in two worlds: a review of the trophic and toxic properties of amyloid-beta.* Brain Res Brain Res Rev, 2003. 43(1): p. 1-16.

[25] Walsh, D.M., et al., *Naturally secreted oligomers of amyloid beta protein potently inhibit hippocampal long-term potentiation in vivo.* Nature, 2002. 416(6880): p. 535-9.

[26] Pearson, H.A. and C. Peers, *Physiological roles for amyloid beta peptides.* J Physiol, 2006. 575(Pt 1): p. 5-10.

[27] Shankar, G.M., et al., *Natural oligomers of the Alzheimer amyloid-beta protein induce reversible synapse loss by modulating an NMDA-type glutamate receptor-dependent signaling pathway.* J Neurosci, 2007. 27(11): p. 2866-75.

[28] Kamenetz, F., et al., *APP processing and synaptic function.* Neuron, 2003. 37(6): p. 925-37.

[29] Garcia-Osta, A. and C.M. Alberini, *Amyloid beta mediates memory formation.* Learn Mem, 2009. 16(4): p. 267-72.

[30] Puzzo, D., et al., *Picomolar amyloid-beta positively modulates synaptic plasticity and memory in hippocampus.* J Neurosci, 2008. 28(53): p. 14537-45.

[31] Kohli, B.M., et al., *Interactome of the amyloid precursor protein APP in brain reveals a protein network involved in synaptic vesicle turnover and a close association with Synaptotagmin-1.* J Proteome Res, 2012. 11(8): p. 4075-90.

[32] Octave, J.N., et al., *From synaptic spines to nuclear signaling: nuclear and synaptic actions of the amyloid precursor protein.* J Neurochem, 2013. 126(2): p. 183-90.

[33] Jung, C.K. and J. Herms, *Role of APP for dendritic spine formation and stability.* Exp Brain Res, 2011. 217(3-4): p. 463-70.

[34] Tyan, S.H., et al., *Amyloid precursor protein (APP) regulates synaptic structure and function.* Mol Cell Neurosci, 2012. 51(1-2): p. 43-52.

[35] Weyer, S.W., et al., *APP and APLP2 are essential at PNS and CNS synapses for transmission, spatial learning and LTP.* EMBO J, 2011. 30(11): p. 2266-80.

[36] Abramsson, A., et al., *The zebrafish amyloid precursor protein-b is required for motor neuron guidance and synapse formation.* Dev Biol, 2013. 381(2): p. 377-88.

[37] Sosa, L.J., et al., *Amyloid precursor protein is an autonomous growth cone adhesion molecule engaged in contact guidance.* PLoS One, 2013. 8(5): p. e64521.

[38] Chen, Q.S., et al., *Impairment of hippocampal long-term potentiation by Alzheimer amyloid beta-peptides.* J Neurosci Res, 2000. 60(1): p. 65-72.

[39] Freir, D.B., C. Holscher, and C.E. Herron, *Blockade of long-term potentiation by beta-amyloid peptides in the CA1 region of the rat hippocampus in vivo.* J Neurophysiol, 2001. 85(2): p. 708-13.

[40] Cleary, J.P., et al., *Natural oligomers of the amyloid-beta protein specifically disrupt cognitive function.* Nat Neurosci, 2005. 8(1): p. 79-84.

[41] Puzzo, D., et al., *Endogenous amyloid-beta is necessary for hippocampal synaptic plasticity and memory.* Ann Neurol, 2011. 69(5): p. 819-30.

[42] Morley, J.E., et al., *A physiological role for amyloid-beta protein:enhancement of learning and memory.* J Alzheimers Dis, 2009. 19(2): p. 441-9.

[43] Cirrito, J.R., et al., *Endocytosis is required for synaptic activity-dependent release of amyloid-beta in vivo.* Neuron, 2008. 58(1): p. 42-51.

[44] Cirrito, J.R., et al., *Synaptic activity regulates interstitial fluid amyloid-beta levels in vivo.* Neuron, 2005. 48(6): p. 913-22.

[45] Smith, D.G., R. Cappai, and K.J. Barnham, *The redox chemistry of the Alzheimer's disease amyloid beta peptide.* Biochim Biophys Acta, 2007. 1768(8): p. 1976-90.

[46] Baruch-Suchodolsky, R. and B. Fischer, *Abeta40, either soluble or aggregated, is a remarkably potent antioxidant in cell-free oxidative systems.* Biochemistry, 2009. 48(20): p. 4354-70.

[47] Kontush, A. and C.S. Atwood, *Amyloid-beta: phylogenesis of a chameleon.* Brain Res Brain Res Rev, 2004. 46(1): p. 118-20.

[48] Nunomura, A., et al., *Oxidative damage is the earliest event in Alzheimer disease.* J Neuropathol Exp Neurol, 2001. 60(8): p. 759-67.

[49] Curtain, C.C., et al., *Alzheimer's disease amyloid-beta binds copper and zinc to generate an allosterically ordered membrane-penetrating structure containing superoxide dismutase-like subunits.* J Biol Chem, 2001. 276(23): p. 20466-73.

[50] Huang, X., et al., *The A beta peptide of Alzheimer's disease directly produces hydrogen peroxide through metal ion reduction.* Biochemistry, 1999. 38(24): p. 7609-16.

[51] Huang, X., et al., *Cu(II) potentiation of alzheimer abeta neurotoxicity. Correlation with cell-free hydrogen peroxide production and metal reduction.* J Biol Chem, 1999. 274(52): p. 37111-6.

[52] Kontush, A., et al., *Amyloid-beta is an antioxidant for lipoproteins in cerebrospinal fluid and plasma.* Free Radic Biol Med, 2001. 30(1): p. 119-28.

[53] Zou, K., et al., *A novel function of monomeric amyloid beta-protein serving as an antioxidant molecule against metal-induced oxidative damage.* J Neurosci, 2002. 22(12): p. 4833-41.

[54] Gibson, G.E., et al., *Differential alterations in antioxidant capacity in cells from Alzheimer patients.* Biochim Biophys Acta, 2000. 1502(3): p. 319-29.

[55] Leutner, S., et al., *Reduced antioxidant enzyme activity in brains of mice transgenic for human presenilin-1 with single or multiple mutations.* Neurosci Lett, 2000. 292(2): p. 87-90.

[56] Guo, Q., et al., *Increased vulnerability of hippocampal neurons from presenilin-1 mutant knock-in mice to amyloid beta-peptide toxicity: central roles of superoxide production and caspase activation.* J Neurochem, 1999. 72(3): p. 1019-29.

[57] Lopez-Toledano, M.A. and M.L. Shelanski, *Neurogenic effect of beta-amyloid peptide in the development of neural stem cells.* J Neurosci, 2004. 24(23): p. 5439-44.

[58] Gage, F.H., J. Ray, and L.J. Fisher, *Isolation, characterization, and use of stem cells from the CNS.* Annu Rev Neurosci, 1995. 18: p. 159-92.

[59] Jimenez, S., et al., *Age-dependent accumulation of soluble amyloid beta (Abeta) oligomers reverses the neuroprotective effect of soluble amyloid precursor protein-alpha (sAPP(alpha)) by modulating phosphatidylinositol 3-kinase (PI3K)/Akt-GSK-3beta pathway in Alzheimer mouse model.* J Biol Chem, 2011. 286(21): p. 18414-25.

[60] Schulte-Herbruggen, O., M.C. Jockers-Scherubl, and R. Hellweg, *Neurotrophins: from pathophysiology to treatment in Alzheimer's disease.* Curr Alzheimer Res, 2008. 5(1): p. 38-44.

[61] Aimone, J.B., W. Deng, and F.H. Gage, *Adult neurogenesis: integrating theories and separating functions.* Trends Cogn Sci, 2010. 14(7): p. 325-37.

[62] Kempermann, G., et al., *Milestones of neuronal development in the adult hippocampus.* Trends Neurosci, 2004. 27(8): p. 447-52.

[63] Kempermann, G., L. Wiskott, and F.H. Gage, *Functional significance of adult neurogenesis.* Curr Opin Neurobiol, 2004. 14(2): p. 186-91.

[64] Kempermann, G., J. Krebs, and K. Fabel, *The contribution of failing adult hippocampal neurogenesis to psychiatric disorders.* Curr Opin Psychiatry, 2008. 21(3): p. 290-5.

[65] Lledo, P.M. and G. Gheusi, *[Adult neurogenesis: from basic research to clinical applications].* Bull Acad Natl Med, 2006. 190(2): p. 385-400; discussion 400-2.

[66] Deng, W., J.B. Aimone, and F.H. Gage, *New neurons and new memories: how does adult hippocampal neurogenesis affect learning and memory?* Nat Rev Neurosci, 2010. 11(5): p. 339-50.

[67] Altman, J. and G.D. Das, *Autoradiographic and histological studies of postnatal neurogenesis. I. A longitudinal investigation of the kinetics, migration and transformation of cells incorporating tritiated thymidine in neonate rats, with special reference to postnatal neurogenesis in some brain regions.* J Comp Neurol, 1966. 126(3): p. 337-89.

[68] Alvarez-Buylla, A. and J.M. Garcia-Verdugo, *Neurogenesis in adult subventricular zone.* J Neurosci, 2002. 22(3): p. 629-34.

[69] Babu, H., et al., *Enriched monolayer precursor cell cultures from micro-dissected adult mouse dentate gyrus yield functional granule cell-like neurons.* PLoS One, 2007. 2(4): p. e388.

[70] Rakic, P., *Neurogenesis in adult primates.* Prog Brain Res, 2002. 138: p. 3-14.

[71] Babu, H., et al., *Synaptic Network Activity Induces Neuronal Differentiation of Adult Hippocampal Precursor Cells through BDNF Signaling.* Front Neurosci, 2009. 3: p. 49.

[72] Heo, C., et al., *Effects of the monomeric, oligomeric, and fibrillar Abeta42 peptides on the proliferation and differentiation of adult neural stem cells from subventricular zone.* J Neurochem, 2007. 102(2): p. 493-500.

[73] Chen, Y. and C. Dong, *Abeta40 promotes neuronal cell fate in neural progenitor cells.* Cell Death Differ, 2009. 16(3): p. 386-94.

[74] Giuffrida, M.L., et al., *Beta-amyloid monomers are neuroprotective.* J Neurosci, 2009. 29(34): p. 10582-7.

[75] Yankner, B.A., L.K. Duffy, and D.A. Kirschner, *Neurotrophic and neurotoxic effects of amyloid beta protein: reversal by tachykinin neuropeptides.* Science, 1990. 250(4978): p. 279-82.

[76] Diaz-Moreno, M., et al., *Abeta increases neural stem cell activity in senescence-accelerated SAMP8 mice.* Neurobiol Aging, 2013. 34(11): p. 2623-38.

[77] Sotthibundhu, A., et al., *Abeta(1-42) stimulates adult SVZ neurogenesis through the p75 neurotrophin receptor.* Neurobiol Aging, 2009. 30(12): p. 1975-85.

[78] Encinas, J.M. and A. Sierra, *Neural stem cell deforestation as the main force driving the age-related decline in adult hippocampal neurogenesis.* Behav Brain Res, 2012. 227(2): p. 433-9.

[79] Villeda, S.A., et al., *The ageing systemic milieu negatively regulates neurogenesis and cognitive function.* Nature, 2011. 477(7362): p. 90-4.

[80] Mirochnic, S., et al., *Age effects on the regulation of adult hippocampal neurogenesis by physical activity and environmental enrichment in the APP23 mouse model of Alzheimer disease.* Hippocampus, 2009. 19(10): p. 1008-18.

[81] Atwood, C.S., et al., *Amyloid-beta: a vascular sealant that protects against hemorrhage?* J Neurosci Res, 2002. 70(3): p. 356.

[82] Robinson, S.R., et al., *Lessons from the AN 1792 Alzheimer vaccine: lest we forget.* Neurobiol Aging, 2004. 25(5): p. 609-15.

[83] Silva, T., et al., *Alzheimer's disease, cholesterol, and statins: the junctions of important metabolic pathways.* Angew Chem Int Ed Engl, 2013. 52(4): p. 1110-21.

[84] Bodovitz, S. and W.L. Klein, *Cholesterol modulates alpha-secretase cleavage of amyloid precursor protein.* J Biol Chem, 1996. 271(8): p. 4436-40.

[85] Ehehalt, R., et al., *Amyloidogenic processing of the Alzheimer beta-amyloid precursor protein depends on lipid rafts.* J Cell Biol, 2003. 160(1): p. 113-23.

[86] Puglielli, L., R.E. Tanzi, and D.M. Kovacs, *Alzheimer's disease: the cholesterol connection.* Nat Neurosci, 2003. 6(4): p. 345-51.

[87] Martins, I.J., et al., *Apolipoprotein E, cholesterol metabolism, diabetes, and the convergence of risk factors for Alzheimer's disease and cardiovascular disease.* Mol Psychiatry, 2006. 11(8): p. 721-36.

[88] Wolozin, B., et al., *Decreased prevalence of Alzheimer disease associated with 3-hydroxy-3-methyglutaryl coenzyme A reductase inhibitors.* Arch Neurol, 2000. 57(10): p. 1439-43.

[89] Park, S.H., et al., *Hypercholesterolemia accelerates amyloid beta-induced cognitive deficits.* Int J Mol Med, 2013. 31(3): p. 577-82.

[90] Casserly, I. and E. Topol, *Convergence of atherosclerosis and Alzheimer's disease: inflammation, cholesterol, and misfolded proteins.* Lancet, 2004. 363(9415): p. 1139-46.

[91] Thirumangalakudi, L., et al., *High cholesterol-induced neuroinflammation and amyloid precursor protein processing correlate with loss of working memory in mice.* J Neurochem, 2008. 106(1): p. 475-85.

[92] Sambamurti, K., et al., *Cholesterol and Alzheimer's disease: clinical and experimental models suggest interactions of different genetic, dietary and environmental risk factors.* Curr Drug Targets, 2004. 5(6): p. 517-28.

[93] Matsuzaki, T., et al., *Association of Alzheimer disease pathology with abnormal lipid metabolism: the Hisayama Study.* Neurology, 2011. 77(11): p. 1068-75.

[94] Sparks, D.L., et al., *Alterations of Alzheimer's disease in the cholesterol-fed rabbit, including vascular inflammation. Preliminary observations.* Ann N Y Acad Sci, 2000. 903: p. 335-44.

[95] Refolo, L.M., et al., *Hypercholesterolemia accelerates the Alzheimer's amyloid pathology in a transgenic mouse model.* Neurobiol Dis, 2000. 7(4): p. 321-31.

[96] Levin-Allerhand, J.A., C.E. Lominska, and J.D. Smith, *Increased amyloid- levels in APPSWE transgenic mice treated chronically with a physiological high-fat high-cholesterol diet.* J Nutr Health Aging, 2002. 6(5): p. 315-9.

[97] Wang, H.Y., et al., *beta-Amyloid(1-42) binds to alpha7 nicotinic acetylcholine receptor with high affinity. Implications for Alzheimer's disease pathology.* J Biol Chem, 2000. 275(8): p. 5626-32.

[98] Demuro, A., et al., *Calcium dysregulation and membrane disruption as a ubiquitous neurotoxic mechanism of soluble amyloid oligomers.* J Biol Chem, 2005. 280(17): p. 17294-300.

[99] Chen, G.J., Z. Xiong, and Z. Yan, *Abeta impairs nicotinic regulation of inhibitory synaptic transmission and interneuron excitability in prefrontal cortex.* Mol Neurodegener, 2013. 8: p. 3.

[100] Bartus, R.T., *On neurodegenerative diseases, models, and treatment strategies: lessons learned and lessons forgotten a generation following the cholinergic hypothesis.* Exp Neurol, 2000. 163(2): p. 495-529.

[101] Zappettini, S., et al., *Beta Amyloid Differently Modulate Nicotinic and Muscarinic Receptor Subtypes which Stimulate in vitro and in vivo the Release of Glycine in the Rat Hippocampus.* Front Pharmacol, 2012. 3: p. 146.

[102] Khachaturian, Z.S., *Hypothesis on the regulation of cytosol calcium concentration and the aging brain.* Neurobiol Aging, 1987. 8(4): p. 345-6.

[103] Berridge, M.J., *Neuronal calcium signaling.* Neuron, 1998. 21(1): p. 13-26.

[104] Berridge, M.J., *Inositol trisphosphate and calcium signalling mechanisms.* Biochim Biophys Acta, 2009. 1793(6): p. 933-40.

[105] Frandsen, A. and A. Schousboe, *Dantrolene prevents glutamate cytotoxicity and Ca2+ release from intracellular stores in cultured cerebral cortical neurons.* J Neurochem, 1991. 56(3): p. 1075-8.

[106] Lira-De Leon, K.I., et al., *Molecular mechanism of tau aggregation induced by anionic and cationic dyes.* J Alzheimers Dis, 2013. 35(2): p. 319-34.

[107] Gomez-Viquez, N.L., et al., *Inhibition of SERCA pumps induces desynchronized RyR activation in overloaded internal Ca2+ stores in smooth muscle cells.* Am J Physiol Cell Physiol, 2010. 298(5): p. C1038-46.

[108] Lukas, R.J., S.A. Norman, and L. Lucero, *Characterization of Nicotinic Acetylcholine Receptors Expressed by Cells of the SH-SY5Y Human Neuroblastoma Clonal Line.* Mol Cell Neurosci, 1993. 4(1): p. 1-12.

[109] Peng, X., et al., *Human alpha 7 acetylcholine receptor: cloning of the alpha 7 subunit from the SH-SY5Y cell line and determination of pharmacological properties of native receptors and functional alpha 7 homomers expressed in Xenopus oocytes.* Mol Pharmacol, 1994. 45(3): p. 546-54.

[110] Exton, J.H., *Role of G proteins in activation of phosphoinositide phospholipase C.* Adv Second Messenger Phosphoprotein Res, 1993. 28: p. 65-72.

[111] Gu, Z., P. Zhong, and Z. Yan, *Activation of muscarinic receptors inhibits beta-amyloid peptide-induced signaling in cortical slices.* J Biol Chem, 2003. 278(19): p. 17546-56.

Section 4

Neurodegenerative Diseases

Chapter 10

Alzheimer Disease: The Role of Aβ in the Glutamatergic System

Victoria Campos-Peña and
Marco Antonio Meraz-Ríos

Additional information is available at the end of the chapter

http://dx.doi.org/10.5772/57367

1. Introduction

The beta amyloid hypothesis is the most accepted theory explaining the pathophysiology of Alzheimer's disease (AD). In general terms, it is known that AD is characterized by a chronic and progressive neurodegenerative process involving the intracellular and extracellular accumulation of fibrillary proteins. The presence of these aggregates leads to synaptic and neuronal loss observed in Alzheimer's patients. Although the precise etiology of AD is unknown, the main risk factor is advanced age. It is also known that a small proportion of AD patients have an autosomal dominant inheritance pattern in three genes – amyloid precursor protein (AβPP), presenilin 1 (PS1) and presenilin 2 (PS2) [1-6]. The presence of specific mutations in these genes leads to the premature development of the disease, known as Early Onset Alzheimer's Disease (EOAD) or Familial Alzheimer's Disease (FAD). The most common mutations are located in the presenilin genes [1, 7-9], mainly in PS1. Currently more than 185 mutations in PS1 have been reported, with only 13 mutations in PS2. While these mutations are located along the length of the protein sequence, the majority is found in the transmembrane area, and affects protein function. To date, approximately 36 different missense mutations in the APP gene have been identified in 85 families and are located near sites that are recognized by alpha, beta and gamma secretases, thus affecting protein processing and increasing the production of amyloid peptides [10]. The presence of these mutations is a causal factor in the development of AD, and, although they are all related to the disruption of the normal functioning of proteins and an increased formation of beta amyloid, together they are present in less than 10% of all Alzheimer's cases, suggesting that there are many other non-genetic factors involved in the development of the pathology. The remaining 90% of AD cases are known as Sporadic Alzheimer's Disease or Late Onset Alzheimer's disease (LOAD). These patients also exhibit genetic risk factors, such as the presence of allele 4 of the Apolipoprotein E (Apoε4), where individuals with one copy of ε4 allele are three times more at risk of developing the disease, while those with two copies (ε4/ε4) are 10–15 times more likely to develop AD [11-14]. While other non-genetic factors are head trauma, hypertension, atherosclerosis, metabolic disorders such as hypercholesterolemia, obesity and diabetes [15-17], the main risk factor is age. It has been reported that the incidence of the disease increases by 5% in people over 65 and 20% in those over 80. Other factors have also been associated with the development of the disease, such as female gender, smoking, educational level, and a low level of physical and mental activity during the early stages of life.

The pathological markers for AD are the presence of neurofibrillary tangles (NFT) and neuritic plaques (NP). NFT are intracellular and insoluble fibril deposits of paired helical filaments (PHF). As these filaments occupy the cytoplasm of the neuron, the nucleus is displaced and the dendrites disappear, in the absence of which, the filaments takes on the pyramidal shape of the soma and then go on to destroy the neuron itself. Each filament is formed from the association of 6-7 Tau protein fragments, and each fragment consists of 93-95 amino acid residues and has a molecular weight of 12.5Kd [18-21]. In normal conditions, Tau stabilizes microtubules in the cytoskeleton of neurons through a cell process that involves the phosphorylation and dephosphorylation of the protein. In pathological conditions, Tau is abnormally hyperphosphorylated and loses its ability to bind to microtubules, generating insoluble aggregates within the neuron, altering the axonal transport and eventually leading to neuronal death. Generally NFT formation begins in the allocortex of the medial temporal lobe (entorhinal cortex and hippocampus) and spreads to the associative isocortex. In this way, the amount and distribution of NFTs correlate with the severity and duration of dementia.

NPs are extracellular deposits of 10-100μm formed by an insoluble fibrillary core surrounded by activated microglia, reactive astrocytes and dystrophic neurites [22]. Unlike NFTs, amyloid plaques accumulate mainly in the isocortex. The main component in the NP is the amyloid-beta peptide (Aβ); a fragment of 39-42 amino acids with a molecular weight of 4KD [23-24], which arises as a result of the normal secretion derived from amyloid-β precursor protein (AβPP) [25]. Aβ formation occurs as a result of the proteolytic processing of AβPP by the sequential action of β- and γ-secretase. Three AβPP isoforms consisting of 695, 770 and 751 amino acids (APP695, APP751 and APP770) are mainly expressed in the Central Nervous System (CNS). The shortest of these isoforms, APP695, is mostly expressed in neurons, whereas isoforms APP770 and APP751 are expressed in glial cells.

It has been proposed that the progressive accumulation of NP and NFT in the brains of AD patients are responsible for the neurodegeneration observed in the hippocampal, cortical and subcortical neurons. This neurodegenerative damage involves the loss of neuropil networks, selective neuron death, decreased synaptic density and alterations in neurotransmitters and the homeostasis of calcium. An important feature of the NFTs is that the density of such lesions directly correlates with the degree of dementia observed in AD patients [26]. Conversely, it is observed that the number of NP present in a particular region does not correlate with neuronal death, synaptic loss or with cognitive impairment [27-29]. However, the presence of Aβ oligomer deposits has a very important role in synaptic loss [30-32] determining the severity of cognitive impairment. Also has been observed to inhibit the normal critical neuron functions, such as long-term potentiation (LTP)[30]. The amyloid βpeptide, also increases Tau phosphorylation [33-35], oxidative stress and altered homeostasis of Ca^{2+} [36-37] and excitotoxicity [38]. It has been documented that these oligomeric forms of Aβ interact with receptors from the glutamatergic system such as the NMDA-receptors, which are responsible for maintaining glutamate homeostasis [39-40].

1.1. β—Amyloid

Aβ comes from the normal proteolytic processing of AβPP, a type 1 transmembrane glycoprotein [25] whose gene is located on chromosome 21 [41-42]. AβPP processing and the "efficiency" of Aβ formation could be affected by the subcellular localization of the protein. AβPP is synthesized in the endoplasmic reticulum (ER) and transported through the constitutive secretory pathway, and only a small fraction of this protein (10%) goes to the plasma membrane. All AβPP isoforms undergo posttranslational modifications involving N and O-glycosylation, phosphorylation and sulfation. Aβpeptide formation is carried out by the action of β- and γ-secretase, in which the peptides formed vary from 39 to 43 amino-acid residues (Aβ39, 40, 42, 43). Although Aβ40 is the most abundant, Aβ42 is the most hydrophobic and is found in a greater proportion of the NPs observed in AD patients [43]. These peptides are continuously released into the extracellular space at possibly low concentrations, and, in soluble form, could carry out normal physiological functions in the cell including those related to plasticity and memory processes [44].

According to the amyloid hypothesis, the Aβ accumulation in the patient's brain is the key event that leads to the development of the disease, while other pathological findings (NFT formation and neuronal death) are secondary events occurring after the amyloid aggregation. Most of the studies reported in the literature have focused on the toxicity and neuronal death induced by the presence of amyloid aggregates. However, in recent years a great importance has been attached to the role of these peptides as responsible in the etiology of synaptic dysfunction[40]. In this sense, it has been widely documented that the presence of soluble oligomeric forms of Aβ responsible for synaptic damage and neurodegeneration [29, 45-46]. The results reported in the literature indicate that Aβoligomers ranging in size from 2 to 12 subunits may be responsible for the synaptic damage and memory loss observed in patients with Alzheimer's disease [47]. These oligomeric forms may be produced through several routes, either in the extracellular space or inside of the cell organelles such as the endoplasmic reticulum and mitochondria, which complicates the analysis and understanding of the pathophysiology [48-50]. Several types of soluble Aβ oligomers have been described in the brains of AD patients and in transgenic mouse models of AD, however it has been reported that the putative dodecamer Aβ*56 correlated with markers of neuronal dysfunction or injury in cognitively normal subjects [51]. In addition, the role of Aβ oligomers (in the absence of amyloid fibers) in neurodegenerative processes was demonstrated in a transgenic model expressing mutant $hAPP_{E693\Delta}$. This mouse has the ability to form high levels of Aβ oligomers without fibrillization, indicating that the intracellular deposits of Aβ oligomers from 8 months of age onwards correlate with the alterations in synaptic plasticity and memory impairment observed in the mouse model. Other results observed were abnormal Tau phosphorylation, present at 8 months, microglial activation at 12 months, astrocytes activation at 18 months and neuronal loss at 24 months. The results suggest that the presence of oligomeric forms of β—amyloid are able to induce many of the changes observed in the brains of patients with AD, even in the absence of NP [52].

1.2. Extracellular Aβ

The extracellular deposits of amyloid are a specific marker for AD and are involved in synaptic dysfunction and neurotoxicity; however, the complete signaling mechanism involved remains unclear. Importantly, the amyloid oligomers interact with a variety of receptors on the surface, activating or inhibiting several neuronal signaling pathways and possibly contributing to neuronal death [35]. Furthermore, it is also known that the damage caused by amyloid is mainly determined by the level of peptide aggregation. In this way, several studies reported in the literature suggest that extracellular Aβ oligomers could be formed by several biocomponents, such as proteins and ganglioside. For example, the distribution of ganglioside GM1 has the ability to affect the spatial arrangement of the oligosaccharide chains in a molecule. In 2007 Yamamoto *et al.* showed that GM1 provides a microenvironment that favors the formation of amyloid oligomers [53]. These oligomers are spherical structures with a 10-20nm diameter and 200-300kDa that form complexes with the GM1, similar to those identified in the tissue of AD patients. Previous studies have shown that, initially, the peptides adopt a random structure, which then changes when interacting with GM1, and enables the transition from α-helix to β-pleated sheets [54]. Similarly, nonfibrillar Aβ can be produced in presence of αB-crystalline and ApoJ [55-56]. These oligomeric forms interact with the nerve growth factor receptor (NGF), triggering a toxic mechanism that causes cell death. Moreover, the oligomeric forms bind to Frizzled (*Fz*) receptors, inhibiting the *Wnt* signaling pathway, and affecting cell proliferation and neuronal differentiation during development of the brain. Furthermore, the inhibition of Wnt signaling by Aβ oligomers causes Tau phosphorylation and the formation of neuro fibrillary tangles, which suggests a Wnt/β-catenin toxicity pathway [35, 57].

On the other hand, it has also been observed that Aβ oligomers are able to destabilize the plasma membrane, forming pores which alter the normal flow of ions and permitting the entry of extracellular Ca^{2+} and leading to neuronal death [58-60]. Another mechanism of neuronal receptor-mediated damage is the binding of Aβ oligomers to N-methyl-D-aspartate (NMDA) type glutamate receptor (NMDAR), which generates altered calcium homeostasis, increased oxidative stress and loss of synapses [61-63].

1.3. Intracellular Aβ

The presence of intracellular Aβ deposits was first observed by Iqbal *et al* in 1989 [64]. They identified the presence of intraneuronal Aβ, by using an antibody against residues 17–24 of Aβ peptide in tissue from AD patients. Importantly, they also observed the presence of these immuno-positive deposits in neurons that preferentially contained NFT [64]. The discovery of the coexistence of amyloid and NFT in the same neuron allowed the development of several lines of research that attempt to show how a protein can induce or accelerate the neurodegenerative process [65]. In 1993, Wertkin and *et. al.* demonstrated that most significantly, the NT2N neurons constitutively generated intracellular Aβ peptide and released it into the culture medium, which demonstrated the intracellular production of Aβ peptide [66]. The presence of mutations in AβPP (AβPPswe), as well as by the duplication of the AβPP gene on chromosome 21 (which has been observed in patients with Down syndrome [67-68]) could be favorable to the accumulation of intracellular amyloid. Although there is evidence to support the assertion that amyloid accumulation precedes the formation of extracellular Aβ deposits and the microtubule-related pathology, the link between Aβ and Tau remains unclear [67-69]. It has also been demonstrated that the pathological accumulation of Aβ and hyperphosphorylation of Tau within synaptic terminals [70] is associated with early changes in MAP2 in neurites and synapses [71]. Finally, the position of soluble oligomers in cellular processes could help to explain their role in the synaptic dysfunction observed in patients with AD [72]. Several reports in the literature have indicated that amyloid can be formed intracellularly [73-75]. Aside from the plasma membrane, it is known that AβPP as well as β- and γ-secretase activity are located in the trans-Golgi network, the endoplasmic reticulum, and the endosomal, lysosomal and mitochondrial membranes. Aβ is generated mostly in the sub-cellular region and then secreted through exocytosis. It has been proposed that production of Aβ42 occurs in the endoplasmic reticulum, while the Aβ40 is formed in the trans-Golgi network. It has also been observed that non-neuronal cells produce both Aβ isoforms on the cell surface [73].

Secreted amyloid forms extracellular deposits and may also be able to enter the cell through transporters and membrane receptors such as the acetylcholine receptor, the low-density lipoprotein receptor (LPR), the N-methyl-D–aspartate receptor (NMDAR), and the scavenger receptor for advanced glycation end products (RAGE) [57, 69]. The interaction between amyloid and these receptors can trigger neurotoxicity and neuronal dysfunction.

1.4. Aβ Toxicity

The neuronal toxicity mediated by Aβ has been documented *in vitro* and in vivo. *In vitro* studies have demonstrated that the direct administration of Aβ to cell cultures has a neurotoxic effect because it increases oxidative stress levels and apoptosis [76-78]. The accumulation of amyloid also leads to proteasomal dysfunction and the consequent accumulation of damaged, misfolded, and aggregated proteins, including Aβ and Tau [79-81]. The reactive oxygen species (ROS) affect membrane proteins, mitochondrial DNA, lipids, and cytoplasmic proteins, and also contribute to the vascular damage observed in AD patients [57, 61, 82-85]. Oxidative stress has been observed in the early stages of AD and has been directly associated with Aβ accumulation. Moreover, $A\beta_{1-42}$, enhanced glutamate toxicity in human cerebral cortical cell cultures and was associated with changes in intracellular Ca^{2+} levels [86].

Importantly, the alterations in these patients were observed in specific brain areas such as the hippocampus, the entorhinal cortex, the amygdala, the neocortex and some sub-cortical areas, such as the cholinergic neurons in the basal forebrain, the serotonergic neurons of the dorsal raphe nucleus and the noradrenergic neurons of the locus coeruleus. The glutamatergic neurons located in the hippocampus and in the frontal, temporal and parietal cortex are severely affected. As we know, the hippocampus and cortex regions are important for the establishment of memory and learning, and so, therefore, the specific loss of glutamatergic neurons could play an important role in the progression of the pathology. Since the 1980's, it has been proposed that Alzheimer's disease may be caused by the over-activity of glutamatergic neurons causing excitotoxic damage in cortical afferent neurons [87-88]. Several studies have shown that Aβ accumulates in certain synapses in micro molar concentrations of Aβ, and has the ability to bind to NMDA receptors, thus inducing the internalization and deregulation of the NMDA signaling pathway [63, 89-91].

2. Glutamatergic system

2.1. Glutamate

Glutamate is a nonessential amino acid that does not cross the blood-brain barrier (BBB), and is produced primarily by neurons and glial cells from local precursors derived from glucose and α-ketoglutarate. Glutamate participates in balance with GABA to modulate the activity of GABAergic and glutamatergic neurons [92]. The majority of excitatory neurons in the CNS are glutamatergic; moreover, it is estimated that over half of nerve-endings release glutamate. Presynaptic depolarization promotes vesicles to release their contents of glutamate into the synapses through exocytosis, where upon the released glutamate binds to post-synaptic ionotropic receptors, stimulating an influx of cations which depolarizes the post-synaptic cell [93]. To prevent over-stimulation, glutamate is removed by astrocytes and converted to L-glutamine through the action of glutamine synthetase, which is released to the extracellular fluid taken up by neurons. Glutamine, normally found in the extracellular space, is, unlike glutamate, a non-toxic molecule and lacks the ability to activate glutamate receptors. The glutamine transferred back to the neuron is recycled by phosphate-activated glutaminase and, once again, forms L-glutamate, which is taken by vesicular transporters into synaptic vesicles to be available for use in the excitatory neurotransmission [93-96]. This trafficking of glutamate and glutamine between astrocytes and neurons is the primary route by which glutamate may be recycled (glutamine–glutamate cycle). The removal of this neurotransmitter from the synaptic cleft is carried out through high-affinity transporters. These transport proteins are the only existing mechanism for extracellular glutamate removal, and are of vital importance in maintaining low and non-toxic concentrations of this neurotransmitter [94]. Both neurons and glial cells express glutamate transporters. Glutamate taken up by cells may be used for metabolic purposes (protein synthesis, energy metabolism, ammonia fixation) or be reused as a neurotransmitter [94]. It is important to clarify that glutamate is not necessarily derived from glutamine nor it is necessarily converted to glutamine by astrocytes, nor does glutamine necessarily acts as a precursor to glutamate. While the mechanisms involved and the resulting metabolites are more complex, they are not mentioned in this chapter.

Glutamate is the major excitatory neurotransmitter in the CNS (approximately 8–10 mM/kg), and is found in more than 80% of all neurons [92, 97-99]. It is involved in most normal brain function, especially in the cortical and hippocampal regions, which deal with cognition, memory and learning [100] among other functions. Glutamate also plays a major role in the development of the central nervous system, as well as synapse induction and elimination, cell migration, differentiation and death [101-102]. Most of the glutamate in the brain is located intracellularly inside nerve terminals and only a tiny fraction of this glutamate is normally present outside or between the cells [103-105]. The extracellular elevation of glutamate causes alterations in the glutamate-mediated neurotransmission, activating receptors and inducing the depolarization of neurons which in turn triggers a sequence of intracellular events that conclude in Ca^{2+} and Na^{2+} influx. This leads to the exocytosis of glutamate and ultimately cell death, which correlates with the loss of memory function and learning ability in AD patients [106-107]. Recently it has been shown that there is a close correlation between reduced glutamatergic presynaptic button density and cognitive deficits. A study of brain tissue from subjects with no cognitive impairment, mild cognitive impairment, or mild/severe-stage Alzheimer's disease; demonstrated that glutamatergic synaptic remodeling, presents a pattern- dependent pathology, according to disease progression by comparing the mini mental status examination scores of healthy individuals to those of individuals with mild or severe Alzheimer's disease [99, 108] (figure 1).

Glutamate excitotoxicity has also been implicated in other neurodegenerative diseases such as Huntington's disease, epilepsy, ischemia, and trauma [109-111]. In this sense, it is crucial to maintain adequate extracellular levels of glutamate, as it is continuously released from the cells and must therefore be continually removed from the extracellular fluid [93-94, 105]. It has been documented that glutamatergic neurotransmission in neocortical regions and the hippocampus is severely disrupted in Alzheimer's disease. So far, it is unknown whether molecular abnormalities observed in patients are a cause or a consequence of other changes that allow the development of neurodegeneration. Another proposed hypothesis is that alterations in the expression of neurotransmitter transporters could contribute to neurotransmission imbalances in the AD brain [112].

2.2. Glutamate transporters

Under normal conditions, the low concentration of glutamate into the extracellular space is regulated by specific transporters, localized in both nerve endings and surrounding glial cells. This transport system prevents cell damage generated by excessive activation of glutamate receptors [105, 112-113]. There are two glutamate transport systems: the Vesicular GluTs (VGLUT) and the Excitatory Amino Acid Transporters (EAAT) located in the plasma membrane. The VGLUTs are crucial for the storage of glutamate in synaptic vesicles. When a neuron is depolarized, glutamate is released into the synaptic cleft where it binds glutamate receptors to pre and post-synaptic neurons. There are three isoforms; VGLUT1, VGLUT2, VGLUT3. The transport of glutamate into secretory vesicles is highly dependent on Cl^- [114]. This anion stimulates glutamate transport, but is inhibitory at higher concentrations. This process is driven by an electrochemical gradient of H^+ established by V-ATPase, which, together with the VGLUT activity, affect vesicular glutamate content and subsequently the glutamatergic signaling [115].

Studies have also identified five different 'high-affinity' glutamate excitatory amino acid (EAATs) transporters (EAAT1, EAAT2, EAAT3, EAAT4 and EAAT5). Residing on postsy-

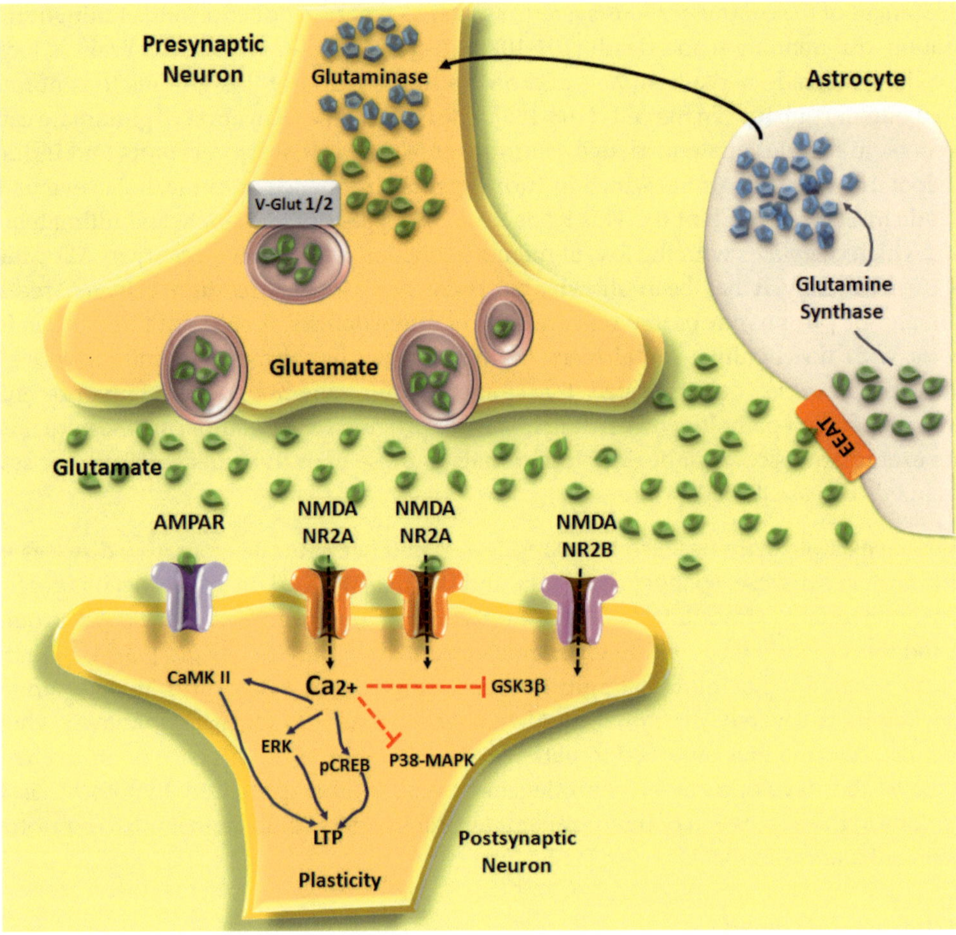

Figure 1. Glutamatergic Transmission in Normal Brain. Glutamate released from presynaptic terminals acts through the activation of glutamate receptors located at the postsynaptic terminal. The interaction between glutamate and NMDA receptor favors the activation of several metabolic pathways such as CaMK, ERK, and CREB, which are responsible for anabolic activation with subsequent activation of long-term potentiation (LTP) mechanisms. Glutamate excess is transported via the EAAT into astrocytes, where is transformed to glutamine by the glutamine synthase. Subsequently, glutamine it is converted into glutamate by glutaminase and packaged into vesicles through specific transporters (VGlut). VGlut (vesicular glutamate transporter); EAAT (excitatory amino acid transporter); NMDANR2A (N-methyl-D-aspartate NR2A subunit); NMDANR2B (N-methyl- D-aspartate NR2B subunit); ERK (extracellular signal-related kinase); CaMKII (calcium calmodulin-dependent kinase II); pCREB (phosphorylated cyclic AMP response element binding protein); GSK3b (glycogen synthase kinase 3b); p38-MAPK (p38 mitogen-activated protein kinase).

naptic GABAergic neurons, EAATs transport glutamate and serve as a precursor for the synthesis of GABA. These two transporter families differ in many of their functional properties, including substrate specificity and ion requirements [113]. EAATs-mediated glutamate transport is Na^+ dependent, where, for each transport cycle, one glutamate molecule is transported together with two or three Na^+ ions and one H^+ in exchange for one K^+ ion. These transporters also interact with other proteins at the plasma membrane and are regulated by protein kinases, growth factors and second messengers [116-117]. Alterations in this regulatory

http://dx.doi.org/10.5772/57367

system as well as genetic mutation in the transporters and enzymes involved in the glutamate metabolism can lead to excitotoxic damage due to an excessive release of glutamate, which in turn can lead to neuronal death.

2.3. Glutamate receptors

Glutamate-mediated neurotransmission occurs through specific receptors. There are 2 families of glutamate receptors located on the plasma membrane of the neurons: ionotropic (iGluR) glutamate receptors, which act as ion channels, and metabotropic (mGluR) glutamate receptors which are linked to the intracellular second messenger systems [92, 99, 118-119].

The iGluR family is divided into three kinds of receptors, depending on their permeability to different cations. NMDA receptors (NR1, NR2A–D and NR3A–B) are predominantly Ca^{2+} ion permeable, whereas α-amino-3-hydroxy-5-methyl-4-isoxazolepropionic acid (AMPA; GluR1–4) and Kainate (KA; GluR5–7, KA1–2) receptors are predominantly permeable to Na^{+} and K^{+} ions [99, 120]. Each of these receptors is composed of four subunits, and variations in the expression of each subunit have different types of response in the receptor function [92, 119]. AMPA receptors have a lower affinity for Glutamate than NMDA receptors, and are responsible for an initial excitatory potential when Glutamate is present in the synapse [92]. Kainate receptors play a role in synaptic neurotransmission, but the exact nature of this role is unclear [119].

NMDA and AMPA receptors are present in most of the synapses in mammalian brains (approximately 70%). This type of receptor is preferentially localized in the cerebral cortex, hippocampus, amygdala, striatum, and septum. The specific location of these receptors is of great importance, since glutamatergic signaling has a very important role in both the plasticity and excitotoxicity processes, and, therefore, changes in their function lead to the development of neurodegenerative processes.

The NMDA receptor is the most important and studied ionotropic receptor to date, and participates in several functions such as synaptogenesis, synaptic plasticity, learning and memory, as well as in the pathogenesis of several central nervous system disorders [121-123]. Calcium influx through the NMDA receptor is capable of modulating physiological and pathological conditions in the neuron. The increase in intracellular Ca^{2+} concentration triggers a cascade of events that dramatically modifies synaptic efficacy and neuronal morphology. Functional NMDA receptors are heterotetrameric complexes composed of different subunits (GluN1, GluN2A-D, GluN3A-B). Typically, each NMDAR comprises two obligatory GluN1 subunits and two GluN2 subunits, which can a form a dimer themselves, or alternatively one GluN2 can combine with one GluN3 subunit to do the same [121, 123-124]. GluN1 occurs as eight distinct isoforms encoded by a single gene [125]. The functional significance of the differential expression of GluN1 isoforms is not clear. GluN2 and GluN3 also exist in several alternatively spliced forms, although the functional differences between them are complex. There are four genes encoding GluN2 subunits and each has a unique spatiotemporal profile. In addition, GluN2A and GluN2B are expressed primarily in the cortex and hippocampus and differ in their kinetic properties, developmental expression pattern, subcellular localization and trafficking regulation. GluN3 subunits also display differential expression patterns, with

GluN3A peaking in early postnatal life and GluN3B increasing throughout development [123]. Finally, although receptor subunits have structural similarities, the composition of the different receptor subtypes confer distinct functional and biophysical properties that are reflected in the ion permeability, protein interactions and membrane localization (synaptic or extrasynaptic). They may also have different roles in modulating synaptic plasticity and development of pathologies [122-123]. In fact, the expression of individual subunits is highly dependent on brain area and developmental stage, thus, alterations in the expression of each subunit can lead to a pathological condition which may be reflected in the development of neurodegenerative diseases.

2.4. Glutamate/NMDAR: Role in learning and memory

In the CNS, it is known that the hippocampus is closely related to learning and memory, and has a very high density of glutamate receptors, particularly the NMDA-type, which are significantly involved in this type of neuronal plasticity. Glutamate is essential for the establishment of new neural networks, forming memory and learning through a process known as long-term potentiation (LTP) or long-term depression (LTD) of synaptic strength, which occurs upon activation of NMDA receptors.

NMDA receptors are characterized by their high Ca^{2+} ions' permeability, their voltage dependent blockade by Mg2+ ions, and their slower gating kinetics. At rest, the NMDA receptor is blocked by Mg^{2+}, while prolonged activation by the presence of glutamate allows the release of the Mg^{2+}, opening the NMDA receptor and allowing the Ca^{2+} ions to freely enter into postsynaptic neuron. Calcium entering through the NMDA receptors activates CaMKII, PKA, PKC and mitogen-activated protein kinase (MAPK), and protein phosphatases. Activated CaMKII phosphorylates the AMPA-type glutamate receptor 1 (GluR1) subunit, which, in turn, promotes synaptic incorporation of GluR1-containing AMPARs, thereby increasing AMPAR number and channel conductance [107, 121, 126]. The fundamental role of the NMDA-receptor system in the establishment of learning and memory has been demonstrated in various animal models [127-131]. However, pharmacological studies and the manipulation of experimental models have shown that, although this system is important in memory induction, it does not participate in the maintenance of memory [132-135] (figure 1).

These features make NMDA receptors quite suitable for mediating plastic changes in the brain, such as learning. However, they may also contribute to the excitotoxicity processes produced by a massive influx of Ca^{2+}. Under these conditions, the continuous presence of glutamate induces constant activation of the NMDA receptor, and the ensuing massive influx of Ca^{2+} may trigger a cascade of events leading to neuronal injury and death[136]. Chronic depolarization of the membrane on vulnerable neurons, as observed in AD patients, is accompanied by other disorders such as neuronal oxidative stress, mitochondrial damage, and inflammation, and the presence of amyloid beta and possibly hyperphosphorylated-tau, which may eventually increase the sensitivity of the glutamatergic system and result in neuronal dysfunction and cell death [97, 106-107].

2.5. Neurotoxicity of Aβ: Synaptic dysfunction in AD

Aside from the above toxic effects, it is known that amyloid has the ability to inhibit normal function of the glutamatergic system. It can also interact with glutamine synthetase (GS) to induce the inactivation of the enzyme [137], chronically depolarize neurons through its action on the metabotropic glutamate receptor 1 [138], and partially relieve the voltage-dependent Mg^{2+} block of NMDA receptors, which allows the continuous entry of calcium into neurons by altering the homeostasis and thus causing cell death. This also causes that neurons to express NMDA receptors selectively and become vulnerable to glutamatergic stimulation. In AD patients, it has been observed that glutamatergic transmission is severely affected by neurons in the cortex and hippocampus (Figure 2).

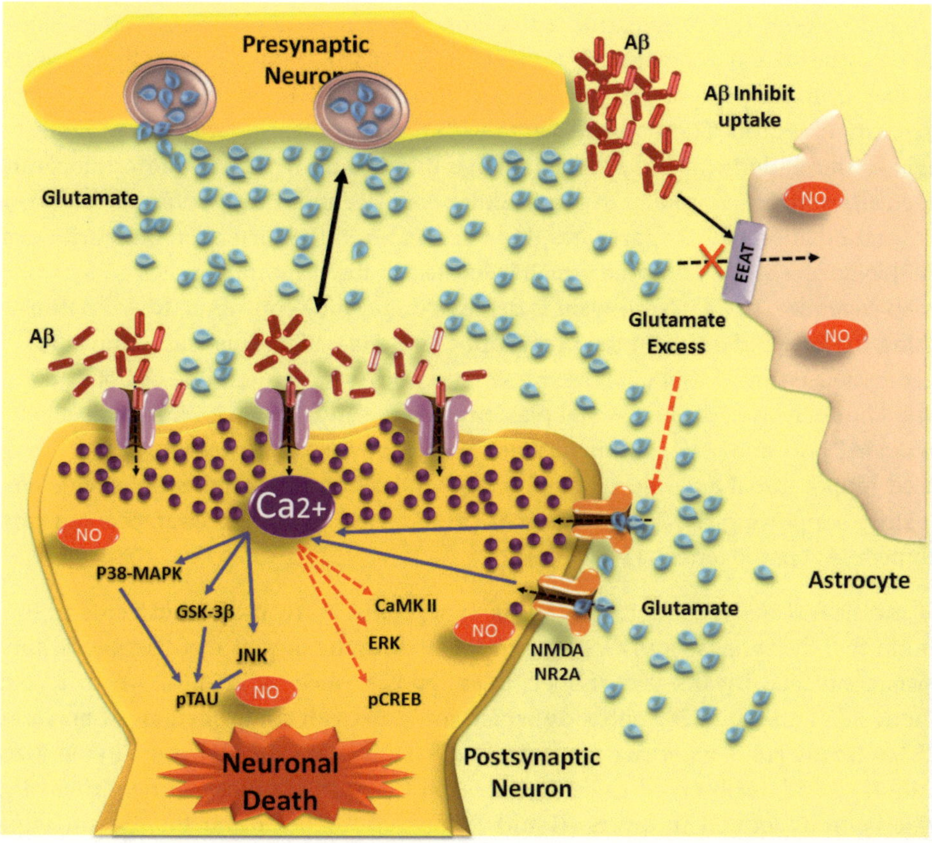

Figure 2. Glutamatergic transmission in Alzheimer's disease. Aβ oligomers enhance the pre-synaptic release of glutamate together with the simultaneous blockade of glutamate uptake by astrocytes through glutamate transporters (EAAT), due to this, glutamate concentration in synaptic cleft increases. In addition, Aβ form complexes with alpha7-nicotinic receptors, increasing levels of glutamate release. Activation of NMDA receptors increases the influx of calcium and activates signaling pathways responsible for neuronal shrinkage and synaptic loss (p38-MbAPK, GSK-3b, JNK), leading to Tau phosphorylation and neuronal death. Finally, there is an inhibition of the survival pathways (CAMK II, ERK, pCREB).

Neurochemical analysis performed on tissue from patients with AD revealed deficits in numerous neurotransmitters. Early symptoms appear to correlate with dysfunction of cholinergic and glutamatergic synapses. Furthermore, morphometric studies of temporal and frontal cortical biopsies from AD have revealed that there is a 25-30% decrease in the density of synapses. In the same way, it has been observed that the degree of cognitive impairment observed correlates with changes in the protein synaptophysin in the hippocampus. In fact, it has also been shown that the presence of soluble amyloid correlates with cognitive deficits and synapse loss [139-140].

In 2005, Kokubo *et al* investigated the ultrastructural localization of soluble Aβ oligomers in human brain tissue. They used post-embedding immunoelectron microscopy (IEM) [72] and an antibody that specifically recognizes soluble oligomers [141]. The results showed that approximately 80% of oligomers are found in active cellular processes. In addition, oligomers were found in both the presynaptic active zone and in postsynaptic densities, and their presence may be related to synaptic dysfunction [72]. This might suggest that the Aβ oligomers are released from the presynaptic site into extracellular space or are synaptically transported from neuron to neuron. These results agree with the hypothesis that the oligomerization of Aβ begins intracellularly [50]. The amyloid that is released from presynaptic terminals and not degraded efficiently accumulates in extracellular deposits and could serve as a seed to induce further accumulation of Aβ aggregates that culminates in the formation of neuritic plaques [142-143]. Neprilysin is an enzyme which is located in the presynaptic sites and participates in the Aβ clearance. In AD, Neprilysin is decreased and may contribute to AD pathogenesis increasing the amyloid levels in the presynaptic sites [144-145]. This was demonstrated in a transgenic mouse model that expressed low levels of APP and had one or both NEP genes silenced. The analysis of the brains and plasma in young and old mice showed elevated levels of human Aβ1-40 and Aβ1-42, an increase in Aβ dimer concentration, and a markedly increased hippocampal amyloid plaque burden, and led to development of severe amyloid angiopathy, supporting the hypothesis that primary defects in Aβ clearance can cause or contribute to AD pathogenesis [146].

In 2012, Koffie *et al* analyzed more than 50,000 synapses in 11 AD brains and 5 control subjects, and found that the synapse loss directly correlated with the presence of oligomeric amyloid. This was confirmed by the use of specific antibodies, such as NAB61, which recognizes oligomeric Aβ, and the R1282 antibody which recognizes all conformations of amyloid and the 82E1 antibody [147]. Extensive neuronal loss is another important feature in the Alzheimer's pathology and, is observed as being restricted to the cell bodies and dendrites of glutamatergic neurons located in layers III and IV of the neocortex and the glutamatergically innervated cortical and hippocampal neurons [38, 148].

The mechanism by which Aβ oligomers induce synaptic dysfunction remains unknown; however, it has been proposed that this alteration in synaptic transmission may be performed through non-excitotoxic glutamatergic mechanisms [149]. In this way, the accumulation of Aβ oligomers in synaptic components, especially in the axon terminal, results in synaptic and cognitive dysfunction seen in AD [72].

2.6. Animal models in AD and synaptic dysfunction

Several studies have shown that amyloid oligomers – both synthetic [150] and those isolated from the brains of patients [63] – have the ability to induce synaptic alterations in neuronal cultures and organotypic hippocampal slice cultures. The transgenic mice models that express different APP mutated forms show extensive neuritic dystrophy and loss of synapses, important features that suggest a neurodegenerative process. In this way, it has been suggested that Aβ oligomers could modulate both pre and post-synaptic structures and functions in a dose and assembly-dependent manner [151-152]. The results indicate that protofibrils and oligomeric forms of Aβ most likely generate neuronal death through a nucleation-dependent process rather than acting as direct neurotoxic ligands [153]. In 2008, Shankar and colleagues showed that the presence of Aβ oligomers in slice cultures blocked the LTP, while NP-derived aggregates had no effect unless they were treated with formic acid. The oligomers potently inhibited long-term potentiation (LTP), enhanced long-term depression (LTD), and reduced dendritic spine density in a normal rodent hippocampus [154].

Animal models overexpressing hAβPP protein also show a decrease in synaptophysin-positive presynaptic terminals, approximately 30% less than that observed in non-transgenic mice. Is important to note that these decreases in presynaptic terminals are dependent on soluble amyloid levels rather than on plaques *per se* [63, 152, 154-156], which would also explain the cognitive deficits observed. In a triple transgenic mice model which presented PS1(M146V), APP(Swe), and tau(P301L) transgenes (3xTg-AD), it was possible to show that the intraneuronal amyloid deposition correlates with the cognitive deficits observed in these mice. At six months, the 3xTg-AD mice showed a profound LTP deficit and intraneuronal Aβ accumulation occurring within pyramidal neurons. This cognitive deficit occurs before the accumulation of extracellular amyloid aggregates, suggesting that cognitive impairment occurs before the formation of neuritic plaques [157-160]. The synaptic dysfunction, including LTP deficits and cognitive alteration manifests in an age-related manner [157].

Moreover, it has also been observed that Aβ oligomers bind to high-affinity cell-surface receptors (cellular prion protein or PrP(C) and block hippocampal long-term potentiation and dendritic spine retraction from pyramidal cells at nanomolar concentrations of oligomers. Anti-PrP antibodies prevent the Aβ-oligomer from binding to PrPC and rescue synaptic plasticity in hippocampal slices from oligomeric Aβ [161]. Other studies also have shown that Aβ/PrPC interaction leads to activation of Fyn kinase. PrPC /Fyn signaling yields phosphorylation of the NR2B subunit of NMDA receptors, which is coupled with an initial increase and then a loss of surface NMDA-receptors. Thus, Aβ generates changes in GluR function and dendritic spine anatomy. Additionally, Fyn activation might suggest correlation with Tau pathology and the epileptiform phenotype observed in some patients with AD [162]. In this sense, it has been reported that oligomers of Aβ lead the activation of AMPK. The increased intracellular Ca^{2+} induced by membrane depolarization or NMDA receptor activation triggers AMP-activated kinase (AMPK) activation in a CAMKK2-dependent manner. CAMKK2 or AMPK overactivation is sufficient to induce dendritic spine loss [163]. The roles of AMPK in the pathogenesis of AD include β-amyloid protein (Aβ) generation and tau phosphorylation [164]. AMPK phosphorylates Tau in S262, while expression of Tau S262A inhibits the synaptotoxic effects of Aβ42 oligomers, which suggests that the CAMKK2-AMPK-Tau pathway could be a critical mediator of the synaptotoxic effects of Aβ42 oligomers [163]

Dendritic spines are certainly the sites with more excitatory synapses, and their loss correlates with the cognitive impairment observed in Alzheimer's patients [165]. A large body of evidence suggests that amyloid oligomers may cause loss of dendritic spines [47, 166-172]. The exposure of cultured pyramidal neurons to Aβ oligomers showed decreased synaptic activity and a decrease in the density of dendritic spines [154]. Multiphoton imaging of GFP-labeled neurons in living Tg2576 APP mice showed disrupted neurite trajectories and reductions in dendritic spine density compared with age-matched control mice. Spine loss is most pronounced near plaques, indicating focal toxicity and also that the decrease in the density of dendritic spines may contribute to the altered neuronal function observed in these mice [166]. It has also been found that Aβ trimmers fully inhibit LTP, whereas dimers and tetramers have an intermediate potency and support the hypothesis that diffusible oligomers of Aβ initiate a synaptic dysfunction that may be an early event in AD [173]. It is known that the presence of oligomers of Aβ induces the loss of synapses, although little is known whether synapse loss precedes or follows plaque formation. In 2012, Bittner *et al* conducted an *in vivo* study using two-photon microscopy through a cranial window in double transgenic APPPS mice. Using this technique, they observed the manner in which the amyloid is deposited to form neuritic plaques and determined the loss of dendritic spines in the vicinity of these deposits. They found that the rate of dendritic spine loss in proximity to plaques is the same in both young and older animals. The plaque size only increases in young animals, while spine loss persists even many months after the initial appearance of the plaque. Finally, they found that spine loss occurs, with a significant time delay, after the birth of new plaques, and persists in the vicinity of amyloid plaques over many months [168].

A key aspect that determines the functionality of dendritic spines is their morphology. It is known that Calcineurin (CaN) activation is critically involved in regulating both the morphology of the spines in response to oligomeric Aβ, and the synaptic plasticity in normal memory. When adding oligomers derived from Tg2576 murine transgenic neurons or human AD brains to wild-type murine primary cortical neurons, CaN activation in spines was observed and led to rapid but reversible morphological changes in spines and postsynaptic proteins, suggesting that Calcineurin might have an important role in regulating the synaptic alterations associated with Alzheimer's disease [174]. Finally, it has been shown that APP has an important role in regulating synaptic and structure function. Analysis of dendritic spines in the primary cultures of hippocampal neurons and the CA1 neurons of hippocampi of APP $^{-/-}$ mice showed a significant decrease in spine density (35%), compared to control cultures. This spine loss was partially restored with sAPPα-conditioned medium. These abnormalities in neuronal morphology were also accompanied by a reduction in long-term potentiation. These results suggest that sAPPα is necessary for the maintenance of dendritic integrity in the hippocampus [172].

The changes in dendritic spines observed in various diseases impact heavily on synapse function and circuit-level connectivity in the form of altered connectivity or changes in connection strength [175]. Changes in the number and morphology of the spines can start a cascade of symptoms and effects that lead to the pathological changes observed in Alzheimer's disease.

2.7. Aβ and synaptic plasticity

Although for many years the theory has been maintained that beta amyloid deposits are the main factor in AD pathology, recent years have seen an increase in the evidence pointing to the fact that its accumulation in certain brain regions may participate importantly in memory and cognition [176]. This dual concept of amyloid, where, at low doses it can positively stimulate the normal physiological processes of the cells, and at high doses it can cause toxic effects has also been observed in a very large number of molecules. This idea has been strongly supported by the observation that APP knock-out mice show long-term potentiation (LTP) and memory impairment [44, 177]. Glutamate, the main excitatory neurotransmitter is undoubtedly another example, as it is known that at low doses, it has the ability to stimulate synaptic plasticity and memory [178], while at high doses it is toxic and favors the development of several neurodegenerative diseases.

We have already mentioned that the amyloid is generated the proteolytic processing of APP through the action of β-and γ-secretases. In recent years, it has been reported that these enzymes are involved in memory and synaptic plasticity. In 2004, Saura and colleagues developed conditional double knockout mice lacking the expression of both presenilins in the postnatal forebrain. The results showed impairments in hippocampal memory and synaptic plasticity. These alterations are associated with decreases in NMDA receptor-mediated responses and the synaptic levels of NMDA receptors and αCaMKII. Also, a decrease was observed in the expression of CBP and CREB/CBP target genes, such as *c-fos* and BDNF, while, increased levels of the Cdk5 activator p25 and hyperphosphorylated Tau were also observed. Finally, these mice develop a process of neurodegeneration, which increases with age. These results indicate that the inhibition of presenilin could accelerate memory loss and neurodegeneration [179]. Other trials have suggested that synaptic plasticity and memory depend on BACE1-mediated APP processing, which may facilitate memory and synaptic plasticity [180]. In the same way, BACE1 null mice exhibit alterations in hippocampal synaptic plasticity as well as in their performance in tests of cognition and emotion [181]. Recently it has been suggested that concentrations of picomolar amyloid are capable of inducing synaptic plasticity and memory in the hippocampus, and that the exposure of amyloid to Aß did not affect the NMDA receptor. The action mechanism of picomolar Aβ42 on synaptic plasticity and memory involves α7-nicotinic acetylcholine receptors [44], suggesting that Aβ42 may be an important modulator of synaptic plasticity and memory in the normal brain. Furthermore it has been observed that many of the effects on amyloid NMDA receptors can be blocked by antagonists of this receptor.

3. Glutamatergic system-targeted treatment in Alzheimer's disease: Focus on memantine

Aβ peptide is able to interact with a whole variety of proteins [97], and this interaction may cause dysfunction of the protein to which Aβ is binding. One group of proteins with which Aβ is able to interact is the glutamatergic NMDA receptors. Texidó *et al.* [182] showed that the Aβ peptide directly binds and activates NMDA receptors expressed in *Xenopus laevis* oocytes, thereby causing an increase in cytosolic calcium concentration. These results are coincident with previous results by McDermott *et al.* [183], who reported increased calcium intracellular concentration in spinal cord mouse neuron cultures, after adding NMDA. Cytosolic calcium overload causes mitochondrial dysfunction and leads to an increase in ROS production, which in turn generates oxidative stress and leads to cell death [184]. For these reasons, the idea was born that NMDAR antagonists could be a promising therapeutic target in AD treatment.

Among all the known NMDAR antagonists, the most widely studied and used in the treatment of AD is the molecule known as memantine. Memantine (1-amine-3, 5, dimethyladamantane) was first synthesized in 1963 [185]. The drug is a derivative of amantadine, an antiviral used in influenza treatment. Like amantadine, memantine has a three ring structure, with an amine group and two methyl groups [186]. Memantine NMDAR antagonist properties remained unknown until Kornhuber et al. [187] reported that memantine had the same properties and same binding site of the well known NMDAR antagonist MK-801. Chen and Lipton [186] observed that memantine affinity towards NMDA receptors was sensitive to NMDA concentration, leading to the conclusion that memantine NMDA receptor antagonism is uncompetitive. It is this uncompetitivity and the fact that his binding is voltage-dependent which makes memantine an effective and safe therapeutic agent. For memantine to be able to exhibit its inhibitory activity, the receptor channel must be in an open state. Memantine blocks NMDAR activity by entering and binding to the cation pore, thus preventing cation flux and inhibiting functional NMDAR activity. Memantine binding to the receptor is voltage-dependant, in such a way that it leaves the channel pore in depolarization conditions, i.e. during excitatory postsynaptic potential, this way allowing synaptic activity to be maintained [188].

Memantine disease-modifying efficacy and safety has been proven in many studies. Most assays using a variety of AD animal models have lead to promising results. Minkeviciene et al. [189] showed that a 4 week oral treatment with memantine (via drinking water) improved the performance in the Morris water maze of mice carrying both a human APP transgene with the Swedish mutation and a human PS1 transgene with the A246E mutation, when compared with placebo-treated mice. In fact, this study showed that memantine-treated transgenic mice performed well in the water maze as well as WT mice, thus revealing a complete rescue of cognitive function due to memantine. Surprisingly, a later study [190] using this same mouse model did not find an effect of memantine treatment on performance in the Morris water maze, but memantine-treated mice performed better in a left-right discrimination task when compared with placebo-treated mice. Another study [191], which used heterozygous APP23 mice (mice carrying one copy of a human APP transgene with the Swedish mutation), reported an increase in spatial accuracy of memantine-treated mice in the Morris water maze, as measured by the time mice spent in the target quadrant of the maze. However, in this study, memantine failed to decrease escape latency (time that takes to mice to reach the target platform of the maze). Martínez-Coria et al. [192], using 3x-TgAD mice (mice that express simultaneously a human APP transgene carrying the Swedish mutation, a PS1 gene carrying the M146V mutation and a human tau transgene carrying a P301L mutation), showed that treatment with memantine caused a significant improvement in mice performance in the

Morris water maze, in an object recognition task and in a passive avoidance task, showing that memantine has an effect on different types of memory.

In contrast, few studies have failed in obtaining a significant cognitive function improvement after memantine treatment. Dong et al. [193], using Tg2576 mice (which also express the Swedish mutation), did not find any treatment effect in a conditioned fear experiment after six months of daily memantine administration. Interestingly, histological analysis revealed that the memantine-treated group exhibited less Aβ plaque deposition, less axonal degeneration and increased synaptic density, when compared with the placebo-treated group.

Because memantine appeared to be effective and safe in animal model assays, clinical trials soon began to be developed. In general, results from these trials showed a modest effect increasing the preservation of cognitive function. Rive et al. [194] classified a group of 252 AD patients in "autonomous" or "dependant" according to their punctuation by the ADCS-ADL (Alzheimer's Disease Cooperative Study-Activities of Daily Living) scale and found that, after a 28-week treatment with memantine or placebo, memantine-treated patients had 3 times more probability of remaining autonomous than placebo-treated patients. Peskind et al. [195] measured the outcomes of 403 AD patients for the ADAS-cog (Alzheimer's Disease Assessment Scale-cognitive subscale), the CIBIC-Plus (Clinician's Interview-Based Impression of Change-Plus caregiver input) scale and the NPI (Neuro-Psychiatric Inventory) scale. Measurements were taken at the beginning of the study and after 24 weeks of memantine or placebo treatment. Results showed that memantine-treated patients exhibited better performance in all of these scales, when compared to placebo treated patients. Another study [196] showed that after 24 weeks of treatment with memantine or placebo, memantine-treated AD patients exhibited significantly slower cognitive decline compared with those treated with placebo, as measured by the SIB (Severe Impairment Battery). Memantine also showed to be moderately effective in the improvement of semantic memory. The study by Ferris et al. [197] found a significant amelioration of language impairment (assessed by the language subscale of the SIB) in AD patients after 28 weeks of memantine treatment. Another study [18] followed 295 AD patients receiving memantine or placebo during 52 weeks. Their results show that memantine-treated patients scored 1.2 points higher in the MMSE (Mini-Mental State Examination) than placebo treated patients.

4. Conclusion

All the aforementioned results point out that memantine is a safe disease-modifying drug to use in AD treatment, and its effectiveness has turned out to be slight, but significant, and comparable to that of other AD treatment drugs, such as cholinesterase inhibitors. Clinical trials in order to assess the effectiveness of combined treatment of memantine with other drugs are currently being implemented.

Finally, studies reported in the literature suggest that Aβ, the glutamatergic system, and in particular NMDA receptors have a major role in the processes of learning and memory. Synaptic plasticity can be regulated positively or negatively, depending on the levels and degrees of amyloid oligomerization. The negative effect of these oligomeric forms may be reversed by the presence of NMDA receptor antagonists. In this regard, it has been reported that the noncompetitive antagonist memantine is able to block the "pathological" receptor activation exerted by these oligomers. In this view, an early pharmacological treatment with memantine, or even a memantine associated treatment combined with AChE inhibitors, might represent a very good option for the treatment of patients with AD.

Author details

Victoria Campos-Peña[1] and Marco Antonio Meraz-Ríos[1*]

*Address all correspondence to: mmeraz@cinvestav.mx

1 Laboratorio Experimental de Enfermedades Neurodegenerativas, Instituto Nacional de Neurología y Neurocirugía, Manuel Velasco Suárez, México City, México

Departamento de Biomedicina Molecular, Centro de Investigación y de Estudios Avanzados del IPN, (CINVESTAV-IPN), México City, México

References

[1] Borchelt, D.R., et al., Familial Alzheimer's disease-linked presenilin 1 variants elevate Abeta1-42/1-40 ratio in vitro and in vivo. Neuron, 1996. 17(5): p. 1005-13.

[2] Chartier-Harlin, M.C., et al., Screening for the beta-amyloid precursor protein mutation (APP717: Val----Ile) in extended pedigrees with early onset Alzheimer's disease. Neurosci Lett, 1991. 129(1): p. 134-5.

[3] Duff, K., et al., Increased amyloid-beta42(43) in brains of mice expressing mutant presenilin 1. Nature, 1996. 383(6602): p. 710-3.

[4] Levy-Lahad, E., et al., A familial Alzheimer's disease locus on chromosome 1. Science, 1995. 269(5226): p. 970-3.

[5] Murrell, J., et al., A mutation in the amyloid precursor protein associated with hereditary Alzheimer's disease. Science, 1991. 254(5028): p. 97-9.

[6] Sisodia, S.S., S.H. Kim, and G. Thinakaran, Function and dysfunction of the presenilins. Am J Hum Genet, 1999. 65(1): p. 7-12.

[7] Pigino, G., et al., Alzheimer's presenilin 1 mutations impair kinesin-based axonal transport. J Neurosci, 2003. 23(11): p. 4499-508.

[8] Sherrington, R., et al., Alzheimer's disease associated with mutations in presenilin 2 is rare and variably penetrant. Hum Mol Genet, 1996. 5(7): p. 985-8.

[9] Sherrington, R., et al., Cloning of a gene bearing missense mutations in early-onset familial Alzheimer's disease. Nature, 1995. 375(6534): p. 754-60.

[10] Kowalska, A., Amyloid precursor protein gene mutations responsible for early-onset autosomal dominant Alzheimer's disease. Folia Neuropathol, 2003. 41(1): p. 35-40.

[11] Corder, E.H., et al., Gene dose of apolipoprotein E type 4 allele and the risk of Alzheimer's disease in late onset families. Science, 1993. 261(5123): p. 921-3.

[12] Schupf, N. and G.H. Sergievsky, Genetic and host factors for dementia in Down's syndrome. Br J Psychiatry, 2002. 180: p. 405-10.

[13] Tang, M.X., et al., Relative risk of Alzheimer disease and age-at-onset distributions, based on APOE genotypes among elderly African Americans, Caucasians, and Hispanics in New York City. Am J Hum Genet, 1996. 58(3): p. 574-84.

[14] Zahs, K.R. and K.H. Ashe, beta-Amyloid oligomers in aging and Alzheimer's disease. Front Aging Neurosci, 2013. 5: p. 28.

[15] Chen, J.H., K.P. Lin, and Y.C. Chen, Risk factors for dementia. J Formos Med Assoc, 2009. 108(10): p. 754-64.

[16] de la Torre, J.C., How do heart disease and stroke become risk factors for Alzheimer's disease? Neurol Res, 2006. 28(6): p. 637-44.

[17] Holscher, C., Diabetes as a risk factor for Alzheimer's disease: insulin signalling impairment in the brain as an alternative model of Alzheimer's disease. Biochem Soc Trans, 2011. 39(4): p. 891-7.

[18] Goedert, M., et al., Cloning and sequencing of the cDNA encoding a core protein of the paired helical filament of Alzheimer disease: identification as the microtubule-associated protein tau. Proc Natl Acad Sci U S A, 1988. 85(11): p. 4051-5.

[19] Jakes, R., et al., Identification of 3- and 4-repeat tau isoforms within the PHF in Alzheimer's disease. EMBO J, 1991. 10(10): p. 2725-9.

[20] Wischik, C.M., et al., Structural characterization of the core of the paired helical filament of Alzheimer disease. Proc Natl Acad Sci U S A, 1988. 85(13): p. 4884-8.

[21] Wischik, C.M., et al., Isolation of a fragment of tau derived from the core of the paired helical filament of Alzheimer disease. Proc Natl Acad Sci U S A, 1988. 85(12): p. 4506-10.

[22] Iversen, L.L., et al., The toxicity in vitro of beta-amyloid protein. Biochem J, 1995. 311 (Pt 1): p. 1-16.

[23] Glenner, G.G., et al., The amyloid deposits in Alzheimer's disease: their nature and pathogenesis. Appl Pathol, 1984. 2(6): p. 357-69.

[24] Selkoe, D.J., Alzheimer's disease: a central role for amyloid. J Neuropathol Exp Neurol, 1994. 53(5): p. 438-47.

[25] Kang, J., et al., The precursor of Alzheimer's disease amyloid A4 protein resembles a cell-surface receptor. Nature, 1987. 325(6106): p. 733-6.

[26] Samuel, W., et al., Hippocampal connectivity and Alzheimer's dementia: effects of synapse loss and tangle frequency in a two-component model. Neurology, 1994. 44(11): p. 2081-8.

[27] Arriagada, P.V., et al., Neurofibrillary tangles but not senile plaques parallel duration and severity of Alzheimer's disease. Neurology, 1992. 42(3 Pt 1): p. 631-9.

[28] Giannakopoulos, P., et al., Tangle and neuron numbers, but not amyloid load, predict cognitive status in Alzheimer's disease. Neurology, 2003. 60(9): p. 1495-500.

[29] Serrano-Pozo, A., et al., Neuropathological alterations in Alzheimer disease. Cold Spring Harb Perspect Med, 2011. 1(1): p. a006189.

[30] Puzzo, D. and O. Arancio, Fibrillar beta-amyloid impairs the late phase of long term potentiation. Curr Alzheimer Res, 2006. 3(3): p. 179-83.

[31] Puzzo, D., A. Palmeri, and O. Arancio, Involvement of the nitric oxide pathway in synaptic dysfunction following amyloid elevation in Alzheimer's disease. Rev Neurosci, 2006. 17(5): p. 497-523.

[32] Prasansuklab, A. and T. Tencomnao, Amyloidosis in Alzheimer's Disease: The Toxicity of Amyloid Beta (A beta), Mechanisms of Its Accumulation and Implications of Medicinal Plants for Therapy. Evid Based Complement Alternat Med, 2013. 2013: p. 413808.

[33] Manczak, M. and P.H. Reddy, Abnormal Interaction of Oligomeric Amyloid-beta with Phosphorylated Tau: Implications to Synaptic Dysfunction and Neuronal Damage. J Alzheimers Dis, 2013. 36(2): p. 285-95.

[34] Reddy, P.H., Amyloid beta-induced glycogen synthase kinase 3beta phosphorylated VDAC1 in Alzheimer's disease: Implications for synaptic dysfunction and neuronal damage. Biochim Biophys Acta, 2013.

[35] Magdesian, M.H., et al., Amyloid-beta binds to the extracellular cysteine-rich domain of Frizzled and inhibits Wnt/beta-catenin signaling. J Biol Chem, 2008. 283(14): p. 9359-68.

[36] Supnet, C. and I. Bezprozvanny, The dysregulation of intracellular calcium in Alzheimer disease. Cell Calcium, 2010. 47(2): p. 183-9.

[37] Supnet, C. and I. Bezprozvanny, Neuronal calcium signaling, mitochondrial dysfunction, and Alzheimer's disease. J Alzheimers Dis, 2010. 20 Suppl 2: p. S487-98.

[38] Hynd, M.R., H.L. Scott, and P.R. Dodd, Glutamate-mediated excitotoxicity and neurodegeneration in Alzheimer's disease. Neurochem Int, 2004. 45(5): p. 583-95.

[39] Crimins, J.L., et al., The intersection of amyloid beta and tau in glutamatergic synaptic dysfunction and collapse in Alzheimer's disease. Ageing Res Rev, 2013.

[40] Boehm, J., A 'danse macabre': tau and Fyn in STEP with amyloid beta to facilitate induction of synaptic depression and excitotoxicity. Eur J Neurosci, 2013. 37(12): p. 1925-30.

[41] Robakis, N.K., et al., Chromosome 21q21 sublocalisation of gene encoding beta-amyloid peptide in cerebral vessels and neuritic (senile) plaques of people with Alzheimer disease and Down syndrome. Lancet, 1987. 1(8529): p. 384-5.

[42] Yoshikai, S., et al., Genomic organization of the human-amyloid beta-protein precursor gene. Gene, 1991. 102(2): p. 291-2.

[43] Jarrett, J.T., E.P. Berger, and P.T. Lansbury, Jr., The carboxy terminus of the beta amyloid protein is critical for the seeding of amyloid formation: implications for the pathogenesis of Alzheimer's disease. Biochemistry, 1993. 32(18): p. 4693-7.

[44] Puzzo, D., et al., Picomolar amyloid-beta positively modulates synaptic plasticity and memory in hippocampus. J Neurosci, 2008. 28(53): p. 14537-45.

[45] Lambert, M.P., et al., Diffusible, nonfibrillar ligands derived from Abeta1-42 are potent central nervous system neurotoxins. Proc Natl Acad Sci U S A, 1998. 95(11): p. 6448-53.

[46] Walsh, D.M. and D.J. Selkoe, Oligomers on the brain: the emerging role of soluble protein aggregates in neurodegeneration. Protein Pept Lett, 2004. 11(3): p. 213-28.

[47] Lacor, P.N., et al., Abeta oligomer-induced aberrations in synapse composition, shape, and density provide a molecular basis for loss of connectivity in Alzheimer's disease. J Neurosci, 2007. 27(4): p. 796-807.

[48] Cuello, A.C., Intracellular and extracellular Abeta, a tale of two neuropathologies. Brain Pathol, 2005. 15(1): p. 66-71.

[49] Selkoe, D.J., et al., The role of APP processing and trafficking pathways in the formation of amyloid beta-protein. Ann N Y Acad Sci, 1996. 777: p. 57-64.

[50] Walsh, D.M., et al., The oligomerization of amyloid beta-protein begins intracellularly in cells derived from human brain. Biochemistry, 2000. 39(35): p. 10831-9.

[51] Lesne, S.E., et al., Brain amyloid-beta oligomers in ageing and Alzheimer's disease. Brain, 2013. 136(Pt 5): p. 1383-98.

[52] Tomiyama, T., et al., A mouse model of amyloid beta oligomers: their contribution to synaptic alteration, abnormal tau phosphorylation, glial activation, and neuronal loss in vivo. J Neurosci, 2010. 30(14): p. 4845-56.

[53] Yamamoto, N., et al., GM1-ganglioside-induced Abeta assembly on synaptic membranes of cultured neurons. Biochim Biophys Acta, 2007. 1768(5): p. 1128-37.

[54] McLaurin, J., et al., Structural transitions associated with the interaction of Alzheimer beta-amyloid peptides with gangliosides. J Biol Chem, 1998. 273(8): p. 4506-15.

[55] Oda, T., et al., Clusterin (apoJ) alters the aggregation of amyloid beta-peptide (A beta 1-42) and forms slowly sedimenting A beta complexes that cause oxidative stress. Exp Neurol, 1995. 136(1): p. 22-31.

[56] Stege, G.J., et al., The molecular chaperone alphaB-crystallin enhances amyloid beta neurotoxicity. Biochem Biophys Res Commun, 1999. 262(1): p. 152-6.

[57] Sakono, M. and T. Zako, Amyloid oligomers: formation and toxicity of Abeta oligomers. FEBS J, 2010. 277(6): p. 1348-58.

[58] Butterfield, S.M. and H.A. Lashuel, Amyloidogenic protein-membrane interactions: mechanistic insight from model systems. Angew Chem Int Ed Engl, 2010. 49(33): p. 5628-54.

[59] Kawahara, M., Neurotoxicity of beta-amyloid protein: oligomerization, channel formation, and calcium dyshomeostasis. Curr Pharm Des, 2010. 16(25): p. 2779-89.

[60] Valincius, G., et al., Soluble amyloid beta-oligomers affect dielectric membrane properties by bilayer insertion and domain formation: implications for cell toxicity. Biophys J, 2008. 95(10): p. 4845-61.

[61] De Felice, F.G., et al., Abeta oligomers induce neuronal oxidative stress through an N-methyl-D-aspartate receptor-dependent mechanism that is blocked by the Alzheimer drug memantine. J Biol Chem, 2007. 282(15): p. 11590-601.

[62] Reddy, P.H. and M.F. Beal, Amyloid beta, mitochondrial dysfunction and synaptic damage: implications for cognitive decline in aging and Alzheimer's disease. Trends Mol Med, 2008. 14(2): p. 45-53.

[63] Shankar, G.M., et al., Natural oligomers of the Alzheimer amyloid-beta protein induce reversible synapse loss by modulating an NMDA-type glutamate receptor-dependent signaling pathway. J Neurosci, 2007. 27(11): p. 2866-75.

[64] Grundke-Iqbal, I., et al., Amyloid protein and neurofibrillary tangles coexist in the same neuron in Alzheimer disease. Proc Natl Acad Sci U S A, 1989. 86(8): p. 2853-7.

[65] Blurton-Jones, M. and F.M. Laferla, Pathways by which Abeta facilitates tau pathology. Curr Alzheimer Res, 2006. 3(5): p. 437-48.

[66] Wertkin, A.M., et al., Human neurons derived from a teratocarcinoma cell line express solely the 695-amino acid amyloid precursor protein and produce intracellular beta-amyloid or A4 peptides. Proc Natl Acad Sci U S A, 1993. 90(20): p. 9513-7.

[67] Gouras, G.K., et al., Intraneuronal beta-amyloid accumulation and synapse pathology in Alzheimer's disease. Acta Neuropathol, 2010. 119(5): p. 523-41.

[68] Gouras, G.K., et al., Intraneuronal Abeta42 accumulation in human brain. Am J Pathol, 2000. 156(1): p. 15-20.

[69] LaFerla, F.M., K.N. Green, and S. Oddo, Intracellular amyloid-beta in Alzheimer's disease. Nat Rev Neurosci, 2007. 8(7): p. 499-509.

[70] Takahashi, R.H., et al., Co-occurrence of Alzheimer's disease ss-amyloid and tau pathologies at synapses. Neurobiol Aging, 2010. 31(7): p. 1145-52.

[71] Takahashi, R.H., et al., Accumulation of intraneuronal beta-amyloid 42 peptides is associated with early changes in microtubule-associated protein 2 in neurites and synapses. PLoS One, 2013. 8(1): p. e51965.

[72] Kokubo, H., et al., Soluble Abeta oligomers ultrastructurally localize to cell processes and might be related to synaptic dysfunction in Alzheimer's disease brain. Brain Res, 2005. 1031(2): p. 222-8.

[73] Hartmann, T., et al., Distinct sites of intracellular production for Alzheimer's disease A beta40/42 amyloid peptides. Nat Med, 1997. 3(9): p. 1016-20.

[74] Skovronsky, D.M., R.W. Doms, and V.M. Lee, Detection of a novel intraneuronal pool of insoluble amyloid beta protein that accumulates with time in culture. J Cell Biol, 1998. 141(4): p. 1031-9.

[75] Wild-Bode, C., et al., Intracellular generation and accumulation of amyloid beta-peptide terminating at amino acid 42. J Biol Chem, 1997. 272(26): p. 16085-8.

[76] Forloni, G., beta-Amyloid neurotoxicity. Funct Neurol, 1993. 8(3): p. 211-25.

[77] Forloni, G., et al., Apoptosis mediated neurotoxicity induced by chronic application of beta amyloid fragment 25-35. Neuroreport, 1993. 4(5): p. 523-6.

[78] Loo, D.T., et al., Apoptosis is induced by beta-amyloid in cultured central nervous system neurons. Proc Natl Acad Sci U S A, 1993. 90(17): p. 7951-5.

[79] Almeida, C.G., R.H. Takahashi, and G.K. Gouras, Beta-amyloid accumulation impairs multivesicular body sorting by inhibiting the ubiquitin-proteasome system. J Neurosci, 2006. 26(16): p. 4277-88.

[80] Oh, S., et al., Amyloid peptide attenuates the proteasome activity in neuronal cells. Mech Ageing Dev, 2005. 126(12): p. 1292-9.

[81] Tseng, B.P., et al., Abeta inhibits the proteasome and enhances amyloid and tau accumulation. Neurobiol Aging, 2008. 29(11): p. 1607-18.

[82] Butterfield, D.A. and R. Sultana, Methionine-35 of abeta(1-42): importance for oxidative stress in Alzheimer disease. J Amino Acids, 2011. 2011: p. 198430.

[83] Christen, Y., Oxidative stress and Alzheimer disease. Am J Clin Nutr, 2000. 71(2): p. 621S-629S.

[84] Ramassamy, C., et al., Oxidative insults are associated with apolipoprotein E genotype in Alzheimer's disease brain. Neurobiol Dis, 2000. 7(1): p. 23-37.

[85] Sultana, R., et al., Increased protein and lipid oxidative damage in mitochondria isolated from lymphocytes from patients with Alzheimer's disease: insights into the role of oxidative stress in Alzheimer's disease and initial investigations into a potential biomarker for this dementing disorder. J Alzheimers Dis, 2011. 24(1): p. 77-84.

[86] Mattson, M.P., et al., beta-Amyloid peptides destabilize calcium homeostasis and render human cortical neurons vulnerable to excitotoxicity. J Neurosci, 1992. 12(2): p. 376-89.

[87] Hardy, J., et al., Region-specific loss of glutamate innervation in Alzheimer's disease. Neurosci Lett, 1987. 73(1): p. 77-80.

[88] Maragos, W.F., et al., Loss of hippocampal [3H]TCP binding in Alzheimer's disease. Neurosci Lett, 1987. 74(3): p. 371-6.

[89] Deshpande, A., et al., A role for synaptic zinc in activity-dependent Abeta oligomer formation and accumulation at excitatory synapses. J Neurosci, 2009. 29(13): p. 4004-15.

[90] Snyder, E.M., et al., Regulation of NMDA receptor trafficking by amyloid-beta. Nat Neurosci, 2005. 8(8): p. 1051-8.

[91] Roselli, F., et al., Soluble beta-amyloid1-40 induces NMDA-dependent degradation of postsynaptic density-95 at glutamatergic synapses. J Neurosci, 2005. 25(48): p. 11061-70.

[92] Frisardi, V., F. Panza, and A.A. Farooqui, Late-life depression and Alzheimer's disease: the glutamatergic system inside of this mirror relationship. Brain Res Rev, 2011. 67(1-2): p. 344-55.

[93] Walton, H.S. and P.R. Dodd, Glutamate-glutamine cycling in Alzheimer's disease. Neurochem Int, 2007. 50(7-8): p. 1052-66.

[94] Danbolt, N.C., Glutamate uptake. Prog Neurobiol, 2001. 65(1): p. 1-105.

[95] Hazell, A.S., et al., Selective down-regulation of the astrocyte glutamate transporters GLT-1 and GLAST within the medial thalamus in experimental Wernicke's encephalopathy. J Neurochem, 2001. 78(3): p. 560-8.

[96] Moriyama, Y. and H. Omote, Vesicular glutamate transporter acts as a metabolic regulator. Biol Pharm Bull, 2008. 31(10): p. 1844-6.

[97] Danysz, W. and C.G. Parsons, Alzheimer's disease, beta-amyloid, glutamate, NMDA receptors and memantine--searching for the connections. Br J Pharmacol, 2012. 167(2): p. 324-52.

[98] Gao, S.F. and A.M. Bao, Corticotropin-releasing hormone, glutamate, and gamma-aminobutyric acid in depression. Neuroscientist, 2011. 17(1): p. 124-44.

[99] Revett, T.J., et al., Glutamate system, amyloid ss peptides and tau protein: functional interrelationships and relevance to Alzheimer disease pathology. J Psychiatry Neurosci, 2013. 38(1): p. 6-23.

[100] Collingridge, G.L. and R.A. Lester, Excitatory amino acid receptors in the vertebrate central nervous system. Pharmacol Rev, 1989. 41(2): p. 143-210.

[101] Komuro, H. and P. Rakic, Modulation of neuronal migration by NMDA receptors. Science, 1993. 260(5104): p. 95-7.

[102] Rossi, D.J. and N.T. Slater, The developmental onset of NMDA receptor-channel activity during neuronal migration. Neuropharmacology, 1993. 32(11): p. 1239-48.

[103] Ottersen, O.P., et al., Ischemic disruption of glutamate homeostasis in brain: quantitative immunocytochemical analyses. J Chem Neuroanat, 1996. 12(1): p. 1-14.

[104] Ottersen, O.P., et al., Molecular organization of a type of peripheral glutamate synapse: the afferent synapses of hair cells in the inner ear. Prog Neurobiol, 1998. 54(2): p. 127-48.

[105] Gasparini, C.F. and L.R. Griffiths, The biology of the glutamatergic system and potential role in migraine. Int J Biomed Sci, 2013. 9(1): p. 1-8.

[106] Wenk, G.L., Neuropathologic changes in Alzheimer's disease: potential targets for treatment. J Clin Psychiatry, 2006. 67 Suppl 3: p. 3-7; quiz 23.

[107] Wenk, G.L., C.G. Parsons, and W. Danysz, Potential role of N-methyl-D-aspartate receptors as executors of neurodegeneration resulting from diverse insults: focus on memantine. Behav Pharmacol, 2006. 17(5-6): p. 411-24.

[108] Bell, K.F., D.A. Bennett, and A.C. Cuello, Paradoxical upregulation of glutamatergic presynaptic boutons during mild cognitive impairment. J Neurosci, 2007. 27(40): p. 10810-7.

[109] Fujikawa, D.G., Prolonged seizures and cellular injury: understanding the connection. Epilepsy Behav, 2005. 7 Suppl 3: p. S3-11.

[110] Won, S.J., D.Y. Kim, and B.J. Gwag, Cellular and molecular pathways of ischemic neuronal death. J Biochem Mol Biol, 2002. 35(1): p. 67-86.

[111] Yi, J.H. and A.S. Hazell, Excitotoxic mechanisms and the role of astrocytic glutamate transporters in traumatic brain injury. Neurochem Int, 2006. 48(5): p. 394-403.

[112] Chen, K.H., et al., Disturbed neurotransmitter transporter expression in Alzheimer's disease brain. J Alzheimers Dis, 2011. 26(4): p. 755-66.

[113] Shigeri, Y., R.P. Seal, and K. Shimamoto, Molecular pharmacology of glutamate transporters, EAATs and VGLUTs. Brain Res Brain Res Rev, 2004. 45(3): p. 250-65.

[114] Kalariti, N., N. Pissimissis, and M. Koutsilieris, The glutamatergic system outside the CNS and in cancer biology. Expert Opin Investig Drugs, 2005. 14(12): p. 1487-96.

[115] Omote, H., et al., Vesicular neurotransmitter transporter: bioenergetics and regulation of glutamate transport. Biochemistry, 2011. 50(25): p. 5558-65.

[116] Kalandadze, A., Y. Wu, and M.B. Robinson, Protein kinase C activation decreases cell surface expression of the GLT-1 subtype of glutamate transporter. Requirement of a carboxyl-terminal domain and partial dependence on serine 486. J Biol Chem, 2002. 277(48): p. 45741-50.

[117] Robinson, M.B., Regulated trafficking of neurotransmitter transporters: common notes but different melodies. J Neurochem, 2002. 80(1): p. 1-11.

[118] Schoepfer, R., et al., Molecular biology of glutamate receptors. Prog Neurobiol, 1994. 42(2): p. 353-7.

[119] Mitchell, N.D. and G.B. Baker, An update on the role of glutamate in the pathophysiology of depression. Acta Psychiatr Scand, 2010. 122(3): p. 192-210.

[120] Kew, J.N. and J.A. Kemp, Ionotropic and metabotropic glutamate receptor structure and pharmacology. Psychopharmacology (Berl), 2005. 179(1): p. 4-29.

[121] Lau, C.G. and R.S. Zukin, NMDA receptor trafficking in synaptic plasticity and neuropsychiatric disorders. Nat Rev Neurosci, 2007. 8(6): p. 413-26.

[122] Mellone, M. and F. Gardoni, Modulation of NMDA receptor at the synapse: Promising therapeutic interventions in disorders of the nervous system. Eur J Pharmacol, 2013.

[123] Sanz-Clemente, A., R.A. Nicoll, and K.W. Roche, Diversity in NMDA receptor composition: many regulators, many consequences. Neuroscientist, 2013. 19(1): p. 62-75.

[124] Traynelis, S.F., et al., Glutamate receptor ion channels: structure, regulation, and function. Pharmacol Rev, 2010. 62(3): p. 405-96.

[125] Horak, M. and R.J. Wenthold, Different roles of C-terminal cassettes in the trafficking of full-length NR1 subunits to the cell surface. J Biol Chem, 2009. 284(15): p. 9683-91.

[126] Luscher, C., et al., Synaptic plasticity and dynamic modulation of the postsynaptic membrane. Nat Neurosci, 2000. 3(6): p. 545-50.

[127] Lozano, V.C., C. Armengaud, and M. Gauthier, Memory impairment induced by cholinergic antagonists injected into the mushroom bodies of the honeybee. J Comp Physiol A, 2001. 187(4): p. 249-54.

[128] Maleszka, R., P. Helliwell, and R. Kucharski, Pharmacological interference with glutamate re-uptake impairs long-term memory in the honeybee, apis mellifera. Behav Brain Res, 2000. 115(1): p. 49-53.

[129] May-Simera, H. and E.D. Levin, NMDA systems in the amygdala and piriform cortex and nicotinic effects on memory function. Brain Res Cogn Brain Res, 2003. 17(2): p. 475-83.

[130] Si, A., P. Helliwell, and R. Maleszka, Effects of NMDA receptor antagonists on olfactory learning and memory in the honeybee (Apis mellifera). Pharmacol Biochem Behav, 2004. 77(2): p. 191-7.

[131] Wong, R.W., et al., Overexpression of motor protein KIF17 enhances spatial and working memory in transgenic mice. Proc Natl Acad Sci U S A, 2002. 99(22): p. 14500-5.

[132] Izquierdo, I. and J.H. Medina, Role of the amygdala, hippocampus and entorhinal cortex in memory consolidation and expression. Braz J Med Biol Res, 1993. 26(6): p. 573-89.

[133] Izquierdo, I., et al., Memory processing by the limbic system: role of specific neurotransmitter systems. Behav Brain Res, 1993. 58(1-2): p. 91-8.

[134] Rickard, N.S., K.T. Ng, and M.E. Gibbs, A nitric oxide agonist stimulates consolidation of long-term memory in the 1-day-old chick. Behav Neurosci, 1994. 108(3): p. 640-4.

[135] Rickard, N.S., et al., Both non-NMDA and NMDA glutamate receptors are necessary for memory consolidation in the day-old chick. Behav Neural Biol, 1994. 62(1): p. 33-40.

[136] Bezprozvanny, I. and P.R. Hiesinger, The synaptic maintenance problem: membrane recycling, Ca2+ homeostasis and late onset degeneration. Mol Neurodegener, 2013. 8: p. 23.

[137] Aksenov, M.Y., et al., Oxidative modification of glutamine synthetase by amyloid beta peptide. Free Radic Res, 1997. 27(3): p. 267-81.

[138] Blanchard, B.J., V.L. Thomas, and V.M. Ingram, Mechanism of membrane depolarization caused by the Alzheimer Abeta1-42 peptide. Biochem Biophys Res Commun, 2002. 293(4): p. 1197-203.

[139] Lue, L.F., et al., Soluble amyloid beta peptide concentration as a predictor of synaptic change in Alzheimer's disease. Am J Pathol, 1999. 155(3): p. 853-62.

[140] McLean, C.A., et al., Soluble pool of Abeta amyloid as a determinant of severity of neurodegeneration in Alzheimer's disease. Ann Neurol, 1999. 46(6): p. 860-6.

[141] Kayed, R., et al., Common structure of soluble amyloid oligomers implies common mechanism of pathogenesis. Science, 2003. 300(5618): p. 486-9.

[142] Kakio, A., et al., Formation of a membrane-active form of amyloid beta-protein in raft-like model membranes. Biochem Biophys Res Commun, 2003. 303(2): p. 514-8.

[143] Lazarov, O., et al., Evidence that synaptically released beta-amyloid accumulates as extracellular deposits in the hippocampus of transgenic mice. J Neurosci, 2002. 22(22): p. 9785-93.

[144] Wang, D.S., et al., Oxidized neprilysin in aging and Alzheimer's disease brains. Biochem Biophys Res Commun, 2003. 310(1): p. 236-41.

[145] Yasojima, K., et al., Reduced neprilysin in high plaque areas of Alzheimer brain: a possible relationship to deficient degradation of beta-amyloid peptide. Neurosci Lett, 2001. 297(2): p. 97-100.

[146] Farris, W., et al., Loss of neprilysin function promotes amyloid plaque formation and causes cerebral amyloid angiopathy. Am J Pathol, 2007. 171(1): p. 241-51.

[147] Koffie, R.M., et al., Apolipoprotein E4 effects in Alzheimer's disease are mediated by synaptotoxic oligomeric amyloid-beta. Brain, 2012. 135(Pt 7): p. 2155-68.

[148] Albin, R.L. and J.T. Greenamyre, Alternative excitotoxic hypotheses. Neurology, 1992. 42(4): p. 733-8.

[149] Hu, N.W., T. Ondrejcak, and M.J. Rowan, Glutamate receptors in preclinical research on Alzheimer's disease: update on recent advances. Pharmacol Biochem Behav, 2012. 100(4): p. 855-62.

[150] Lacor, P.N., et al., Synaptic targeting by Alzheimer's-related amyloid beta oligomers. J Neurosci, 2004. 24(45): p. 10191-200.

[151] Palop, J.J. and L. Mucke, Amyloid-beta-induced neuronal dysfunction in Alzheimer's disease: from synapses toward neural networks. Nat Neurosci, 2010. 13(7): p. 812-8.

[152] Selkoe, D.J., Alzheimer's disease is a synaptic failure. Science, 2002. 298(5594): p. 789-91.

[153] Wogulis, M., et al., Nucleation-dependent polymerization is an essential component of amyloid-mediated neuronal cell death. J Neurosci, 2005. 25(5): p. 1071-80.

[154] Shankar, G.M., et al., Amyloid-beta protein dimers isolated directly from Alzheimer's brains impair synaptic plasticity and memory. Nat Med, 2008. 14(8): p. 837-42.

[155] Mucke, L. and D.J. Selkoe, Neurotoxicity of amyloid beta-protein: synaptic and network dysfunction. Cold Spring Harb Perspect Med, 2012. 2(7): p. a006338.

[156] Cullen, W.K., et al., Block of LTP in rat hippocampus in vivo by beta-amyloid precursor protein fragments. Neuroreport, 1997. 8(15): p. 3213-7.

[157] Oddo, S., et al., Triple-transgenic model of Alzheimer's disease with plaques and tangles: intracellular Abeta and synaptic dysfunction. Neuron, 2003. 39(3): p. 409-21.

[158] Hsia, A.Y., et al., Plaque-independent disruption of neural circuits in Alzheimer's disease mouse models. Proc Natl Acad Sci U S A, 1999. 96(6): p. 3228-33.

[159] Tseng, B.P., M. Kitazawa, and F.M. LaFerla, Amyloid beta-peptide: the inside story. Curr Alzheimer Res, 2004. 1(4): p. 231-9.

[160] LaFerla, F.M. and S. Oddo, Alzheimer's disease: Abeta, tau and synaptic dysfunction. Trends Mol Med, 2005. 11(4): p. 170-6.

[161] Lauren, J., et al., Cellular prion protein mediates impairment of synaptic plasticity by amyloid-beta oligomers. Nature, 2009. 457(7233): p. 1128-32.

[162] Um, J.W., et al., Alzheimer amyloid-beta oligomer bound to postsynaptic prion protein activates Fyn to impair neurons. Nat Neurosci, 2012. 15(9): p. 1227-35.

[163] Mairet-Coello, G., et al., The CAMKK2-AMPK kinase pathway mediates the synaptotoxic effects of Abeta oligomers through Tau phosphorylation. Neuron, 2013. 78(1): p. 94-108.

[164] Cai, Z., et al., Roles of AMP-activated protein kinase in Alzheimer's disease. Neuromolecular Med, 2012. 14(1): p. 1-14.

[165] Scheff, S.W., et al., Synaptic alterations in CA1 in mild Alzheimer disease and mild cognitive impairment. Neurology, 2007. 68(18): p. 1501-8.

[166] Spires, T.L., et al., Dendritic spine abnormalities in amyloid precursor protein transgenic mice demonstrated by gene transfer and intravital multiphoton microscopy. J Neurosci, 2005. 25(31): p. 7278-87.

[167] Lacor, P.N., Advances on the understanding of the origins of synaptic pathology in AD. Curr Genomics, 2007. 8(8): p. 486-508.

[168] Bittner, T., et al., Amyloid plaque formation precedes dendritic spine loss. Acta Neuropathol, 2012. 124(6): p. 797-807.

[169] Selkoe, D.J., Soluble oligomers of the amyloid beta-protein impair synaptic plasticity and behavior. Behav Brain Res, 2008. 192(1): p. 106-13.

[170] Kirkwood, C.M., et al., Dendritic Spine Density, Morphology, and Fibrillar Actin Content Surrounding Amyloid-beta Plaques in a Mouse Model of Amyloid-beta Deposition. J Neuropathol Exp Neurol, 2013. 72(8): p. 791-800.

[171] Sivanesan, S., A. Tan, and J. Rajadas, Pathogenesis of Abeta oligomers in synaptic failure. Curr Alzheimer Res, 2013. 10(3): p. 316-23.

[172] Tyan, S.H., et al., Amyloid precursor protein (APP) regulates synaptic structure and function. Mol Cell Neurosci, 2012. 51(1-2): p. 43-52.

[173] Townsend, M., et al., Effects of secreted oligomers of amyloid beta-protein on hippocampal synaptic plasticity: a potent role for trimers. J Physiol, 2006. 572(Pt 2): p. 477-92.

[174] Wu, H.Y., et al., Distinct dendritic spine and nuclear phases of calcineurin activation after exposure to amyloid-beta revealed by a novel fluorescence resonance energy transfer assay. J Neurosci, 2012. 32(15): p. 5298-309.

[175] Penzes, P., et al., Dendritic spine pathology in neuropsychiatric disorders. Nat Neurosci, 2011. 14(3): p. 285-93.

[176] Puzzo, D., L. Privitera, and A. Palmeri, Hormetic effect of amyloid-beta peptide in synaptic plasticity and memory. Neurobiol Aging, 2012. 33(7): p. 1484 e15-24.

[177] Seabrook, G.R., et al., Mechanisms contributing to the deficits in hippocampal synaptic plasticity in mice lacking amyloid precursor protein. Neuropharmacology, 1999. 38(3): p. 349-59.

[178] Rezvani, A.H., Involvement of the NMDA System in Learning and Memory. 2006.

[179] Saura, C.A., et al., Loss of presenilin function causes impairments of memory and synaptic plasticity followed by age-dependent neurodegeneration. Neuron, 2004. 42(1): p. 23-36.

[180] Ma, H., et al., Involvement of beta-site APP cleaving enzyme 1 (BACE1) in amyloid precursor protein-mediated enhancement of memory and activity-dependent synaptic plasticity. Proc Natl Acad Sci U S A, 2007. 104(19): p. 8167-72.

[181] Laird, F.M., et al., BACE1, a major determinant of selective vulnerability of the brain to amyloid-beta amyloidogenesis, is essential for cognitive, emotional, and synaptic functions. J Neurosci, 2005. 25(50): p. 11693-709.

[182] Texido, L., et al., Amyloid beta peptide oligomers directly activate NMDA receptors. Cell Calcium, 2011. 49(3): p. 184-90.

[183] MacDermott, A.B., et al., NMDA-receptor activation increases cytoplasmic calcium concentration in cultured spinal cord neurones. Nature, 1986. 321(6069): p. 519-22.

[184] Peng, T.I. and M.J. Jou, Oxidative stress caused by mitochondrial calcium overload. Ann N Y Acad Sci, 2010. 1201: p. 183-8.

[185] Gerzon, K., et al., The Adamantyl Group in Medicinal Agents. I. Hypoglycemic N-Arylsulfonyl-N' -Adamantylureas. J Med Chem, 1963. 6: p. 760-3.

[186] Chen, H.S. and S.A. Lipton, Mechanism of memantine block of NMDA-activated channels in rat retinal ganglion cells: uncompetitive antagonism. J Physiol, 1997. 499 (Pt 1): p. 27-46.

[187] Kornhuber, J., et al., Memantine displaces [3H]MK-801 at therapeutic concentrations in postmortem human frontal cortex. Eur J Pharmacol, 1989. 166(3): p. 589-90.

[188] Rogawski, M.A. and G.L. Wenk, The neuropharmacological basis for the use of memantine in the treatment of Alzheimer's disease. CNS Drug Rev, 2003. 9(3): p. 275-308.

[189] Minkeviciene, R., P. Banerjee, and H. Tanila, Memantine improves spatial learning in a transgenic mouse model of Alzheimer's disease. J Pharmacol Exp Ther, 2004. 311(2): p. 677-82.

[190] Filali, M., R. Lalonde, and S. Rivest, Subchronic memantine administration on spatial learning, exploratory activity, and nest-building in an APP/PS1 mouse model of Alzheimer's disease. Neuropharmacology, 2011. 60(6): p. 930-6.

[191] Van Dam, D. and P.P. De Deyn, Cognitive evaluation of disease-modifying efficacy of galantamine and memantine in the APP23 model. Eur Neuropsychopharmacol, 2006. 16(1): p. 59-69.

[192] Martinez-Coria, H., et al., Memantine improves cognition and reduces Alzheimer's-like neuropathology in transgenic mice. Am J Pathol, 2010. 176(2): p. 870-80.

[193] Dong, H., et al., Effects of memantine on neuronal structure and conditioned fear in the Tg2576 mouse model of Alzheimer's disease. Neuropsychopharmacology, 2008. 33(13): p. 3226-36.

[194] Rive, B., et al., Memantine enhances autonomy in moderate to severe Alzheimer's disease. Int J Geriatr Psychiatry, 2004. 19(5): p. 458-64.

[195] Peskind, E.R., et al., Memantine treatment in mild to moderate Alzheimer disease: a 24-week randomized, controlled trial. Am J Geriatr Psychiatry, 2006. 14(8): p. 704-15.

[196] Reisberg, B., et al., A 24-week open-label extension study of memantine in moderate to severe Alzheimer disease. Arch Neurol, 2006. 63(1): p. 49-54.

[197] Ferris, S., et al., Treatment effects of Memantine on language in moderate to severe Alzheimer's disease patients. Alzheimers Dement, 2009. 5(5): p. 369-74.

Chapter 11

Genetics of Alzheimer´S Disease

Victoria Campos-Peña, Rocío Gómez and
Marco Antonio Meraz Ríos

Additional information is available at the end of the chapter

http://dx.doi.org/10.5772/58286

1. Introduction

Alzheimer's disease, which was first described in 1907 by Alois Alzheimer, is a progressive neurodegenerative disorder characterized by memory loss and other cognitive functions, and is the most common cause of dementia in old age. Histopathologically, AD is defined by the presence of two specific features: neuritic plaques (NP), containing beta amyloid (Aβ) deposits and neurofibrillary tangles (NTF), containing hyperphosphorylated tau protein [1-3] (Figure 1). The pathological changes observed in the brains of AD patients are not distributed uniformly over the cerebral cortex. Instead, these changes are located in specific cortical areas, indicating a relationship between disease progression and the connectivity of affected areas [2, 4-5]. These changes follow a pattern that correspond to the information transmission routes between cortical and subcortical areas of the brain, suggesting a direct correlation between anatomical damage and the clinical phases of the disease.

There are two subtypes of AD: 1) familial Alzheimer´s disease which is associated with mutations in three different genes and 2) sporadic Alzheimer´s disease, which is much more common and the causes for it, are not yet completely understood. In recent decades, numerous genome-wide association studies (GWAS) have been performed in an attempt to identify new risk loci related with the development of sporadic cases. In this regard, genetic association studies of cases and controls, have proven the existence of polymorphic variants in genes which could be interpreted as genetic susceptibility factors contributing to the development of LOAD. However, these results are not replicated in all populations, suggesting the importance of geographical and environmental factors in the phenotypic expression of the disease. For this purpose and in order to validate the data obtained, it is necessary to take in account confounding factors as genetic admixture in population-based genetic association studies. This review, describe the genetics of Alzheimer´s disease and some of the most relevant GWAS conducted to date.

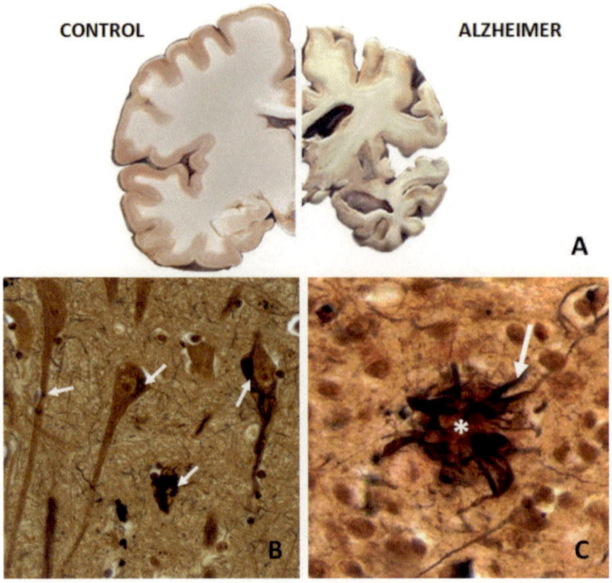

Figure 1. Pathological changes observed in AD patients brains. (A) Cross-section on the left represents a normal brain and the one on the right represents a brain with Alzheimer's disease. The picture shows the generalized brain atrophy in AD, characterized by widening in sulcus, ventricles dilatation and extensive cell loss. **(B)** Silver stain showing the presence of neurofibrillary tangles (NFT) the Tau protein aggregates are indicated by white arrows. We observe the formation of these deposits at different stages of neurodegeneration. **(C)** Double staining showing a neuritic plaque (NP), amyloid deposits are seen in red and marked with an asterisk; neurofibrillary aggregates surrounding the amyloid are marked with the arrow.

2. Diagnosis

There are currently several clinical tools for the diagnosis of AD, including the minimum mental state examination (MMSE) [6] and the Diagnostic and Statistical Manual of Mental Disorders (Fourth Edition [DSM-IV]). In general terms, these tools consist of a semi-structured interview with an appropriate reporter and the patient with damage being described as loss of two or more of the following cognitive areas: memory, orientation, calculation and language. Other aspects are similarly evaluated, such as problem solving, social relationships, work, hobbies and personal care. Another commonly used criterion for diagnosis is that of the National Institute of Neurological and Communicative Disorders and Stroke-Alzheimer´s Disease and Related Disorders Association (NINCDSADRDA). Under this criterion, the state of dementia is clinically determined based on the loss of two cognitive areas and the absence of other systemic disorders, accompanied by a progressive loss of memory. These criteria are sufficient to determine *probable Alzheimer´s disease.* However, diagnosis of AD requires exclusion of other neurodegenerative diseases, such as frontotemporal dementia, Parkinson's disease and Lewy Body disease. Discrimination between AD and other types of dementia are usually achieved based on clinical history and through neurological examinations that require imaging studies. Nevertheless, definitive diagnosis of AD requires postmortem confirmation by histopathological examination to demonstrate the presence of NP and NFT (Figure 1).

2. Neuritic plaques and the β-amyloid precursor protein

Neuritic plaques are extracellular deposits of 10-100 μm in diameter, contain an insoluble core consisting of a peptide known as amyloid-β (Aβ), surrounded by microglia, reactive astrocytes and dystrophic neurites [7]. Aβ is a peptide of 39-42 amino acids [8-9] that originates as a normal secretory product derived from amyloid-β precursor protein (AβPP) [10]. AβPP is an integral membrane protein that is widely expressed in epithelial cells of various organs, such as the thyroid gland, skin and the central nervous system. AβPP is a type I integral membrane glycoprotein that resembles a signal-transduction receptor [10]. This protein is conformed by a large extracellular domain, a hydrophobic transmembrane domain and a short cytoplasmic carboxyl terminus (Figure 2). The gene is located on chromosome 21q21 and consists of 18 exons. Alternative splicing generates several isoforms with lengths varying between 365 and 770 amino acid residues. In the central nervous system, four isoforms are expressed: APP695, APP714, APP751 and APP770. Amyloid-β is present only in APP695, APP751 and APP770 (Figure 3A, 3B). The APP695 isoform is mainly expressed in neuronal cells [11], while the APP751 and APP770 isoforms are expressed in glial cells [12-13]. To date, the primary function of the protein has not been defined yet, but it has been proposed that it could participate as a growth factor in cultured fibroblasts [14] and play role in cell adhesion [15], intraneuronal calcium regulation [16], neural plasticity [17] and act as a regulator of synapse formation [18]. AβPP, is posttranslationally modified by N-and O-glycosylation, phosphorylation and tyrosine sulphation and undergoes two types of proteolytic processing [19] through three

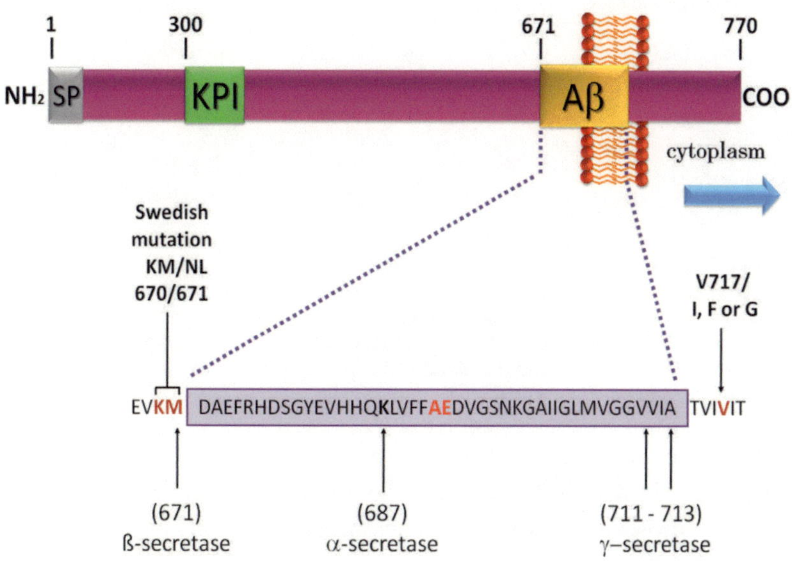

Figure 2. Schematic representation of AβPP. AβPP is a member of a family of conserved type I membrane proteins, consists of a large extracellular domain, a hydrophobic transmembrane domain, and a short cytoplasmic carboxyl terminus. Amyloid sequence contains 40-and 43-amino acid residues that extend from the ectodomain into the transmembrane domain of the protein. The Aβ sequence lies partially outside the cell membrane (amino acids 1–17 of Aβ) and the some identified mutations in the protein are indicated in bold.

enzyme activities α-secretase, β-secretase which cleave AβPP within the luminal domain, and a third activity, termed γ-secretase which cleaves APP within the transmembrane domain. All three AβPP secretases are transmembrane proteases.

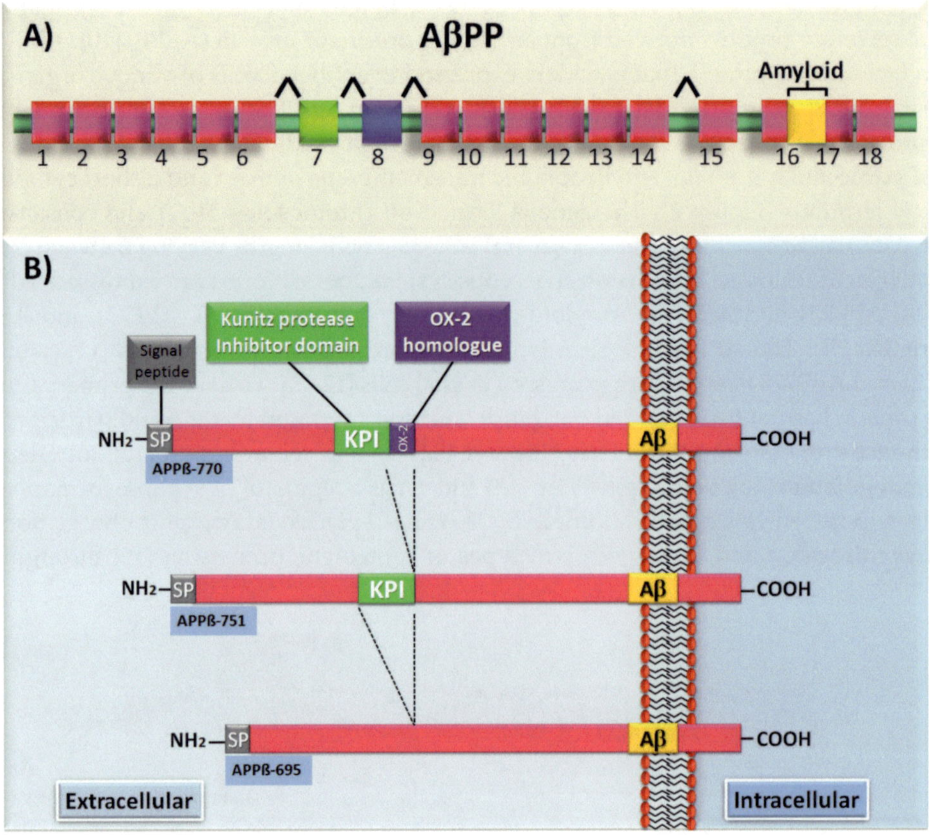

Figure 3. Human APP gene structure. (A) The APP gene consist of 18 exons, is located on chromosome 21 (21q21.2-3). The region encoding the amyloid sequence comprises part of exons 16 and 17 (yellow box). **(B)** APP is alternatively spliced into several products, named according to their length in amino acids (ie, APP695, APP714, APP751, APP770, and APP563) that are expressed differentially by tissue type. The major APP derivatives in the CNS are APP695, APP751 and APP770. Some isoforms contain a 57 amino acid KPI domain and a 19 aminoacid MRC OX-2 antigen in the extracellular sequences (pink box).

It is believed that the principal proteolytic cleavage of AβPP is non-amyloidogenic pathway, which is performed by the action of a protease known as alpha-secretase. This protease cleaves, at residues 612-613 corresponding to the middle portion Aβ (Lys16 and Leu17 in Aβ peptide), thereby preventing amyloid formation [20-21]. α-secretase (ADAM10) generates two products: a soluble fragment (sAPPα) that is released into the extracellular space and a carboxyl terminal membrane-anchored product, called C83. Finally, the C83 fragment is cut by γ-secretase generating a 6 KDa fragment, called AICD (APP intracellular domain-) and a ~3kDa peptide (p3) that is released into the extracellular space (Figure 4A).

The first step of amyloidogenic processing is carried out by the action of β-secretase, (BACE1), which generates the formation of two products: 1) a soluble product (sAβPP) that is released into the extracellular space and 2) a carboxyl terminal membrane-anchored called C99. In the same way C99 is cut by the γ-secretase, generating the AICD fragment into the cytoplasm and the neurotoxic fragment amyloid beta (Aß) (Figure 4B) [22].

Although AβPP metabolism and amyloid peptide accumulation represent central events in the pathogenesis of AD, in animal models, it has not been possible to demonstrate that their occurrence *per se* is capable of generating the complete pathology of the disease.

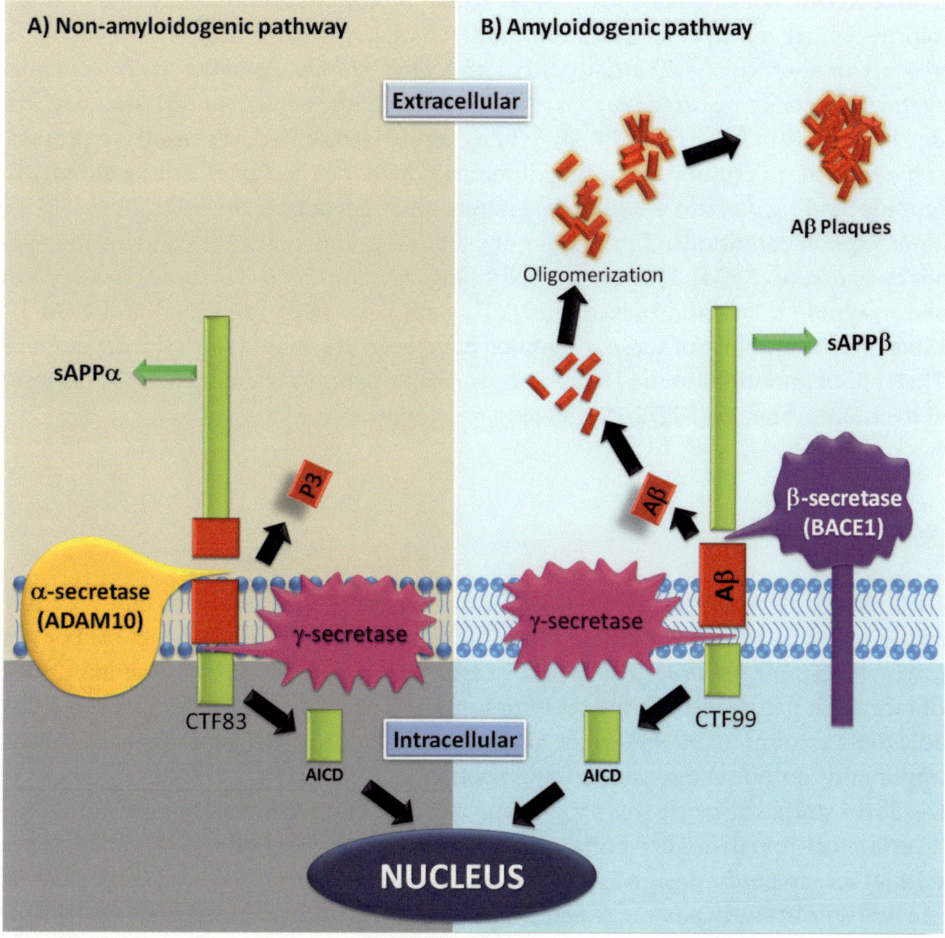

Figure 4. AβPP Processing. The AβPP is an integral membrane protein, is sequentially processed by the three proteases α-, β-, and γ-secretase. **(A)** The non amyloidogenic pathway involves the α-secretase, which made the cut at the middle portion of the fragment corresponding to the amyloid sequence; preventing the amyloid peptides generation. **(B)** The amyloidogenic pathway involves β-secretase, leading to the formation of C-terminal fragments (CTFs) that are subsequently cleaved by the "γ-secretase-complex" which is responsible for the formation of Aβ (40 or 42 amino acids in length) and the AβPP intracellular domain peptide (AICD) of 58 or 56 amino acids.

3. Neurofibrillary tangles and tau

Neurofibrillary tangles are simpler and yet more enigmatic than neuritic plaques. Unlike NP, the density of NFT in the brains of AD patients is closely related to the severity of dementia [23-24]. In particular, neurofibrillary degeneration is a prerequisite for the clinical expression of AD pathology, i.e., *dementia,* whereas amyloid accumulation in the absence of neurofibrillary tangles does not produce the AD pathology. The structural units of NFT are paired helical filaments (FHA), which are formed by the association of five to six6 fragments of the microtubule binding protein Tau. The gene that encodes this protein is located on chromosome 17 and comprises 16 exons of which-1 and 14 exons, can be transcribed but not translated [25-27]. Alternative RNAm splicing of exons 2, 3 and 10, of the *MAPT* gene generates the formation of six isoforms which are expressed in adult brain [28]. Each isoform differs from each other by the presence or absence of a 29-aminoacid or 58-aminoacid inserts in the amino-terminal half and by the inclusion or not in the carboxy-terminal half of the protein of a 31-aminoacid repeat encoded by exon 10 of *MAPT* [25, 29-30]. When exon 10 is excluded, the result is a protein with three repeats of the microtubule-binding domain (3RMBD). When exon 10 is included, a fourth microtubule binding domain is added to generate four-repeat tau (4RMBD) [28, 31-32] (Figure 5). Under normal conditions, Tau is a highly soluble protein, since it contains no apparent secondary structure [33-34]. However, in pathological conditions, Tau tends to self-assemble into the insoluble filament structures [32]. To date have been identified and MAPT gene mutations, however, none of these mutations have been associated with the development of AD. This type of mutations in the Tau gene cause frontotemporal dementia with Parkinsonism linked to chromosome 17 (FTDP-17) [35-39]

4. Genetics of AD

Conventionally, AD is divided into two forms depending on the age of onset: early onset Alzheimer´s disease (EOAD) and late onset Alzheimer´s disease (LOAD). EOAD or familial cases, which account for only 5-10% of all cases, exhibit an autosomal dominant mode of inheritance, high penetrance of clinical symptoms and onset before 55 years of age. LOAD or sporadic cases account for 90-95% of all AD cases, usually present a later onset age (≥ 65 years) and apparently do not show familial aggregation associated with the development of the disease. Twin studies provide insight into the relative contributions of genetic and environmental influences for Alzheimer´s disease and other types of dementia [40-42]. It has long been argued that a twin study design is advantageous for identifying risk and protective factors because this type of study has suggested the existence of a genetic component associated with the development of LOAD cases [43]. The results of these studies have shown that the pairwise concordance rate for Alzheimer´s disease is 78% (7/9) among monozygotic and 39% (9/23) among dizygotic twin pairs [40]. In 2006, Gatz adjusted their findings for age and also included like-and unlike-sex pairs, and the results showed that the age–adjusted heritability for AD was estimated to be 58-79%, and there were no significant differences between men and women regarding prevalence or heritability after controlling for age [41]. Nevertheless, it was observed

http://dx.doi.org/10.5772/58286

that among patients who develop LOAD, approximately 40-65% present an indirect genetic agent in the form of the 4 allele of apolipoprotein E (ApoE/4) [44-47]. However, the effect of APOEe4 as a genetic risk factor is not sufficient or necessary for developing the disease [48-49].

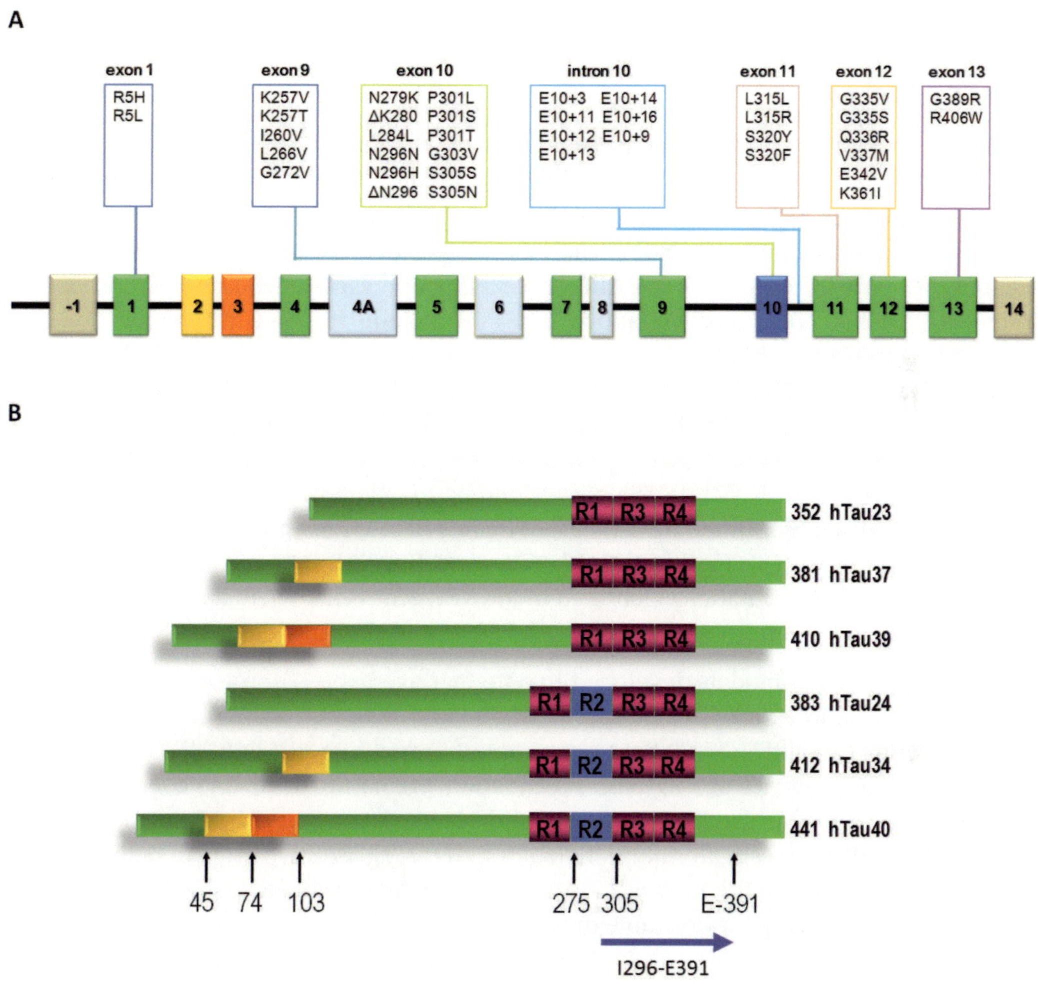

Figure 5. Human Tau-protein. (A) Schematic representation human tau gene (MAPT). The human gene comprises 16 exons of which exons-1 and 14, can be transcribed but not translated. In central nervous system are expressed 6 isoforms, which are obtained by alternative splicing of exons 2, 3 and 10; the exons 1, 4, 5, 7, 9, 11, 12 and 13 are expressed in all isoforms. In boxes, are indicated the mutations found in the gene which have been associated with FTDP-17. **(B)** Representation of the 6 Tau isoforms. The different isoforms differ from each other by the presence of one or two inserts located in the region N (yellow and orange boxes) and the presence of 3 or 4 repeated domains, located in C-terminus of the molecule (blue box) and termed microtubule binding domain (MTBD). The expression of the different isoforms is regulated during development; in fetal stages are expressed only isoforms containing 3 repeated whereas adult stages, all isoforms are expressed.

5. Early onset alzheimer´s disease

While the vast majority of cases of AD occur late in life and are sporadic, approximately 5–10% of cases exhibit an early onset. EOAD or Familial Alzheimer´s disease is associated with mutations in proteins such as presenilin 1 and 2 (PS1 and PS2) and amyloid precursor protein (APP) [50-58]. Currently, more than 200 distinct disease-causing mutations have been identified across these genes, which exhibit an autosomal dominant transmission pattern.

5.1. APP mutations

To date, approximately 36 different missense mutations in the APP gene have been identified among 85 families (Table 1). AβPP mutations account for 0.1% of AD patients, all missense mutations influence APP processing since they are positioned in or near the Aβ coding exons 16-17, in the transmembranal domain, where the sites recognized by the α, β and γ-secretases are found (Figure 2). This alters the APPβ processing and causes the accumulation of Aβ42 fragments [54-55]. The major mutations in APPβ include the Swedish double mutation (APPSW: APPK670N, APPM671L) [59] and the London mutation (V717I) [55]. The Swedish mutation is located just outside the N-terminus of the Aβ domain of APP, favors β-secretase cleavage and it is associated with increased levels and deposition of Aβ1-42 in the brains of AD patients [60-61]. London mutation is located in exon 17 and leads to a valine to isoleucine change at amino acid 717 (V717I) [55], corresponding to the transmembrane domain near the γ-secretase cleavage site. Other mutations in APP linked to EOAD include the Dutch (E693Q) [62], Indiana (V717F) [58], Florida (I716V) [63], Iowa (D694N) [64] and Arctic (E693G) [65] mutations. Besides the mutations identified in the APP gene is known that duplication of APP regions containing several genes [66-68] or APP [69] were clinically linked to EOAD.

The transgenic animal models developed to date that overexpress these mutations have the potential to develop extracellular deposits of amyloid beta and exhibit different types of neurological abnormalities [55, 70-73]. For example, transgenic mouse line APP/V717I displays deficits in the maintenance of long-term potentiation, premature death and cognitive impairment, which is directly correlated with amyloid plaque formation [74]. Another transgenic mouse line used to investigate the pathology of AD is Tg2576, which carries the Swedish mutation. These mice exhibit memory loss starting at 6 months of age, which coincides with the appearance of detergent-insoluble amyloid aggregates [73]. Overexpression of mutated AβPP in cell cultures induces DNA synthesis and apoptosis [75], suggesting that APPβ could induce the apoptotic events observed in Alzheimer´s disease patients via activation of specific pathways of neuronal signaling.

5.2. Presenilin mutation

Presenilin represent the catalytic component of the gamma-secretase complex, which also includes nicastrin, anterior pharynx-defective 1 (Aph-1) and presenilin enhancer 2 (Pen-2) [76]. Presenilins are expressed in several tissues and in the brain, where are mainly expressed in neurons [52]. Presenilins localize into the endoplasmic reticulum (ER), Golgi apparatus, endosomes, lysosomes, phagosome plasma membranes and mitochondria [77-79]. During

Mutation	Phenotype	Age of Onset	References
E665D	AD, but may not be pathogenic	86?	Peacock, et al., 1994
KM670/671NL (Swedish)	AD	52 (44-59)	Mullan, et al. 1992
H677R	AD	55 (55-56)	Janssen, et al. 2003
D678N (Tottori)	FAD	60	Wakutani, et al. 2004
E693Δ	AD		Tomiyama et al., 2008
D694N (Iowa)	AD or Cerebral Hemorrhage	69	Grabowski, et al. 2001
A713T	AD, but may not be pathogenic	59	Carter, et al., 1992
T714A (Iranian)	AD	52 (40-60)	Pasaler, et al., 2002
T714I (Austrian)	Affects γ-secretase cleavage directly, 11X increase in Aβ(42)/Aβ(40) ratio in vitro.		Kumar-Singh, et al.
V715A (German)	AD	47	De Jonghe, et al., 2001; Cruts, et al., 2003
V715M (French)	AD	52 (40-60)	Ancolio, et al., 1999
I716T	AD	55	Terrini, et al., 2002
I716V (Florida)	AD	55	Eckman, et al., 1997
V717F (Indiana)	AD	47 (42-52)	Murrell, et al. 1991
V717G	AD	55 (45-62)	Chartier-Harlin, et al. 1991
V717I (London)	AD	55 (50-60)	Goate, et al. 1991
T719P	AD	46	Ghidoni et al., 2009
L723P (Australian)	AD	56 (45-60)	Kwok JB, 2000

Table 1. Amyloid Precursor Protein Mutations

assembly and maturation of the complex, presenilin undergoes endoproteolitic processes generating stable N-and C-terminal fragments (NTF and CTF, respectively). Both fragments (NTF and CTF) contribute with one of the two catalytic aspartates that are, the active site which is responsible for the intramembranal proteolysis of AβPP and some other proteins as well [60, 80-85]. Both presenilins (PS1 and PS2) possess these conserved aspartate residues required for γ-secretase activity [85]. In addition, presenilins directly or indirectly regulate the trafficking and metabolism of select membrane proteins in neurons [86], as well as having a role in synaptic function [87-88], learning and memory [89], neuronal survival in the adult brain, regulation of calcium homeostasis [90-91] and presynaptic neurotransmitter release [92].

PS1 is an integral membrane protein with eight transmembranal domains and a hydrophilic domain between the 6 and 7 domains. The PSEN1 gene is located on chromosome 14q24.2, comprises 12 exons and generates a protein with a length of 467 amino acids. To date, more than 180 mutations in PSEN1 have been described in 405 families (http://www.molgen.ua.ac.be/ADmutations), all of which are related to the appearance of the disease at younger ages (Figure 6A) [93-94]. The PSEN2 gene is located on chromosome 1q42.13 and comprises 12 exons, of which only 10 are translated to generate a protein with a length of 448 amino acid residues. This protein exhibits 9 transmembrane domains and displays tissue-specific alternative splicing [95]. Only 13 mutations in PS2 have been described among 22 families (Figure 6B). (http://www.molgen.ua.ac.be/ADmutations)

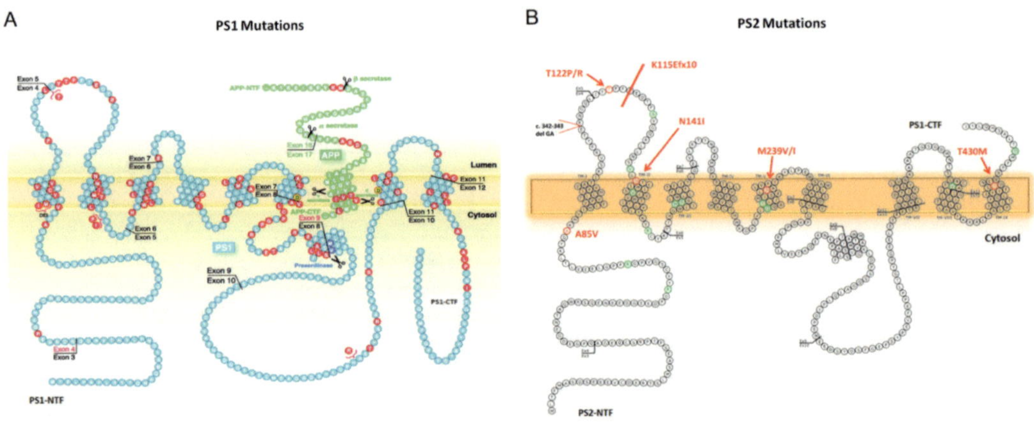

Figure 6. Schematic representation of Presenilis. (A) Presenilins are membrane proteins that form the catalytic core of the γ-secretase complex. The PSEN1 gene is located on chromosome 14q24.2 and comprises 12 exons. PS1 is an integral membrane protein with eight transmembrane domains and a hydrophilic domain between domains 6 and 7. Two aspartate residues in transmembrane domains (TMs) 6 and 7 constituting the catalytic site. To date, more than 185 mutations in PSEN1 have been described in 405 families all of which are related to the appearance of the disease at younger ages. Although mutations are found throughout the protein, most are located in the transmembrane region. **(B)** The PSEN2 gene is located on chromosome 1q42.13 and comprises 12 exons, of which only 10 are translated to generate a protein with a length of 448 amino acid residues. This protein exhibits 9 transmembrane domains and displays tissue-specific alternative splicing, major mutations found in the protein are identified.

Most familial cases of Alzheimer´s disease are associated with mutations in presenilins [50, 53, 96], the majority of PSEN mutations are single-nucleotide substitutions, but small deletions and insertions have been described as well. It has been suggested that these mutations induce overproduction of β-amyloid, apparently by increasing γ-secretase activity [51, 53, 97-102]. Although transgenic mice expressing presenilin mutations do not develop the formation of neuritic plaques, these animals showed changes similar to those observed in AD patients, such as neuronal damage, synaptic loss and vascular disease. The most severe mutation in *PSEN1* is a donor-acceptor splice mutation that causes a two-aminoacid substitution and an in-frame deletion of exon 9. However, the biochemical consequences of these mutations for γ-secretase assembly seem to be limited [103-104]. PS1 also appears to modulate GSK3β activity and the release of kinesin-I from membrane-bound organelles at sites of vesicle delivery and membrane insertion. These findings suggest that mutations in PS1 may compromise neuronal function, affecting GSK-3 activity and kinesin-I-based motility and, thus, leading to neurodegeneration [105]. Although PS2 shows close homology to PS1, PS2 is less efficient with respect to amyloid peptide production [106]. *In vitro* expression of PSEN2 V393M cDNA did not result in a detectable increase in the secreted Aβ42/40 peptide ratio. However, patients heterozygous for this missense mutation are characterized by profound language impairment [107]. Although mutations are found throughout the protein, most are located in the transmembrane region.

6. Late onset alzheimer´s disease

6.1. Apoe risk gene

Allele 4 of apolipoprotein E (ApoE4) has been reported to represent the main identified risk factor for sporadic AD [44, 49, 108]. This gene has been associated with EOAD and LOAD in multiple ethnic groups, and carriers of APOE4 exhibit an earlier age of onset for AD [44, 109-110]. The frequency of the APOE4 allele varies among ethnic groups and it has been shown that ApoE4 is determinant for AD risk in white's individuals; however, in Hispanic and African populations, there is no correlation between the presence of the pathology and this allele. These results suggest that other genes or risk factors may contribute to the increased risk of AD in African and Hispanics [111-114].

The ApoE4 gene is located at chromosome 19q13.2 [115] and consists of 4 exons encoding a protein of 299 amino acid residues with a molecular weight of 34 kDa. APOE is a glycoprotein exhibiting variable levels of posttranslational sialylation due to O-linked glycosylation at threonine 194 [116]. The gene contains several single-nucleotide polymorphisms (SNPs) [117] leading to changes in the amino acid sequence of the protein, resulting in the production of three isoforms: ApoE2, ApoE3 and ApoE4, which are associated with different alleles (ε2, ε3, ε4). The three isoforms differ only by one or two amino acids, with the changes occurring at amino acid residues 112 and 158: ApoE2 (cys112, cys158), ApoE3 (cys112, arg158) and ApoE4 (arg112, arg158) [118-120]. The allelic distribution varies among ethnic groups, although it has generally been observed that allele 3 is the most frequent (77%), followed by allele 4 (15%), while allele 2 is less frequently observed (8%).

ApoE is a plasma protein that plays an important role in lipid metabolism and cholesterol transport in various tissues [108, 121-122]. The amino acid changes observed in the different isoforms of ApoE alter the 3-dimensional structure of the protein, affecting its lipid-binding properties, indicating that each isoform is metabolically different and varies in its affinity to bind to lipoprotein particles [123-124]. Apolipoproteins are synthesized primarily in the liver but can be processed and secreted in the brain by astrocytes and microglia. They are involved in neuronal regeneration [125], an increase in the synthesis of these proteins has been observed in the central and peripheral nervous system during neuronal damage. The distinct human ApoE isoforms differ significantly in their long-term effects on neuronal integrity as well as in their ability to protect against exocitotoxicity [126-128]. When ApoE isoforms are expressed in brain cells of ApoE-knockout (APOE-/-) mice, it can be observed that ApoE3 has a protective effect against age-related Aβ toxicity and neurodegeneration [129-130]. These differences in the neuroprotective capacities of apoE3 and apoE4 could contribute to the increased susceptibility of human ApoE4 carriers to AD [131]. Cholesterol homeostasis in hippocampal neurons is affected by the presence of apoE4, while the presence of ApoE2 and ApoE3 is not associated with any alterations in homeostasis [132]. Other roles of APOE isoforms include proliferation, synaptogenesis, myelination and amyloid elimination and tau phosphorylation.

6.2. Apoe and amyloid

Overexpression of a mutated form of human APP has shown that the levels of amyloid and ApoE increase in the brain with age, which is associated with decreasing Aβ levels in plasma [133]. It is possible that ApoE increases Aβ sequestration, deregulating the clearance of amyloid and leading to cognitive impairment in transgenic mice expressing a mutant form of human APP [134-135]. Recent studies have shown that apolipoprotein E (ApoE) receptor 2 and other members of the low-density lipoprotein receptor family (LRP, LRP1B, SorLA/LR11) interact with AβPP and regulates its endocytic trafficking [136-137]. Stable expression of human APP in B103 rat neuroblastoma cells (B103-APP); demonstrated that the isoform-specific effects of ApoE on Aβ production result from an alteration of AβPP recycling due to more pronounced stimulation of AβPP recycling by apoE4 than ApoE3 [138]. However, other authors have noted that there is no clear evidence upon which to base conclusions regarding the isoform-specific effects on AβPP processing [127, 139].

Although clearance of Aβ by ApoE has not been extensively studied, ApoE may modulate the removal of Aβ from the brain (Figure 7). Nevertheless, it has been suggested that clearance of Aβ is regulated by low-density lipoprotein receptor related protein-1 (LRP) and the receptor for advanced glycation end products (RAGE); this function is compromised in AD, which may contribute to elevation of the levels of amyloid in the brain [135, 140-141].

6.3. Apoe and tau

Neither the mechanisms by which the tau and ApoE4 proteins confer pathogenicity nor the nature of the interaction between these proteins has yet been established. Some authors have suggested that there is a relationship between the dosage of the ApoE4 allele and the density of NTFs [142-143]. It is known that ApoE3 has the ability to form a stable complex with Tau protein, and this association is believed to decrease Tau phosphorylation, preventing abnormal phosphorylation of Tau protein and their aggregation into paired helical filaments (PHF) [144]. When tau is phosphorylated, it loses its ability to interact with ApoE3. In contrast, ApoE4 does not interact with Tau.

It has recently been shown that the expression of a carboxy-terminal truncated fragment of the ApoE4 protein (Δ272-299 carboxyl terminal) is sufficient to elicit AD-like neurodegeneration

http://dx.doi.org/10.5772/58286

and behavioral deficits *in vivo* [145]. Transgenic mice expressing apoE4Δ272–299 displayed AD-like neurodegenerative alterations in the cortex and hippocampus, including abnormally phosphorylated tau (p-tau) and Gallyas silver-positive neurons that contained cytosolic straight filaments with diameters of 15–20 nm, resembling pre-neurofibrillary tangles [145]. Similarly, overexpression of human ApoE4 in neurons results in hyperphosphorylation of the tau protein, which increases with age [146-147].

Finally, although the presence of allele 4 of ApoE is not a deterministic factor for AD, it has been observed that this allele may favor the development of the disease at younger ages [148].

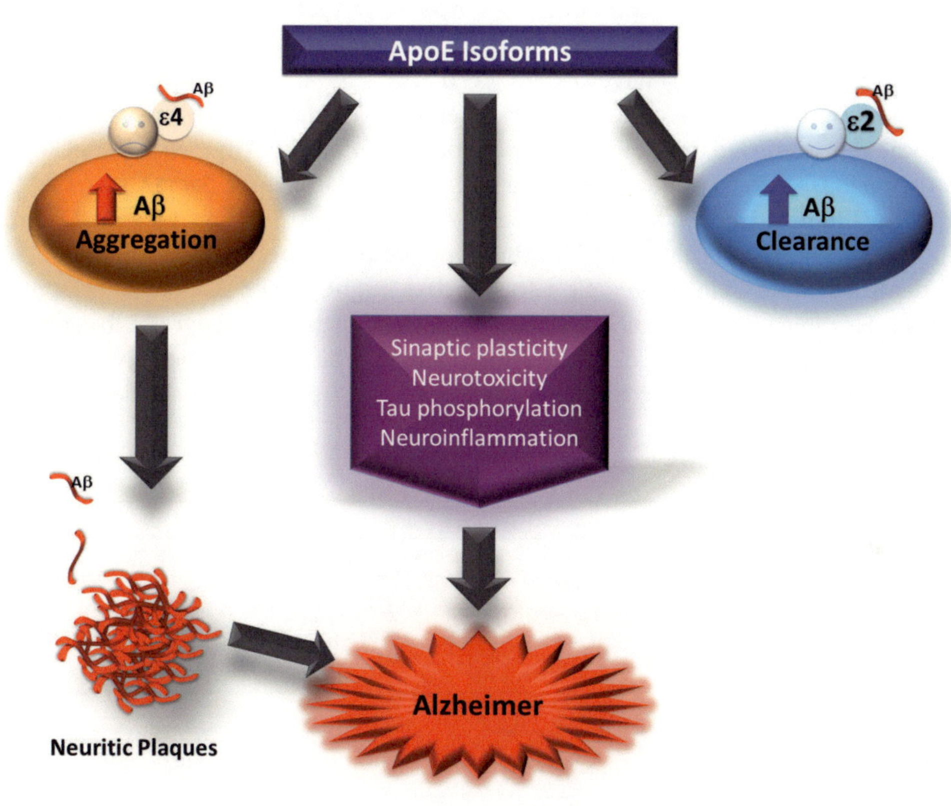

Figure 7. Interaction of Amyloid and ApoE. The ApoE4 gene is located on chromosome 19q13.2. It has been suggested that ApoE, could be involved in the Aβ aggregation and clearance. This process can be regulated of ApoE isoform and thereby promote the onset of Aβ aggregation. In this way other pathologic mechanisms could be favored

7. Genome-wide association studies (gwas)

The genetic causes of AD can be highly variable, even for familial forms. While EOAD is characterized by the presence of mutations with high penetrance in specific genes, the genetics of sporadic cases (LOAD) are more complex. LOAD susceptibility is determined by an uncertain number of genetic risk factors exhibiting low penetrance that are present at a high frequency. This is particularly important because although patients who develop this subtype of the disease have been considered to represent *sporadic cases*, the genetic component of these cases is a feature that has not been established. A possible explanation for the difficulty involved in the identification of genetic risk factors is that LOAD is a multifactorial complex disorder that involves both genetic and environmental components.

In the last thirty years, a considerable number of studies have been developed aimed at identifying risk factors that confer susceptibility for developing AD. In this regard, genome-wide association studies (GWAS) represent a powerful approach for identifying putative candidate genes for common complex diseases, such as LOAD. These studies simultaneously analyze a large number of genetic markers, typically consisting of single-nucleotide polymorphisms (SNPs). Although they have also involved arrays for assessing copy-number variants (deletions or multiplications of chromosomal segments), other GWAS arrays only contain SNPs located in predicted or known coding regions (cSNPs). The Affymetrix GeneChip 500K platform exhibits 60% coverage of the phase II HapMAp (Affymetrix, Santa Clara, CA, USA), whereas the Illumina Hap300 platform presents 77% coverage (Illumina, Inc., San Diego, CA, USA). At least 12 GWAS addressing Alzheimer's disease have been published to date, which have identified more than 40 genetic variants that might confer risk for developing this pathology. However, much remains to be learned regarding the pathology and the genetic risk factors associated with late onset Alzheimer's disease. The main studies investigating the associations between cases and controls with LOAD using such platforms are described below (Table 2).

Genome-Wide Association Studies (GWAS)

Study	Design	Type	Population	# of SNPs	AD Cases			Normal Controls		Featured Genes
					DX	# Subjects GWAS	# Subjects (follow-up)	# Subjects GWAS	# Subjects (follow-up)	
CAUSASIAN										
Abraham, 2008	CC	GWAS pooled	Overlaps with Harold, 2009	561494	C	1082	-	1239	1400	APOE, LRAT
Beecham, 2009	CC	GWAS	USA (CAP)	532000	M	492	238	496	220	APOE, FAM113B
Bertram, 2008	FBAT	GWAS	USA (NIMH)	484522	M	941	1767	404	838	APOE ATXN1 CD33 GWA 14q31.2
Carrasquillo, 2009	CC	GWAS	USA (Mayo)	313504	M	844	1547	1255	1209	APOE PCDH11X
Coon, 2007	CC	GWAS	USA, Netherlands (TGEN1)	502627	N	664	-	422	-	APOE
Grupe, 2007	CC	GWAS	USA & UK	17343	M	380	1428	396	1666	ACAN, APOE, BCR, CTSS, EBF3, FAM63A, GALP, GWA_14q32.13,

Genome-Wide Association Studies (GWAS)										
					AD Cases			Normal Controls		
Study	Design	Type	Population	# of SNPs	DX	# Subjects GWAS	# Subjects (follow-up)	# Subjects GWAS	# Subjects (follow-up)	Featured Genes
										GWA_7p15.2, LMNA, LOC651924, MY13, PCK1, PGBD1, TNK1, TRAK2, UBD
Harold, 2009	CC	GWAS	Europe & USA (GERAD1)	529205	M	3941	2023	7848	2340	APOE, CLU, PICALM
Heinzen, 2009	CC	GWAS +CNV	USA (CAP, DUKE)	n.g.	U	331	-	368	-	
Hollingworth, 2011	CC	GWAS	Europe & USA (GERAD1+2, EADI1+2, ADNI, TGEN1, MAYO2, CHARGE)	496763	M	6688	13182	13685	26261	ABCA7, BIN1, CD2AP, CD33, CR1, EPHA1, MS4A4E, MS4A6A
Hu, 2011	CC	GWAS	USA (Pfizer, ADNI), Canada (GenADA, Genizon)	509376	C	1831	751	1764	751	APOE, BIN1
Lambert, 2009	CC	GWAS	Europe (EADI1)	537029	C	2032	3978	5328	3297	APOE, CLU, CR1
Li, 2008	CC	GWAS	Canada (GenADA)	469438	C	753	418	736	249	APOE, GOLM1, GWA_15q21.2, GWA_9p24.3
Naj, 2011	CC	GWAS	USA (ADGC)	2,324,889 (imputed)	M	8309	3531	7366	3565	APOE, BIN1, CD2AP, CD33, CLU, CR1, EPHA1, MS4A4A, PICALM
Poduslo, 2009	CC, FBAT	GWAS	USA	489218	C	9	199	10	225	TRCP4AP
Potkin, 2009	CC, QT	GWAS	USA (ADNI)	516645	C	172	-	209	-	APOE, ARSB, CAND1, EFNA5, MAG12, PRUNE2 TOMM40
Reiman, 2007	CC	GWAS	USA, Netherlands (TGEN1)	312316	M	446	415	290	260	GAB2
Seshadri, 2010	CC	GWAS + meta-analysis	Europe & USA (CHARGE, EADI1, GERAD1)	2,540,000 (imputed)	M	3006	6505	22604	13532	APOE, BIN1, CLU, EXOC3L2, PICALM
Sherva, 2011	CC	GWAS	Israel (Wadi Ara)	2,540,000 (imputed)	C	124	-	142	-	AGPAT1, ATPVOA4, GLOD4, RGS6, TMEM132C
Wijsman, 2011	CC, FBAT	GWAS	USA (NIA, NCRAD)	565336	M	1848	617	1991	573	APOE, CELF2

Table 2. Genome-Wide Association Studies in Alzheimer's Disease.

7.1. Grupe 2007

The first GWAS addressing Alzheimer´s disease was reported in 2007 by Grupe *et al.* A total of 17, 343 SNPs, located in 11 221 unique genes were tested for an association with LOAD in a case–control discovery sample from the UK (1808 LOAD cases and 2062 controls) [149]. These researchers reported the identification of several candidate SNPs showing a significant association with LOAD. Three of these SNPs (**rs157581, rs405509** and **rs1132899**) are located on chromosome 19, close to the APOE gene, and exhibit genome-wide significance (P value=6.94E-81 to 0.0001) and linkage disequilibrium (LD) with the APOE4 and 2/3 variants (0.09 < D0 < 1). Furthermore, sixteen additional SNPs showed evidence of an association with LOAD [P=0.0010-0.00006; odds ratio (OR)=1.07–1.45].

Of these SNPs, one was a missense mutation (**rs3745833**) located in the galanin-like peptide precursor (**GALP**) gene. The associated SNP encodes a non-synonymous substitution (Ili72Met) in exon 4. In the Caucasian population, the common minor C-allele increases the risk for AD in 10% of individuals. The galanin gene has been implicated in neuronal survival, regeneration and neuroprotection as well as the inhibition of cholinergic neurotransmission and suppression of long-term potentiation [150-151]. In limbic brain regions of AD patients, galanin expression is upregulated and could conceivably worsen the symptoms of the disease. Transgenic mice overexpressing galanin display cognitive and neurochemical deficits similar to those observed in AD patients [152].

Another important SNP was found to be located in PGBD1 (piggyBack transposable element derived 1). The associated SNP (**rs3800324**) encodes a non-synonymous substitution (Gly244Glu) in exon 5, and the presence of the minor A (Glu) allele significantly increases the risk of AD by 20%. The function of this protein is not known, but it is specifically expressed in the brain. Finally, in this study, the authors showed that four additional SNPs showed evidence of association with LOAD. These variants include SNPs located in TNK1 and PCK1 as well as an intergenic SNP near SERPINA13.

TNK1 is a non-receptor tyrosine kinase that mediates phospholipid signal transduction. In addition, together with TRAK2, TNK1 may be involved in protein trafficking and signal transduction [153] and participate in the processing of amyloid precursor protein and amyloid β-production [154-155]. Aberrant TNK1 activity may increase the risk of LOAD [156].

7.2. Coon 2007, Reiman 2007

In the same year, Coon *et al.* employed an ultra-high-density whole-genome association analysis, demonstrating the ability to identify the APOE locus as a major susceptibility gene for late onset AD [157]. This study used the Affymetrix 500K platform, including 502,627 SNPs, and was performed in a population of 1086 histopathologically verified AD cases and controls. The results obtained showed that the APOE locus is the major susceptibility gene for late onset AD in the human genome, with an OR significantly greater than any other locus in the human genome (Bonferroni corrected OR=4.01). The polymorphism identified in this study (**rs4420638**) is located on chromosome 19 and is 14 kilobase pairs distal to the APOE epsilon variant.

In a subsequent study, the same group of researchers divided each cohort of LOAD cases and controls into two subgroups: allelic APOE ε4 carriers and APOE ε4 noncarriers. The results showed an association with six SNPs of the GRB-associated binding protein 2 (GAB2) gene and a common haplotype encompassing the entire **GAB2** gene [158]. SNP **rs2373115** was associated with an odds ratio of 4.06 (confidence interval 2.81–14.69) and interacts with APOE ε4 to further modify risk.

The GAB2 protein is involved in a number of different pathways, and thus, it is possible that GAB2 could affect mechanisms involved in cell survival, Tau phosphorylation and NFT formation. Additionally, GAB2 may be involved in the production of Aβ [158], contributing to the development of AD pathology. Finally, GAB2 has been found to be coexpressed with other putative AD-related genes [159].

7.3. Abraham 2008

The GWAS conducted by Abraham in 2008 differs from all other currently published GWAS addressing AD in that, in the initial screening in this study, DNA pools were utilized for genotyping rather than individual DNA samples [160]. DNA samples were collected from 1,082 individuals with LOAD and 1,239 control subjects. The age at onset ranged from 60 to 95 years, and controls were matched for age (mean=76.53 years, SD=33), gender and ethnicity. The construction of the pools was validated using the SNaPshot method. The pools were genotyped using Illumina HumanHap300 and Illumina Sentrix HumanHap240S arrays, testing 561,494 SNPs. The results showed an association of several SNPs close to the *APOE* locus with LOAD, including 7 SNPs within 71 kb, with allele frequency differences of between 6% – 14%. Five of the seven SNPs were individually genotyped and were confirmed to present highly significant associations with LOAD. Although these studies using pooled DNA samples considerably reduce costs, their results may not accurately represent real allele frequency distributions.

7.4. Bertram 2008.

Another GWAS addressing AD was performed by Bertram *et al.* in 2008. This study represented the first to employ family-based methods for the initial screening. This case, a genome-wide association (GWA) analysis was performed using 484,522 single-nucleotide polymorphisms (SNPs) on a large (1,376 samples from 410 families) sample of AD families of self-reported European descent. All 10,388 X chromosome markers were eliminated, as also were 5,758 SNPs that did not pass genotype quality assessment or showed a minor allele frequency (MAF). A total of 404,604 (80.8%) SNPs were finally used for screening [161].

In this study, five SNPs were identified as showing either a significant or marginally significant genome-wide association with a multivariate phenotype combining affection status and onset age. Four of these markers were not related to APOE4. The first marker, **rs4420638**, is located 340 bp 3′ of APOC1 on chromosome 19q13 and very likely reflects the effects of the APOE4 allele (**rs429358**). The other markers are **rs11159647** (located in predicted gene NT_026437.1360 on chromosome 14q31.2), **rs179943** (located in **ATXN1** [MIM 601556] on chromosome 6p22.3,

rs3826656 (located in predicted gene NT_011109.848 on 19q13.33), and **rs2049161** (located in cDNA BC040718 on 18p11.31). These four SNPs were tested in three additional independent AD family samples composed of nearly 2700 individuals from almost 900 families. SNP **rs11159647** on chromosome 14q31 was primarily associated with age of onset (p=0.006), with a median reduction in onset age of 1.1 years being observed. Evidence of an association with this allele was also found in GWA data generated in an independent sample of ~1,400 AD cases and controls (p=0.04). None of these markers were previously described as modifiers of AD risk or onset age (Bertram 2008). The SNP **rs179943** on chromosome 6p22.3 is located within an intron of the ataxin 1 (ATXN1) gene. Although the function of ataxin1 is not known, it has been proposed to be associated with spinocerebellar ataxia type 1 (**SCA1**), a progressive neurodegenerative disease. The SNP **rs3826656** on 19q33 is located less than 2 kb proximal of the transcription initiation site of **CD33**. This protein is a cell-surface receptor on cells of monocytic or myeloid lineages. Additionally, it is a member of the SIGLEC family of lectins that bind sialic acid and regulate the innate immune system via the activation of caspase-dependent and caspase-independent cell death pathways.

7.5. Beecham 2009

Another GWAS was carried out by Beecham in 2009. This GWAS included 998 individuals of European descent, including 492 LOAD cases and 496 cognitive controls, using Illumina's HumanHap550 BeadChip. An additional 238 cases and 220 controls were also used in this study as a validation dataset for single-nucleotide polymorphisms (SNPs) that met the genome-wide significance criteria. The results showed associations of 38 SNPs with LOAD with uncorrected p values < 0.00005, six of which were in or near the APOE gene [162].

The most significant non-APOE SNP was rs11610206 on chromosome 12q13 (45.92 Mb), which presented an uncorrected $p=1.93X10^{-6}$. This SNP was genotyped in an independent replication dataset of 238 cases and 220 controls, resulting in a p value of $3.452X10^{-7}$, which was more significant than in the initial dataset. This SNP is not located in a known gene but is less than 10 kb from the FAM113B gene. Additionally, there are a number of nearby candidate genes, such as the *vitamin D* (1,25-dihydroxyvitamin D3) *receptor* (*VDR* [MIM 601769]) and *adhesion molecule with Ig-like domain 2* (*AMIGO2*) genes.

These authors also compared their results with those obtained by Reiman, and four polymorphisms were found that showed an association in both studies. Two of these SNPs, 1q42 and 19q13, are located within genes; the two other signals replicated in both datasets are not in known genes. The 1q42 SNP (rs12044355) resides in the DISC1 gene, which has been associated with schizophrenia and is linked to bipolar disorder, depression, and cognitive function. The 19q13 signal is located in and near exon 6 of *zinc finger protein 224* (*ZNF224* [MIM 194555]); two of the associated markers (rs4508518 and rs3746319) are within the exon. The first SNP (rs4508518) is a coding but synonymous polymorphism, whereas the second (rs3746319) leads to a missense mutation.

Finally, nine candidate genes from the over 500 genes in the AlzGene candidate gene list present SNPs with a nominal association in both GWASs. These genes (**ADAM12, CSF1, GBP2,**

KCNMA1, NOS2A, SORCS2, SORCS3, SORL1, and **WWC1)** exhibited p values ranging from 0.003 to 0.05 in the individual GWAS and from 0.0001 to 0.01 in the joint analysis.

Of these genes, the main candidate associated with the development of LOAD in several populations is the *sortlin-related receptor* (**SORL1**) gene. The mechanism by which SORL1 affects the development of Alzheimer´s disease is unknown, but it has been established to have the ability to interact with APP and APOE, possibly affecting the formation and accumulation of amyloid beta peptides.

7.6. Carrasquillo 2009

This genome-wide association study was performed in two stages using the Illumina Human-Hap300 array. In stage I, 313,504 SNPs were analyzed in 844 cases and 1,255 controls (2100 subjects from the Mayo clinic), and only six *APOE*-linked SNPs showed genome-wide significance in this stage of study. Of these polymorphisms, only rs2075650 (located on chromosome 19) showed genome-wide significance, and this SNP shows strong linkage disequilibrium (LD) with APOE (P value $4.8x10^{-46}$). In stage II, the 25 SNPs showing the most significant associations in stage I were genotyped in an additional 845 cases and 1,000 controls. These 25 SNPs included 10 SNPs in the APOE region on chromosome 19, all of which presented *P* values ranging from $9.5X10^{-79}$ to 0.05. The other 15 SNPs are located on other chromosomes. One of two SNPs on the X chromosome, rs5984894 (P value 0.0006), is located within the gene encoding protocadherin 11, X-linked (**PCDH11X**) in the Xq21.3/Yp11.2 region. To extend the analysis of *PCDH11X*, three *PCDH11X* SNPs (rs5941047, rs4568761 and rs2573905) residing in the same haplotype block as rs5984894 were genotyped in all stages. Highly significant associations were observed for all three SNPs, with *P* values of 1.6×10^{-7} (rs2573905), 8.0×10^{-5} (rs5941047) and 0.001 (rs4568761) being obtained. rs2573905 is located 8,483 bp 3′ of rs5984894 and is in strong linkage disequilibrium with rs5984894 (r2=0.98, D'=0.99). Analysis of rs5984894 by multivariable logistic regression adjusted by sex showed that the association was stronger in female homozygotes (OR=1.75, P=$2.0x^{10-7}$) and heterozygotes (OR=1.26, P=0.01). For hemizygous males, a similar trend was observed (OR=1.18), although this did not reach statistical significance (P-value 0.07) [163].

The ***PCDH11X*** gene contains at least 17 exons spanning over 700 kb. Alternative splicing of *PCDH11X* produces several isoforms that are mainly expressed in the brain, with particularly strong expression being detected in the cortex and hippocampus and weaker expression being observed in the cerebellum. The PCDH11X protein plays a fundamental role in cell-cell recognition and it is essential for the segmental development and function of the central nervous system. However, among all published and reported AD GWASs, this is the only one that reports involvement of an X chromosome locus, which, if confirmed, could at least partially explain the well-established increased disease prevalence in women versus men.

7.7. Harold 2009

In the first stage of this study, an association with the APOE locus (rs2075650, $p=1.8\times10^{-157}$) was established in 3,941 patients and 7,848 controls. Additionally, this GWA analysis identified strong associations of SNPs in two new loci: rs11136000, which is located in the ***CLU***, or ***APOJ***, gene ($p=1.4\times10^{-9}$), and rs3851179, a SNP 5′ to the *PICALM* gene ($p=1.9\times10^{-8}$). rs11136000 is located within an intron of the clusterin (*CLU*, also known as *APOJ*) gene on chromosome 8, and rs3851179 is found 88.5 kb 5′ of ***PICALM*** on chromosome 11. In stage 2, these new SNPs were genotyped in 2,023 AD cases and 2,340 age-matched controls from an independent sample. Associations were found for both polymorphisms, with p=0.017 and OR=0.905 for rs11136000 and p=0.014 and OR=0.897 for rs3851179. A meta-analysis of stages 1 and 2 was also conducted in this study, and the results showed highly significant evidence of associations for the *CLU* and *PICALM* loci (rs11136000 $p=8.5\times10^{-10}$ and rs3851179 $p=1.3\times10^{-9}$, respectively). Finally, no significant interactions of novel SNPs associated with *APOE* status were observed to influence AD risk (rs11136000x*APOE*4 interaction p=0.674; rs3851179x*APOE*4 interaction p=0.735) [164].

CLU is a secreted chaperone that can also be found in the cytosol under some stress conditions. It has been suggested that CLU is involved in several basic biological events, including cell death, tumor progression, and neurodegenerative disorders. The genetic risk allele (C) of CLU gene variant rs11136000 is carried by ~88% of Caucasians; the C allele confers 1.16 greater odds of developing late onset AD than the T allele [165].

PICALM is a phosphatidylinositol-binding clathrin assembly protein. This protein plays a role in altering synaptic vesicle cycling or APP endocytosis. Although the presence of polymorphism rs3851179 was associated with high significance related to the development of AD in the Caucasian population, these results could not be replicated in Chinese or Italian populations [166-167]. The results obtained in recent studies by Piaceri showed that the segregation of the PICALM rs3851179 variant did not show a statistically significant difference between LOAD cases and controls, suggesting a reduced risk of developing late onset Alzheimer′s disease (LOAD).

7.8. Han 2010

Unlike the studies described above, this study additionally established a relationship between the allelic variants found by GWAS and cerebrospinal fluid (CSF) levels of amyloid Ab1-42, T-tau, and P-tau181P [168]. The data used in this study was obtained from the Alzheimer′s Disease Neuroimaging Initiative (ADNI). This database consists of approximately 800 adults with ages between 55-90 years, 243 of whom were normal subjects, while 235 presented mild cognitive impairment, and 340 had been diagnosed with Alzheimer′s disease. These participants were genotyped using Illumina Human Genome 610 Quad BeadChips, and the CSF levels of amyloid Ab1-42, T-tau, and P-tau181P were determined in 410 subjects (119 normal, 115 MCI and 247 AD), of which 247 were men and 163 were women. An association analysis using age and APOE4 genotype as covariates was also performed, but did not incorporate principal component analysis.

The results showed that T-Tau levels are higher in AD patients than in control subjects. When the results were adjusted using APOE and the age of individuals as covariates, it was not possible to observe an association between SNPs and CSF levels among patients. This study also identified polymorphisms associated with the development of AD that had been already reported in previous studies: CYP19A1 (rs2899472, p=1.90 × 10-7) and NCAM2 (rs1022442, p=2.75 × 10-7).

8. Population genetics and genetic association studies: crucial issues to enhance the transparency of results.

Although efforts to obtain genetic biomarkers that help in anticipate diagnostic of Alzheimer disease, present-day the clinical research not have the results that expected. The publications that relate genes with Alzheimer disease has increased exponentially however, numerous lines of evidence have demostrated discrepant results among populations. These findings suggest that it is neccesary diminish the confounder factors and focus on identify the cause [169]. Once the causes are established, could integrated in practice of medicine helping with anticipate diagnostic.

In order to avoid spurious associations Little J. et al published an initiative that pretends increase the quality of reporting genetic association studies dissemining this information in different journals (epidemiology, clinical investigation, internal medicine and basic research) [170-176]. The publication refered as STREGA report (STrenghthening the REporting of Geenetic Association studies) provides additional comments to 22 items reported previously by STROBE (STrengthening the Reporting of OBservational Studies in Epidemiology) [177]. These comments include different items, however population genetics topics are crucial issues whose depreciation, increase statistical mistakes type I and II [173].

One of the most important topics in genetic association studies (GAS) is Hardy-Weinberg equilibrium. Hardy-Weinberg equilibrium (HWE) is represented by the equation $(p+q)^2=1$, whose perfect square binomial equation it is represented by $p^2+2pq+q^2=1$, where p^2 and q^2 represented homozygous state, whereas 2pq represented heterozygous state. Under random maiting and non-overlapping, homozygous and heterozygous states are in equal proportions (0.5 each one) maintaining the HWE. This equilibrium are also maintained when evolutionary forces are absents (mutation, random drift, genetic flow, natural selection), the population size it is nearby to the infinitum, and when frequencies of alleles in both sexes are equal [178]. However, some conditions could modify these proportions provoking a Hardy-Weinberg departure (HWD). HWD is related with an excess of homozygous individuals (with subsequent heterozygous deficit) or heterozygous individuals (with subsequent homozygous deficit). Therefore, Hardy-Weinberg model is an essential element used to analyze genetic data, and is the initial step for check the quality of genotyping, because genotyping errors due to poor quality provoke HWD as a consequence of distort in genotype distribution [179]. Nevertheless, HWD are not only related with genotyping mistakes because some factors as demographic events, young population, founder effect, inbreeding, and population stratification may provoke HWD.

Population stratification is the consequence of populations with a recent miscegenation. Admixture populations show different allele frequencies among different subpopulations that conform the whole population, which consequently is not a homogeneous population [180].

Indeed, admixture population is an heterogeneous population with dissimilar ancestry proportions. Consequently, the population stratification may lead to spurious associations because each subpopulation are not equally represented [169, 179]. Applying these premises to GAS, the differences of frequencies between cases and controls populations could be related with dissimilar frequencies among different population strata rather than association of genes with disease. Therefore, population stratification is the most common problem and one of the most important confounder factors in GAS [180-181].

At first glance could appear that HWD are only related with false associations nevertheless, HWD could also be a signature of disease association, principally in case-control studies, because if some allele is associated with a disease this association break the random maiting provoking HWD [182-183]. This HWD is the result of differences between allele frequencies, where one allele are overrepresented in cases group (excess of homozygous), whereas the same allele are underrepresented in control cases (excess of heterozygous). In order to suport these findings it is neccesary to know the frequency of distribution of this allele in the general population. If the allele show a high frequency in the general population, this finding could be not related with the disease [182, 184-185]. Conversely, if the prevalence of the allele is low in the general population, these data may support a relationship between the allele and the disease suggesting the allele could be a risk allele. As a consequence, the HWD is particularly relevant in GAS.

In light of these evidence, several methods have been developed to detect HWD. The most used method is chi square, however this statistic only must be used in homogeneous population [186]. Other approach is detect the intrapoblational variance (F_{is}), where $F_{is} > 0$ means a homozygous excess, whereas $F_{is} < 0$ means heterozygous deficit [187]. Recently, Li M and Li C have developed a likelihood test that allows assessment of HWD taking into account potential association with the disease [182]. This method can differentitate HWD caused by disease association, diminishing the over estimation of type I error and avoiding the false exclusion of associated markers. Hence, is necessary diminish the effect of genetic structure in order to detect susceptibility loci for complex disease. Studies to date suggest different methods, among which are:

- Genomic control. This method diminish the population heterogeneity due to cryptic relatedmess or correlation across individuals, correcting the variance inflation, which is previously detected with unlinked null markers [188].
- Infer the number of populations. This Bayesian analysis inferrers the number of subpopulations (*k*) and correct them, decreasing the effect of admixture over GAS [189].
- Summarize the genetic background using hierarchical clustering through principal component analysis (PCA) and its variants enable the detecction of differences between samples, detect clinal distributions and suggest other demographic events as isolation-by-distance [190-191].

All of these bioinformatic models have been an excelent help to clarify the genetic associations in population-based genetic associations increasing the statistical power. These methods have detected limitations or errors in assessments genotypes (20-70%) [192], as well as spurious association rates (40%) [193]. However, these methods help to identify rare variants that could have a role in common disease etiology [194]. Hence, all of these variants have an implications in desing, analysis and interpretation of GAS, and are a good strategy for developing markers to elucidate the origins of many human genetic diseases. This alternative approach of anticipated diagnosis can significantly reduce treatment costs by providing preventive medicine

9. Conclusions

Alzheimer´s disease is one of the main causes of dementia. This disease is clinically characterized by the irreversible and progressive loss of memory and it is histopathologically characterized by the presence of neuritic plaques (NP) and neurofibrillary tangles (NFT). Both types of lesions are formed due to the accumulation of insoluble protein aggregates, consisting of beta amyloid peptide and the microtubule binding protein Tau, respectively. Studies performed in the last thirty years have provided important advances in understanding the molecular mechanisms involved in the pathology of AD. Through genetic studies, it has been possible to identify the presence of mutations in the APP, PS1 and PS2 genes as causal factors for early onset Alzheimer´s disease (EOAD). These mutations are associated with beta amyloid peptide accumulation, which generates a series of molecular events that lead to a neurodegenerative process. With respect to late onset Alzheimer´s disease (LOAD), the results obtained to date do not support amyloid overproduction as a cause; in this case, it has been proposed that alterations in the mechanisms responsible for peptide clearance indirectly favor the amyloid accumulation. Amyloids have the ability to interact with several different receptor types, including the Frizzled, insulin, NMDA and NGF receptors, triggering events leading to neuronal death. Additionally, it is known that molecules such as APOE play an important role in the clearance and aggregation of amyloid beta and other risk factors that may eventually determine the conformational changes that allow amyloids to aggregate and form neuritic plaques. For LOAD, APOE is the single most important risk factor. However, a recent GWAS identified several susceptibility loci associated with disease development in different populations, although these studies provide a better understanding of the pathophysiology of the disease, these new genetic markers seem to have a weak genetic effect. Therefore, it is necessary to consider using other tools to detect genotyping errors that can be caused among other reasons, by population stratification.

Author details

Victoria Campos-Peña[1], Rocío Gómez[2] and Marco Antonio Meraz Ríos[3*]

*Address all correspondence to: mmeraz@cinvestav.mx

1 Laboratorio Experimental de Enfermedades Neurodegenerativas, Instituto Nacional de Neurología y Neurocirugía Manuel Velasco Suárez. Mexico City, Mexico

2 Centro de Investigación y de Estudios Avanzados del Instituto Politécnico Nacional, Departamennto de Toxicología, Mexico

3 Centro de Investigación y de Estudios Avanzados del Instituto Politécnico Nacional, Departamento de Biomedicina Molecular. México City, Mexico

References

[1] Tomlinson, B.E.C., JAN, *Ageing and the dementias*. Greenfield's Neuropathology, ed. J.C. Hume Adams, JAN; Duchen, L.W.. 1984, London Edward Arnold.

[2] Roberts, G.W., et al., *On the origin of Alzheimer's disease: a hypothesis.* Neuroreport, 1993. 4(1): p. 7-9.

[3] Terry, R.D., et al., *Physical basis of cognitive alterations in Alzheimer's disease: synapse loss is the major correlate of cognitive impairment.* Annals of neurology, 1991. 30(4): p. 572-80.

[4] Heyman, A., et al., *Early-onset Alzheimer's disease: clinical predictors of institutionalization and death.* Neurology, 1987. 37(6): p. 980-4.

[5] McKhann, G., et al., *Clinical diagnosis of Alzheimer's disease: report of the NINCDS-ADRDA Work Group under the auspices of Department of Health and Human Services Task Force on Alzheimer's Disease.* Neurology, 1984. 34(7): p. 939-44.

[6] Folstein, M.F., S.E. Folstein, and P.R. McHugh, *"Mini-mental state". A practical method for grading the cognitive state of patients for the clinician.* Journal of psychiatric research, 1975. 12(3): p. 189-98.

[7] Iversen, L.L., et al., *The toxicity in vitro of beta-amyloid protein.* The Biochemical journal, 1995. 311 (Pt 1): p. 1-16.

[8] Glenner, G.G., et al., *The amyloid deposits in Alzheimer's disease: their nature and pathogenesis.* Applied pathology, 1984. 2(6): p. 357-69.

[9] Selkoe, D.J., *Alzheimer's disease: a central role for amyloid.* Journal of neuropathology and experimental neurology, 1994. 53(5): p. 438-47.

[10] Kang, J., et al., *The precursor of Alzheimer's disease amyloid A4 protein resembles a cell-surface receptor.* Nature, 1987. 325(6106): p. 733-6.

[11] Sandbrink, R., C.L. Masters, and K. Beyreuther, *Beta A4-amyloid protein precursor mRNA isoforms without exon 15 are ubiquitously expressed in rat tissues including brain, but not in neurons.* The Journal of biological chemistry, 1994. 269(2): p. 1510-7.

[12] Graebert, K.S., et al., *Localization and regulated release of Alzheimer amyloid precursor-like protein in thyrocytes.* Laboratory investigation; a journal of technical methods and pathology, 1995. 72(5): p. 513-23.

[13] Hoffmann, J., et al., *A possible role for the Alzheimer amyloid precursor protein in the regulation of epidermal basal cell proliferation.* European journal of cell biology, 2000. 79(12): p. 905-14.

[14] Schmitz, A., et al., *The biological role of the Alzheimer amyloid precursor protein in epithelial cells.* Histochemistry and cell biology, 2002. 117(2): p. 171-80.

[15] Schubert, D., et al., *The regulation of amyloid beta protein precursor secretion and its modulatory role in cell adhesion.* Neuron, 1989. 3(6): p. 689-94.

[16] Crowther, R.A. and C.M. Wischik, *Image reconstruction of the Alzheimer paired helical filament.* The EMBO journal, 1985. 4(13B): p. 3661-5.

[17] Turner, P.R., et al., *Roles of amyloid precursor protein and its fragments in regulating neural activity, plasticity and memory.* Progress in neurobiology, 2003. 70(1): p. 1-32.

[18] Priller, C., et al., *Synapse formation and function is modulated by the amyloid precursor protein.* The Journal of neuroscience : the official journal of the Society for Neuroscience, 2006. 26(27): p. 7212-21.

[19] De Strooper, B. and W. Annaert, *Proteolytic processing and cell biological functions of the amyloid precursor protein.* J Cell Sci, 2000. 113 (Pt 11): p. 1857-70.

[20] Esch, F.S., et al., *Cleavage of amyloid beta peptide during constitutive processing of its precursor.* Science, 1990. 248(4959): p. 1122-4.

[21] Sisodia, S.S., et al., *Evidence that beta-amyloid protein in Alzheimer's disease is not derived by normal processing.* Science, 1990. 248(4954): p. 492-5.

[22] Dries, D.R. and G. Yu, *Assembly, maturation, and trafficking of the gamma-secretase complex in Alzheimer's disease.* Curr Alzheimer Res, 2008. 5(2): p. 132-46.

[23] Blessed, G., B.E. Tomlinson, and M. Roth, *The association between quantitative measures of dementia and of senile change in the cerebral grey matter of elderly subjects.* The British journal of psychiatry : the journal of mental science, 1968. 114(512): p. 797-811.

[24] Braak, H. and E. Braak, *Staging of Alzheimer-related cortical destruction.* International psychogeriatrics / IPA, 1997. 9 Suppl 1: p. 257-61; discussion 269-72.

[25] Andreadis, A., W.M. Brown, and K.S. Kosik, *Structure and novel exons of the human tau gene.* Biochemistry, 1992. 31(43): p. 10626-33.

[26] Neve, R.L., et al., *Identification of cDNA clones for the human microtubule-associated protein tau and chromosomal localization of the genes for tau and microtubule-associated protein 2.* Brain Res, 1986. 387(3): p. 271-80.

[27] Neve, R.L., et al., *A cDNA for a human microtubule associated protein 2 epitope in the Alzheimer neurofibrillary tangle.* Brain Res, 1986. 387(2): p. 193-6.

[28] Goedert, M., et al., *Multiple isoforms of human microtubule-associated protein tau: sequences and localization in neurofibrillary tangles of Alzheimer's disease.* Neuron, 1989. 3(4): p. 519-26.

[29] Goedert, M. and R. Jakes, *Expression of separate isoforms of human tau protein: correlation with the tau pattern in brain and effects on tubulin polymerization.* EMBO J, 1990. 9(13): p. 4225-30.

[30] Spillantini, M.G. and M. Goedert, *Tau pathology and neurodegeneration.* Lancet Neurol, 2013. 12(6): p. 609-22.

[31] Ennulat, D.J., et al., *Two separate 18-amino acid domains of tau promote the polymerization of tubulin.* The Journal of biological chemistry, 1989. 264(10): p. 5327-30.

[32] Goedert, M. and A. Klug, *Tau protein and the paired helical filament of Alzheimer's disease.* Brain research bulletin, 1999. 50(5-6): p. 469-70.

[33] Cleveland, D.W., S.Y. Hwo, and M.W. Kirschner, *Physical and chemical properties of purified tau factor and the role of tau in microtubule assembly.* Journal of molecular biology, 1977. 116(2): p. 227-47.

[34] Schweers, O., et al., *Structural studies of tau protein and Alzheimer paired helical filaments show no evidence for beta-structure.* The Journal of biological chemistry, 1994. 269(39): p. 24290-7.

[35] Buee, L. and A. Delacourte, *Comparative biochemistry of tau in progressive supranuclear palsy, corticobasal degeneration, FTDP-17 and Pick's disease.* Brain pathology, 1999. 9(4): p. 681-93.

[36] Poorkaj, P., et al., *Tau is a candidate gene for chromosome 17 frontotemporal dementia.* Annals of neurology, 1998. 43(6): p. 815-25.

[37] Spillantini, M.G., T.D. Bird, and B. Ghetti, *Frontotemporal dementia and Parkinsonism linked to chromosome 17: a new group of tauopathies.* Brain pathology, 1998. 8(2): p. 387-402.

[38] Hutton, M., *Molecular genetics of chromosome 17 tauopathies.* Annals of the New York Academy of Sciences, 2000. 920: p. 63-73.

[39] Hutton, M., et al., *Association of missense and 5'-splice-site mutations in tau with the inherited dementia FTDP-17.* Nature, 1998. 393(6686): p. 702-5.

[40] Bergem, A.L., K. Engedal, and E. Kringlen, *The role of heredity in late-onset Alzheimer disease and vascular dementia. A twin study.* Archives of general psychiatry, 1997. 54(3): p. 264-70.

[41] Gatz, M., et al., *Role of genes and environments for explaining Alzheimer disease.* Archives of general psychiatry, 2006. 63(2): p. 168-74.

[42] Raiha, I., et al., *Alzheimer's disease in Finnish twins.* Lancet, 1996. 347(9001): p. 573-8.

[43] Gatz, M., et al., *Dementia in Swedish twins: predicting incident cases.* Behavior genetics, 2010. 40(6): p. 768-75.

[44] Corder, E.H., et al., *Gene dose of apolipoprotein E type 4 allele and the risk of Alzheimer's disease in late onset families.* Science, 1993. 261(5123): p. 921-3.

[45] Saunders, A.M., et al., *Association of apolipoprotein E allele epsilon 4 with late-onset familial and sporadic Alzheimer's disease.* Neurology, 1993. 43(8): p. 1467-72.

[46] Aleshkov, S., C.R. Abraham, and V.I. Zannis, *Interaction of nascent ApoE2, ApoE3, and ApoE4 isoforms expressed in mammalian cells with amyloid peptide beta (1-40). Relevance to Alzheimer's disease.* Biochemistry, 1997. 36(34): p. 10571-80.

[47] Strittmatter, W.J. and A.D. Roses, *Apolipoprotein E and Alzheimer disease.* Proceedings of the National Academy of Sciences of the United States of America, 1995. 92(11): p. 4725-7.

[48] Ertekin-Taner, N., *Genetics of Alzheimer's disease: a centennial review.* Neurologic clinics, 2007. 25(3): p. 611-67, v.

[49] Kim, J., J.M. Basak, and D.M. Holtzman, *The role of apolipoprotein E in Alzheimer's disease.* Neuron, 2009. 63(3): p. 287-303.

[50] Levy-Lahad, E., et al., *A familial Alzheimer's disease locus on chromosome 1.* Science, 1995. 269(5226): p. 970-3.

[51] Duff, K., et al., *Increased amyloid-beta42(43) in brains of mice expressing mutant presenilin 1.* Nature, 1996. 383(6602): p. 710-3.

[52] Kovacs, D.M., et al., *Alzheimer-associated presenilins 1 and 2: neuronal expression in brain and localization to intracellular membranes in mammalian cells.* Nature medicine, 1996. 2(2): p. 224-9.

[53] Borchelt, D.R., et al., *Familial Alzheimer's disease-linked presenilin 1 variants elevate Abeta1-42/1-40 ratio in vitro and in vivo.* Neuron, 1996. 17(5): p. 1005-13.

[54] Scheuner, D., et al., *Secreted amyloid beta-protein similar to that in the senile plaques of Alzheimer's disease is increased in vivo by the presenilin 1 and 2 and APP mutations linked to familial Alzheimer's disease.* Nature medicine, 1996. 2(8): p. 864-70.

[55] Goate, A., et al., *Segregation of a missense mutation in the amyloid precursor protein gene with familial Alzheimer's disease.* Nature, 1991. 349(6311): p. 704-6.

[56] Sisodia, S.S., S.H. Kim, and G. Thinakaran, *Function and dysfunction of the presenilins.* American journal of human genetics, 1999. 65(1): p. 7-12.

[57] Chartier-Harlin, M.C., et al., *Screening for the beta-amyloid precursor protein mutation (APP717: Val----Ile) in extended pedigrees with early onset Alzheimer's disease.* Neuroscience letters, 1991. 129(1): p. 134-5.

[58] Murrell, J., et al., *A mutation in the amyloid precursor protein associated with hereditary Alzheimer's disease.* Science, 1991. 254(5028): p. 97-9.

[59] Mullan, M., et al., *A pathogenic mutation for probable Alzheimer's disease in the APP gene at the N-terminus of beta-amyloid.* Nature genetics, 1992. 1(5): p. 345-7.

[60] Nunan, J. and D.H. Small, *Regulation of APP cleavage by alpha-, beta-and gamma-secretases.* FEBS letters, 2000. 483(1): p. 6-10.

[61] Perez, R.G., S.L. Squazzo, and E.H. Koo, *Enhanced release of amyloid beta-protein from codon 670/671 "Swedish" mutant beta-amyloid precursor protein occurs in both secretory and endocytic pathways.* The Journal of biological chemistry, 1996. 271(15): p. 9100-7.

[62] Levy, E., et al., *Mutation of the Alzheimer's disease amyloid gene in hereditary cerebral hemorrhage, Dutch type.* Science, 1990. 248(4959): p. 1124-6.

[63] Eckman, C.B., et al., *A new pathogenic mutation in the APP gene (I716V) increases the relative proportion of A beta 42(43).* Human molecular genetics, 1997. 6(12): p. 2087-9.

[64] Grabowski, T.J., et al., *Novel amyloid precursor protein mutation in an Iowa family with dementia and severe cerebral amyloid angiopathy.* Annals of neurology, 2001. 49(6): p. 697-705.

[65] Nilsberth, C., et al., *The 'Arctic' APP mutation (E693G) causes Alzheimer's disease by enhanced Abeta protofibril formation.* Nature neuroscience, 2001. 4(9): p. 887-93.

[66] Kasuga, K., et al., *Identification of independent APP locus duplication in Japanese patients with early-onset Alzheimer disease.* J Neurol Neurosurg Psychiatry, 2009. 80(9): p. 1050-2.

[67] Rovelet-Lecrux, A., et al., *APP locus duplication in a Finnish family with dementia and intracerebral haemorrhage.* J Neurol Neurosurg Psychiatry, 2007. 78(10): p. 1158-9.

[68] Rovelet-Lecrux, A., et al., *APP locus duplication causes autosomal dominant early-onset Alzheimer disease with cerebral amyloid angiopathy.* Nat Genet, 2006. 38(1): p. 24-6.

[69] Sleegers, K., et al., *APP duplication is sufficient to cause early onset Alzheimer's dementia with cerebral amyloid angiopathy.* Brain, 2006. 129(Pt 11): p. 2977-83.

[70] Higgins, G.A. and H. Jacobsen, *Transgenic mouse models of Alzheimer's disease: phenotype and application.* Behavioural pharmacology, 2003. 14(5-6): p. 419-38.

[71] Mineur, Y.S., et al., *Genetic mouse models of Alzheimer's disease.* Neural plasticity, 2005. 12(4): p. 299-310.

[72] Irizarry, M.C., et al., *APPSw transgenic mice develop age-related A beta deposits and neuropil abnormalities, but no neuronal loss in CA1.* Journal of neuropathology and experimental neurology, 1997. 56(9): p. 965-73.

[73] Westerman, M.A., et al., *The relationship between Abeta and memory in the Tg2576 mouse model of Alzheimer's disease.* The Journal of neuroscience : the official journal of the Society for Neuroscience, 2002. 22(5): p. 1858-67.

[74] Moechars, D., et al., *Transgenic mice expressing an alpha-secretion mutant of the amyloid precursor protein in the brain develop a progressive CNS disorder.* Behavioural brain research, 1998. 95(1): p. 55-64.

[75] McPhie, D.L., et al., *DNA synthesis and neuronal apoptosis caused by familial Alzheimer disease mutants of the amyloid precursor protein are mediated by the p21 activated kinase PAK3.* The Journal of neuroscience : the official journal of the Society for Neuroscience, 2003. 23(17): p. 6914-27.

[76] Wolfe, M.S., *The gamma-secretase complex: membrane-embedded proteolytic ensemble.* Biochemistry, 2006. 45(26): p. 7931-9.

[77] Rechards, M., et al., *Presenilin-1 exists in both pre-and post-Golgi compartments and recycles via COPI-coated membranes.* Traffic, 2003. 4(8): p. 553-65.

[78] Chyung, J.H., D.M. Raper, and D.J. Selkoe, *Gamma-secretase exists on the plasma membrane as an intact complex that accepts substrates and effects intramembrane cleavage.* The Journal of biological chemistry, 2005. 280(6): p. 4383-92.

[79] Vetrivel, K.S., et al., *Association of gamma-secretase with lipid rafts in post-Golgi and endosome membranes.* The Journal of biological chemistry, 2004. 279(43): p. 44945-54.

[80] Kulic, L., et al., *Separation of presenilin function in amyloid beta-peptide generation and endoproteolysis of Notch.* Proceedings of the National Academy of Sciences of the United States of America, 2000. 97(11): p. 5913-8.

[81] Vassar, R. and M. Citron, *Abeta-generating enzymes: recent advances in beta-and gamma-secretase research.* Neuron, 2000. 27(3): p. 419-22.

[82] Ebinu, J.O. and B.A. Yankner, *A RIP tide in neuronal signal transduction.* Neuron, 2002. 34(4): p. 499-502.

[83] Marambaud, P., et al., *A presenilin-1/gamma-secretase cleavage releases the E-cadherin intracellular domain and regulates disassembly of adherens junctions.* The EMBO journal, 2002. 21(8): p. 1948-56.

[84] Li, T., et al., *Nicastrin is required for assembly of presenilin/gamma-secretase complexes to mediate Notch signaling and for processing and trafficking of beta-amyloid precursor protein in mammals.* The Journal of neuroscience : the official journal of the Society for Neuroscience, 2003. 23(8): p. 3272-7.

[85] Yu, G., et al., *Nicastrin modulates presenilin-mediated notch/glp-1 signal transduction and betaAPP processing.* Nature, 2000. 407(6800): p. 48-54.

[86] Naruse, S., et al., *Effects of PS1 deficiency on membrane protein trafficking in neurons.* Neuron, 1998. 21(5): p. 1213-21.

[87] Saura, C.A., E. Servian-Morilla, and F.G. Scholl, *Presenilin/gamma-secretase regulates neurexin processing at synapses.* PloS one, 2011. 6(4): p. e19430.

[88] Pratt, K.G., et al., *Presenilin 1 regulates homeostatic synaptic scaling through Akt signaling.* Nature neuroscience, 2011. 14(9): p. 1112-4.

[89] Toda, T., et al., *Presenilin-2 mutation causes early amyloid accumulation and memory impairment in a transgenic mouse model of Alzheimer's disease.* Journal of biomedicine & biotechnology, 2011. 2011: p. 617974.

[90] Supnet, C. and I. Bezprozvanny, *Presenilins function in ER calcium leak and Alzheimer's disease pathogenesis.* Cell calcium, 2011. 50(3): p. 303-9.

[91] Zhang, H., et al., *Role of presenilins in neuronal calcium homeostasis.* The Journal of neuroscience : the official journal of the Society for Neuroscience, 2010. 30(25): p. 8566-80.

[92] Zhang, C., et al., *Presenilins are essential for regulating neurotransmitter release.* Nature, 2009. 460(7255): p. 632-6.

[93] Campion, D., et al., *A novel presenilin 1 mutation resulting in familial Alzheimer's disease with an onset age of 29 years.* Neuroreport, 1996. 7(10): p. 1582-4.

[94] Wisniewski, T., et al., *A novel Polish presenilin-1 mutation (P117L) is associated with familial Alzheimer's disease and leads to death as early as the age of 28 years.* Neuroreport, 1998. 9(2): p. 217-21.

[95] Prihar, G., et al., *Structure and alternative splicing of the presenilin-2 gene.* Neuroreport, 1996. 7(10): p. 1680-4.

[96] Sherrington, R., et al., *Cloning of a gene bearing missense mutations in early-onset familial Alzheimer's disease.* Nature, 1995. 375(6534): p. 754-60.

[97] Citron, M., et al., *Mutant presenilins of Alzheimer's disease increase production of 42-residue amyloid beta-protein in both transfected cells and transgenic mice.* Nature medicine, 1997. 3(1): p. 67-72.

[98] Busciglio, J., et al., *Neuronal localization of presenilin-1 and association with amyloid plaques and neurofibrillary tangles in Alzheimer's disease.* The Journal of neuroscience : the official journal of the Society for Neuroscience, 1997. 17(13): p. 5101-7.

[99] Jacobsen, H., et al., *The influence of endoproteolytic processing of familial Alzheimer's disease presenilin 2 on abeta42 amyloid peptide formation.* The Journal of biological chemistry, 1999. 274(49): p. 35233-9.

[100] Storey, E. and R. Cappai, *The amyloid precursor protein of Alzheimer's disease and the Abeta peptide.* Neuropathology and applied neurobiology, 1999. 25(2): p. 81-97.

[101] Wolfe, M.S., et al., *Are presenilins intramembrane-cleaving proteases? Implications for the molecular mechanism of Alzheimer's disease.* Biochemistry, 1999. 38(35): p. 11223-30.

[102] Wolfe, M.S., et al., *Two transmembrane aspartates in presenilin-1 required for presenilin endoproteolysis and gamma-secretase activity.* Nature, 1999. 398(6727): p. 513-7.

[103] Steiner, H., et al., *A loss of function mutation of presenilin-2 interferes with amyloid beta-peptide production and notch signaling.* J Biol Chem, 1999. 274(40): p. 28669-73.

[104] Bentahir, M., et al., *Presenilin clinical mutations can affect gamma-secretase activity by different mechanisms.* J Neurochem, 2006. 96(3): p. 732-42.

[105] Pigino, G., et al., *Alzheimer's presenilin 1 mutations impair kinesin-based axonal transport.* The Journal of neuroscience : the official journal of the Society for Neuroscience, 2003. 23(11): p. 4499-508.

[106] Bentahir, M., et al., *Presenilin clinical mutations can affect gamma-secretase activity by different mechanisms.* Journal of neurochemistry, 2006. 96(3): p. 732-42.

[107] Lindquist, S.G., et al., *A novel presenilin 2 mutation (V393M) in early-onset dementia with profound language impairment.* European journal of neurology : the official journal of the European Federation of Neurological Societies, 2008. 15(10): p. 1135-9.

[108] Holtzman, D.M., J. Herz, and G. Bu, *Apolipoprotein E and apolipoprotein E receptors: normal biology and roles in Alzheimer disease.* Cold Spring Harb Perspect Med, 2012. 2(3): p. a006312.

[109] Schupf, N. and G.H. Sergievsky, *Genetic and host factors for dementia in Down's syndrome.* The British journal of psychiatry : the journal of mental science, 2002. 180: p. 405-10.

[110] Tang, M.X., et al., *Relative risk of Alzheimer disease and age-at-onset distributions, based on APOE genotypes among elderly African Americans, Caucasians, and Hispanics in New York City.* American journal of human genetics, 1996. 58(3): p. 574-84.

[111] Farrer, L.A., et al., *Association between bleomycin hydrolase and Alzheimer's disease in caucasians.* Annals of neurology, 1998. 44(5): p. 808-11.

[112] Tang, M.X., et al., *The APOE-epsilon4 allele and the risk of Alzheimer disease among African Americans, whites, and Hispanics.*JAMA : the journal of the American Medical Association, 1998. 279(10): p. 751-5.

[113] Graff-Radford, N.R., et al., *Association between apolipoprotein E genotype and Alzheimer disease in African American subjects.* Archives of neurology, 2002. 59(4): p. 594-600.

[114] Murrell, J.R., et al., *Association of apolipoprotein E genotype and Alzheimer disease in African Americans.* Archives of neurology, 2006. 63(3): p. 431-4.

[115] Weisgraber, K.H., *Apolipoprotein E: structure-function relationships.* Advances in protein chemistry, 1994. 45: p. 249-302.

[116] Wernette-Hammond, M.E., et al., *Glycosylation of human apolipoprotein E. The carbohydrate attachment site is threonine 194.* The Journal of biological chemistry, 1989. 264(15): p. 9094-101.

[117] Nickerson, D.A., et al., *Sequence diversity and large-scale typing of SNPs in the human apolipoprotein E gene.* Genome research, 2000. 10(10): p. 1532-45.

[118] Seripa, D., et al., *The genetics of the human APOE polymorphism.* Rejuvenation Res, 2011. 14(5): p. 491-500.

[119] Persico, A.M., et al., *Enhanced APOE2 transmission rates in families with autistic probands.* Psychiatr Genet, 2004. 14(2): p. 73-82.

[120] Avramopoulos, D., *Genetics of Alzheimer's disease: recent advances.* Genome Med, 2009. 1(3): p. 34.

[121] Davignon, J., R.E. Gregg, and C.F. Sing, *Apolipoprotein E polymorphism and atherosclerosis.* Arteriosclerosis, 1988. 8(1): p. 1-21.

[122] Mahley, R.W. and Z.S. Ji, *Remnant lipoprotein metabolism: key pathways involving cell-surface heparan sulfate proteoglycans and apolipoprotein E.* Journal of lipid research, 1999. 40(1): p. 1-16.

[123] Fullerton, S.M., et al., *Apolipoprotein E variation at the sequence haplotype level: implications for the origin and maintenance of a major human polymorphism.* American journal of human genetics, 2000. 67(4): p. 881-900.

[124] Hui, D.Y., T.L. Innerarity, and R.W. Mahley, *Defective hepatic lipoprotein receptor binding of beta-very low density lipoproteins from type III hyperlipoproteinemic patients. Importance of apolipoprotein E.* The Journal of biological chemistry, 1984. 259(2): p. 860-9.

[125] Strittmatter, W.J., et al., *Binding of human apolipoprotein E to synthetic amyloid beta peptide: isoform-specific effects and implications for late-onset Alzheimer disease.* Proceedings of the National Academy of Sciences of the United States of America, 1993. 90(17): p. 8098-102.

[126] Buttini, M., et al., *Cellular source of apolipoprotein E4 determines neuronal susceptibility to excitotoxic injury in transgenic mice.* The American journal of pathology, 2010. 177(2): p. 563-9.

[127] Cedazo-Minguez, A., M. Huttinger, and R.F. Cowburn, *Beta-VLDL protects against A beta(1-42) and apoE toxicity in human SH-SY5Y neuroblastoma cells.* Neuroreport, 2001. 12(2): p. 201-6.

[128] Wilhelmus, M.M., et al., *Apolipoprotein E genotype regulates amyloid-beta cytotoxicity.* J Neurosci, 2005. 25(14): p. 3621-7.

[129] Buttini, M., et al., *Expression of human apolipoprotein E3 or E4 in the brains of Apoe-/- mice: isoform-specific effects on neurodegeneration.* The Journal of neuroscience : the official journal of the Society for Neuroscience, 1999. 19(12): p. 4867-80.

[130] Keller, J.N., et al., *Amyloid beta-peptide effects on synaptosomes from apolipoprotein E-deficient mice.* Journal of neurochemistry, 2000. 74(4): p. 1579-86.

[131] Deane, R., et al., *apoE isoform-specific disruption of amyloid beta peptide clearance from mouse brain.* The Journal of clinical investigation, 2008. 118(12): p. 4002-13.

[132] Rapp, A., B. Gmeiner, and M. Huttinger, *Implication of apoE isoforms in cholesterol metabolism by primary rat hippocampal neurons and astrocytes.* Biochimie, 2006. 88(5): p. 473-83.

[133] Kuo, Y.M., et al., *Elevated A beta and apolipoprotein E in A betaPP transgenic mice and its relationship to amyloid accumulation in Alzheimer's disease.* Molecular medicine, 2000. 6(5): p. 430-9.

[134] Nilsson, L.N., et al., *Cognitive impairment in PDAPP mice depends on ApoE and ACT-catalyzed amyloid formation.* Neurobiology of aging, 2004. 25(9): p. 1153-67.

[135] Castellano, J.M., et al., *Human apoE isoforms differentially regulate brain amyloid-beta peptide clearance.* Sci Transl Med, 2011. 3(89): p. 89ra57.

[136] Cam, J.A. and G. Bu, *Modulation of beta-amyloid precursor protein trafficking and processing by the low density lipoprotein receptor family.* Molecular neurodegeneration, 2006. 1: p. 8.

[137] Marzolo, M.P. and G. Bu, *Lipoprotein receptors and cholesterol in APP trafficking and proteolytic processing, implications for Alzheimer's disease.* Seminars in cell & developmental biology, 2009. 20(2): p. 191-200.

[138] Ye, S., et al., *Apolipoprotein (apo) E4 enhances amyloid beta peptide production in cultured neuronal cells: apoE structure as a potential therapeutic target.* Proceedings of the National Academy of Sciences of the United States of America, 2005. 102(51): p. 18700-5.

[139] Irizarry, M.C., et al., *Apolipoprotein E affects the amount, form, and anatomical distribution of amyloid beta-peptide deposition in homozygous APP(V717F) transgenic mice.* Acta neuropathologica, 2000. 100(5): p. 451-8.

[140] Deane, R., et al., *Clearance of amyloid-beta peptide across the blood-brain barrier: implication for therapies in Alzheimer's disease.* CNS & neurological disorders drug targets, 2009. 8(1): p. 16-30.

[141] Sagare, A., et al., *Clearance of amyloid-beta by circulating lipoprotein receptors.* Nature medicine, 2007. 13(9): p. 1029-31.

[142] Ohm, T.G., et al., *Apolipoprotein E polymorphism influences not only cerebral senile plaque load but also Alzheimer-type neurofibrillary tangle formation.* Neuroscience, 1995. 66(3): p. 583-7.

[143] Polvikoski, T., et al., *Apolipoprotein E, dementia, and cortical deposition of beta-amyloid protein.* The New England journal of medicine, 1995. 333(19): p. 1242-7.

[144] Strittmatter, W.J., et al., *Hypothesis: microtubule instability and paired helical filament formation in the Alzheimer disease brain are related to apolipoprotein E genotype.* Experimental neurology, 1994. 125(2): p. 163-71; discussion 172-4.

[145] Harris, F.M., et al., *Carboxyl-terminal-truncated apolipoprotein E4 causes Alzheimer's disease-like neurodegeneration and behavioral deficits in transgenic mice.* Proceedings of the National Academy of Sciences of the United States of America, 2003. 100(19): p. 10966-71.

[146] Brecht, W.J., et al., *Neuron-specific apolipoprotein e4 proteolysis is associated with increased tau phosphorylation in brains of transgenic mice.* The Journal of neuroscience : the official journal of the Society for Neuroscience, 2004. 24(10): p. 2527-34.

[147] Tesseur, I., et al., *Expression of human apolipoprotein E4 in neurons causes hyperphosphorylation of protein tau in the brains of transgenic mice.* The American journal of pathology, 2000. 156(3): p. 951-64.

[148] Leoni, V., *The effect of apolipoprotein E (ApoE) genotype on biomarkers of amyloidogenesis, tau pathology and neurodegeneration in Alzheimer's disease.* Clinical chemistry and laboratory medicine : CCLM / FESCC, 2011. 49(3): p. 375-83.

[149] Grupe, A., et al., *Evidence for novel susceptibility genes for late-onset Alzheimer's disease from a genome-wide association study of putative functional variants.* Human molecular genetics, 2007. 16(8): p. 865-73.

[150] Counts, S.E., et al., *Galanin hyperinnervation upregulates choline acetyltransferase expression in cholinergic basal forebrain neurons in Alzheimer's disease.* Neuro-degenerative diseases, 2008. 5(3-4): p. 228-31.

[151] Lang, R., A.L. Gundlach, and B. Kofler, *The galanin peptide family: receptor pharmacology, pleiotropic biological actions, and implications in health and disease.* Pharmacology & therapeutics, 2007. 115(2): p. 177-207.

[152] Steiner, R.A., et al., *Galanin transgenic mice display cognitive and neurochemical deficits characteristic of Alzheimer's disease.* Proceedings of the National Academy of Sciences of the United States of America, 2001. 98(7): p. 4184-9.

[153] Felschow, D.M., C.I. Civin, and G.T. Hoehn, *Characterization of the tyrosine kinase Tnk1 and its binding with phospholipase C-gamma1.* Biochemical and biophysical research communications, 2000. 273(1): p. 294-301.

[154] Emmerling, M.R., et al., *Phospholipase A2 activation influences the processing and secretion of the amyloid precursor protein.* Biochemical and biophysical research communications, 1993. 197(1): p. 292-7.

[155] Wolf, B.A., et al., *Muscarinic regulation of Alzheimer's disease amyloid precursor protein secretion and amyloid beta-protein production in human neuronal NT2N cells.* The Journal of biological chemistry, 1995. 270(9): p. 4916-22.

[156] Arvanitakis, Z., et al., *Diabetes mellitus and risk of Alzheimer disease and decline in cognitive function.* Archives of neurology, 2004. 61(5): p. 661-6.

[157] Coon, K.D., et al., *A high-density whole-genome association study reveals that APOE is the major susceptibility gene for sporadic late-onset Alzheimer's disease.* The Journal of clinical psychiatry, 2007. 68(4): p. 613-8.

[158] Reiman, E.M., et al., *GAB2 alleles modify Alzheimer's risk in APOE epsilon4 carriers.* Neuron, 2007. 54(5): p. 713-20.

[159] Li, K.C., et al., *A system for enhancing genome-wide coexpression dynamics study.* Proceedings of the National Academy of Sciences of the United States of America, 2004. 101(44): p. 15561-6.

[160] Abraham, R., et al., *A genome-wide association study for late-onset Alzheimer's disease using DNA pooling.* BMC medical genomics, 2008. 1: p. 44.

[161] Bertram, L., et al., *Genome-wide association analysis reveals putative Alzheimer's disease susceptibility loci in addition to APOE.* American journal of human genetics, 2008. 83(5): p. 623-32.

[162] Beecham, G.W., et al., *Genome-wide association study implicates a chromosome 12 risk locus for late-onset Alzheimer disease.* American journal of human genetics, 2009. 84(1): p. 35-43.

[163] Carrasquillo, M.M., et al., *Genetic variation in PCDH11X is associated with susceptibility to late-onset Alzheimer's disease.* Nature genetics, 2009. 41(2): p. 192-8.

[164] Harold, D., et al., *Genome-wide association study identifies variants at CLU and PICALM associated with Alzheimer's disease.* Nature genetics, 2009. 41(10): p. 1088-93.

[165] Braskie, M.N., et al., *Common Alzheimer's disease risk variant within the CLU gene affects white matter microstructure in young adults.* The Journal of neuroscience : the official journal of the Society for Neuroscience, 2011. 31(18): p. 6764-70.

[166] Piaceri, I., et al., *Implication of a genetic variant at PICALM in Alzheimer's disease patients and centenarians.* Journal of Alzheimer's disease : JAD, 2011. 24(3): p. 409-13.

[167] Yu, J.T., et al., *Genetic association of PICALM polymorphisms with Alzheimer's disease in Han Chinese.* Journal of the neurological sciences, 2011. 300(1-2): p. 78-80.

[168] Han, M.R., G.D. Schellenberg, and L.S. Wang, *Genome-wide association reveals genetic effects on human Abeta42 and tau protein levels in cerebrospinal fluids: a case control study.* BMC neurology, 2010. 10: p. 90.

[169] Jiang, Y., M.P. Epstein, and K.N. Conneely, *Assessing the Impact of Population Stratification on Association Studies of Rare Variation.* Hum Hered, 2013. 76(1): p. 28-35.

[170] Little, J., et al., *STrengthening the REporting of Genetic Association studies (STREGA)--an extension of the STROBE statement.* Eur J Clin Invest, 2009. 39(4): p. 247-66.

[171] Little, J., et al., *STrengthening the REporting of Genetic Association Studies (STREGA)--an extension of the STROBE statement.* Genet Epidemiol, 2009. 33(7): p. 581-98.

[172] Little, J., et al., *Strengthening the reporting of genetic association studies (STREGA): an extension of the strengthening the reporting of observational studies in epidemiology (STROBE) statement.* J Clin Epidemiol, 2009. 62(6): p. 597-608 e4.

[173] Little, J., et al., *STrengthening the REporting of Genetic Association Studies (STREGA): an extension of the STROBE statement.* PLoS Med, 2009. 6(2): p. e22.

[174] Little, J., et al., *STrengthening the REporting of Genetic Association studies (STREGA): an extension of the STROBE Statement.* Ann Intern Med, 2009. 150(3): p. 206-15.

[175] Little, J., et al., *Strengthening the reporting of genetic association studies (STREGA): an extension of the STROBE statement.* Eur J Epidemiol, 2009. 24(1): p. 37-55.

[176] Little, J., et al., *Strengthening the reporting of genetic association studies (STREGA): an extension of the STROBE Statement.* Hum Genet, 2009. 125(2): p. 131-51.

[177] Noah, N., *The STROBE initiative: STrengthening the Reporting of OBservational studies in Epidemiology (STROBE).* Epidemiol Infect, 2008. 136(7): p. 865.

[178] Schaap, T., *The applicability of the Hardy-Weinberg principle in the study of populations.* Ann Hum Genet, 1980. 44(Pt 2): p. 211-5.

[179] Zang, Y. and Y. Yuan, *A Shrinkage Method for Testing the Hardy-Weinberg Equilibrium in Case-Control Studies.* Genet Epidemiol, 2013.

[180] Pritchard, J.K. and P. Donnelly, *Case-control studies of association in structured or admixed populations.* Theor Popul Biol, 2001. 60(3): p. 227-37.

[181] Voight, B.F. and J.K. Pritchard, *Confounding from cryptic relatedness in case-control association studies.* PLoS Genet, 2005. 1(3): p. e32.

[182] Li, M. and C. Li, *Assessing departure from Hardy-Weinberg equilibrium in the presence of disease association.* Genet Epidemiol, 2008. 32(7): p. 589-99.

[183] Deng, H.W., W.M. Chen, and R.R. Recker, *Population admixture: detection by Hardy-Weinberg test and its quantitative effects on linkage-disequilibrium methods for localizing genes underlying complex traits.* Genetics, 2001. 157(2): p. 885-97.

[184] Sha, Q. and S. Zhang, *A test of Hardy-Weinberg equilibrium in structured populations.* Genet Epidemiol, 2011. 35(7): p. 671-8.

[185] Ryckman, K. and S.M. Williams, *Calculation and use of the Hardy-Weinberg model in association studies.* Curr Protoc Hum Genet, 2008. Chapter 1: p. Unit 1 18.

[186] Chen, W., et al., *A rapid association test procedure robust under different genetic models accounting for population stratification.* Hum Hered, 2013. 75(1): p. 23-33.

[187] Rousset, F. and M. Raymond, *Testing heterozygote excess and deficiency.* Genetics, 1995. 140(4): p. 1413-9.

[188] Devlin, B. and K. Roeder, *Genomic control for association studies.* Biometrics, 1999. 55(4): p. 997-1004.

[189] Falush, D., M. Stephens, and J.K. Pritchard, *Inference of population structure using multilocus genotype data: linked loci and correlated allele frequencies.* Genetics, 2003. 164(4): p. 1567-87.

[190] Athanasiadis, G. and P. Moral, *Spatial principal component analysis points at global genetic structure in the Western Mediterranean.* J Hum Genet, 2013.

[191] Matsen, F.A.t. and S.N. Evans, *Edge principal components and squash clustering: using the special structure of phylogenetic placement data for sample comparison.* PLoS One, 2013. 8(3): p. e56859.

[192] Salanti, G., et al., *Hardy-Weinberg equilibrium in genetic association studies: an empirical evaluation of reporting, deviations, and power.* Eur J Hum Genet, 2005. 13(7): p. 840-8.

[193] O'Connor, T.D., et al., *Fine-scale patterns of population stratification confound rare variant association tests.* PLoS One, 2013. 8(7): p. e65834.

[194] He, H., et al., *Effect of population stratification analysis on false-positive rates for common and rare variants.* BMC Proc, 2011. 5 Suppl 9: p. S116.

Chapter 12

Accumulation of Abnormally Processed Tau Protein in Neuronal Cells as a Biomarker for Dementia

J. Luna-Muñoz, A. Martínez-Maldonado,
V. Ibarra-Bracamontes, M. A. Ontiveros-Torres,
I. Ferrer, B. Floran-Garduño,
M. del C. Cárdenas-Aguayo, R. Mena and
M.A. Meraz Ríos

Additional information is available at the end of the chapter

http://dx.doi.org/10.5772/58305

1. Introduction

Among neurodegenerative diseases, dementias are an heterogeneous group in terms of their symptoms and pathological findings. One of the main risk factors for developing neurodegenerative disease is aging. Currently there is no cure for these diseases, mainly due to the lack of knowledge of the causes and mechanisms of the accumulation of abnormal protein aggregates within the cellular or extracellular body. This is a common characteristic pathological feature in several neurodegenerative diseases. Pathological protein accumulations not only define the characteristics of a particular neurodegenerative disease, but also are associated with clinical progression, including cognitive impairment or motor disorders [1].

Research in this field had been focused on finding potential highly specific biomarkers that correlates with the disease and can be detected at early stages of the pathology. In medicine, a biomarker is defined as a featured specific somatic or measurable biological change related to a health condition or disease [2]. A biomarker can be measured and objectively evaluated as an indicator of normal biological processes or disease, as well as the pharmacological response to treatment. In general, we can say that a biomarker can be used to diagnose the disease, or to establish its severity and allow monitoring its progression and response [1, 3, 4]. A biomarker must adhere to the following statements: 1) detect a fundamental feature of the neuropathology of the disease, 2) must be validated in cases confirmed by neuropathological examination, 3) have a high sensitivity and specificity, above 80% for discriminating the neuropathology in question, 4) must be reliable. [3] In clinical studies, the biochemical analyse of cerebrospinal fluid, plasma and urine, constitute the preferred samples to search for biomarkers [5]. On the other hand neuroimaging studies and detection of genetic markers are also useful for tracking the progression of the disease [6-8]. However, these studies remain in an experimental phase and need to be further investigated. The challenge is to find the correlation between the biomarker expression, the cognitive decline and the onset of the neuropsychiatric symptoms. It is also important to emphasize that the diagnosis of neurodegenerative diseases is mainly clinical and in most of the cases it is done when the dementia syndrome has already been established. To this day, the more accurate confirmation of the diagnosis is the post-mortem pathological study. This greatly limits the early therapeutic interventions. Optimally, it is expected that biomarker studies will focus at four levels: 1) biomarkers of risk, which will help identify risk populations with mutations or changes in gene sequence, 2) diagnostic biomarkers in the early differential diagnosis would be useful to confirming the occurrence of the neurodegenerative disease, and thus allow the possibility of an early therapeutic intervention. An example of this type of biomarker approach are the neuroimaging studies, associated with the positron emission tomography, taking into consideration the measurement of the degree of atrophy of the cortex, the amplitude of the ventricles, as well as of hippocampus, 3) biomarkers of progression, these markers could predict the evolution of the disease. Finally, 4) neuropathological-molecular biomarkers are the abnormal neuropathological lesions that constitute the features of the disease. For example, the abnormal processing and deposits of hallmark proteins (such as of tau protein, amyloid-β peptide and α-synuclein) of neurodegenerative diseases.

In this chapter we will focus on the description and abnormal processing of tau protein, amyloid β peptide and α-synuclein, and its implication as specific biomarkers of neurodegeneration. First we will talk about abnormal processing and pathological aggregates of tau protein. The group of diseases characterized by abnormal tau processing and deposits, are known as tauopathies. Tauopathies include fronto temporal dementia (FTD), progressive supranuclear palsy (PSP), neurofibrillary tangle-predominant dementia (NFTD) and Alzheimer's disease (AD); these neurodegenerative diseases are characterized by the presence of neurofibrillary tangles (NFTs), consisting of paired helical filaments (PHFs). These filaments are mainly comprised of tau protein, and constitute specific markers of this kind of neurodegeneration. Better understanding the process that lead to protein aggregations and its abnormal processing in pathological conditions, could improve the differential diagnosis and would allow tracking the progression of the neurodegenerative disease.

2. Alzheimer's disease

Alzheimer's disease (AD) is the most common cause of dementia in older adults. Characterized for a severe cerebral atrophy that is associated to the presence of two types of structures, the neuritic plaques (NPs) and neurofibrillary tangles (NFTs). The density of these structures correlates with the clinical state of dementia and their presence offers a definitive diagnosis of AD at post mortem.

http://dx.doi.org/10.5772/58305

2.1. Neuritic plaques

NPs, that could be found in normal aging brain, but in lower amount (approximately 1000 times less that in AD), are composed of a core of β amyloid fibrils (Aβ) closely associated with dystrophic neuritis distributed to the periphery of the amyloid core (Fig 1A). The biological Aβ peptide is a product of Amyloid precursor protein (APP) processed by several proteases (Fig 2).

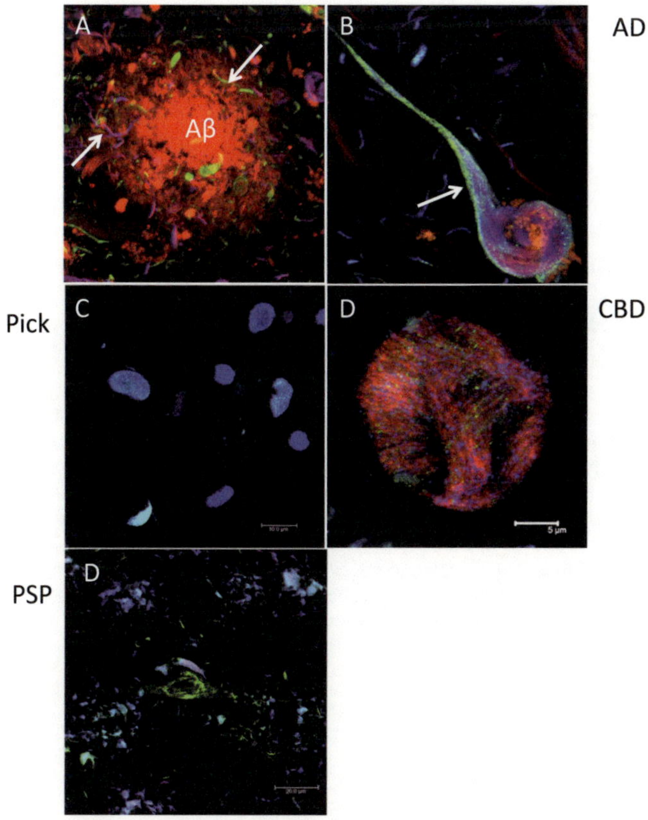

Figure 1. Histopathological lesions of human brain with dementia. A, B) Alzheimer´s disease, C) Pick's dementia, C) corticobasal degeneration D) progressive supranuclear palsy neurodegeneration. Triple inmunolabelling with antibodies raised against phosphorylated tau protein. A) neuritic plaque, amyloid beta peptide is evidenced by thiazine red dye, this dye recognized extracellular deposits of Aβ fibrillar. The dystrophic neurites are evidenced by antibodies raised against phosphorylated tau protein. B) Neurofibrillary tangles, evidenced by antibodies raised against phosphorylated tau protein at Thr231 (green channel) thiazine red (red channel) and phosphorylated tau at Ser396 (Blue channel). C) Pick Bodies in neuronal cells (Molecular layer of hippocampus) are detected by antibodies against phosphorylated tau protein at Thr231 (green) and phosphorylated tau at Ser396 (blue), thiazine red did not have affinity to this accumulation of tau protein. C) Ballooned neurons. Immunoreactivity to antibodies raised against phosphorylated tau at Thr231 (red channel), and tau pSer396 (blue channel). The expression of truncated tau protein at Asp423 (detected by antibody TauC3) showed a weak staining in a doted patter in the NFTs (green Channel). D) Immunureactivity of oligodendroglial coiled bodies and tufted astrocyes to phosphorylated tau protein at Ser202 and Ser205 (AT8 antibody, green channel) and phosphorylated tau at Ser396 (blue channel). Thiazine red showed a strong affinity for accumulations of tau protein in astrocytes and microglia.

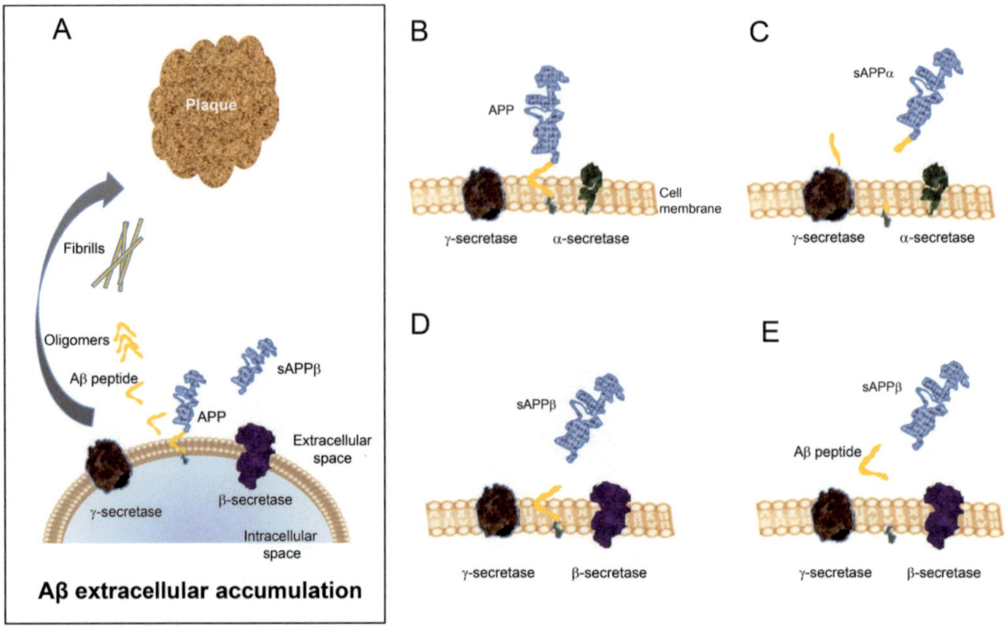

Figure 2. Processing of amyloid precursor protein. A) APP processing is the starting point of the formation of amyloid plaques. APP is a transmembranal protein that is processed by a series of proteolytical enzymes, releasing several fragments among themis the Aβ fragment that is released into the extracellular space which accumulates and forms amyloid-β plaques. B, C) APP processing to generate sAPPa fragment. C) non-amyloidogenic pathway of APP processing by α-secretase, generating a fragment called sPPAα, which is secreted into the extracellular space, subsequently proteolyzed by γ-secretase fragment remains in the membrane, leading to a small fragment called p3. D-E) amyloidogenic pathway. Alternative processing of APP, which generates the amyloid-β peptide, initiated by β-secretase, releasing a fragment called sPPAβ, being liberated into the extracellular space, the γ-secretase subsequently proteolyzed a fragment that is enclosed within the cell membrane releasing amyloid-β fragment into the extracellular space, that later could form amyloid-β plaques.

3. Amyloid precursor protein

The amyloid precursor protein (APP) is a type I transmembrane glycoprotein of approximately 120 kDa. APP has several isoforms derived from differential splicing, where the predominant variants are APP695, APP770 APP751(the numbers correspond to the number of amino acids (aa.) in each isoform). These three isoforms have in common the transmembrane region and the intracellular domain, however, in the brain, APP695 is the predominant APP specie present in neurons, while APP770 and APP751 and are primarily expressed in glial cells [9].

The human gene encoding APP, is located on chromosome 21, and was first identified in 1987 [10]. More than 76 mutations have been identified in APP, that cause the inherited form of AD and a related condition hereditary known as cerebral amyloid angiopathy. These mutations consist in amino acid substitutions within or adjacent the Aβ domain. However, even though

APP mutations are found only in rare cases of AD, they are important because they provide evidence that Aβ and APP play a central role in the pathogenesis of AD.

The APP is mainly located in the cell membrane, but has also been localized in the trans-Golgi, endoplasmic reticulum (ER) and endosomal and lysosomal membranes [11]. Aβ peptide release occurs where the secretase complex is precent and, therefore, is likely to be produced in various cell compartments. Most tissues and cells has the enzymatic machinery necessary to produce and degrade Aβ. This suggests that the production of Aβ from APP has a normal biological function. Since the discovery of the APP, a number of physiological functions have been attributed to this molecule, some of them unique to certain isoforms, but their actual functions remain unclear. It is important to mention that a number of functional domains have been assigned to the extracellular and intracellular APP regions. Most of these domains are binding sites for metals (copper and zinc), extracellular matrix components (heparin, collagen and laminin), neurotrophins and adhesion molecules, and protease inhibition domain (the protease inhibitor domain Kunitz present in the isoforms APP751 and APP770) [12].

APP processing by the complex of secretase enzymes, occurs thru two pathways: The non-amyloidogenic (Fig. 2 B, C) and amyloidogenic (Fig. 2 D, E). In the non-amyloidogenic pathway, APP is cleaved by the α-secretase, a membrane-associated zinc metalloprotease that belongs to the ADAM family (an enzyme in the family of metalloproteases and disintegrins such as ADAM9, ADAM10 and ADAM17). The cleavage by α-secretase occurs at amino acid position 83, counting from the carboxyl terminal domain of APP, where is a large ectodomain called sPPAα which is secreted into the extracellular milieu [13]. The resulting fragment of 83 amino acids, known as C83, is retained in the membrane and subsequently cut by the γ-secretase, resulting in a shorter fragment called p3, which is considered non-amyloidogenic although it is deposited in diffuse plaques [14]. The γ-secretase has been identified as an enzyme complex comprised of presenilin 1 or 2 (PS1 and PS2), nicastrin, APH-1 (anterior pharynx defective 1) and PEN-2 (presenilin enhancer 2). Importantly, the cleavage made by α-secretase occurs within Aβ sequence, between residues 16 and 17, which excludes the formation of this peptide (Fig. 2 B, C).

The amyloidogenic pathway is an alternative processing for APP resulting in the generation of Aβ. Initial proteolysis is mediated by β-secretase, the enzyme known as BACE1 (β-site APP-cleaving enzyme), at aminoacid position 99, counting from the C-terminus. This cut results in the release of a fragment called sPPAβ to the extracellular space and leaves the fragment C99 within the membrane, and generates the amino terminus for Aβ[15]. Subsequently, γ-secretase cuts at different points of the carboxyl terminus of the Aß, between amino acid residues 38 and 43, finally releasing the Aβ peptides [16]. (Fig. 2 D and E).

4. B-amyloid peptide

Most of the secreted Aβ peptide consist of 40 amino acid residues (Aβ40), while a small proportion, about 10%, comprise 42 amino acid residues (Aβ42) [11]. Because Aβ42 is more hydrophobic, aggregates rapidly and is more prone to form fibrils, which explains why this isoform is predominantly found in brain plaques of AD patients. Historically, Aβ (1-40 aa.) and Aβ (1-42aa.) are the the main focus of research in the neurodegeneration field, because they are the most frequently found in NPs of AD brains. However, it is well established that Aβ truncated or modified forms at the N-and C-terminus are also present in AD brains. The Aβ C-terminus truncation may be due to the action of different γ-secretases. Furthermore, it has been confirmed a greater heterogeneity of species of Aβ truncated at the amino terminus in the core of the NPs [17].

5. N-terminal truncated species of amyloid β

The loss of the hydrophilic part located at Aβ amino terminus increases the hydrophobicity of this peptide, which favors their propensity to aggregate and deposit. It has been proposed that Aβ species truncated at the N-terminus play an important role in the pathogenesis of AD. In this respect, with mass spectrometry it has been identified in NPs, besides isoforms 40 and 42, two other peptideswith truncations at the amino terminus, one in the amino acid 3 of Aβ (3-42 aa.) and another at amino acid residue 11 of Aβ (11-42 aa.), with relative molecular masses of 4.2 kDa and 3.5 kDa, respectively [17]. Other in vitro studies have shown that a small increase in the physiological production of these species may be sufficient to trigger the formation of neuronal processes which induce changes in cytoskeletal proteins, moreover, It has been proposed that these amino-terminus truncated Aβ peptides might act as a center of aggregation of other Aβ neurotoxic species, that predominate in the core of the NPs [18]. Truncated species may be generated from APP through alternative processing by the BACE enzyme or produced from the full-length Aβ peptide (1-42 aa.) by extracellular amino peptidases. It is known that two isoforms of BACE are involved in the production of Aβ: BACE1 and BACE2, however it is established that the main neuronal protease BACE1 is required to cut an APP in sites 1 and 11 of the Aβ peptide. BACE1 is a transmembranal glycoprotein type I, that exhibits all the Properties of β-secretase. For example, the optimum pH is slightly acidic, is located in cell compartments where Aβ is generated, and cleaves APP in the β cleavage site with a high affinity for the swedish APP (swAPP), which is a mutated APP, associated with familial AD, known to increase the production of Aβ. Finally, BACE1 is present in the secretory cells (i.e. microglia) of Aβ and is highly expressed in neurons.

6. Aggregation of amyloid β

A common feature among several neurodegenerative diseases is that some mutations associated to them, lead to the expression of protein variants with an increased tendency to aggregate. Thus, conformational changes and aggregation of Aβ peptide are central features in AD.

Currently, there is evidence that Aβ monomers are not toxic to the cells and have a protective effects on neurons against oxidative stress [19]. However, there are many reports that indicate that the oligomers of Aβ, also known as soluble oligomeric ligands of amyloid-β peptide

(ADDLs) could be even more toxic than Aβ fibrils. The ADDLs mediated toxicity was described by Klein and colleagues, which found that the oligomers cause neuronal death in hippocampal slices at nanomolar concentrations [20].

The polymerization of Aβ monomers in the extracellular space of the brain appears to correlate with the presence of metals [21]. These same metals may generate reactive oxygen species (ROS), oxidative stress-producing agents. Iron, for example, is in the NPs. This could indicate that this metal has a toxic effect due to the promotion of ROS, but could also promote Aβ assembly [18]. It is known that transition metals produce oxidative stress through the generation of reactive oxygen species (ROS) and recently was noted that the presence of these metals may be related to the polymerization of the monomers of Aβ in the brain neuropil space [21]. Thus iron in NPs, seems to have toxic effects because it promotes the formation of ROS as it enhances Aβ assembly [18].

7. Tau protein – AD brains

7.1. Normal tau

The interaction between the microtubule motor proteins and microtubules is regulated by tau protein, which operates and controls the movement of axonal organelles such as mitochondria and vesicles favoring the function and viability of neuronal cells [22] (Fig 3A). Proline-rich region at the N-terminus, interact with proteins containing an SH3 domain and with FYN tyrosine kinase. FYN interaction is highly relevant for routing toward the postsynaptic region, since this kinase phosphorylates the NMDA receptor 2B subunit [23]. This phosphorylation enables interaction of NMDA receptor with the postsynaptic density protein 95 (PSD95) and this interaction is required for the excitotoxic signaling[24].

Two main regions characterize the tau molecule, the N-terminal portion that accounts for two-thirds of the molecule, and the proline-rich region. The N-terminus region is subdivided into two subregions: one acidic, which has been proposed as a possible binding site for metals [25]. The other region is the proline-rich region. This site has a high amount of amino acids potentially susceptible to phosphorylation and appears to be important for the binding of tau to microtubules [26]. Other important regions in tau protein are: the microtubule binding domains including the repeats 3 or 4 with 31 or 32 aa's. and theC-terminal region, that also contains a proline rich region and an acidic region (Fig 3).

tau is encoded by a single gene located on chromosome 17q21. The gene has 16 exons, in which through alternative splicing 6 isoforms are generated in the Central Nervous System (CNS). These isoforms vary in length by including exons 2, 3 and 10, with a maximum length of 441 amino acids in the largest protein isoform. In sporadic AD, no mutations of the tau protein have been reported.

The tau protein is susceptible to posttranslational modifications that have direct effects on their function (Fig. 3B). The most important modification is the phosphorylation of certain residues that regulate microtubule binding. The coordinated activity of kinases and phosphatases

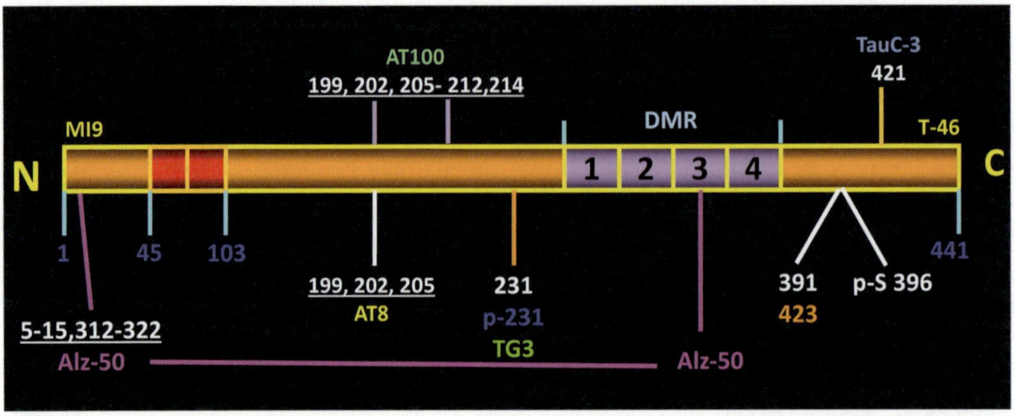

Figure 3. Schematic representation of the functional domains of the longest tau isoform. The projection domain, including an acidic and a proline-rich region, interacts with cytoskeletal elements between microtubules in axons. The N-terminal region is also involved in signal transduction pathways by interacting with proteins as PLC-γ and Src-kinases. The C-terminus part, referred to as microtubules binding domain, regulates the rate of microtubules polymerization. In this schematic diagram it is depicted the site were some tau antibodies specifically recognize tau protein epitopes.

regulate the phosphorylated state of the protein, which decreases when the level of phosphorylation promotes microtubule binding. Otherwise, the increased phosphorylation of the protein in these residues facilitates disassembly of the microtubule. tau protein has 85 potential phosphorylation sites, of which a large amount is not involved in the normal regulation of its association with microtubules [27].

tau protein may undergo other posttranslational modifications such as glycosylation, nitration, poliamination, ubiquitination and SUMOlyzation [28], which role is not well understood. These changes seem to be more involved in the deregulation of the normal function of the tau protein favouring other effects such as loss of function and promotion of abnormal aggregation characteristic of the large group of diseases with tau alterations (tauopathies), including AD.

7.2. Abnormal post-translational modification of tau

Several studies have confirmed the importance of tau abnormalities as a mechanism that alters its microtubule binding capability, and promotes abnormal aggregation [29, 30]. Phosphorylation is a major post-translational modification of tau that regulates microtubule binding and release. Tau protein is equipped with 85 phosphorylation sites, 45 serines, 35 threonines, and 5 tyrosines [28]. Increased phosphorylation reduces its affinity for microtubules, resulting in disruption of the cytoskeleton, particularly phosphorylation at threonine 231 and serine 293, 324 and 356. It has been described 30 phosphorylation sites related to AD. *In vivo*, the kinases that are more associated with tau phosphorylation are glycogen synthase kinase-3β (GSK3β), cyclin-dependent kinase 5 (CDK5) and the microtubule-affinity regulating kinase (MARK) [28, 31].

http://dx.doi.org/10.5772/58305

Kinases that contribute mainly in the abnormal phosphorylation of tau protein are: GSK3β, CDK5 and MARK. In AD and other tauopathies an alteration in the expression or in the activity of these kinases has been reported [32, 33].

Moreover, tau protein is a substrate for various proteases such as calpain, caspase 6 and caspase-3, shown by *in vitro* experiments [34, 35]. However, this effect has not been recognized as a normal mechanism and it has been proposed that endogenous proteolysis contributes tau aggregation process and abnormal toxicity. The most relevant truncations in AD are those occurring in the Asp421 and Glu391 of tau C-terminus [34, 36-38]. There is controversy about the genesis of these truncations, and it has even been postulated that they are mutually exclusive, but occur in a continuous process along AD porogression [39-41] and contribute to the formation of NFTs [40]. Moreover, it has also been proposed that such truncations occur very early in the disease and do not necessarily participate in tau assembled, thus these truncations can be observed in the unassembled amorphous aggregates of tau protein [42]. Notwithstanding these studies it has been found that there is a pathological effect of these truncations, reflected in an increased cytotoxicity when they are overexpressed in cultured neuronal cells *in vitro*. Finally, the accumulation of these truncated forms in brain tissue of subjects with AD, seems to correlate with AD clinical diagnosis and progression [40], which makes the truncation of tau protein an important biomarker in the diagnosis AD.

The truncated form of tau protein in the Glu391, is characterized as a 12 kDa fragment, with a length of 92 to 95 amino acids corresponding to the region of the microtubule binding domain. This fragment is known as paired helical filament minimum core (PHFcore) [43]. tau PHFcore has high affinity for the intact tau protein. The association of tau full length with the PHF core, triggers a molecular mechanism of phosphorylation and subsequent truncations that could induce the formation of a new tau fragment truncated at Glu391 that would have affinity for more intact tau molecules, thus inducing phosphorylations and truncations of these intact full length tau molecules, self-propagating this capture-breaking process generating more aggregated PHFcores that forms stable insoluble filaments [36]. The PHFcore fragment is recognized by antibody 423 [44]. So far the PHFcore seems to be the only peptide whose cytotoxicity has been demonstrated by Fasulo et al [45], in COS cells co-transfected with the cDNA of full length tau protein and the sequence for the PHFcore, reporting that these cells died by apoptosis. This showed the high toxicity of tau truncated at Glu391. This finding in a cell model, together with molecular neuropathology studies, which showed that tau truncation at Glu391 correlates with AD pathology and other tauopathies, suggests that this PHF core could be used as an accurate marker for this type of neurodegenerative disease. This type of propagation of the pathological tau specie (PHFcore), resembles prions disease "infectious process", thus modified tau could induce pathological changes in normal tau, which in turn would modify more normal tau molecules. This new approach to understanding AD pathology in terms of protein seeding had been proposed by several groups [46-48], however, since 1993, the group of Novak [43], had already called the PHFcore as "tauon", considering its prion like behaviour.

Glycation is a non-enzymatic glycosylation observed during aging, and its modified products cannot be degraded or eliminated by the normal clearance mechanisms. These products also contribute to the generation of free radicals. tau is a substrate of glycation and this modification increases the capability of tau to form aggregates and stabilize the formation of polymers of this protein [49]. O-GlcNAcylation may regulate phosphorylation of tau in a site-specific manner. Moreover O-GlcNAcylation at Ser356 greatly slows down the aggregation speed of tau and also reduces its phosphorylation by GSK3β and CDK5 [50].

Other dementias known as tauopathies, such as Pick's disease, hereditary frontotemporal dementia with Parkinsonism linked to chromosome 17, sporadic corticobasal degeneration and progressive supranuclear palsy, are also associated with post-translational modifications of tau protein. In these neurological disorders, it has been described that tau protein is aggregated in characteristic lesions that include pick bodies (Fig 1D), the NFTs, granulo-vacuolar degenerations, the threads of neuropil, and dystrophic neurites. In most of these lesions, it has been reported that tau protein undergoes the same posttranslational modifications that occur in AD, mainly hyperphosphorylation at various domains [51]. However, in other diseases characterized by the presence of filamentous tau protein, known as tauopathies, several mutations of this gene occur, mainly the P301L mutation, which is associated with the frontotemporal degeneration with parkinsonism linked to chromosome 17 (FTLD17). This mutation is the most widely studied in various *in vivo* models [52]. Apart from mutations, there are truncations in tau protein that are associated to this disease, such as endogenous truncation and mainly the C-terminus truncation at the Asp421 [51].

8. α-synuclein and Parkinson's disease

In elder adults, Parkinson's disease (PD) is a major cause of movement disorders. This disease is characterized by loss of dopaminergic neurons of the compact substantia nigra, which results in lowering of dopamine in the striatum. PD belongs to a group of neurodegenerative disorders called Lewy bodies diseases (ECL) [53] (Fig 1 C). The major components of Lewy bodies are aggregates of filamentous α-synuclein (αS) protein (Fig 5C). The human α-S is a 140 amino acid protein. This protein consists of three regions: an amphipathic N-terminal (amino acids residues 1-60), non-β-amyloid component (NAC) hydrophobic central region (amino acids residues 61-95) and an acidic C-terminal region (amino acids 96-140) [54].

αS belongs to the family of Synuclein included beta-synuclein (β-S), and γ-synuclein (γ-S) [54]. The Synuclein genes are highly conserved between species. Synuclein family was found in vertebrates and has never been observed in unicellular organisms. In invertebrates it has been observed an homologous to the synuclein protein.

With regard to the normal function of the αS, little is known. However, it is reported that αS is expressed at high levels in the brain, specifically associated to neurons, and also has been observed expression in other tissues such as hematopoietic cells. αS can be associated to lipids, in neurons it has been observed associated with synaptic vesicles modulating its activity, suggesting that under normal conditions αS could be involved in various functions associated

http://dx.doi.org/10.5772/58305

with neurotransmission and synaptic plasticity [55]. Also, it was shown that αS participates in synaptic plasticity during development and learning [54] and in the regulation of synaptic vesicle mobilization in nerve terminals [56].

Immunostaining with antibodies recognizing αS in normal human brain, shown a diffuse pattern in the neuropil-like synaptic region. However, in PD brains, αS immunoreactivity is also strong in some of the Lewy bodies and neuronal processes [57]. Currently, ubiquitin immunostaining and eosin staining, are the most widely used technique to demonstrate Lewy bodies in PD brains. Biochemical studies have shown that αS is the most abundant protein in Lewy bodies and it is located in the fibrous material contained in this structure. αS pathological deposits are less soluble than the normal synuclein. This is possibly due to posttranslational modifications such as truncations, nitrations, and phosphorylations, ubiquitination. αS undergoes pathological modifications in PD. It should be emphasized that although αS is a neuropathological marker of PD as well as dementia with Lewy bodies (DLB), there is no evidence that αS is related to the cause of these disease.

In vitro studies suggest that the hydrophobic region of αS NAC is essential for the aggregation and toxicity of the molecule [58]. This region is partially absent in β-Synuclein (βS), which may explain why the βS has a low ability to auto-aggregate and form oligomers and fibrils [59, 60]. Hashimoto et al (2001), demonstrated, that βS interacts with αS and it is capable of preventing αS aggregation *in vitro* and *in vivo* [59]. *In vitro* studies have shown that βS by itself tends to associate strongly with αS to form aggregates [61][58]. Studies suggest that the aggregates are formed from intermediate forms (with unchanged conformation) partially folded structures, which would give rise to the fibrils. Previous structures of these fibrils are oligomers and annular protofibrils forming pore-like structures [62]. However, the mechanisms by which they form oligomers and then fibrils are not yet understood.

Some changes in αS protein are posttranslational, which have been associated with a role as mediators of the cytotoxicity of this protein.

Furthermore, the pathological αS is characterized by phosphorylation at Ser129 which is detected by immunohistochemistry in Lewy bodies in PD human brain. The Kinase responsible for this phosphorylation is casein kinase II and GRK2/5, which phosphorylates αS *in vitro*. Originally, the Ser129 phosphorylation was found in a Drosophila model, which generated a pseudophosphorilation (S129A) from the regular αS. This modification resulted in a tendency to intracellular accumulation of this protein (αS), compared with wildtype organisms. This change was not associated with any toxicity, although this still is controversial and it is need to clarify the role of phosphorylation at Ser129 αS in the molecular pathology of PD.

The truncation of αS has been associated with its high capacity of aggregation. Ttransgenic mice expressing truncated αS have substantial cell loss especially in the brain. Truncated species of αS were found in the lysosome suggesting its proteolysis in these organelles, nonetheless α-synuclein is also a substrate for cytoplasmic calpains [57].

In the pathogenesis of diseases with Lewy Bodies, interactions between β-amyloid protein and αS are crucial. For example, Aβ worsens associated deficit coused by αS accumulation and also promotes oligomerization of αS [63]. It has also been demonstrated that in pathological conditions both aggregates of αS and Aβ, are membrane-associated. It is suggested that lipid rafts can be a suitable site for abnormal interactions between the aggregated forms of α-S and Aβ. These aggregated forms are also described in various intracellular membranous structures [59].

To elucidate how the interactions between αS and Aβ influence its aggregation properties, *in vitro* studies were done. Evidence, demonstrated that β-amyloid promotes αS aggregation *in vivo*, on the other hand, in APP transgenic mice, it was observed an accumulation of αS. Therefore, It was hypothesized that β-amyloid, αS, and tau protein promote the accumulation of each other [64], in recent years, there have been a number of studies that support this hypothesis.

The αS has become one of the key proteins in the aetiology and pathogenesis of some of the most common neurodegenerative diseases, such asPD.

It is suggested that the Lewy bodies (LB) constitute an histpopathological marker that correlates with the onset of symptoms of dementia. In 10-20% of the cases of dementia with LB it is observed also the presence of NFTs and NPs at Braak stages V and VI, suggesting that this type of neurodegeneration could share pathologic features with AD. The molecular analysis of LB in PD and dementia associated with Parkinson's disease are indistinguishable, however the difference is based on the localization of these lesions. Using double immunostaining it is possible to observed the presence of epitopes of phosphorylated and non-phosphorylated tau protein, in the periphery of the LB or colocalizing with these structure and with αS aggregates. *in vitro* studies had shown that alpha synuclein preformed fibrils may promote the formation of fibrils of phosphorylated recombinant tau protein, that is insoluble and thioflavin-S positive.

9. Taupathies

The Tauopathies are classified according to the predominant species of tau that accumulates: tau proteins containing 3 (3R) or 4 repeats (4R) of microtubule binding domain. In Pick's disease (PiD), 3R tau predominates, whereas 4R tau is characteristic of corticobasal degeneration (CBD) and progressive supranuclear palsy (PSP) [65].

PiD is the least common FTLD-tau characterized by neuronal Pick bodies in a stereotypic neuroanatomical distribution. PSP and CBD are more common than PiD and have extensive clinical and pathologic overlap, with no distinctive clinical syndrome or biomarker that permits their differentiation. The hallmark's to diagnosis rests upon postmortem analysis of the human brain and demonstration of the presence of tangles, oligodendroglial coiled bodies and tufted astrocytes in PSP or threads, pretangles and astrocytic plaques in CBD. The anatomical distribution of tau pathology determines the clinical presentation of PSP and CBD, as well as PiD

10. Pick's disease

In Pick's disease the first symptoms occur in emotional and social functioning. It is the mood changes, often biased towards euphoria, disinhibition and deterioration in social skills that are so noticeable. Pick's disease generally occurs between the ages of forty and sixty years of age. In PiD brain tissue changes and neuronal loss occurs in focal areas rather than the generalized damage of Alzheimer's. Pick's disease affects the frontal and temporal lobes of the brain. Marked shrinkage, called atrophy, of the frontal lobes of the brain occurs that can be seen on brain scans. Pick's disease is marked by the presence of abnormalities in brain cells called Pick's bodies. These are found in the affected areas as well as elsewhere in the brain. Pick's bodies are fibres that look very different from the neurofibrillary tangles found in Alzheimer's disease. Pick's bodies are straight rather than paired and helical. Pick bodies, are characterized by the presence of distinct argyrophilic (silver staining) spherical inclusions called Pick bodies and globose neurons. Pick bodies are composed of tau protein enriched in 3R tau, which can be evidenced with biochemical studies [66] or more recently with antibodies specific to tau isoforms. Mondragon-Rodriguez et al (2008) [51], conducted an immunohistochemical study and confocal microscopy analysis of brains section of Pick body dementia, and showed phosphorylation epitopes and conformational changes of tau protein that are described in AD.

11. Cortico basal degeneration

CBD is a progressive neurological disorder characterized by neuronal cell loss and *atrophy* (shrinkage) of multiple areas of the brain including the cerebral cortex and the basal ganglia. CBD progresses gradually. Initial symptoms, which typically begin at or around age 60, may first appear on one side of the body (unilateral), but eventually affect both sides as the disease progresses. Symptoms are similar to those found in Parkinson disease, such as poor coordination, *akinesia* (an absence of movements), *rigidity* (a resistance to imposed movement), *disequilibrium* (impaired balance); and limb *dystonia* (abnormal muscle postures). Other symptoms such as cognitive and visual-spatial impairments, apraxia (loss of the ability to make familiar, purposeful movements), hesitant and halting speech, *myoclonus* (muscular jerks), and *dysphagia* (difficulty swallowing) may also occur. An individual with CBD eventually becomes unable to walk.

CBD is a sporadic neurodegenerative process related to abnormal aggregation of hyperphosphorylated tau protein. This disease is associated with abnormal insoluble tau isoforms with four conserved repeat sequences (4R tau). Neuropathological criteria for CBD emphasize the histopathological findings of tau-immunoreactive lesions in addition to ballooned neurons, cortical atrophy, and nigral degeneration. The ballooned achromatic neurons, were once emphasized as a major component of the histopathology and gave the disorder its original name. Abnormal tau immunoreactivity is found in both the neurons and the glia. In neurons, tau immunohistochemistry reveals diffuse or granular cytoplasmic staining, pre-tangles, and small neurofibrillary tangles. These probably account for the corticobasal inclusions found in subcortical gray matter regions including the substantia nigra. tau immunoreactive threads in both neurons and glia are numerous in gray and white matter. CBD pathology includes astrocytic plaques with tau deposition largely in the distal processes of astrocytes. These astrocytic plaques are distinct from tufted astrocytes found in PSP, where tau is deposited more proximally to the cell body as well as in distal processes. Both CBD and PSP had in common oligodendroglial inclusions, coiled bodies, and threads, although the astrocytic changes can distinguish between the two disease (CBD or PSD). In addition, while threads are numerous and diffuse in CBD, they are rarely seen in the cerebral cortices in PSP, although they may be dense in other areas. A recent neuropathological study has discovered the presence of TAR-DNA-binding protein 43 (TDP-43) in a subset of patients with CBD pathology. There was no clear clinical correlation with the presence of TDP-43 inclusions in CBD [67].

12. Progressive supranuclear palsy

Progressive supranuclear palsy affects men and women equally and in most cases it appears as a atypical parkinsonism with axial rigidity, postural instability and unexplained falls, with most patients also developing progressive vertical gaze palsy (for which the disorder is named), dysarthria and dysphagia [68] PSP has asymmetric cortical atrophy and can clinically mimic CBS. The pathologic diagnosis is made by the microscopic findings of globose neurofibrillary tangles and variable neuron loss with gliosis of the globus pallidus, subthalamic nucleus, periaqueductal grey matter of pons, and substantia nigra. Mutant tau protein is present in inclusions [69, 70].

Whereas 4R tau is characteristic of corticobasal degeneration (CBD) and progressive supranuclear palsy. Diagnosis rests upon postmortem examination of the brain and demonstration of globose tangles, oligodendroglial coiled bodies and tufted astrocytes. The core neuroanatomical regions affected in all cases of PSP include the basal ganglia, subthalamic nucleus and the substantia nigra. Cortical involvement is greatest in motor and premotor cortices. Pathology of the cerebellar dentate nucleus and the cerebellar outflow pathway (dentato-rubrothalamic pathway) is usually severe and associated with profound atrophy of the superior cerebellar peduncle.

13. Conclusion

This review, gives a neuropathological approach towards finding biomarkers for dementia. However, finding the optimal biomarker for each neurodegenerative disease is still in an experimental face. In the case of AD, it is required far deeper molecular and immunohistochemical studies of abnormal tau posttranslational modifications (i.e. phosphorylation and truncation) and better understanding of its contribution to the development of dementia, particularly, it is important to understand the role of the paired helical filaments, that accumulate in the neuronal soma, promoting degeneration and cell death. Of relevance is to consider that in other dementias such as tauopathies, tau protein processing resembles the initial steps in AD, although there is no well-defined neuropathological impact of tau aggregation in lesions such as Pick bodies, Lewy bodies, as well as the presence of tau in NFTs and glial cells in CBD and PSP. Therefore, all efforts should be focused on determining reliable biomarkers for each of the dementias with the aim of generating new improved diagnostic approaches for early detection of these neurodegenerative diseases.

Acknowledgements

The authors wish to express their gratitude to the Mexican families who donate the brain of their loved ones affected with AD, and made possible our research. We also want to thank Ms. Maricarmen De Lorenz for her outstanding technical and secretarial support and Mrs. Amparo Viramontes Pintos, for her support in the maintenance of brain tissue. This work was supported by the Grant from CONACYT, No. 142293.

Author details

J. Luna-Muñoz[1], A. Martínez-Maldonado[2], V. Ibarra-Bracamontes[2], M. A. Ontiveros-Torres[3], I. Ferrer[4], B. Floran-Garduño[2], M. del C. Cárdenas-Aguayo[5], R. Mena[1,2] and M.A. Meraz Ríos[5]

1 National Brain Bank, Laboratorio Nacional de Servicios experimentales (LaNSE), Centro de Investigación y de Estudios Avanzados del IPN, (CINVESTAV-IPN), México City, México

2 Department of Physiology, Biophysics and Neuroscience, Centro de Investigación y de Estudios Avanzados del IPN, (CINVESTAV-IPN), México City, México

3 Department of Cell Biology, Centro de Investigación y de Estudios Avanzados del IPN, (CINVESTAV-IPN), México City, México

4 CIBERNED (Centro de Investigación Biomédica en Red de enfermedades neurodegenerativas), Institut de Neuropatologia, IDIBELL-Hospital Universitari de Bellvitge, Universitat de Barcelona, Hospitalet de Llobregat, Spain

5 Department of Molecular Biomedicine, Centro de Investigación y de Estudios Avanzados del IPN, (CINVESTAV-IPN), México City, México

References

[1] Shaw, L.M., et al., *Biomarkers of neurodegeneration for diagnosis and monitoring therapeutics.* Nat Rev Drug Discov, 2007. 6(4): p. 295-303.

[2] Atkinson, A.J., Jr. et al., *Biomarkers and surrogate endpoints: preferred definitions and conceptual framework.* Clin Pharmacol Ther, 2001. 69(3): p. 89-95.

[3] Anoop, A., et al., *CSF Biomarkers for Alzheimer's Disease Diagnosis.* Int J Alzheimers Dis, 2010. 2010.

[4] Blennow, K., *CSF biomarkers for Alzheimer's disease: use in early diagnosis and evaluation of drug treatment.* Expert Rev Mol Diagn, 2005. 5(5): p. 661-72.

[5] Mossello, E., et al., *Biomarkers of Alzheimer's disease: from central nervous system to periphery?* Int J Alzheimers Dis, 2011. 2011: p. 342980.

[6] Allan, C.L. and K.P. Ebmeier, *The influence of ApoE4 on clinical progression of dementia: a meta-analysis.* Int J Geriatr Psychiatry, 2011. 26(5): p. 520-6.

[7] Allan, C.L., et al., *Imaging and biomarkers for Alzheimer's disease.* Maturitas, 2010. 65(2): p. 138-42.

[8] Tanzi, R.E., et al., *The gene defects responsible for familial Alzheimer's disease.* Neurobiol Dis, 1996. 3(3): p. 159-68.

[9] Selkoe, D.J., *The cell biology of beta-amyloid precursor protein and presenilin in Alzheimer's disease.* Trends Cell Biol, 1998. 8(11): p. 447-53.

[10] Tanzi, R.E., et al., *Amyloid beta protein gene: cDNA, mRNA distribution, and genetic linkage near the Alzheimer locus.* Science, 1987. 235(4791): p. 880-4.

[11] LaFerla, F.M., K.N. Green, and S. Oddo, *Intracellular amyloid-beta in Alzheimer's disease.* Nat Rev Neurosci, 2007. 8(7): p. 499-509.

[12] Thinakaran, G. and E.H. Koo, *Amyloid precursor protein trafficking, processing, and function.* J Biol Chem, 2008. 283(44): p. 29615-9.

[13] Kojro, E. and F. Fahrenholz, *The non-amyloidogenic pathway: structure and function of alpha-secretases.* Subcell Biochem, 2005. 38: p. 105-27.

[14] Haass, C., et al., *beta-Amyloid peptide and a 3-kDa fragment are derived by distinct cellular mechanisms.* J Biol Chem, 1993. 268(5): p. 3021-4.

[15] Vassar, R., et al., *Beta-secretase cleavage of Alzheimer's amyloid precursor protein by the transmembrane aspartic protease BACE.* Science, 1999. 286(5440): p. 735-41.

[16] Jarrett, J.T., E.P. Berger, and P.T. Lansbury, Jr., *The carboxy terminus of the beta amyloid protein is critical for the seeding of amyloid formation: implications for the pathogenesis of Alzheimer's disease.* Biochemistry, 1993. 32(18): p. 4693-7.

[17] Larner, A.J., *Hypothesis: amyloid beta-peptides truncated at the N-terminus contribute to the pathogenesis of Alzheimer's disease.* Neurobiol Aging, 1999. 20(1): p. 65-9.

[18] Manzano-Leon, N. and J. Mas-Oliva, *[Oxidative stress, beta-amyloide peptide and Alzheimer's disease].* Gac Med Mex, 2006. 142(3): p. 229-38.

[19] Kontush, A., *Alzheimer's amyloid-beta as a preventive antioxidant for brain lipoproteins.* Cell Mol Neurobiol, 2001. 21(4): p. 299-315.

[20] Klein, W.L., *Abeta toxicity in Alzheimer's disease: globular oligomers (ADDLs) as new vaccine and drug targets.* Neurochem Int, 2002. 41(5): p. 345-52.

[21] Duce, J.A., et al., *Iron-export ferroxidase activity of beta-amyloid precursor protein is inhibited by zinc in Alzheimer's disease.* Cell, 2010. 142(6): p. 857-67.

[22] Hong, M., et al., *Mutation-specific functional impairments in distinct tau isoforms of hereditary FTDP-17.* Science, 1998. 282(5395): p. 1914-7.

[23] Lee, G., R.L. Neve, and K.S. Kosik, *The microtubule binding domain of tau protein.* Neuron, 1989. 2(6): p. 1615-24.

[24] Amadoro, G., et al., *NMDA receptor mediates tau-induced neurotoxicity by calpain and ERK/MAPK activation.* Proc Natl Acad Sci U S A, 2006. 103(8): p. 2892-7.

[25] Perez, M., et al., *Ferritin is associated with the aberrant tau filaments present in progressive supranuclear palsy.* Am J Pathol, 1998. 152(6): p. 1531-9.

[26] Goode, B.L., et al., *Functional interactions between the proline-rich and repeat regions of tau enhance microtubule binding and assembly.* Mol Biol Cell, 1997. 8(2): p. 353-65.

[27] Hanger, D.P., B.H. Anderton, and W. Noble, *Tau phosphorylation: the therapeutic challenge for neurodegenerative disease.* Trends Mol Med, 2009. 15(3): p. 112-9.

[28] Martin, L., X. Latypova, and F. Terro, *Post-translational modifications of tau protein: implications for Alzheimer's disease.* Neurochem Int, 2011. 58(4): p. 458-71.

[29] Johnson, G.V. and W.H. Stoothoff, *Tau phosphorylation in neuronal cell function and dysfunction.* J Cell Sci, 2004. 117(Pt 24): p. 5721-9.

[30] Iqbal, K., et al., *Mechanisms of tau-induced neurodegeneration.* Acta Neuropathol, 2009. 118(1): p. 53-69.

[31] Gendron, T.F. and L. Petrucelli, *The role of tau in neurodegeneration.* Mol Neurodegener, 2009. 4: p. 13.

[32] Chung, S.H., *Aberrant phosphorylation in the pathogenesis of Alzheimer's disease.* BMB Rep, 2009. 42(8): p. 467-74.

[33] Noble, W., et al., *Inhibition of glycogen synthase kinase-3 by lithium correlates with reduced tauopathy and degeneration in vivo.* Proc Natl Acad Sci U S A, 2005. 102(19): p. 6990-5.

[34] Gamblin, T.C., et al., *Caspase cleavage of tau: linking amyloid and neurofibrillary tangles in Alzheimer's disease.* Proc Natl Acad Sci U S A, 2003. 100(17): p. 10032-7.

[35] Park, S.Y., et al., *Caspase-3- and calpain-mediated tau cleavage are differentially prevented by estrogen and testosterone in beta-amyloid-treated hippocampal neurons.* Neuroscience, 2007. 144(1): p. 119-27.

[36] Wischik, C.M., et al., *Structural characterization of the core of the paired helical filament of Alzheimer disease.* Proc Natl Acad Sci U S A, 1988. 85(13): p. 4884-8.

[37] Wischik, C.M., et al., *Isolation of a fragment of tau derived from the core of the paired helical filament of Alzheimer disease.* Proc Natl Acad Sci U S A, 1988. 85(12): p. 4506-10.

[38] Garcia-Sierra, F., et al., *Conformational changes and truncation of tau protein during tangle evolution in Alzheimer's disease.* J Alzheimers Dis, 2003. 5(2): p. 65-77.

[39] Mondragon-Rodriguez, S., et al., *Cleavage and conformational changes of tau protein follow phosphorylation during Alzheimer's disease.* Int J Exp Pathol, 2008. 89(2): p. 81-90.

[40] Basurto-Islas, G., et al., *Accumulation of aspartic acid421- and glutamic acid391-cleaved tau in neurofibrillary tangles correlates with progression in Alzheimer disease.* J Neuropathol Exp Neurol, 2008. 67(5): p. 470-83.

[41] Garcia-Sierra, F., S. Mondragon-Rodriguez, and G. Basurto-Islas, *Truncation of tau protein and its pathological significance in Alzheimer's disease.* J Alzheimers Dis, 2008. 14(4): p. 401-9.

[42] Luna-Munoz, J., et al., *Earliest stages of tau conformational changes are related to the appearance of a sequence of specific phospho-dependent tau epitopes in Alzheimer's disease.* J Alzheimers Dis, 2007. 12(4): p. 365-75.

[43] Novak, M., J. Kabat, and C.M. Wischik, *Molecular characterization of the minimal protease resistant tau unit of the Alzheimer's disease paired helical filament.* EMBO J, 1993. 12(1): p. 365-70.

[44] Novak, M., et al., *Characterisation of the first monoclonal antibody against the pronase resistant core of the Alzheimer PHF.* Prog Clin Biol Res, 1989. 317: p. 755-61.

[45] Fasulo, L., et al., *Tau truncation in Alzheimer's disease: expression of a fragment encompassing PHF core tau induces apoptosis in COS cells.* Alzheimer's Rep., 1998. 1: p. 25-32.

[46] Walker, L.C., et al., *Mechanisms of Protein Seeding in Neurodegenerative Diseases.* Arch Neurol, 2012: p. 1-7.

[47] Walker, L.C., et al., *Mechanisms of protein seeding in neurodegenerative diseases.* JAMA Neurol, 2013. 70(3): p. 304-10.

[48] Jucker, M. and L.C. Walker, *Pathogenic protein seeding in Alzheimer disease and other neurodegenerative disorders.* Ann Neurol, 2011. 70(4): p. 532-40.

http://dx.doi.org/10.5772/58305

[49] Ledesma, M.D., M. Medina, and J. Avila, *The in vitro formation of recombinant tau polymers: effect of phosphorylation and glycation.* Mol Chem Neuropathol, 1996. 27(3): p. 249-58.

[50] Yu, C.H., et al., *O-GlcNAcylation modulates the self-aggregation ability of the fourth microtubule-binding repeat of tau.* Biochem Biophys Res Commun, 2008. 375(1): p. 59-62.

[51] Mondragon-Rodriguez, S., et al., *Conformational changes and cleavage of tau in Pick bodies parallel the early processing of tau found in Alzheimer pathology.* Neuropathol Appl Neurobiol, 2008. 34(1): p. 62-75.

[52] Gotz, J., et al., *A decade of tau transgenic animal models and beyond.* Brain Pathol, 2007. 17(1): p. 91-103.

[53] Goedert, M., *Alpha-synuclein and neurodegenerative diseases.* Nat Rev Neurosci, 2001. 2(7): p. 492-501.

[54] Clayton, D.F. and J.M. George, *The synucleins: a family of proteins involved in synaptic function, plasticity, neurodegeneration and disease.* Trends Neurosci, 1998. 21(6): p. 249-54.

[55] Cheng, F., G. Vivacqua, and S. Yu, *The role of alpha-synuclein in neurotransmission and synaptic plasticity.* J Chem Neuroanat, 2010. 42(4): p. 242-8.

[56] Cabin, D.E., et al., *Synaptic vesicle depletion correlates with attenuated synaptic responses to prolonged repetitive stimulation in mice lacking alpha-synuclein.* J Neurosci, 2002. 22(20): p. 8797-807.

[57] Cookson, M.R., *alpha-Synuclein and neuronal cell death.* Mol Neurodegener, 2009. 4: p. 9.

[58] Kim, E.M., et al., *Effects of intrahippocampal NAC 61-95 injections on memory in the rat and attenuation with vitamin E.* Prog Neuropsychopharmacol Biol Psychiatry, 2009. 33(6): p. 945-51.

[59] Hashimoto, M., et al., *beta-Synuclein inhibits alpha-synuclein aggregation: a possible role as an anti-parkinsonian factor.* Neuron, 2001. 32(2): p. 213-23.

[60] Uversky, V.N., et al., *Biophysical properties of the synucleins and their propensities to fibrillate: inhibition of alpha-synuclein assembly by beta- and gamma-synucleins.* J Biol Chem, 2002. 277(14): p. 11970-8.

[61] Gao, H.M., et al., *Neuroinflammation and oxidation/nitration of alpha-synuclein linked to dopaminergic neurodegeneration.* J Neurosci, 2008. 28(30): p. 7687-98.

[62] Ding, T.T., et al., *Annular alpha-synuclein protofibrils are produced when spherical protofibrils are incubated in solution or bound to brain-derived membranes.* Biochemistry, 2002. 41(32): p. 10209-17.

[63] Mandal, P.K., et al., *Interaction between Abeta peptide and alpha synuclein: molecular mechanisms in overlapping pathology of Alzheimer's and Parkinson's in dementia with Lewy body disease.* Neurochem Res, 2006. 31(9): p. 1153-62.

[64] Giasson, B.I., et al., *Initiation and synergistic fibrillization of tau and alpha-synuclein.* Science, 2003. 300(5619): p. 636-40.

[65] Dickson, D.W., et al., *Neuropathology of frontotemporal lobar degeneration-tau (FTLD-tau).* J Mol Neurosci, 2011. 45(3): p. 384-9.

[66] Buee, L. and A. Delacourte, *Comparative biochemistry of tau in progressive supranuclear palsy, corticobasal degeneration, FTDP-17 and Pick's disease.* Brain Pathol, 1999. 9(4): p. 681-93.

[67] Kouri, N., et al., *Corticobasal degeneration with olivopontocerebellar atrophy and TDP-43 pathology: an unusual clinicopathologic variant of CBD.* Acta Neuropathol, 2013. 125(5): p. 741-52.

[68] Steele, J.C., J.C. Richardson, and J. Olszewski, *Progressive Supranuclear Palsy. A Heterogeneous Degeneration Involving the Brain Stem, Basal Ganglia and Cerebellum with Vertical Gaze and Pseudobulbar Palsy, Nuchal Dystonia and Dementia.* Arch Neurol, 1964. 10: p. 333-59.

[69] Bigio, E.H., *Making the diagnosis of frontotemporal lobar degeneration.* Arch Pathol Lab Med, 2013. 137(3): p. 314-25.

[70] Boeve, B.F., *Parkinson-related dementias.* Neurol Clin, 2007. 25(3): p. 761-81, vii.

Chapter 13

Energy-Dependent Mechanisms of Cholinergic Neurodegeneration

Agnieszka Jankowska-Kulawy, Anna Ronowska and Andrzej Szutowicz

Additional information is available at the end of the chapter

http://dx.doi.org/10.5772/58339

1. Introduction

Dementia is a typical symptom of many neurodegenerative diseases. The characteristic feature of this pathology is preferential loss of cholinergic neurons in the brain septum, that are responsible for almost all cognitive functions in humans and animals. Alzheimer disease (AD) is one of the most common neurodegenerative diseases in elderly populations. There are estimations that 30 million people worldwide are suffering from AD. Incidency of AD continues to grow, becoming not only a medical but also a socio-economical problem, especially when number of patients by 2050 will triple in connection with the lengthening of the human life span. The human brain constitutes only 2% of body weight, but consumes about 20% of the total body energy output under resting conditions. In contrast to other tissues, glucose is an almost exclusive energy substrate for the brain. In hypoxia or ketonemia brain may consume certain amounts of lactate and beta-hydroxybutyrate, which, however, cannot fully replace glucose to meet brain demands for energy. That is due to the fact that neurons, constituting 10% of all brain cells, produce and consume about 80% of its energy. In addition they have no capacity to store an inventory of high energy compounds. Therefore, the effective functioning of neurons is dependent on the continuous supply of equivalent amounts of glucose and oxygen. Most of the energy produced in the neurons, (60-70%) is consumed for the maintenance and restoration of the pre-and postsynaptic membrane potentials.

Energy homeostasis of the brain is a very complex process due to the high sensitivity of neurons to metabolic stress, isolation of the brain due to the existence of the blood brain barrier, high energy requirements of the brain, and finally due to limited glycogen stores, as a dynamic source of energy. However the first step in neurodegeneration is mitochondrial dysfunction. This appears during some pathologic conditions such as: hypoxia, hypoglycemia, amyloid β accumulation, Zn, Fe, Al excess, free radicals formation and thiamine deficiency. All these pathologic signals strongly inhibited activity of the key enzymes engaged in energy metabolism.

In some cholinergic encephalopathies an impairment of brain energy metabolism occurs, a process known as hypometabolism. Studies of brain PET using [^{18}F] fluorodeoxyglucose reveal impaired glucose uptake and metabolism in different regions of an encephalopathic brain. The extent of these deficits correlates with the degree of cognitive impairment in the AD patients. On the other hand, PET combined with Pittsburgh compound-B application, can specifically determine the amyloid-β accumulation in the patient's brain. Hence, it is possible to diagnose the AD in the early stages. Another characteristic feature of neurodegeneration of AD type, is inhibition of tricarboxylic acid cycle and the respiratory chain enzymes activities. Thus, there is a reduction in the synthesis and utilization of acetyl-CoA resulting from significant decreases in pyruvate dehydrogenase (PDHC) and α-ketoglutarate dehydrogenase (KDHC) complex activities. Marked inhibition of aconitase and isocitrate dehydrogenase (IDH) activities was also reported in brain regions affected by AD pathology. This particular susceptibility of cholinergic neurons to several neurotoxic signals may be caused by the fact that they use acetyl-CoA not only to produce energy but also to synthesize acetylcholine. Thus the changes observed in AD brains concern he loss of several cholinergic markers including choline acetyltransferase (ChAT), acetylcholine esterase (AChE), high affinity choline uptake system (HACU), vesicular acetylcholine transporter (VAChT) and resulting from them reductions in ACh content and its quantal release. As a consequence, an impairment of signal transduction processes caused by a loss of muscarinic (M_{AChR}) and nicotinic (N_{AChR}) receptors and a decrease in the acetylcholine level take effect. The decrease of different cholinergic markers and protein levels were also observed *post mortem* in affected areas of human brain. It gives rise to a suggestion that impairment of cholinergic neurons in AD may precede later stages of the neurodegeneration process. These observations support the idea the key role of cholinergic dysfunction in triggering the process of AD dementia. It is widely proven that neuroinflammation is a prominent feature in AD brains and that inflammatory responses play a significant role in progression of the disease. Prolonged and spread activation of microglia in AD brain correlates with the extent of brain atrophy and cognitive decline. However the role of microglia in the development of AD is controversial. There are some data about impairment of energy metabolism in astrocytes in AD and other neurodegenerative conditions.

Astrocytes play several important functions in the metabolism of the brain including intercompartmental turnover of amino acid neurotransmitters and energy substrates. Among others, these cells provide neurons with lactate, glutamine and aspartate for energy production as well as with the precursors for neurotransmitter. The end-feet of astrocytes occupy a strategically special location in brain between capillary endothelial cells and neurons. In addition, astrocytes as a member of the tripartite synapse remove efficiently neurotransmitters such as glutamate from the synaptic cleft and have important functions in regulating extracellular ion homeostasis. Due to the extensive contacts with both blood vessels and neurons astrocytes play a key role in the control of cerebral energy and transmitter metabolism. Astrocyte function and astrocyte-neuronal interactions are very important for synaptic

http://dx.doi.org/10.5772/58339

plasticity. Thus impairment of astrocyte metabolism in various brain pathologies also has its negative influence on neuronal functions.

2. Brain energy metabolism

Particular cellular compartments of the brain differ markedly in their rates of energy generation and consumption. Among them, neurons constituting only 10% of the brain cells, consume up to 80% of its total energy output. Neuronal cells have no capacity to store any meaningful reserves of high energy compounds. Therefore, the effective functioning of neurons is dependent on the permanent supply of equivalent amounts of glucose and oxygen. About 60-70% of the energy produced in the neurons is consumed for the maintenance and restoration of the pre-and postsynaptic membrane potentials after the functional depolarization taking place with frequency from several to tens of Hz. Furthermore, the synthesis of neurotransmitters, particularly acetylcholine (ACh), also consumes fraction of pyruvate derived acetyl-CoA, a key substrate for tricarboxylic acid cycle (TCA). Neurotransmission requires a transmembrane lipid asymmetry and the constant rearrangement of phospholipids. The amount of energy consumed in these processes is constitutes about 25% of the total pool [1]. Therefore, the energy expenditures for maintenance metabolic activity of the brain are very high and can be a factor limiting the number of neurons that can be fully active at any given time [2].

Glucose from brain vascular compartment is transported across the blood brain barrier and astrocytes extensions by transporters GLUT1 of high-density and medium affinity for glucose (Km 5-10 mmol/L). Their expression in endothelium is reduced by chronic hyperglycemia [3]. On the other hand, neurons on their plasma membranes contain high density of transporters GLUT3 of high affinity to glucose (Km 1-2 mmol/L), expression of which may increase during chronic hypoglycemia [3-4]. In turn, astrocytes, take up glucose through the transporter GLUT1. The high rate of glucose uptake by neurons and astrocytes makes its concentration in extracellular spaces of the brain to be one third lower than in the blood plasma. Thus, under physiological conditions, the transport of glucose into neurons is the maximum a rate of about 6.5 μmol/s in the whole brain [3]. It should be noted that GLUT1 transporters are insensitive to hypoglycemia, whereas GLUT3 to hyperglycemia [5]. These properties make the transport of glucose into neurons optimized, which assures a relatively constant supply of this energy substrate, despite large fluctuations in blood glucose concentrations under physiological and pathological conditions.

An additional fraction of energy substrates is provided by astrocytes, which by their extensions take up the glucose directly from the circulation and display a high rate of glycolytic cycle. Therefore, they synthesize and release large amounts of lactate, which may be taken up by neurons through their monocarboxylic acids transporters MCT1 and MCT4. Lactate is transported into neurons serving as a source of pyruvate, the direct precursor of acetyl-CoA [6-7]. There are claims, that the lactate under certain physiologic and pathologic conditions may provide up to 25% of the energy in neurons [5,8-10]. In addition, high-fat diets, starvation, as well as diabetic ketoacidosis can activate uptake of BHB, through the beta-hydroxybutyrate dehydrogenaseacetoacetyl-CoA synthetase-beta-ketothiolase steps. The level of BHB in extracellular compartment is about 3.4 mmol/L. After being taken up into the cells by MCT1/MCT4 it becomes a source of acetyl-CoA independent of pyruvate dehydrogenase complex (PDHC) [4]. Therefore ketogenic diet is used to treat syndromes of congenital deficiency of PDHC, although the effectiveness of this treatment is limited [1,11-13]. Patients improvement is limited to the general conditions including alleviation of seizures. Deep losses of cognitive functions remain uncorrected. Hence, neither lactate nor ketoacids can't completely replace glucose as energy substrate for neurons.In this respect, there is no explanation why under *in vitro* conditions pyruvate/lactate remain better energy/acetyl-CoA sources than the glucose [9,14].

3. Cholinergic neurons and their role in central nervous system

Cholinergic neurons constitute only 1-10% of the total pool of neurons depending on the region of the brain, but are indispensable for its basic function-cognition. With other transmitter systems (glutamatergic, GABAergic etc.) they form structural networks for short-and long-term memory formation as well as multiple associative functions [15]. The cholinergic neurotransmission is linked with cognition, higher feelings, the analysis of visual stimuli, olfactory and auditory processes, sustain attention, recall previously stored memory traces and the regulation of behavior. The cholinergic system regulates cerebral blood flow and controls the level of activity of the cerebral cortex, including the sleep-wake cycle [30] [15,17,30]. It also modulates cognitive functions plasticity processes in the brain [16,18]. Cholinergic motor neurons innervating neuro-muscular junctions are indispensable for contraction of all groups of striated muscles [16,19].

The prevalence of neurodegenerative pathologies increases with age. Many of them, including Alzheimer's disease (AD) or Wernicke or hypoxic encephalopathies, are connected with decay of cholinergic innervation in the regions of brain cortex responsible for diverse cognitive functions. *Post mortem* examinations reveal decrease in their number, atrophy, loss of arborization and the reduction of the level and activity of cholinergic markers such as choline acetyltransferase (ChAT) vesicular acetylcholine transporter (VAChT) or high affinity choline uptake system (HACU). They are linked with the impairment of cholinergic neurotranssmition. They correlate with results of the cognitive status of the patients shortly before their death in a progressive physiological age-associated memory impairment and cognitive function [19-20]. Recent reports indicate that accelerated and excessive cholinergic neuron atrophy and loss of their connections are the main feature of cellular pathology underlying AD [21]. Reductions of the number of septal cholinergic neurons were reported to vary from 10% to 90% [22-23].

4. Selective vulnerability of cholinergic neurons

Cholinergic neurons compared to other types of neurons exhibit significantly higher sensitivity to various pathogenic agents [7,16,24-26]. Different groups of cholinergic neurons in the central nervous system are characterized by the different sensitivity to similar, harmful active signals and factors. In AD first of all cholinergic neurons of septum are found to be damaged. This type of neurons have nerve endings in the hippocampus and different regions of cerebral cortex. On the other hand, cholinergic interneurons in the striatum and motor neurons in anterior horns of medulla oblongata remain intact, sometimes to the final stages of the disease. Pathological changes were observed in the cholinergic terminals in medial temporal lobe [27]. Early, selective changes in cholinergic neurons are also observed in the olfactory cortex, amygdala, CA-1 region and subiculum. Recent studies have shown that early amyloid overload in the amygdalar regions was associated with appearance of neurofibrillary tangles inside the neurons. These areas of the brain are known to be responsible for the formation of declarative and long-term memory [28-30]. Abundant deposits of amyloid-β (Aβ) also occur in the frontal, temporal and parietal lobes. In the final stages of AD up to 60-65% losses of cholinergic neurons in different areas of the hippocampus, and the accumulation of neurofibrillary tangles in other neurons have been reported [24]. Abundance of neurofibrillary tangles correlated with gravity of clinical symptoms of dementia. On the contrary, the presence of senile plaques was also found in several older patients, who were free from cognitive deficits [31]. Selective neurodegeneration of specific areas of the hippocampus leads to the functional isolation and contributes to the short term memory impairment, which can be seen particularly in the initial stage of the disease. Variable sensitivity of brain regions rich in cholinergic neurons to neurodegeneration may be due to the influence of other regionally characteristic, diverse neurotransmitter networks, as well as the variable interactions with astrocytic and microglial cells. It can also result from phenotypic diversity of individual groups of cholinergic neurons. The underlying cause of the varying sensitivity of different groups of cholinergic neurons may be the level of their cholinergic neurotransmission, the presence of different classes of glutamatergic receptors as well as the frequency of their basic electrophysiological activity. Studies on different whole brain and cell lines indicate, that particular sensitivity of cholinergic neurons to cytotoxic stimuli may be due to the fact that they are using acetyl-CoA, not only, as the other group of neurons, to produce energy, but also for the synthesis of the neurotransmitter, which is ACh [7,26,32].

5. Alzheimer's disease

Alzheimer disease (AD) is one of the most common neurodegenerative diseases in elderly populations. It is estimated that 30 millions people are suffering from AD around the world. The number of cases of AD continues to grow, it is anticipated that the number of patients by 2050 will triplicate as a result of increasing longevity in modern societies.

AD is characterized by a decrease in the number of neurons and their interconnections, linked with progressive impairments of memory and cognitive functions, disorientation and the appearance of neurodegenerative alterations in affected areas of the brain. Disruption of axonal transport in cholinergic neurons is one of the earliest signs of AD observed both in humans and in experimental studies using transgenic mice [33]. The typical hallmark of AD is preferential loss of cholinergic neurons and their extensions in the olfactory bulbs, hippocampus, frontal, occipital and parietal lobes [34]. Differential sensitivity of between particular groups of cholinergic neurons may be due to their highly variable phenotypes as well as functional status (septal and motor neurons as an example) [35]. Clinical and animal studies demonstrated that loss of septal cholinergic neurons occurred well before those of other groups of neuronal and glial cells. Particular susceptibility of cholinergic neurons may be caused by the fact that in pathological neurodegenerative conditions, their demand for acetyl units for ACh synthesis overlaps with inhibition of PDHC [7,26,32]. This conclusion remains in accord with studies on human AD brains, that revealed a decrease of PDHC, α-ketoglutarate dehydrogenase (KDHC) and aconitase activities in areas affected by this pathology [7,35-36].

Accumulation of Aβ/senile plaques in extracellular compartment and hyperphosphorylated *tau* protein inside the neurons are characteristic histopathological findings in AD brains [37].

The process of Aβ peptide accumulation and its polymerization under favorable conditions is very slow. It gave rise to the hypothesis that amyloidosis is just an outcome but not the cause of AD degeneration [38-40]. Aβ synthesized mainly as 40 amino acid peptide, with minute fractions of 39, 41 and 43 amino acid peptides, all of none or limited neurotoxicity. The 42 aminoacid Aβ is apparently most toxic peptide in its mono-and oligomeric forms [30,41-42]. Amyloid peptides are formed by proteolytic processing of amyloid precursor protein (APP) in sequential reactions catalysed by β-and γ-secretase, respectively. Amyloid polymers are thought to disrupt the neuronal cells through formation high flow uncontrollable Ca-cation channels in their plasma membranes [41-42]. That triggers intensive red-ox processes being the source of excessive amounts of free radicals. Peroxidation of membrane phospholipids disrupts ions transport across cell membranes, including calcium homeostasis and causes changes in the functioning of the cell membrane receptor proteins. Aggregation and polymerization of Aβ peptide and the accumulation of paired helical filaments in neurons and the synaptic endings impairs axonal transport leading to degeneration and death of neurons.

Biochemical alterations observed in the AD brains are associated with decreased activities of enzymes involved in energy metabolism as well as in those responsible for the biosynthesis, release and breakdown of ACh, such as ChAT, acetylcholine esterase (AChE), HACU or VAChT. The impairment of signal transduction processes caused by decreased densities in muscarinic (M_{AChR}) and nicotinic (N_{AChR}) receptors and inhibition of the ACh synthesis and quantal release were also reported [7,30,42].

AChE is an enzyme present both in the axons and nerve ending of cholinergic neurons and in postsynaptic neurons in the cerebral cortex. Therefore its activity/level is also decreased in parallel with the loss of cholinergic neurons taking place in AD and other encephalopathies, [43-44]. These changes were also accompanied by impaired axonal transport, which is one of the earliest functional alterations in cholinergic neurons of AD brains [43]. The decrease of activities/levels different cholinergic markers were also observed *post mortem* in affected brain areas [45-46]. It gave rise to the suggestion that impairment of cholinergic neurons in AD may precede later stages of neurodegeneration process [30]. These observations support the hypothesis of the pivotal role of cholinergic dysfunction in the pathomechanisms of AD dementia.

6. Hypometabolism in Alzheimer's disease

Energy homeostasis of the brain is a very complex process. This is due to the high sensitivity of neurons to metabolic stress, existence of the blood brain barrier, high-energy requirements of the brain, and finally due to limited reserves of energy precursor substrates. In AD an impairment of brain energy metabolism occurs, a process known as hypometabolism [1,47-48]. Studies with positron emission tomography (PET) using [^{18}F] fluorodeoxyglucose exhibit impaired glucose metabolism in brain regions of both sides in the temporal, parietal and cingulate cortex. The extent of these changes correlates with cognitive impairment in the affected patients. These changes are one of the well established diagnostic criteria for AD. PET combined with marking Pittsburgh blue (Pittsburgh compound-B) can specifically determine the Aβ deposits in the brain, so it is possible to diagnose the AD in its early stages [49-54]. Disturbances in glucose metabolism are associated with the reduction in the density of glucose transporters GLUT1 and GLUT3 in the neurons. Also activity of phosphofructokinase and glyceraldehyde-3-phosphate are diminished yielding suppression of the glycolytic metabolism, and facilitation of amyloidogenic transformation of APP and apoptosis [55-56].

However, the most important alteration in AD brains seems to be suppression of acetyl-CoA synthesis and TCA as well as the respiratory chain proteins. Reductions of PDHC, KDHC complex activities may be key factor in this pathomechanism due to reduction of acetyl-CoA synthesis and its utilization in TCA cycle, respectively. Studies of cholinergic septal neuronal cell lines have shown, that neurotoxins associated with AD pathomechanisms caused direct/instant inhibition of aconitase, PDHC, KDHC and suppressed synthesis and utilization of acetyl-CoA in mitochondria yielding increased mortality in septal cholinergic SN56 neuronal cells with high expression of the cholinergic phenotype [7,32]. One of the main changes observed an early stage of AD is the impairment of oxidative phosphorylation, which leads to decrease of electron transport in the respiratory chain, mainly in complex IV, which is associated with inhibition/decreased expression of cytochrome oxidase and ATP synthase. In this way, in the AD brains reduced of ATP level occurs. At this stage of the disease morphological changes of mitochondria were also observed. Disturbances in membrane fluidity and structure, reduction of the mitochondrial combs, density of mitochondria were also observed [57-59].

7. Pivotal role of acetyl-CoA

The principal, immediate source of acetyl-CoA in the brain is pyruvate formed from the glycolytic metabolism of glucose. The reaction of the oxidative decarboxylation of pyruvate supplying acetyl-CoA is catalyzed by PDHC, located in the mitochondria. More than 97% of acetyl residues *via* citrate synthase is metabolized to citrate and consumed in TCA cycle to produce the energy needed to restore the membrane potential during depolarization-repolarization cycles of several Hz frequency. Only 3% of the pool of generated acetyl-CoA is used in the synthesis of ACh, which takes place in the cytoplasmic compartment [60-63]. However, under resting conditions acetyl-CoA molecules practically do not pass through the inner mitochondrial membrane into the cytoplasm. Therefore acetyl moiety for ACh synthesis must be transported to the cytoplasm through the intermediate metabolites, such as citrate, acetyl-L-carnitine, for which the inner mitochondrial membrane has a suitable transport systems [64]. In cytoplasm, acetyl-CoA is resynthesized from these compounds. It has been found, that in brain nerve terminals about 30-50% of acetyl-CoA pool is transported from the mitochondria to synaptoplasm, as citrate [65-67]. In cholinergic neurons and nerve terminals the metabolic flow through this pathway is facilitated by the preferential localization of ATP-citrate lyase (ACL) [67-70].

In various forms of dementia including AD, thiamine deficiency, hypoxia or dialysis evoked encephalopathies in humans and animal models of dementia, loss of cognitive functions correlated with preferential deficits of cholinergic markers. Another striking feature in all of these pathologies was the decrease in energy metabolism in the affected regions of the brain [7,21,35,57-58,71]. The decreases in glucose metabolism and reduced stores of phosphocreatine and ATP have been shown during the life of the patients, by PET investigations [51-52,54]. This is confirmed by *post mortem* studies, which show that the cause of these changes may be decreased activity of PDHC, aconitase and KDHC in pathologically altered regions of the central nervous system [26,71-74]. These changes correlated with both the loss of cholinergic markers and the degree of degreased cognitive scores, before the death of the patient [19,30,75]. Studies on isolated cholinergic murine septal neuronal cell lines displayed strong inverse correlations between rates of cell death and PDHC activities or acetyl-CoA levels in their mitochondrial compartment under various neurodegenerative and neuroprotective conditions [7,40,76-80]. On the other hand, ChAT activity, ACh level and synthesis as well as quantal release correlated directly with levels of acetyl-CoA in cytoplasmic compartment of the cholinergic neurons [7,81].

8. Acute and chronic neurotoxicity

Cognitive deficits, the main clinical symptoms of cholinergic encephalopathies may in some cases combine with motor disability [82]. These changes correlate well with the degree of functional and structural losses of basal forebrain cholinergic neurons projecting axons to hippocampus and different cortical areas, motor neurons innervating different groups of striated muscles [45]. In these cases suppression of energy metabolism, correlates with losses of cholinergic markers in affected areas of brain cortex or spinal cord segments. Dysfunction of brain mitochondria is thought to be both the consequence of pathologic insults as well as a source of signals triggering neurodegeneration. Therefore, alterations in PDHC synthesized acetyl-CoA metabolism in the cholinergic neurons should be considered both as a source of disturbances in their transmitter functions and viability (Fig. 1) [7,32]. Several pathologic disturbances of aging brain cause excessive depolarization and overload of neuronal cells with $Ca^{2+}$and other divalent cations yielding diverse cytotoxic reactions.

http://dx.doi.org/10.5772/58339

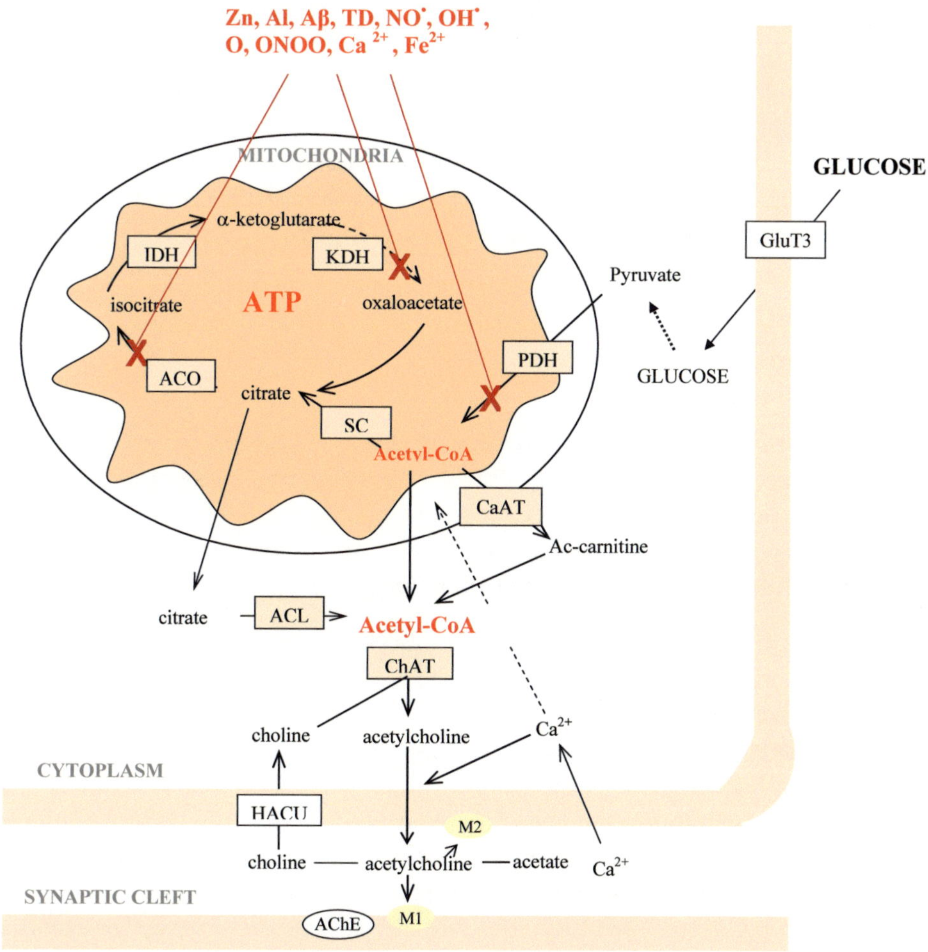

Figure 1. Putative neurotoxic signals affecting pathways acetyl-CoA and energy metabolism in brain cells and their specific interactions with cholinergic neurons.

Glutamateric neurotransmitter system constitutes 50% of all brain neurons and synaptic terminals. Prolonged pathologic depolarization yields an excessive co-release of glutamate and Zn from brain terminals triggering action potentials through NMDA, AMPA receptors and other voltage gated Ca channels located on postsynaptic neurons including cholinergic ones [83-85]. They cause dysfunction of postsynaptic neurons that may lead to apoptosis and necrosis [86-87]. Energy deficits also inhibit uptake of glutamate by adjacent astrocytes, due to the down-regulation of EAA, GLAST and GLT1 transporters and inhibition of their glutamine synthetase [88]. Sustained elevations of glutamate and Zn levels within the synaptic clefts, yield prolonged depolarization of postsynaptic neurons, as well as astroglial and microglial cells [89]. The disruption of Ca^{2+}homeostasis affects enzymes linked with pathways involved in energy, neurotransmitter, and NO metabolism. The Ca^{2+}excess in the mitochondria compartment may lead to PDHC activity inhibition due to activation of PDH kinase. That may cause acetyl-CoA deficits in subcellular compartments of cholinergic neuronal cells [40,90-91]. During brain hypoxic/ischemic episodes the earliest event is excitotoxic activation caused by prolonged release of glutamate and Zn from glutaminergic nerve terminals. The excess of glutamate/Zn in the synaptic cleft results in, through multiple receptors and transporters, excitotoxic depolarization of postsynaptic neurons and adjacent glial cells as well. These alterations pave the road to subsequent chronic steps of neurodegeneration yielding characteristic histopathologic picture of amyloidosis-β and tauopathy [92-93].

9. Amyloid-β toxicity

It has been found that AD frequently combines with stroke and cerebral vessel thrombosis and other defects of capilary circulation [94]. Transient hypoxic and hypoperfusion conditions, frequent in eldery people brains, may also augment Aβ accumulation by activation of γ and β-secretases. They catalyze amyloidogenic cleavage of APP and increase Aβ accumulation in extra-and intracellular compartments of the brain [95].

There is a common view that different extra-and intracellular deposits of Aβ are the main cause of neuronal injury in the course of AD. Neurotoxic properties of Aβ have been demonstrated in several experimental paradigms. It has been shown, that Aβ added to the cell cultures inhibited the key enzymes of TCA cycle, as well as PDHC [77, 92,96]. It resulted in depletion of acetyl-CoA yielding supression of respiratory chain and ATP levels in affected neuronal cells [76-77,97]. These alterations could be aggravated by Aβ-evoked disruption of endogenous metal homeostasis, including calcium, iron, zinc and copper [98]. Accumulation of these metals as well as xenobiotic. Espesially aluminium, has been found in AD amyloid lesions. Each of these metals may aggravate inhibitory effects of Aβ on oxidative/energy metabolism and cholinergic neurotransmission, yielding increased mortality of cholinergic neurons both in cultures and in brain tissue *in situ* [32]. Aβ fibrilar polymers were reported to form high conductance Ca-channels in cell plasma membranes, with apparent impairment of energy metabolism and activation catabolic pathways [99-100]. Subtoxic levels of Aβ were found to directly inhibit PDHC activity in brain nerve terminals [96]. Accumulation of extracellular Aβ aggravated suppressive effect of NGF mediated by p75 receptors abundantly expressed in septal cholinergic neurons, yielding different suppressive and neurotoxic reactions [32,101]. Aβ also facilitaed inflammatory responses of microglial cells, that promote neurodegenerative processes through excessive production of inflammatory cytokines [102]. However, a recent report reveals that Aβ accumulation in sensitive regions of human cortex correlated neither with loss of cholinergic innervation nor with impairment of respective cognitive functions [103]. That supports earlier notions that Aβ should be considered rather as an outcome than the cause of AD encephalopathy. Nevertheless, that does not rule out the possibility that accumulated Aβ may combine with preceding cytotoxic signals, yielding augmentation of neurodegeneration processes.

10. Zinc neurotoxicity

Zinc is an essential trace element for living organisms, being the component of active centers of about 300 enzymes and proteins including: carboxypeptidase, aspartate carbamoyltransferase, alcohol dehydrogenases, peroxide dismutase, zinc finger structures of transcription factors and several others [104-105]. It down-regulates the activity of NMDA receptors and other transporter proteins. As a crucial structural element in zinc-fingers, Zn is a regulator of transcription and other adaptative reactions of the organism [106-107]. It inhibits the opening of NMDA channels [108], that during sustained depolarization may take up the excess of this metal from-the synaptic cleft into the postsynaptic neurons [108].

Zinc concentration in synaptic vesicles of glutaminergic terminals may reach levels of few hundred mmol/L as it forms complex with L-glutamate to assure isoosmolality of the vesicular fluid. In accordance with this the highest whole tissue concentration of Zn, about 0.15 mmol/L, was found in the grey matter. During pathologic brain depolarization glutamate is released with zinc from glutaminergic terminals to synaptic clefts, where it can reach concentrations as high as 0.3 mmol/L. Under physiological conditions Zn is quickly cleared from the synaptic cleft mainly by astrocytes and postsynaptic neurons.

There are three groups of proteins specifically regulating Zn distribution in brain cells. They include: ZnT1, located in the neuronal plasma membranes; ZnT2 in endoplasmic reticulum and ZnT3 in synaptic vesicles of nerve terminals [109]. These proteins are activated when zinc concentration in the cytoplasm is elevated. Apart from that, the neuron-specific membrane transporters Zip1, 4, 6 participate in zinc turnover [110]. Zip 1 and 4 remove zinc from the cell, whereas Zip 6 accumulates this cation in the intracellular compartment [111]. It is however not known how ZnTs functions combine with various Ca-channel/transporter activities in the regulation of Zn levels and compartmentalization in the neuronal cells.

Several pathologic conditions cause excessive release of zinc from presynaptic glutamatergic vesicles. High amounts of free Zn are taken-up by postsynaptic neurons and adjacent glial cells. There is no evidence whether large amounts of Zn can be released from other locations apart synaptic vesicles. There was increasing Zn^{2+}accumulation in degenerating neurons after excitotoxic stimulation of transgenic mice, lacking ZnT3 transporter that results in no zinc accumulation in vesicles [112]. Our earlier study revealed that high zinc accumulation in cultured neurons caused inhibition of key enzymes of energy metabolism [40,80]. Namely, Zn^{2+}directly inhibited PDHC and KDHC as well as aconitase activities which led to reduction of acetyl-CoA and ATP levels [40,80]. These Zn/glutamate induced energy deficits along with sustained depolarization along may cause Ca and free radical overloads. That triggers excessive synthesis of nitric oxide (NO), by nNOS and iNOS present in adjacent postsynaptic neuronal and glial cells, respectively. As a result excess of highly toxic peroxynitrite radicals accumulate in affected area. NO excess was reported to cause irreversible inhibition of aconitase and isocitrate dehydrogenase and the reversible one PDHC and KDHC [32,77,98]. These effects apparently aggravated cytotoxic effects of Zn, triggering vicious cycle of cholinergic neurodegeneration [76,80-81]. There are evidences that aberrant Zn homeostasis is involved in the pathogenesis of AD [113]. Zn may be directly involved in the process of amyloidogenesis as APP protein was found to contain Zn binding motif [113] located within the cysteine-rich region of its ectodomain. This points out that Zn may play a role in yet unknown functions of APP.

High dietary intake of Zn significantly increased the Zn and APP levels in transgenic APP/P1 mouse brains. It also enhanced amyloidogenic cleavage of APP protein both under *in vivo* and *in vitro* conditions [114]. In mouse brain Zn inhibited α-sectetase activity, elevating the β and γ-secretase activities promoting accumulation of Aβ(1-40), the main component of Aβ plaques [108,115]. There was accompanied by the impairment of learning capacity in the Morris water maze test [114]. Zinc cytotoxic effects were observed not only in AD but also in several other brain pathologies including: epilepsy, mechanical trauma, ischemic stroke, hypoglycemia, hypoxia, thiamine deficits and other inherited or acquired metabolic blocks [115].

Besides, chronic pathological conditions may down-regulate expression of different classes of ZnT in astrocytes. In the same conditions Zn may be released to perisynaptic compartments [116]. Hence, Zn excitotoxicity would not be caused by overall increase of its concentration in the brain, but by its aberrant redistribution between different extra-and intracellular compartments of the brain [117].

Increased Zn concentrations in extracellular space may induce oligomerization of Aβ, aggravating its cytotoxic effect in AD brains. That is why short-time elevation of Zn concentrations in extracellular fluid (ECF) might trigger the long-term amyloidogenetic process. These signals were found to exert negative influence on cholinergic neurons that are responsible for cognitive functions and short-time memory formation [32]. It seems that high expression of the cholinergic phenotype in neurons (SN56) of septal origin makes them particularly susceptible to Zn-cytotoxic signaling [7,40,80].

There was also reported that xenobiotic metal Al may also accumulate in the brains in age-dependent manner [118-119]. It could inhibit calcium channels and Na/Ca exchanger in mitochondrial membranes what might increase mitochondrial and decrease cytoplasmic calcium levels in nerve terminals and cholinergic neuronal cells [32,74]. All these pathogens either alone or in combination were found to cause the decrease acetyl-CoA synthesis in neuronal mitochondria and reduction of energy production yielding increased cholinergic neuron susceptibility to degeneration [32,80]. In addition, lowering the cytoplasmic level of calcium could reduce direct transport of acetyl-CoA from mitochondria to cytoplasm through permeability transition pores (PTP) [32,74]. Shortages of acetyl-CoA in cytoplasmic compartment cause inhibition of acetylcholine synthesis and release [40].

On the other hand, primary or secondary Zn deficits could also induce neurodegenerative brain injury. Such conditions were found in the elderly people who maintained themselves on Zn-deficient diet [41]. Some life periods such as intensive growth, pregnancy, lactation, intensive physical exercises increase demand for Zn facilitating appearance of its deficits. That is why numerous therapeutical and schedules recommend taking supplements that contain Zn organic complexes: zinc bisglicine, or zinc bisaspartate. They are claimed to be safer in use than nonchelatable inorganic Zn salts. However, there is no convincing data that would support this claim. Zn deficits in experimental animals were reported to cause to have increased oxidative stress and/or had greater rate of lipid peroxidation [120].

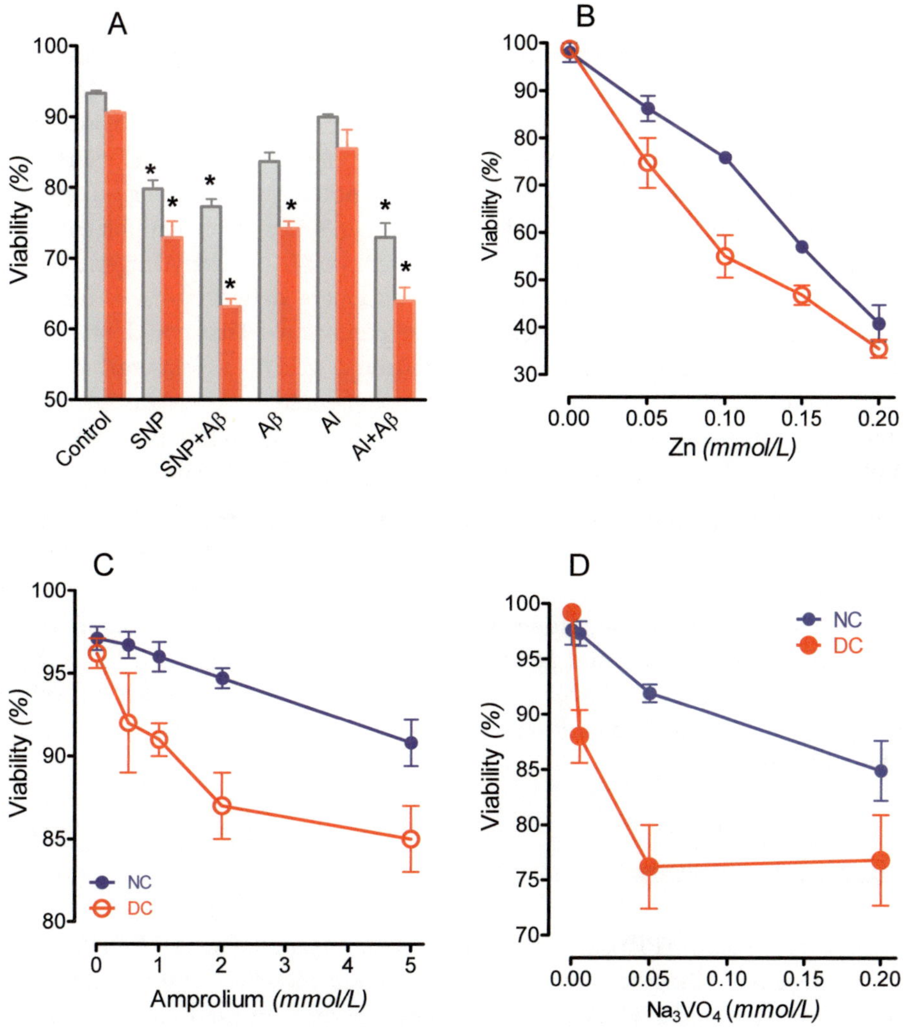

Figure 2. Differential neurotoxicities in nondifferentiated and differentiated cholinergic SN56 neuroblastoma cells. Recalculated from: [32,40,81,158-159].

11. NO excess

Glutamate-Zn evoked increases of [Ca^{2+}]/[calmodulin-Ca] in cytoplasmic compartments of postsynaptic neurons and adjacent glial cells activated nNOS and iNOS, respectively. It seems however, that only increased expression of Ca-independent iNOS in the microglial/astroglial cells may contribute significantly to neurodegeneration. It has been demonstrated, that only iNOS-dependent activation may elevate the NO levels in the brain up to low micromolar, pathologically relevant, concentrations [121]. In fact, bacterial lipopolysaccharides could induce several-fold increase of NO synthesis by microglia [121]. On the other hand, fraction of NO produced by nNOS/eNOS may reach levels two orders of magnitude lower, and is likely to play a physiologic roles of "volume transmitter" and guanyl cyclase activator [89]. Peroxynitrite radicals were found to react with wide range of intracellular biomolecules linked with energy and glycolytic metabolism and several regulatory and transport or neurotransmitter pathways, as well as with antioxidant systems. Excess of endogenous NO exerts rapid but reversible inhibition of cytochrome c oxidase and less potent one for other proteins of respiratory chain and ATP-synthetase, as well [122]. However, NO may also inhibit earlier steps of energy metabolism including: PDHC, aconitase, isocitrate NADP-dehydrogenase, as well as KDHC [40,76,77]. Other enzymes of TCA cycle: succinate dehydrogenase, fumarase, and malate dehydrogenase were not affected by these conditions. That could cause deficits of acetyl-CoA and ATP in NO/ONOO-exposed neuronal [32,76]. Cholinergic neurons with residual expression of the cholinergic phenotype appeared to be more resistant to NO neurotoxicity than those with high expression of the cholinergic phenotype, apparently due to negligible demand for acetyl-CoA to support ACh synthesis in the former.

Lipoic acid or acetyl-L-carnitine were found to exert positive effects on viability in NO or Zn-exposed cholinergic SN56 cells through preservation of acetyl-CoA availability in their mitochondrial and cytoplasmic compartments [32,77]. However, delay in cytoprotectant application markedly diminished their efficacy, apparently due to instant, irreversible inactivation of aconitase by Zn and $NO/ONOO^-$[40,123]. ChAT appeared to be resistant to direct, acute exposition to NO-excess. However, its expression was adaptatively down-regulated by chronic cytotoxic conditions decreasing acetyl-CoA provision into cytoplasmic compartment [124].

12. Thiamine deficiency

Thiamine pyrophosphate (TPP) is a cofactor for E1 subunits of PDHC and KDHC, that are key rate limiting steps regulating acetyl-CoA synthesis and its metabolic flux through TCA cycle, respectively [61,71,118,125-126]. Activities of these enzymes in the brain mitochondria are several times higher than in nonneuronal tissues, due to high demand for energy in this tissue. Therefore, thiamine pyrophosphate deficits (TD) evoked by chronic alcoholism, starvation or thiamine depleting diets caused dramatic clinical symptoms of motor, cognitive and metabolic disturbances in the form of Wernicke–Korsakoff encephalopathy, muscular dystonia, edema and lactic acidosis, with frequently fatal outcomes [125,127-128]. On the other hand, early supplementation of TPP deficient subjects with thiamine, reversed symptoms of these pathologies [129]. The majority of TD-evoked neurologic and cognitive disturbances may be explained by the impairment of cholinergic neurotransmission. In TD brains there are two major mechanisms that are responsible for dysfuctioning and loss of cholinergic neurons: the primary limitation of acetyl-CoA provision and excytotoxic Zn overload. The first one is caused

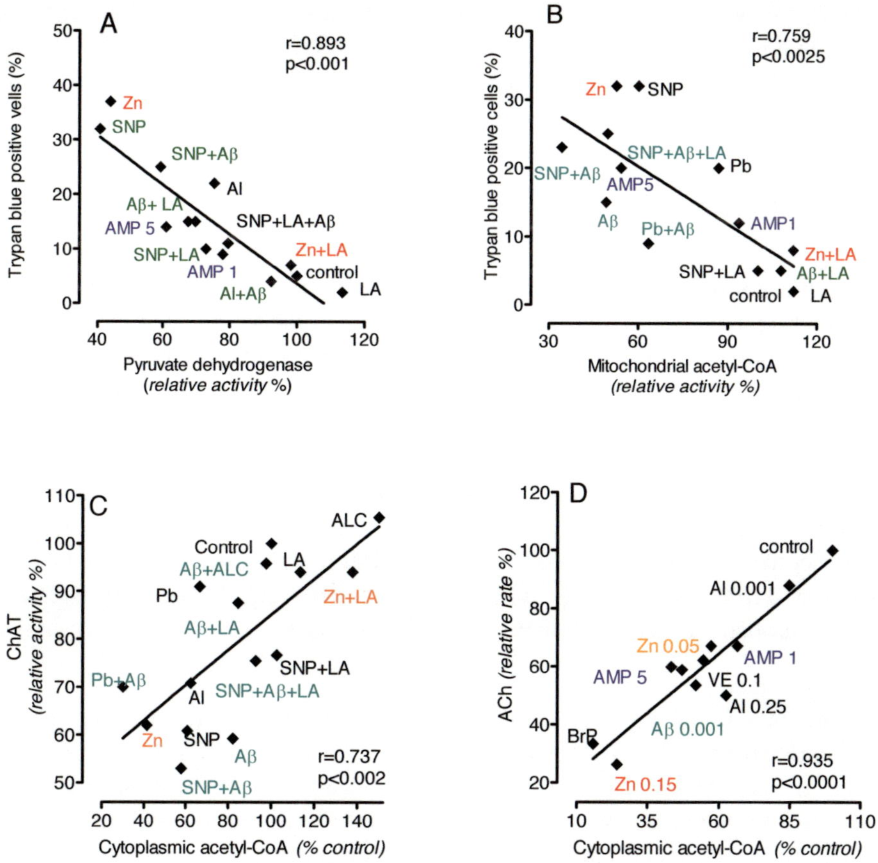

Figure 3. Existence of significant correlations between: intramitochondrial acetyl-CoA metabolism and cholinergic neuronal cell injury (AB) and cytoplasmic acetyl-CoA levels and transmitter functions (CD) of cholinergic neuronal cells of septal origin. Data collected from: [32,40,81,124].

by the impaired synthesis of acetyl-CoA by PDHC, what strightly leads to the excytotoxic release of glutamate-Zn from energy depleted glutamatergic neurons [108]. In whole brain and cellular models of TD, the reduction of mitochondrial levels of acetyl-CoA correlated with losses of cholinergic markers and viability of the neurons [81,119,130-131].

The decreases of cytoplasmic acetyl-CoA in amprolium-induced TD SN56 cells and brain nerve terminals, from pyrythiamine treated rats, resulted from limited synthesis of this metabolite in the mitochondrial compartment by TD-deficient PDHC. In consequence, lower rates of ACh synthesis and its quantal release in TD cholinergic neurons positively correlated with decreased concentration of acetyl-CoA in their cytoplasmic compartment [81,130]. These findings fit to a general rule that the rate of ACh synthesis/release depends on the availability of acetyl-CoA in cytoplasmic/synaptoplasmic compartment of cholinergic neurons, irrespective of the type of neurotoxic signal [7,32]. However, unlike for AD or other neurotoxic conditions, acute

TD altered ChAT activity neither in pyrithiamine-rat brain synaptosomes nor in amprolium-SN56 cells [132]. These data prove that, at least in early stages of TD, the structure of cholinergic neurons remained well preserved and that inhibition of ACh quantal release is exclusively due to the inhibition of acetyl-CoA provision to the site of its synthesis.

13. Glia and neurotoxicity

Astrocytes play several important functions in the metabolism of the brain including inter-compartmental turnover of aminoacid neurotransmitters and energy substrates. They supply neurons with lactate, glutamine and aspartate for energy production neurotransmitter synthesis [133]. The end-feet of astrocytes occupy a strategic sites between capillary endothelial cells and neurons. In addition, astrocytes as a member of the tripartitie synapse remove efficiently neurotransmitters such as glutamate from the synaptic cleft and have important functions in maintenance of ion homeostasis in the extracellular compartments of the brain [134]. Due to the extensive contact with both blood vessels and neurons, astrocytes play the key role in the control of cerebral energy and transmitter metabolism. Astrocyte viability and astrocyte-neuronal interactions take part in processes of synaptic plasticity. Thus impairment in astrocyte metabolism in various brain pathologies also has its negative influence on neuronal functions.

There are some data about impairment of energy metabolism in astrocytes in AD and other neurodegenerative diseases [135]. However, most of them have been collected using isolated astroglial cells or whole brain models without taking into account subcellular distribution of energy metabolism. Therefore, like in the neuronal cells [7] putative aberrations of acetyl-CoA metabolism in the cytoplasmic and mitochondrial compartments of astrocytes, should be investigated in different models of AD and other cholinergic encephalopathies. The main role of astrocytes is to protect and support neurons. Astrocytes are capable to produce net lactate, L-glutamine and accumulate glycogen. They consume about 15-20% of the glucose in the brain [136,137]. Thanks to this they can deliver lactate to neurons, through monocarboxylate transporters MCT1, MCT 2. Lactate, after conversion to pyruvate may serve as an alternative to glucose source of acetyl-CoA under hypoglycaemic or hypoxic conditions. During physiologic activation of glutamatergic endings Na^{+}dependent transport of glutamate into astrocytes by GLT1 and GLAST transporters was found to be enhanced. Subsequently glutamate was converted there to L-glutamine [136]. There are no Zip transporters on the surface of astrocyte's cellular membrane. Therefore uptake of zinc from synaptic cleft occurs through high density divalent metal transporters: DMT1. Except of Zn ions astrocytes may take up also iron and copper [138]. Apart from that, astrocytes contain high levels of metalothioneins (MTs). In consequence they can take up Zn from synaptic cleft and bind it forming complexes with MTs [139]. That is why impairment of astrocytes under cytotoxic conditions may limit their neuroprotective functions and indirectly facilitate neurodegenerative processes.

There are several therapeutic and preventive approaches to AD and other cholinergic encephalopathies of advanced age. However, now days only cholinomimetics and GABA-antagonists are approved for treatment of AD and related dementive disorders. They, however neither prevent nor slow down the progress of cognitive loses [102]. Other, therapeutic approaches such as choline supplementation, provision of acetyl-CoA precursors, or free radical scavengers, neurotrophin supply, antiinflamatory drugs application, inhibition of Aβ synthesis or reduction of its overload appeared to be ineffective.

Neuroinflammation is one of principal pathomechanisms of AD which significantly contributes to the progress of the disease [102]. Prolonged and widely spread activation of microglia in AD brain correlates with the extent of brain atrophy and cognitive decline. However, the role of microlglia in the development of AD is a subject of discrepant reports. On one hand, microglial fagocytosis of Aβ is belived to be a protective mechanism againts neurodegeneration [140]. Both atrocytes and microglia release both pro-and anti-inflammatory cytokines and prostaglandins, as well as oxygen, nitrosyl radicals. Cytokines through TLR-4 receptors were found to stimulate variety of intracellular signaling pathways that have been implicated in neuronal damage in AD. Therefore, people taking chronically nonsteroid anti-inflammatory drugs displayed lower prevalence of this pathology [141]. Microglial activation by many endogenous and signaling compounds such as L-glutamate, ATP, 7-ketocholesterol, cAMP were reported to cause inhibition of several enzymes of their energy metabolism [32,141]. Both Zn and Aβ oligomers are capable of microglia activation. This results in release of soluble neurotoxic compounds that compromise integrity of neurons and synapses [142]. Also Zn in rather low concentrations (30-50 micromol/L) activates microglia through mechanism dependent on activation of transcription factor NF-kappaB [143]. Simultaneously active compounds derived from activated microglia augment Zn release from glutamatergic neuronal endings what may accelerate neurodegenerative processes [144].

The activation of both astrocytes and microglial cells is associated with the induction of major proinflammatory pathways [145]. Gene expression profile analysis confirmed the prominent upregulation of genes associated with the immune/inflammatory pathways, including several chemokines and pro-inflammatory cytokines [146]. Activation the IL-1β pathway has been revealed both, in glial as well as in neuronal cells in brains of chronically epileptic rats [147]. Both the complement pathway and the plasminogen system are also activated within the hippocampus affected by multiple-sclerosis [148-149]. Both IL-1β, complement components and plasminogen activators were found to increase the permeability of the blood brain barrier (BBB) [150,151]. Toll-like receptor (TLR) signaling pathways in brains affected by various pathologies such as epilepsy, ischemia or AD, may contribute to neuronal injury [152]. Moreover microRNAs (miRNA) also play a role in the regulation of the innate and adaptive immune responses. In particular, miR-146a, which can be induced by different pro-inflammatory stimuli such as IL-1β and TNF-α, has been shown to critically modulate innate immunity through regulation of TLR signaling and cytokine responses [153]. Interestingly, this miRNA is upregulated in TLR as well as in experimental models of epilepsy. These observations suggest miRNA as potential targets to modulate inflammatory pathways.

Moreover activation of microglia is the well known source of nitric oxide and other reactive oxygen species (ROS) [154]. There are data showing that NO produced by activated microglia inhibits the activity KDHC [155].

Numberous data proved that prolonged activation of microglia leads to excessive secretion of NO, ROS and proinflamatory cytokines [156]. Lypopolysacharide (LPS) derived from bacteria exerts the capacity to activate microglial cells. In such conditions the cells secrete augmented levels of Il-1β, Il-6, TNF-α. TNF-α in nonactivated microglia is produced in insignificant concentration whereas in LPS-activated cells the level of its release is several times expanded [157]. Microglia may be also stimulated by Aβ what in consequence conducts to excessive release of TNF-α, that becomes the neurotoxic factor. However some data reports that low Il-1β concentrations may have positive effect on highly differentiated cholinergic neurons by increasing the ChAT expression and activity in cholinergic neurons treated by neurotoxic concentrations of Aβ [124]. In consequence the level of ACh was also elevated. Moreover these data also proved that added Il-1β reversed the inhibitory effect of cytotoxic factors on acetyl-CoA level in cytoplasmic compartment. These changes in cholinergic phenotype correlated well with cell viability and morphology. From the other hand Il-1β-activation was completely inhibited by IL-6 or TNF-α.

The other data proves that in the cocultures of neuronal cells with microglial cells the last ones protect neurons from death caused by some cytotoxic factors such as elevated Zn or NO levels (Gul-Hinc et al. unpublished). The cytoprotective effect may be caused by the restoration by microglia the proper level of Il-6 in cholinergic neurons and restoration of the high activity of PDHC and acetyl-CoA level. From the other hand LPS-induced excessive release of TNF-α by microglia exerts the cytotoxic effect that is independent on acetyl-CoA level.

14. Conclusions

There is some data concerning the mechanism of cholinergic encephalopathies in particular Alzheimer disease. They are mainly focused on disturbances in Aβ metabolism and only little of them reflect changes in energy metabolism particularly after various cytotoxic factors. However there is the existence of significant correlation between components of pyruvate-acetyl-CoA-acetycholine pathway. Cytotoxic insults that are responsible for AD such as: Aβ, Zn, Al, NOO·, TD directly or indirectly inhibits the activity of PDHC and KDHC what leads to acetyl-CoA synthesis. Consequently, there is inhibition of activity of three carboxylic acid cycle what causes the development of neurodegenerative changes in brain. Characterictic feature of some neurodegenerative diseases in preferential loss of cholinergic neurons what correlates with the degree of energy metabolism inhibition. Some data proved that survival of cholinergic neurons is limited by the level of acetyl-CoA in mitochondrial compartment. Moreover it is independent in the reason. The particular susceptibility of cholinergic neurons to various cytotoxic insults is triggered by relative shortage of this metabolite in mitochondria and used for acetylcholine synthesis. That is why it might be said that PDHC activity strait determine acetyl-CoA level in mitochondria what limits its utilization for energy production and acetylcholine synthesis under cytotoxic insults.

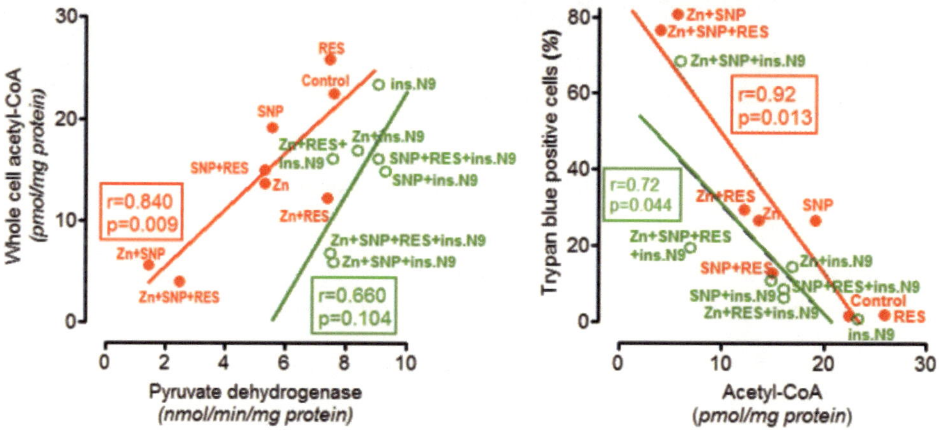

Figure 4. Parcrine effects of microglial N9 cells rescuing cholinergic SN56 neurons under excititocic conditions. A. Microglial effect preserving PDHC activity. B. Microglial effect decreasing mortality without affecting acetyl-CoA levels in cholinergic neurons. *(Gul-Hinc, unpublished).*

Acknowledgements

Supported by the Ministry of Research and Higher Education projects: NN401 1029937, IP 2010 035370 and IP 2011 046071.

Author details

Agnieszka Jankowska-Kulawy, Anna Ronowska and Andrzej Szutowicz

Department of Clinical Biochemistry Medical University of Gdansk, Poland

References

[1] Cunnane S, Nugent S, Roy M, Courchesne-Loyer A, Croteau E, Tremblay S, Castellano A, Pifferi F, Bocti Ch, Paquet N, Begdouri H, Bentourkia M, Turcotte E, Allard M, Barberger-Gateau P, Fulop T, Rapoport S. Brain fuel metabolism, aging, and Alzheimer's disease. Nutrition 2011;27 3–20.

[2] Torrealdea FJ, Sarasola C, d'Anjou A. Energy consumption and information transmission in model neurons. Chaos, Solitions and Fractals 2009;40 60–68.

[3] Duelli R, Kuschinsky W. Brain glucose transporters: relationship to local energy demand. News Physiol Sci 200;16 71–76.

[4] Simpson IA, Carruthers A, Vannucci SJ. Supply and demand in cerebral energy metabolism: the role of nutrient transporters. J Cereb Blood Flow Metab 2007;27 1766–1791.

[5] Barros LF, Deitmer JW. Glucose and lactate supply to the synapse. Brain Res Rev 2010; 63 149–159.

[6] Pierre K, Pellerin L. Monocarboxylate transporters in the central nervous system: distribution, regulation and function. J Neurochem 2005;94 1–14.

[7] Szutowicz A, Bielarczyk H, Jankowska-Kulawy A, Pawełczyk T, Ronowska A. Acetyl-CoA the key factor for survival or death of cholinergic neurons in course of neurodegenerative diseases. Neurochem Res 2013;38 1523-1542.

[8] Aubert A, Costalat R, Magistretti PJ, Pellerin L. Brain lactate kinetics: modeling evidence for neuronal lactate uptake upon activation. Proceedings of the National Academy of Science of the United States of America 2005;102(45) 16448–16453.

[9] Rasmussen P, Wyss MT, Lundby C. Cerebral glucose and lactate consumption during cerebral activation by physical activity in humans. FASEB J 2011;25 2865– 2873.

[10] Xiang Y, Shen J. Simultaneous detection of cerebral metabolism of different substrates by in vivo^{13}C isotopomer MRS. J Neurosci Methods 2011;198 8-15.

[11] Freeman JM, Kossoff EH. Ketosis and the ketogenic diet, 2010: advances in treating epilepsy and other disorders. Adv Pediatr 2010;57 315–329.

[12] Leigh D. Subacute necrotizing encephalomyelopathy in an infant. J Neurol Neurosurg Psychiatry 1951;14 216.

[13] Uziel G, Ghezzi D, Zeviani M. Infantile mitochondria encephalopathy. Arch Dis Child Seminars in Fetal and Neonatal Medicine 2011;16 205–215.

[14] Herzog RI, Jiang L, Herman P, Zhao Ch, Sanganahalli BG, Mason GF, Hyder F, Rothman DL, Shervin RS, Behar KL. Lactate preserves neuronal metabolism and function following antecedent recurrent hypoglycemia. J Clin Invest 2013;123 1988-1998.

[15] Lucas-Meunier E, Fossier P, Baux G, Amar M. Cholinergic modulation of the cortical neuronal network. Pflugers Arch 2003;446 17–29.

[16] McKinney. Brain cholinergic vulnerability: relevance to behavior and disease. Biochem Pharmacol 2005;70 1115–1124.

[17] Sato A, Sato Y, Uchida S. Activation of the intracerebral cholinergic nerve fibers originating in the basal forebrain increase regional cerebral blood flow in the rat's cortex and hippocampus. Neurosci Lett 2004;361 90–93.

[18] Schliebs R, Rossner S, Bigl V. Immunolesion by 192IgG-saporin of rat basal forebrain cholinergic system – a useful tool to produce cortical cholinergic dysfunction. Progr Brain Res 1996;109 253–264.

[19] Schliebs R, Arendt T. The significance of the cholinergic system in the brain during aging and in Alzheimer's disease. J Neural Transm 2006;113 1625–1644.

[20] Tucek S. Short-therm control of synthesis of acetylcholine. Prog Biophys Mol Biol 1993;60 59–69.

[21] Swaab DF, Bao AM. (Re-)activation of neurons in aging and dementia: lessons from the hypothalamus. Exp Gerontol 2011;46 178–184.

[22] Pakkenberg B, Gundersen HJ. Neocortical neuron number in humans: effect of sex and age. J Comp Neurol 1997;384 312–320.

[23] Swaab DF, Dubelaar EJ, Hofman MA, Scherder EJ, van Someren EJ, Verwer RW. Brain aging and Alzheimer's disease; use it or lose it. Prog Brain Res 2002;138 343–373.

[24] Double KL, Reyes S, Werry EL, Halliday GM. Selective cell death in neurodegeneration: why are some neurons spared in vulnerable regions? Prog Neurobiol 2010;92 316–329.

[25] Szutowicz A, Tomaszewicz M, Jankowska A, Madziar B, Bielarczyk H. Mechanizmy selektywnej wrażliwości neuronów cholinergicznych na bodźce neurotoksyczne. Postępy Hig Med Dośw 1999;53 263–275.

[26] Szutowicz A, Tomaszewicz M, Jankowska A, Madziar B, Bielarczyk H. Acetyl-CoA metabolism in cholinergic neurons and their susceptibility to neurotoxic inputs. Metab Brian Dis 2000;15 29–44.

[27] Braak H, Braak E. Neuropathological staging of Alzheimer-related changes. Acta Neuropathol, 1991; 82 239–259.

[28] Mohamed NV, Herrou T, Plouffe V, Piperno N, Leclerc N. Spreading of tau pathology in Alzheimer's disease by cell-to-cell transmission. Eur J of Neurosci 2013;37 1939-1948.

[29] Rodriguez-Martin T, Cuchillo-Ibanez I, Noble W, Nyenya F, Anderton BH, Hanger DP. Tau phosphorylation affects its axonal transport and degeneration. Neurobiol of Aging 2013;34 2146-2157.

[30] Schliebs R, Arendt T. The cholinergic system in aging and neuronal degeneration. Behavioral Brain Res 2011;221 555–563.

[31] Driscoll I, Resnick SM, Troncoso JC. Impact of Alzheimer's pathology on cognitive trajectories in nondemended elderly. Ann Neurol 2006;60 688–695.

[32] Szutowicz A, Bielarczyk H, Gul S, Ronowska A, Pawełczyk T, Jankowska-Kulawy A. Phenotype-dependent susceptibility of cholinergic neuroblastoma cells to neurotoxic inputs. Metab Brain Dis 2006;21 149–161.

[33] Herholz K, Weisenbach S, Kalbe E. Deficits of the cholinergic system in early AD. Neuropsychologia 2008;46 1642-1647.

[34] Serrano-Pozo A, Frosch MP, Masliah E, Hyman BT. Neuropathological alterations in Alzheimer disease. Cold Spring Harb Perspect Med 2011;1(1) 1-23.

[35] Bubber P, Haroutunian V, Fisch G, Blass JP, Gibson GE. Mitochondrial abnormalities in Alzheimer brain: mechanistic implications. Ann Neurol 2005;57 695-703.

[36] Sheu KF, Blass JP. The alpha-ketoglutarate dehydrogenase complex. Ann N Y Acad Sci 1999;893 61-78.

[37] Ouerfurth HW, LaFerla FM. Alzheimer's disease. N Engl J Med 2010;362 329-344.

[38] Cameron B, Landreth GE. Inflammation, microglia, and Alzheimer's disease. Neurobiol Dis 2010;37 503–509.

[39] Heneka MT, O'Banion MK, Terwel D, Kummer MP. Neuroinflammatory processes in Alzheimer's disease. J Neural Transm 2010;117 919–947.

[40] Ronowska A, Dyś A, Jankowska-Kulawy A, Klimaszewska-Łata J, Bielarczyk H, Romianowski P, Pawełczyk T, Szutowicz A. Short-term effects of zinc on acetylcholine metabolism and viability of SN56 cholinergic neuroblastoma cells. Neurochem Int 2010;56 143-51.

[41] Blennow K, de Leon M, Zetterberg H. Alzheimer disease. Lancet 2006;368 387– 403.

[42] Schliebs R. Basal forebrain cholinergic dysfunction in Alzheimer's disease – interrelationship with β-amyloid, inflammation and neurotrophin signaling. Neurochem Res 2005;30 895–908.

[43] Herholz K. Acetylcholine esterase activity in mild cognitive impairment and Alzheimer's disease. Eur J Nucl Med Mol Imaging 2008;35(1) 25–29.

[44] Jazi R, Lalonde R, Qian S, Strazielle C. Regional brain evaluation of acetylcholinesterase activity in PS1/A246E transgenic mice. Neurosci Res 2009;63 106–114.

[45] Pappas BA, Bayley PJ, Bui BK, Hansen LA, Thal LJ. Choline acetyltransferase activity and cognitive domain scores of Alzheimer's patients. Neurobiol Aging 2000;21 11-17.

[46] Terwel D, Bothmer J, Wolf E, Meng F, Jolles J. Affected enzymes activity in Alzheimer's disease are sensitive to antemortem hypoxia. J Neurol Sci 1998;161 47-56.

[47] Mosconi L. Glucose metabolism in normal aging and Alzheimer's disease: methodological and physiological considerations for PET studies. Clin Transl Imaging 2013, DOI 10.1007/s40336-013-0026-y.

[48] Teipel S. Risk and resilience: a new perspective on Alzheimer's disease. Geriatr Ment Health Care 2013;1 47-55.

[49] Ballard C, Gauthier S, Corbett A, Brayne C, Aarsland D, Jones E. Alzheimer's disease. Lancet 2011;377 1019–1031.

[50] Britschgi M, Wyss-Coray T. Blood protein signature for the early diagnosis of Alzheimer disease. Arch Neurol 2009; 66 161–165.

[51] Herholz K. Amyloid PET: Its diagnostic potential compared to FDG. Med Nucléaire 2011;35 322–326.

[52] Kossowska B, Dudka I, Gancarz R, Antonowicz-Juchniewicz J. Analiza proteomiczna profili białkowych w niektórych stanach patologicznych ludzkiego organizmu. Postępy Hig Med Dośw 2009;63 549–563.

[53] Mosconi L, Brys M, Glodzik-Sobanska L, De Santi S, Rusinek H, de Leon J. Early detection of Alzheimer's disease using neuroimaging. Exp Gerontol 2007;42 129– 138.

[54] Price JC, Klunk WE, Lopresti BJ, Lu X, Hoge JA, Ziolko ST, Holt DP, Meltzer CC, DeKosky ST, Mathis CA. Kinetic modeling of amyloid binding in humans using PET imaging and Pittsburgh Compound-B. J Cereb Blood Flow Metab 2005;25 1528–1547.

[55] Liu Y, Iqbal K, Grundke-Iqbal I, Gong ChX. Decreased glucose transporters correlate to abnormal hyperphosphorylation of tau in Alzheimer disease. FEBS Lett 2008;582 359–364.

[56] Mazzola JL, Sirover M. Subcellular alteration of glyceraldehyde-3-phosphate dehydrogenase in Alzheimer's disease fibroblasts. J Neurosci Res 2003;71 279–285.

[57] Ferreira IL, Resende R, Ferreiro E, Rego AC, Pereira CF. Multiple deficits in energy metabolism in Alzheimer's disease. Curr Drug Targets 2010;11 1–14.

[58] Maruszak A, Żekanowski C. Mitochondrial dysfunction and Alzheimer's disease. Prog Neuropsychopharmacol Biol Psychiatry 2011;35 320–330.

[59] Tereni B, Boada J, Portero-Otin M, Pamplona R, Ferrer I. Mitochondrial ATP-synthase in the entorhinal cortex is a target of oxidative stress at stages I/II of Alzheimer's disease pathology. Brain Pathol 2010;20 222–233.

[60] Gibson GE, Jope R, Blass JP. Decreased synthesis of acetylcholine accompanying impaired oxidation of pyruvic acid in rat brain minces. Biochem J 1975;148 17–23.

[61] Lefresne P, Guyenet P, Głowiński J. Acetylcholine synthesis from [2-^{14}C] pyruvate in rat striatal slices. J Neurochem 1973;20 1083–1097.

[62] Lefresne P, Hamon N, Beaujouan C, Głowiński J. Origin of acetyl moiety of acetylcholine synthesized in rat striatal synaptosomes. Biochimie 1977;59 197–215.

[63] Tucek S. Acetylcoenzyme-A and the synthesis of acetylcholine in neurons. Review of recent progress. Gen Physiol Biophys 1983;2 313–324.

[64] Srere PA. The molecular physiology of citrate. Nature, Lond 1965;766–770.

[65] Gibson GE, Shimada M. Studies on the metabolic pathway of the acetyl group for acetylcholine synthesis. Biochem Pharmacol 1980;29 167–174.

[66] Szutowicz A, Stępień M, Łysiak W, Angielski S. Effect of (-)hydroxycitrate on the activities of ATP citrate lyase and the enzymes of acetyl-CoA metabolism in rat brain. Acta Biochim Pol 1976;22 227–234.

[67] Szutowicz A, Łysiak W, Angielski S. The effect of (-)hydroxycitrate on pyruvate metabolism in rat brain synaptosomes. J Neurochem 1977;29 375–378.

[68] Szutowicz A, Bielarczyk H, Łysiak W. The role of citrate derived from glucose in the acetylcholine synthesis in rat brain synaptosomes. Int J Biochem 1981a;13 887–892.

[69] Szutowicz A, Stępień M, Piec G. Determination of pyruvate dehydrogenase and acetyl-CoA synthase activities using citrate synthase. Anal Biochem 1981b;115 81–87.

[70] Szutowicz A, Tomaszewicz M, Bielarczyk H. Disturbances of acetyl-CoA, energy and acetylcholine metabolism in some encephalopathies. Acta Neurobiol Exp 1996;56 323–339.

[71] Bubber P, Ke ZJ, Gibson GE. Tricarboxylic acid cycle enzymes following thiamine deficiency. Neurochem Int 2004;45 1021–1028.

[72] Butterworth RF, Giguere JF, Besnard AM. Activities of thiamine-dependent enzymes in two experimental models of thiamine-deficiency encephalopathy: 1. The puryvate dehydrogenase complex. Neurochem Res 1985;10 1417–1428.

[73] Szutowicz A, Bielarczyk H, Skulimowska H. Effect of dichloroacetate on acetyl-CoA content and acetylcholine synthesis in rat brain synaptosomes. Neurochem Res 1994;19(9) 1107–1112.

[74] Szutowicz A, Bielarczyk H, Kisielevski Y, Jankowska A, Madziar B, Tomaszewicz M. Effects of aluminium and calcium on acetyl-CoA metabolism in rat brain mitochondria. J Neurochem 1998;71(6) 2447-2453.

[75] Niewiadomska G, Baksalerska-Pazera M, Riedel G. The septo-hippocampal system, learning and recovery of function. Prog Neuropsychopharmacol Biol Psychiatry 2009;33(5) 791–805.

[76] Bielarczyk H, Jankowska A, Madzar B, Matecki A, Michno A, Szutowicz A. Differential toxicity of nitric oxide, aluminium and amyloid beta peptide in SN56 cholinergic cells from mouse septum. Neurochem Int 2003;42 323-331.

[77] Bielarczyk H, Gul S, Ronowska A, Bizon-Zygmanska D, Pawełczyk T, Szutowicz A. RS-alpha-lipoic acid protects cholinergic cells against sodium nitroprusside and amyloid-beta neurotoxicity through restoration of acetyl-CoA level. J Neurochem 2006;98 1242-51.

[78] Jankowska A, Blusztajn JK, Szutowicz A. Activities of enzymes of acetyl-CoA and acetylcholine metabolism in SN56 hybrid cholinergic cell line differentiated by dibutyryl cyclic AMP and all-trans retinoic acid. Folia Neuropathol 1997;35 247–249.

[79] Jankowska A, Madziar B, Tomaszewicz M, Szutowicz A. Acute and chronic effects of aluminum on acetyl-CoA and acetylcholine metabolism in differentiated and nondifferentiated SN56 cholinergic cells. J Neurosci Res 2000;62 615-22.

[80] Ronowska A, Gul-Hinc S, Bielarczyk H, Pawełczyk T, Szutowicz A. Effects of zinc on SN56 cholinergic neuroblastoma cells. J Neurochem 2007;103(3) 972-83.

[81] Bizon-Zygmańska D, Jankowska-Kulawy A, Bielarczyk H, Pawełczyk T, Ronowska A, Marszałł M, Szutowicz A. Acetyl-CoA metabolism in amprolium-evoked thiamine pyrophosphate deficits in cholinergic SN56 neuroblastoma cells. Neurochem Int 2011;59, 208–216.

[82] Crochemore C, Peña-Altamira E, Virgili M, Monti B, Contestabile A. Disease-related regressive alterations of forebrain cholinergic system in SOD1 mutant transgenic mice. Neurochem Int 2005;(5) 357-68.

[83] Frederickson CJ, Maret W, Cuajungco MP. Zinc and excitotoxic brain injury: a new model. Neuroscientist 2004;10(1) 18-25.

[84] Hynd MR, Scott HL, Dodd PR. Glutamate-mediated excitotoxicity and neurodegeneration in Alzheimer's disease. Neurochem Int 2004;45(5) 583-95.

[85] Mocchegiani E, Bertoni-Freddari C, Marcellini F, Malavolta M. Brain, aging and neurodegeneration: role of zinc ion availability. Prog Neurobiol 2005;75(6) 367-90.

[86] Supnet C, Bezprozvanny I. Neuronal calcium signaling, mitochondrial dysfunction, and Alzheimer's disease. J Alzheimers Dis 2010;20,Suppl2 487-98.

[87] Yu JT, Chang RC, Tan L. Calcium dysregulation in Alzheimer's disease: from mechanisms to therapeutic opportunities. Prog Neurobiol 2009;89(3) 240-55.

[88] Jhala SS, Hazell AS. Modeling neurodegenerative disease pathophysiology in thiamine deficiency: consequences of impaired oxidative metabolism. Neurochem Int 2011;58(3) 248-60.

[89] Steinert JR, Chernova T, Forsythe ID. Nitric oxide signaling in brain function, dysfunction, and dementia. Neuroscientist 2010;16(4) 435-52.

[90] Lai JC, DiLorenzo JC, Sheu KF. Pyruvate dehydrogenase complex is inhibited in calcium-loaded cerebrocortical mitochondria. Neurochem Res 1988;13(11) 1043-8.

[91] Malloch GD, Munday LA, Olson MS, Clark JB. Comparative development of the pyruvate dehydrogenase complex and citrate synthase in rat brain mitochondria. Biochem J 1986;15 238(3) 729-36.

[92] Selkoe DJ. Amyloid beta-protein precursor: new clues to the genesis of Alzheimer's disease. Curr Opin Neurobiol 1994;4(5) 708-16.

[93] Sensi SL, Paoletti P, Bush AI, Sekler I. Zinc in the physiology and pathology of the CNS. Nat Rev Neurosci 2009;10(11) 780-91.

[94] Torre JC. Alzheimer's disease prevalence can be lowered with non-invasive testing. J Alzheimers Dis 2008;14(3) 353-9.

[95] Guglielmotto M, Tamagno E, Danni O: Oxidative stress and hypoxia contribute to Alzheimer's disease pathogenesis: two sides of the same coin. The Scientific World J 2009;9 781–791.

[96] Hoshi Y, Hazeki O, Kakihana Y, Tamura M. Redox behavior of cytochrome oxidase in the rat brain measured by near-infrared spectroscopy. J Appl Physiol 1997;83 1842-81.

[97] Pereira C, Santos MS, Oliveira C. Involvement of oxidative stress on the impairment of energy metabolism induced by A beta peptides on PC12 cells: protection by antioxidants. Neurobiol Dis 1999;6(3) 209-19.

[98] Sensi SL, Yin HZ, Weiss JH. Glutamate triggers preferential Zn^{2+}flux through Ca^{2+}permeable AMPA channels and consequent ROS production. Neuroreport 1999;10(8) 1723-1727.

[99] Berridge MJ. Calcium signalling and Alzheimer's disease. Neurochem Res 2011;36(7) 1149-56.

[100] Ueda K, Shinohara S, Yagami T, Asakura K, Kawasaki K. Amyloid-protein potentiates Ca^{2+}influx through L-type voltage-sensitive Ca2+channels: a possible involvement of free radicals. J Neurochem 1997;68 265–271.

[101] Coulson EJ. Does the p75 neurotrophin receptor mediate Aβ-induced toxicity in Alzheimer's disease? J Neurochem 2006; 98 654-660.

[102] Mizuno T. The biphasic role of microglia in Alzheimer's disease. Int J Alzheimers Dis 2012;37846 1-9.

[103] Furst AJ, Rabinovici GD, Rostomian AH, Steed T, Alkalay A, Racine C, Miller BL, Jagust WJ. Cognition, glucose metabolism and amyloid burden in Alzheimer's disease. Neurobiol Aging 2012;33(2) 215-25.

[104] Fernandez LL, de Lima MN, Scalco F, Vedana G, Miwa C, Hilbig A, Vianna M, Schröder N. Early post-natal iron administration induces astroglial response in the brain of adult and aged rats. Neurotox Res 2011; 20(2) 193-9.

[105] Vallee BL, Falchuk KH. Zinc and gene expression. Philos Trans R Soc Lond B Biol Sci 1981;294(1071) 185-97.

[106] Imanishi M, Imamura Ch, Higashi C, Yan W, Negi S, Futaki S, Sugiura Y. Zinc finger–zinc finger interaction between the transcription factors, GATA-1 and Sp1. Biochemical and Biophysical Research Communications 2010;400 4 625-630.

[107] Nagaoka M, Sugiura Y. Artificial zinc finger peptides: creation, DNA recognition, and gene regulation. J Inorg Biochem 2000;82(1-4) 57-63.

[108] Takeda A. Zinc signaling in the hippocampus and its relation to pathogenesis of depression. Mol Neurobiol 2011;44(2) 166-74.

[109] Colvin RA. Characterization of a plasma membrane zinc transporter in rat brain. Neurosci Lett 1998;247(2-3) 147-50.

[110] Guerinot ML. The ZIP family of metal transporters. Biochim Biophys Acta 2000;1465(1-2) 190-8.

[111] Szewczyk B, Pałucha-Poniewiera A, Poleszak E, Pilc A, Nowak G. Investigational NMDA receptor modulators for depression. Expert Opin Investig Drugs 2012;21(1) 91-102.

[112] Lee SH, Huang JW, Hung KY, Leu LJ, Kan YT, Yang CS, Chung Wu D, Huang CL, Chen PY, Chen JS, Chen WY. Trace Metals' abnormalities in hemodialysis patients: relationship with medications. Artif Organs 2000;24(11) 841-4.

[113] Maynard C, Bush A, Masters C, Cappai R, Li Q. Metals and amyloid-beta in Alzheimer's disease. Int J Exp Pathol 2005;86 147–159.

[114] Wang CY, Wang T, Zheng W, Zhao BL, Danscher G, Chen YH, Wang ZY. Zinc overload enhances APP cleavage and Aβ deposition in the Alzheimer mouse brain. PLoS One 2010;5(12) e15349.

[115] Takeda A. Insight into glutamate excitotoxicity from synaptic zinc homeostasis. Int J Alzheimers Dis 2010;Vol. 2011, Article ID: 491597.

[116] Bertoni-Freddari C, Fattoretti P, Casoli T, Di Stefano G, Solazzi M, Perna E, De Angelis C. Reactive structural dynamics of synaptic mitochondria in ischemic delayed neuronal death. Ann N Y Acad Sci 2006;1090 26-34.

[117] Gil-Bea FJ, García-Alloza M, Domínguez J, Marcos B, Ramírez MJ. Evaluation of cholinergic markers in Alzheimer's disease and in a model of cholinergic deficit. Neurosci Lett 2005;375(1) 37-41.

[118] Szutowicz A: Aluminum, NO, and nerve growth factor neurotoxicity in cholinergic neurons. J Neurosci Res 2001;66 1009–1018.

[119] Szutowicz A, Jankowska-Kulawy A, Bielarczyk H. Disturbances in acetyl-CoA metabolism. A key factor in pre clinical and overt thiamine deficiency encephalophaty. Food and Nutritional Components in Focus: Chemistry, Analysis, Function and Effects, The Royal Society of Chemistry, edited by professor Victor Preedy, Chapter 33, 553-571, 2013a.

[120] Taysi S, Cikman O, Kaya A, Demircan B, Gumustekin K, Yilmaz A, Boyuk A, Keles M, Akyuz M, Turkeli M. Increased oxidant stress and decreased antioxidant status in erythrocytes of rats fed with zinc-deficient diet. Biol Trace Elem Res 2008;161-7.

[121] Doherty GH. Nitric oxide in neurodegeneration: potential benefits of non-steroidal anti-inflammatories. Neurosci Bull 2011;27(6) 366-82.

[122] Moncada S, Bolaños JP. Nitric oxide, cell bioenergetics and neurodegeneration. J Neurochem 2006;97(6) 1676-89.

[123] Paradies G, Petrosillo G, Paradies V, Ruggiero FM. Mitochondrial dysfunction in brain aging: role of oxidative stress and cardiolipin. Neurochem Int 2011;58(4) 447-57.

[124] Bielarczyk H, Jankowska-Kulawy A, Gul S, Pawełczyk T, Szutowicz A. Phenotype dependent differential effects of interleukin-1beta and amyloid-beta on viability and cholinergic phenotype of T17 neuroblastoma cells. Neurochem Int 2005;47(7) 466-73.

[125] Gibson GE, Starkov A, Blass JP, Ratan RR, Beal MF. Cause and consequence: mitochondrial dysfunction initiates and propagates neuronal dysfunction, neuronal death and behavioral abnormalities in age-associated neurodegenerative diseases. Biochim Biophys Acta 2010;1802(1) 122-34.

[126] Szutowicz A, Tomaszewicz M, Bielarczyk H. Key role of acetyl-CoA in cytoplasm of nerve terminals in disturbances of acetylcholine metabolism in brain. Folia Neuropathol 1997;35(4) 241-3.

[127] Anzalone S, Vetreno RP, Ramos RL, Savage LM. Cortical cholinergic abnormalities contribute to the amnesic state induced by pyrithiamine-induced thiamine deficiency in the rat. Eur J Neurosci 2010;32(5) 847-58.

[128] Butterworth RF, Spahr L, Fontaine S, Layrargues GP. Manganese toxicity, dopaminergic dysfunction and hepatic encephalopathy. Metab Brain Dis 1995;10(4) 259-67.

[129] Bettendorff L. Thiamine homeostasis in neuroblastoma cells. Neurochem Int 1995;26(3) 295-302.

[130] Jankowska-Kulawy A, Bielarczyk H, Pawełczyk T, Wróblewska M, Szutowicz A. Acetyl-CoA and acetylcholine metabolizm in nerve terminal compartment of thiamine deficient rat brain. J Neurochem 2010;115 333-42.

[131] Jankowska-Kulawy A, Bielarczyk H, Pawełczyk T, Wróblewska M, Szutowicz A. Acetyl-CoA deficyt in braim mitochondria in experimental thiamine deficiency encephalopathy. Neurochem Int 2010a;57 851-856.

[132] Zhao N, Zhong C, Wang Y, Zhao Y, Gong N, Zhou G, Xu T, Hong Z. Impaired hippocampal neurogenesis is involved in cognitive dysfunction induced by thiamine deficiency at early pre-pathological lesion stage. Neurobiol Dis 2008;29(2) 76-85.

[133] Grass D, Pawlowski PG, Hirrlinger J, Papadopoulos N, Richter DW, Kirchhoff F, Hülsmann S. Diversity of functional astroglial properties in the respiratory network. J Neurosci 2004;11 1358-65.

[134] Allen NJ, Barres BA. Neuroscience: Glia-more than just brain glue. Nature 2009;457(7230) 675-7.

[135] Gibbs ME, Gibbs Z, Hertz L. Rescue of Aβ(1-42)-induced memory impairment in day-old chick by facilitation of astrocytic oxidative metabolism: implications for Alzheimer's disease. J Neurochem 2009;109 Suppl 1 230-6.

[136] McKenna MC, Waagepetersen HS, Schousboe A, Sonnewald U. Neuronal and astrocytic shuttle mechanisms for cytosolic-mitochondrial transfer of reducing equivalents: current evidence and pharmacological tools. Biochem Pharmacol 2006;14,71 399-407.

[137] Jakoby P, Schmidt E, Ruminot I, Gutiérrez R, Barros LF, Deitmer JW. Higher transport and metabolism of glucose in astrocytes compared with neurons: a multiphoton study of hippocampal and cerebellar tissue slices. Cereb Cortex 2013 (in press)

[138] Bishop GM, Dang TN, Dringen R, Robinson SR. Accumulation of non-transferrin-bound iron by neurons, astrocytes, and microglia. Neurotox Res 2011;19(3) 443-51.

[139] Dineley KT, Kayed R, Neugebauer V, Fu Y, Zhang W, Reese LC, Taglialatela G. Amyloid-beta oligomers impair fear conditioned memory in a calcineurin-dependent fashion in mice. Neurosci Res 2010;88(13) 2923-32.

[140] Simard A, Soulet D, Gowing G, Julien J, Rivest S. Bone marrow-derived microglia play a critical role in restricting senile plaques formation in Alzheimer disease. Neuron 2006;49 489-502.

[141] Block ML, Zecca L, Hong JS. Microglia-mediated neurotoxicity: uncovering the molecular mechanisms. Nat Rev Neurosci 2007; 8(1) 57-69.

[142] Maezawa I, Zimin P, Wulf H, Jin L. Amyloid-beta protein oligomer at low nanomolar concenrations activates microglia and induces microglial neurotoxicity. J Biol Chem 2011;286 3693-3706.

[143] Kauppinen TM, Higashi Y, Suh SW, Escartin C, Nagasawa K, Swanson RA. Zinc triggers microglial activation. J Neurosci 2008;28(22) 5827-35.

[144] Knoch ME, Hartnett KA, Hara H, Kandler K, Aizenman E. Microglia induce neurotoxicity via intraneuronal Zn(2+) release and a K(+) current surge. Glia 2008;56(1) 89-96.

[145] Vezzani A, French J, Bartfai T, Baram TZ. The role of inflammation in epilepsy. Nat Rev Neurol 2011;7 31–40.

[146] Aronica E, Gorter JA. Gene expression profile in temporal lobe epilepsy. Neuroscientist 2007;13 100–108.

[147] Ravizza SM, Lucas S, Balosso L, Bernardino G, Ku F, Noé J, Malva JC, Randle S, Allan A. Inactivation of caspase-1 in rodent brain: a novel anticonvulsive strategy. Epilepsia 2006;47 1160–1168.

[148] Aronica K, Boer EA, van Vliet S, Redeker JC, Baayen WG, Spliet PC, van Rijen D, Troost FH, da Silva WJ, Wadman JA, Gorter JA. Complement activation in experimental and human temporal lobe epilepsy. Neurobiol Dis 2007;26 497–511.

[149] Iyer AM, Zurolo E, Boer K, Baayen JC, Giangaspero, F, Arcella A, Di Gennaro GC, Esposito V, Spliet WGM, van Rijen PC, Troost D, Gorter JA, Aronica E. Tissue plasminogen activator and urokinase plasminogen activator in human epileptogenic pathologies. Neuroscience 2010;19 929–945.

[150] Ballabh P, Braun A, Nedergaard M. The blood–brain barrier: an overview: structure, regulation, and clinical implications. Neurobiol Dis 2004;16 1–13.

[151] Lucas SM, Rothwell NJ, Gibson RM. The role of inflammation in CNS injury and disease. Br J Pharmacol 2006;147(Suppl. 1) 232–240.

[152] Maroso M, Balosso S, Ravizza T, Liu J, Aronica E, Iyer AM, Rossetti C, Molteni M, Casalgrandi M, Manfredi AA, Bianchi ME, A. Toll-like receptor 4 and high-mobility group box-1 are involved in ictogenesis and can be targeted to reduce seizures. Nat Med 2010;16(4) 413–419.

[153] Sheedy FJ, O'Neill LA. Adding fuel to fire: microRNAs as a new class of mediators of inflammation. Ann Rheum Dis 2008;67(Suppl. 3) 50–55.

[154] Colton CA, Gilbert DL. Production of superoxide anions by a CNS macrophage, the microglia. FEBS Lett 1987;223(2) 284-8.

[155] Park JK, Williams BP, Alberta JA, Stiles CD. Bipotent cortical progenitor cells process conflicting cues for neurons and glia in a hierarchical manner. J Neurosci 1999;19(23) 10383-9.

[156] Stoll G, Müller HW. Nerve injury, axonal degeneration and neural regeneration: basic insights. Brain Pathol 1999;9(2) 313-25.

[157] Feinstein DL, Galea E, Reis DJ. Suppression of glial iNOS expression by tyrosine kinase inhibitors. Ann N Y Acad Sci 1994;17(738) 325-8.

[158] Suwalsky M, Fierro P, Villena F, Aguilar LF, Sotomayor CP, Jemiola-Rzeminska M, Strzalka K, Gul-Hinc S, Ronowska A, Szutowicz A. Human erythrocytes and neuroblastoma cells are in vitro affected by sodium orthovanadate. Biochim Biophys Acta 2012;1818(9) 2260-70.

[159] Suwalsky M, Fierro P, Villena F, Gallardo MJ, Jemiola-Rzeminska M, Strzalka K, Gul-Hinc S, Ronowska A, Zysk M, Szutowicz A. Effects of sodium metavanadate on in vitro neuroblastoma and red blood cells. Arch Biochem Biophys 2013;535(2) 248-56.